Target Discovery and Validation Reviews and Protocols
Volume 2, Emerging Molecular Targets and Treatment Options

METHODS IN MOLECULAR BIOLOGY™

John M. Walker, SERIES EDITOR

METHODS IN MOLECULAR BIOLOGY™

Target Discovery and Validation Reviews and Protocols

VOLUME 2

*Emerging Molecular Targets
and Treatment Options*

Edited by

Mouldy Sioud

*Department of Immunology,
Institute for Cancer Research,
The Norwegian Radium Hospital,
University of Oslo, Oslo, Norway*

HUMANA PRESS ✳ TOTOWA, NEW JERSEY

Cover design by Patricia F. Cleary
Cover illustrations: *Foreground:* Joint damage in human tumor necrosis factor (hTNF)α-transgenic mice (Chapter 13, Fig. 2; *see* complete caption on p. 269). *Background:* Overexpression of green fluorescent protein-tagged centrosome/spindle pole-associated protein in HEK293T cells (Volume 1, Chapter 1, Fig. 1; *see* complete caption on p. 3).

For additional copies, pricing for bulk purchases, and/or information about other Humana titles, contact Humana at the above address or at any of the following numbers: Tel.: 973-256-1699; Fax: 973-256-8341; E-mail: orders@humanapr.com; or visit our Website: www.humanapress.com

Photocopy Authorization Policy:
Authorization to photocopy items for internal or personal use, or the internal or personal use of specific clients, is granted by Humana Press Inc., provided that the base fee of US $30.00 per copy is paid directly to the Copyright Clearance Center at 222 Rosewood Drive, Danvers, MA 01923. For those organizations that have been granted a photocopy license from the CCC, a separate system of payment has been arranged and is acceptable to Humana Press Inc. The fee code for users of the Transactional Reporting Service is: [978-1-58829-890-4 • 1-58829-890-6/06 $30.00].

Printed in the United States of America. 10 9 8 7 6 5 4 3 2 1

eISBN 1-59745-208-4

ISSN 1064-3745

Library of Congress Cataloging-in-Publication Data
Target discovery and validation : reviews and protocols / edited by
Mouldy Sioud.
      p. ; cm. -- (Methods in molecular biology, ISSN 1064-3745 ; 360-361)
   Includes bibliographical references and index.
   ISBN-13: 978-1-58829-656-6 (v. 1 : alk. paper)
   ISBN-10: 1-58829-656-3 (v. 1 : alk. paper)
   ISBN-13: 978-1-58829-890-4 (v. 2 : alk. paper)
   ISBN-10: 1-58829-890-6 (v. 2 : alk. paper)
   1. Tumor markers. 2. Biochemical markers--Therapeutic use. 3.
DNA microarrays. 4. Drug targeting. 5. Drugs--Design. 6.
Molecular pharmacology. I. Sioud, Mouldy. II. Series: Methods in
molecular biology (Clifton, N.J.) ; v. 360-361.
   [DNLM: 1. Antineoplastic Agents. 2. Drug Design. 3. Tumor
Markers, Biological. W1 ME9616J v.360-361 2007 / QV 269 T185 2007]
   RC270.3.T84T37 2007
   616.99'4075--dc22
                                                                  2006020032

Preface

During the last few years we have seen fundamental changes in the way scientists approach the identification and validation of new drug targets. These novel strategies for target validation are expected to maximize the likelihood of achieving target-selective inhibition with minimal in vivo side effects. For example, by the use of small interfering RNAs (siRNAs) to down regulate expression of known genes, a number of therapeutic targets have been validated both in vitro and in vivo. The technologies developed to do this have not only yielded a significant number of drug targets but have influenced our understanding of gene function, the molecular mechanisms of diseases, and the design of new therapeutic interventions. Specific gene and protein targets—on which, for example, cancer cells depend—can now be identified, along with the therapeutic agents directed against them. Several relevant examples that have been validated, and some that have reached the clinic, are featured in Volume 2, *Emerging Molecular Drug Targets and Treatment Options,* of *Target Discovery and Validation Reviews and Protocols.*

Despite knowing the molecular mechanisms of most drugs, patients vary in their responses to a medication's efficacy and side effects. Indeed, the sequence of the human genome has shown that there is extensive genetic variation among individuals that would be expected to affect the response to medication. Thus, a better understanding of the molecular mechanisms that lead to an improved treatment response should play an important role in the development of *individualized* medicine. DNA sequence alterations and the expression profiles of mRNA molecules and proteins can be used to predict drug response. These genetic and epigenetic changes may be used in turn to develop treatment algorithms adjusted for use in individual patients. Several examples of such individualized treatment, aimed at increasing drug efficacy as well as decreasing toxicity, are discussed in this edition.

In systemic autoimmune diseases, current clinical practice calls for immunosuppressive drug therapy. However, some drugs are not target-specific and some carry a high risk of side effects. New immunosuppressive strategies, such as monoclonal antibodies and receptor antagonists, are now emerging as potentially valuable discriminating agents for use in innovative combinations. Such novel opportunities for therapeutic targeting in systemic autoimmune diseases are described in Volume 2.

MicroRNAs (miRNAs) are a family of short noncoding regulatory RNA molecules expressed in a variety of different cell types. These tiny RNAs have been shown to play important biological functions and may regulate the expression of more than 30% of human genes. Presently, evidence is emerging that particular miRNAs may play a role in human cancer pathogenesis. Thus, the identification of miRNA expression signatures in patients with cancer may help to identify subjects who are at high risk of developing cancer or those who have an early stage of cancer. In order to interfere with miRNA expression, modified antisense oligonucleotides targeting individual miRNAs have been developed and these agents have the potential to eventually progress into a new class of therapeutic agents.

Volume II, *Emerging Molecular Drug Targets and Treatment Options,* was written by leading experts in the field and presents a unique source of current information. Along with Volume I, *Emerging Strategies in Drug Targets and Biomarker Discovery,* this work will be of interest to researchers, pharmaceutical companies, clinicians, and students of biology, medicine, or pharmacy.

I would like to thank the authors for their contributions, Anne Dybwad for critical reading of the manuscripts, and all those involved in the production of the book.

***Mouldy Sioud**withparity*

Contents

Contributors

Dietmar Abraham • *Laboratory for Cardiovascular Research, Center for Anatomy and Cell Biology, Vienna Medical University, Vienna, Austria*

Seyedhossein Aharinejad • *Laboratory for Cardiovascular Research, Center for Anatomy and Cell Biology, Vienna Medical University, Vienna, Austria*

Vincent Boissoneault • *Centre de Recherche en Rhumatologie et Immunologie, Université Laval, Québec, Canada*

Howard E. Boudreau • *Departments of Radiation Medicine and Biochemistry and Molecular Biology, Lombardi Comprehensive Cancer Center, Georgetown University Medical Center, Washington, DC*

Martha Chekenya • *Department of Biomedicine, Section of Anatomy and Cell Biology, University of Bergen, Bergen, Norway*

Laura Cerchia • *Instituto per l'Endocrinologia el'Oncologia Sperimentale del CNR Gaetano Salvatore, Napoli, Italia*

Vittorio de Franciscis • *Instituto per l'Endocrinologia el'Oncologia Sperimentale del CNR Gaetano Salvatore, Napoli, Italia*

Manel Esteller • *Cancer Epigenetic Laboratory, Molecular Pathology Program, Spanish National Cancer Centre, Madrid, Spain*

Marco Folini • *Department of Experimental Oncology and Laboratories, National Cancer Institute, Milan, Italy*

Lise-Andrée Gobeil • *Centre de Recherche en Rhumatologie et Immunologie, Université Laval, Québec, Canada*

Prafulla C. Gokhale • *Departments of Radiation Medicine and Biochemistry and Molecular Biology, Lombardi Comprehensive Cancer Center, Georgetown University Medical Center, Washington, DC*

Andreas Herbst • *Clinical Research Unit for Gastrointestinal Cancers and Department of Medicine II, Klinikum Grosshadern, Ludwig-Maximilians-University, Munich, Germany*

Michel Herranz • *Cancer Epigenetic Laboratory, Molecular Pathology Program, Spanish National Cancer Centre, Madrid, Spain*

Sergey E. Ilyin • *Johnson and Johnson Pharmaceutical Research and Development, Spring House, PA*

Heike Immervoll • *The Gade Institute, Department of Pathology, Haukeland University Hospital, Bergen, Norway*

FRANK THOMAS KOLLIGS • *Clinical Research Unit for Gastrointestinal Cancers and Department of Medicine II, Klinikum Grosshadern, Ludwig-Maximilians-University, Munich, Germany*

USHA N. KASID • *Departments of Radiation Medicine and Biochemistry and Molecular Biology, Lombardi Comprehensive Cancer Center, Georgetown University Medical Center, Washington, DC*

STEFAN KUBICKA • *Department of Gastroenterogy, Hepatology and Endocrinology, Medical School Hannover, Hannover, Germany*

DEEPAK KUMAR • *Departments of Radiation Medicine and Biochemistry and Molecular Biology, Lombardi Comprehensive Cancer Center, Georgetown University Medical Center, Washington, DC*

MARIANNE LEIRDAL • *Molecular Medicine Group, Institute of Cancer Research, Oslo, Norway*

TREVOR LUCAS • *Laboratory for Cardiovascular Research, Center for Anatomy and Cell Biology, Vienna Medical University, Vienna, Austria*

ØYVIND MELIEN • *Clinical Research Unit, Section of Clinical Pharmacology, Rikshospitalet University Hospital, Oslo, Norway*

YUKI NAITO • *Department of Biophysics and Biochemistry, Graduate School of Science, University of Tokyo, Tokyo*

MERYEM OUARZANE • *Inserm U606 and University of Paris 7; Centre Viggo Petersen, l'Hôpital Lariboisière, Paris, France*

DOMINIQUE L. OUELLET • *Centre de Recherche en Rhumatologie et Immunologie, Université Laval, Québec, Canada*

WILLIAM PARRISH • *North Shore University Hospital, Manhasset, NY*

JIN PEI • *Departments of Radiation Medicine and Biochemistry and Molecular Biology, Lombardi Comprehensive Cancer Center, Georgetown University Medical Center, Washington, DC*

MARZIA PENNATI • *Department of Experimental Oncology and Laboratories, National Cancer Institute, Milan, Italy*

MARJORIE P. PERRON • *Centre de Recherche en Rhumatologie et Immunologie, Université Laval, Québec, Canada*

CARLOS R. PLATA-SALAMÁN • *Global External Researchand Development, Lilly Research Laboratories, Lilly Corporate Centre, Indianapolis, IN*

PATRICK PROVOST • *Department of Anatomy and Physiology, Université Laval Centre de Recherche en Rhumatologie et Immunologie, Québec, Canada*

KAORU SAIGO • *Department of Biophysics and Biochemistry, Graduate School of Science, University of Tokyo, Tokyo*

ISAMU SAKABE • *Departments of Radiation Medicine and Biochemistry and Molecular Biology, Lombardi Comprehensive Cancer Center, Georgetown University Medical Center, Washington, DC*

MOULDY SIOUD • *Department of Immunology, Institute for Cancer Research, The Norwegian Radium Hospital, University of Oslo, Oslo, Norway*

KUMIKO UI-TEI • *Department of Biophysics and Biochemistry, Graduate School of Science, University of Tokyo, Tokyo*

LUIS ULLOA • *North Shore University Hospital, Manhasset, New York*

RICHARD O. WILLIAMS • *Kennedy Institute of Rheumatology Division, Imperial College London, London, UK*

NADIA ZAFFARONI • *Department of Experimental Oncology and Laboratories, National Cancer Institute, Milan, Italy*

LARS ZENDER • *Cold Spring Harbor Laboratory, Cold Spring Harbor, NY*

CHUANBO ZHANG • *Departments of Radiation Medicine and Biochemistry and Molecular Biology, Lombardi Comprehensive Cancer Center, Georgetown University Medical Center, Washington, DC*

MONCEF ZOUALI • *Inserm U606 and University of Paris 7; Centre Viggo Petersen, l'Hôpital Lariboisière, Paris, France*

Contents of Volume 1:
Emerging Strategies for Targets and Biomarker Discovery

1

Druggable Signaling Proteins

Mouldy Sioud and Marianne Leirdal

Summary

In normal cells, signaling pathways are tightly regulated. However, when they are aberrantly activated, certain pathways are capable of causing diseases. In many tumors, the aberrantly activated signaling proteins include members of the epidermal growth factor receptor family, the Ras proteins, protein kinase C isoenzymes, BCR-ABL fusion protein as well as transcription factors such as signal transducers and activators of transcriptions and Myc. Accordingly, deregulation of these signaling proteins holds promise for the development of new anticancer drugs. Studies in vitro and in disease-relevant models demonstrated that blocking the activation of a key target in a constitutively activated signaling pathway could reverse disease phenotype. Moreover, constitutive activation of the target alone is sufficient to induce relevant disease phenotype. Notably, the most dramatic therapeutic advances in cancer therapy during the last decade have come from agents targeted against active thyrosine kinases. These include imatinib (anti-BCR-ABL), gefitinib (anti-EGF receptor), and herpetin (anti-ErbB-2). Here, some selected validated and drugable targets are summarized.

Key Words: Signaling pathways; Ras proteins; BCR-ABL kinase; STAT proteins; PKC; EGF receptor; MAP kinases.

1. Introduction

Cancer is a multistep process driven by progressive accumulation of genetic alterations, each of which contributes to the breakdown of mechanisms that control cell growth. During the last years both genetic and epigenetic changes associated with malignant transformation and progression in a wide variety of human cancers have been identified *(1)*. Activation of multiple oncogenes, inactivation mutations in tumor-suppressor genes, and defects in DNA repair genes are the hallmarks of the disease. Cancer cells are often dependent on the continued activation of growth-promoting genes for maintenance of their malignant

From: *Methods in Molecular Biology, vol. 361, Target Discovery and Validation Reviews and Protocols*
Volume 2, Emerging Molecular Targets and Treatment Options
Edited by: M. Sioud © Humana Press Inc., Totowa, NJ

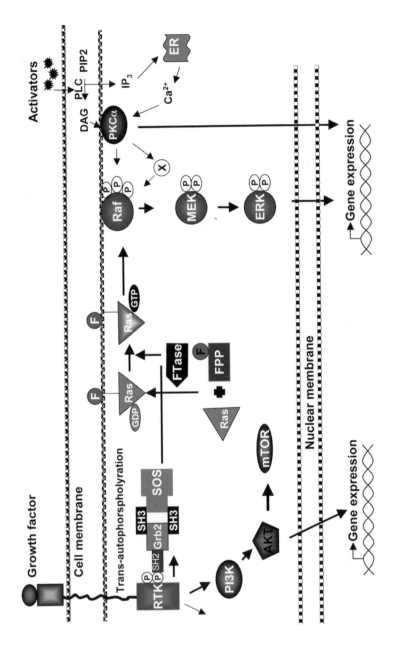

phenotype *(2,3)*. Among the best-studied growth factor receptor systems has been the epidermal growth factor (EGF) receptor family and the platelet-derived growth factor receptor. These receptors contain an extracellular binding domain, a transmembrane lipophilic domain, and intracellular protein tyrosine kinase domain. Interaction of a growth factor with its receptor tyrosine kinase would activate several signaling proteins that ultimately lead to cell proliferation *(4,5)*. Thus, one way to inhibit cell proliferation is to use receptor antagonists.

The initial step of selecting an appropriate target for pharmaceutical development is of fundamental importance. The primary criterion for target selection is now established as disease relevance based on functional data in vitro and in vivo. However, before embarking on target validation it is important to investigate whether the selected candidate gene products are druggable. This would increase the rate of developing new drugs. As illustrated in **Fig. 1**, several receptor tyrosine kinases and cytokine receptors activate Ras protein, which is a major contributor to human cancer. Constitutive activation of Ras via mutations has been found in 30% of all cancer types, establishing a potential causal relation between the target (Ras) and cancer in humans *(6)*. Models organisms also confirmed the importance of Ras activation. Thus, Ras is a viable drug target.

Subsequent to activation, Ras interacts with and activates the serine/threonine protein kinase Raf-1, which in turn phosphorylates and activates mitogen-activated protein kinase (MEK). Activated MEK then phosphorylates extracellular signal-regulated protein kinase (ERK)-1 and ERK-2. Raf mutations have been identified in a range of human tumors and constitutive activation of MEK resulted in cellular transformation. Because of their important roles, both Raf and MEK kinases represent attractive targets in cancer. In addition to Ras, Raf-1 can

---

Fig. 1. *(Opposite page)* Schematic overview of the receptor tyrosine-kinase-RAS-ERK signaling pathway. The binding of a growth factor to its receptor tyrosine kinase (RTK) results in auto phosphorylation and activation of signaling proteins. The Src-homology 2 (SH2) domain on the adaptor molecule growth factor binding protein-2 (Grb2) binds to phosphorylated tyrosine residues on the RTK. Grb2 via its SH3 domain binds to Sos, which translocates to the plasma membrane and binds to Ras. Ras is post-translationally modified in to order to translocate into the plasma membrane. Activated Ras recruits and activates Raf to the plasma membrane. Activated Raf phosphorylates activate MEK, which further phosphorylates and activates extracellular signal regulated protein kinase (ERK). ERK translocates to the nucleus where it can regulate gene expression by phosphorylation of transcription factors. Protein kinase C (PKC) is activated by diacyl glycerol (DAG) and Ca2+. Phospholipase C (PLC) hydrolyses phospho-inositol diphosphate (PIP2) to DAG and inositol triphosphate (IP3). Cytosolic IP3 induces endoplasmatic reticulum to release Ca2+. PKCα can either directly or indirectly activate Raf kinase. Nuclear translocation of PKCα into the nucleus cans active gene expression.

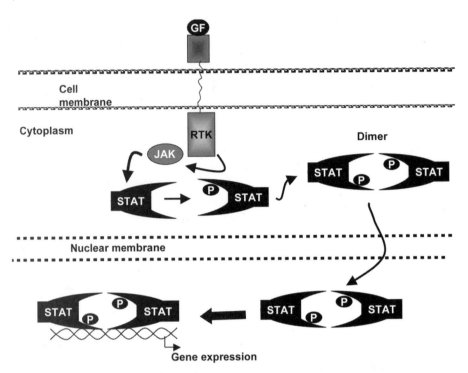

Fig. 2. Schematic representation of signal transducers and activators of transcription (STAT) signaling. STAT activation is initiated by tyrosine phosphorylation that is mediated by growth factor receptors and/or cytoplasmic protein tyrosine kinases (cPTKs), such as JAKs and Src. Phosphorylation of STAT induces dimerization, which allows STATs to translocate to the nucleus where they bind to consensus STAT-binding sequences of target genes and thereby activate gene transcription. Serine phosphorylation by protein serine kinases allows maximal transcriptional activity.

be activated by either protein kinase C (PKC)-α or the antiapoptotic protein Bcl-2. Theoretically, it could be argued that all the components of the RTK signaling pathway could represent a viable strategy to interfere with tumor growth *(7)*.

In addition to MAPK activation *(8)*, growth factor receptors also activate a family of cytoplasmic proteins known as signal transducers and activators of transcription (STAT) **(Fig. 2)**. STAT proteins are also activated by cytoplasmic tyrosine kinases, particularly Janus kinase (JAK) and Src kinase families *(9)*. Because of their diverse biological functions, aberrations in STAT signaling are predicted to have a wide variety of consequences. Abnormal activity of certain STAT family members, particularly STAT-3 and STAT-5, is associated with a wide range of human malignancies, including breast and prostate cancers. And constitutive STAT-3 activation is required for oncogenic transformation by v-Src *(10)*. Importantly, a constitutively activated STAT-3 mutant alone is sufficient to induce transformation *(11)*, thus confirming the oncogenic function of STAT-3. Based upon these findings, STAT3 is a viable target in cancers.

Defects in Wnt signaling pathways are associated with several cancer types *(12)* (*see* Chapter 3). Wnt signaling acts as a positive regulator by inhibiting β-catenin degradation, which stabilizes β-catenin, and causes its accumulation and translocation to the nucleus. The mechanism by which β-catenin translocates into the nucleus is not completely clear, as it does not contain a nuclear localization signal and thus may be transported by other binding proteins. A key event in cancer is the loss of control over β-catenin levels, which can be the consequences of loss-of-function mutations in APC, originally discovered because they predispose to colorectal cancer *(13)*. Around 80% of colorectal tumors have APC gene mutations *(9)*. In addition to its role as a transcription factor, β-catenin is also involved in the control of cellular adhesion. It binds to the cytoplasmic domain of type I cadherins and plays an essential role in the structural organization and function of cadherins by binding to α-catenin, which in turn binds to actin cytoskeleton. Because β-catenin is the critical component of Wnt signaling, it represents an appropriate target in Wnt-causing cancers.

Several of evidences suggest that the level of PKC activity is important for certain cancer types *(14)*. PKC is member of a family of cytoplasmic serine-threonine kinases, which are activated by several growth factors and lipid derivitives. Notably, many of the effectors molecules in inflammation are generated from phospholipids in the cell membrane. This makes the phospholipids not only building blocks in a membrane, but also very important reservoir from which cells generate intracellular and intercellular messengers. These include the oxidized fatty acids, platelet-activating factor, diacyl glycerol, and phosphatodic acid, which all are generated by a group of enzymes, the phospholipases. Phospholipase C uses phosphatidylinositol-4, 5-bis-phosphate to generate IP3 and diacyl glycerol, which lead to the activation of several PKC isoenzymes (**Fig. 1**). In addition to being involved in tumor growth, certain PKC isoenzymes were found to play an important role in the neoplastic progression of tumors and drug-resistant phenotype *(15)*. Thus, modulation of PKC activity may improve therapies in some cancer types.

Despite some encouraging results with some therapeutic strategies, most tumors develop resistance to drug- and radiation-induced apoptosis. This resistance is mainly mediated by high expression of Bcl-2 family proteins, which can contribute to cancer cell expansion by preventing normal cell turnover initiated by physiological cell death pathways *(16–18)*. High expression of Bcl-2 was found in a wide range of human cancers. Therefore, Bcl-2 and related proteins might be an effective therapeutic target in some cancers where altered expression profile contributes to the disease. Herein, we summarize recent work on targeting signaling pathways, a new optimism for cancer therapeutics.

2. Anticancer Drugs Targeting Receptor Tyrosine Kinase Pathways

Receptor tyrosine kinases are a family of proteins that signal cells through tyrosine phosphorylation reactions, and are the first part of a signaling pathway, which connects the signaling from membrane receptors to transcription factors that control gene expression. Hunter et al. *(7)* identified 478 typical and 40 atypical protein kinase genes in humans that correspond to approx 2% of all human genes. The family includes 385 serine/threonine kinases, 90 protein-tyrosine kinases, and 43 tyrosine-kinase-like proteins. Of the 90 protein-tyrosine kinases, 58 are receptor kinases *(7,8)*. The receptor tyrosine kinase signaling pathways play an important role in the control of fundamental cellular processes such as cell cycle, migration, survival, proliferation, and differentiation *(4)*. Examples of tyrosine kinase receptors are epidermal growth factor receptor (EGFR) and platelet-derived growth factor receptor *(4)*. Given their involvement in several cellular functions, RTK are tightly regulated *(4)*. Protein-tyrosine phosphatases have an important role in this control by dephosphorylating phospho-tyrosine residues and thereby inhibiting the activity of the receptor. In cancer, however, the receptor tyrosine kinases are often constitutively active owing to mutations, therefore leading to ligand-independent signaling *(7)*.

Among the best-studied growth factor receptor systems has been the EGF receptor family, which contains four homologous receptors: the epidermal growth factor receptor (ErbB1/EGFR/HER-1), ErbB2 (HER2/neu), ErbB3 (HER3), and ErbB4 (HER4). These receptors become activated by dimerization between two identical receptors or between different receptors of the same family *(5)*. The mechanisms that promote the formation of receptor dimers include ligand binding as well as high receptor density as a result of overexpression. The most widely studied and best-understood ErbB receptors are ErbB1 and ErbB2. Both display abnormal or enhanced expression in many types of cancer, suggesting their involvement in tumorigenesis *(19–21)*. Moreover overexpression has been shown to correlate with disease progression, survival, stage, and response to therapy. The exact mechanisms that are responsible for tumorigenic activity arising from these receptors in different types of cancer are not fully understood. EGFR seems to have a role in normal astrocyte differentiation and survival of the neural stem cell compartment. It is entirely possible that increased EGFR pathway activation may interfere with the normal differentiation process and serve to enhance malignant potential in gliomas *(22)*. Preclinical data suggest that EGFR regulates a number of important signaling pathways, including the Ras-RAF-MAPK cascade as well as the PI3K/AKT pathway, which, when upregulated via EGFR amplification/overexpression, lead to increased cellular proliferation, migration, and invasion. It is also becoming clear that upregulation of EGFR may contribute to the intrinsic radioresistance of glioma cells *(22)*.

Approximately 40% of the GBMs with EGFR amplification express a mutant form of EGFR, referred to as EGFRvIII. The EGFRvIII mutant lacks a portion of the extracellular ligand-binding domain as the result of genomic deletions of exons 2–7 in the EGFR mRNA. This results in constitutive phosphorylation, or activation, of the EGFR pathway *(23,24)*.

The *ErbB2* gene encodes a growth factor receptor with tyrosine kinase activity that is amplified in 10–40% of breast cancer resulting in overexpression of the *ErbB2* gene. In addition to breast and ovarian cancer, overexpression has also been found in lung, gastric, and oral cancers. ErbB2 overexpression is associated with particularly aggressive disease and poor patient prognosis *(25,26)*. A point mutation at the transmembrane domain and gene amplification are both believed to result in activation of the receptor. This is likely a result of the enhanced formation and stabilization of the receptor dimers, allowing the protein to remain in an active state. As previously mentioned, MAPK pathway has been strongly believed to participate in growth and transformation in many cell types *(21)*. Autophosphorylation of ErbB2, leading to the activation of Ras/Raf/ERK/MAPK pathway, appears to be very important for this process of transformation *(22)*. Another signaling molecule downstream of ErbB2 is PI3-kinase, which contains a 110-kDa catalytic and an 85-kDa regulatory subunit. Activation of this pathway is mediated by activated Ras or directly by some tyrosine kinase receptors that are under several growth factors and cytokines. Although ErbB2 protein has no p85-binding site, it may associate with PI3K, probably through heterodimerization with ErbB3. PI3-kinase is very often activated in cancer and contributes to cell cycle progression, cell survival, and metastasis. PI3-kinase activates Akt, a serine and threonine kinase, which in turn phosphorylates BCL2-antagonist of cell death (BAD) protein and inhibits apoptosis. The PI3K and AKT are considered proto-oncogenes, and the tumor-suppressor gene PTEN inhibits the pathway. Other evidence supports the interaction between the c-Src and ErbB2. Indeed, a high c-Src activity was found in ErbB2-induced mammary tumors than in the adjacent epithelium *(21)*. The activation of c-Src correlated with its ability to form complexes with tyrosine-phosphorylated ErbB2. Also, the PI3/AKT signaling pathway is a key modulator pathway by which growth factor receptors activate a protein kinase termed mammalian target of rapamycin (mTOR). Akt indirectly activates mTOR via TSC, which in turn phosphorylates and activates several target genes **(Fig. 1)**. Agents (e.g., CCI-779) targeting the rapamycin-sensitive signal transduction pathways have been developed for cancer therapy *(27)*.

Over the last decade, several approaches were used to interfere with TKR signaling. These include the modulation of downstream signaling from the receptor by inhibiting or attenuating the activity of secondary messenger proteins, blockage of receptor expression or activity, and reducing the amount of

Table 1
Anticancer Agents Targeting Receptor Tyrosine Kinases

Drug	Type	Target	Malignancies	Development phase
Iressa® (ZD1839)	Tyrosine kinase inhibitor (quinazoline)	ErbB1 (EGFr), competitive with ATP	NSCLC, prostate, head/neck, glioma	II-III, approved for NSCLC
Tarceva® (OSI774)	Tyrosine kinase inhibitor (quinazoline)	ErbB1, competitive with ATP	NSCLC, pancreas, ovarian	II-III
Herceptin®	Monoclonal antibody	ErbB2	Breast	III/IV
Cetuximab (IMC-C225)	Monoclonal antibody	ErbB1	Colorectal, breast	II/III
Erbitux®	Monoclonal antibody	ErbB1	Colorectal, HNSCC	II/III
CI1033 (PD183805)	Tyrosine kinase inhibitor (quinizalone)	ErbB1 competitive with ATP	Squamous cell skin cancer, NSCLC, breast	I
GW2016	Tyrosine kinase inhibitor (quinazoline)	ErbB1, competitive with ATP	Lung	I

available ligands. Most progress has been made with the first two approaches (**Tables 1** and **2**). Small-molecule tyrosine kinase inhibitors represent the largest and most promising class of agents in development *(28)*. The pharmacological characteristics of Iressa® (ZD1839), a quinazoline, were first described in 1996 as a potent and selective inhibitor of the EGFR tyrosine kinase, acting as an adenosine triphosphate (ATP)-competitive inhibitor of the EGFR tyrosine kinase *(28)*. Iressa exhibited in vivo activity in a diverse human tumor xenograft models. Multiple phase I trials with Iressa have been conducted and the data showed reasonable pharmacokinetics and clinical efficacy when used as single agents in patients with advanced disease. Ireassa is now approved for NSCLC. Other selective-quinazoline-based inhibitors of the EGFR function have been developed such as CP-358, 774 which have more than 500-fold selectivity against other tyrosine kinases, such as the closely related ErbB2 kinase *(28)*. Clinical studies showed that this new generation of drugs is well tolerated at doses required for antitumor efficacy.

Table 2
Anticancer Drugs Targeting Ras

Drug	Type	Target	Malignancies	Development phase
SCH66336	Farnesyl transferase inhibitor	Farnesyl transferase	Pancreas, bladder, hematologic malignancies, gastrointestinal cancers, breast	II
R115777	Farnesyl transferase inhibitor	Farnesyl transferase	Hematologic malignancies, gastrointestinal cancers, breast	II-III
BMS214662	Farnesyl transferase inhibitor	Farnesyl transferase	Hematologic malignancies	I
ISIS2503	Antisense	Inhibiting Ha-Ras protein expression	Breast, pancreatic, NSCLC	I/II

In addition to quinazoline compounds, monoclonal antibodies (mAb), which block receptor activation, were developed. These antibodies bind to the receptors with affinity comparable to the natural ligands, compete with ligand binding, and thereby block the tyrosine kinase-receptor activity *(5)*. Cetuximab (IMC-225) and Erbitux are two anti-EGFR (ErbB1) mAb, which are in phase II/III studies. mAb 225 induces antibody-mediated receptor dimerization (without activation of the tyrosine kinase), resulting in receptor downregulation. One of the most potent inhibitory anti-ErbB-2 antibodies was humanized for clinical applications. The resulting antibody trastuzumab (Herceptin®) exhibited a higher binding affinity for ErbB2 *(19)*. In addition, to receptor modulations, the developed antibody also induced antibody-dependent cell-mediated cytotoxicity against ErbB2-expressing tumor cells in animal models. An early phase II with trastuzumab was conducted in 46 patients with metastatic breast carcinoma overexpressing ErbB2 resulted in one complete remission and four partial remissions, and additional 14 patients showed minimal response. A phase III clinical trial in combination with cisplatin was also conducted in patients with advanced breast cancers. An enhanced survival was obtained and the antibody is generally well tolerated *(5)*. Laboratory data from cell cultures suggest synergism between trastuzumab and a range of chemotherapeutic agents, including docetaxel, cisplatin, and etoposide. Another

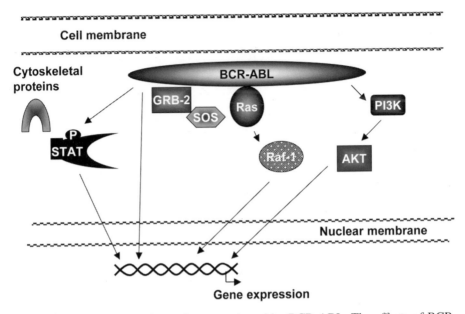

Fig. 3. Signal transduction pathways activated by BCR-ABL. The effects of BCR-ABL are mediated through its interaction with various signaling proteins leading to the activation of Ras signaling pathway, PI3K/AKT signaling pathway, and STAT proteins.

targeting approach is the use of synthetic growth factor antagonists *(23)*. One example is GFB-111, which binds to the platelet-derived growth factor receptor and was shown to inhibit glioblastoma tumor growth in mice up to 80% *(29,30)*.

As illustrated in **Fig. 1**, adaptor molecules are recruited to the active tyrosine kinase receptor. These proteins connect tyrosine kinase receptors to intracellular signaling pathways by functioning as an adapter between phosphotyrosine residues on the tyrosine kinase receptor and a proline-rich area on Sos protein *(6)*. Grb2 is an adaptor protein, which through its Src homology 2 (SH2)-domain recognizes phosphotyrosine residues on the RTK, and through its SH3-domaine recognizes Sos. Subsequently, Sos translocates to the cell membrane and binds to Ras, which are activated by exchange of GDP by GTP. Therefore, interfering with Grb2–SH2-receptor interaction or Grb2–SH3–Sos interaction could potentially inhibit the growth of malignant cells that are dependent upon activated Ras proteins. In this respect, several inhibitors have been developed *(30)*.

It is worth to note that some of the signaling proteins involved in TRK signaling also transduce the oncogenic effect of BCR-ABL kinase *(31)*. For example, by binding to BCR-ABL kinase Grb2 activates several downstream signaling pathways **(Fig. 3)**. The key pathways implicated so far are those involving Ras, mitogen-activated protein kinases, PI3K/AKT as well as transcription factors such as STATs and MYC. The BCR-ABL fusion gene encodes a constitutively activated protein tyrosine kinase that is a hallmark for chronic myeloid leukemia. Notably, BCR-ABL protein is one of the best targets in cancer because it is exclusive to the leukemic cells. During the 1990s, a number of tyrosine kinase inhibitors were purified from natural substances (e.g., herbimycin A and genistein) or chemically synthesized (e.g., tyrphostins). However, only imatinib mesylate (Glivec®, formerly known as STI 571) has resulted in excellent hematologic and cytogenetic responses in for chronic myeloid leukemia patients *(32)*.

3. Anticancer Drugs Targeting Ras

"A number of novel therapies are currently showing promising in preclinical and clinical studies (**Table 2**). These include inhibitors targeting specific branches of TKR activated. As shown in **Fig. 1**, the main activated pathways are those involving Ras and mitogen-activated protein kinases. Ras functions as a membrane-associated biological switch that links signal from ligand-stimulated receptors to cytoplasmatic MAPK cascades. These receptors include G protein-coupled receptors, tyrosine kinase receptors (e.g., EGFR, EGF), and cytokine receptors. As previously mentioned, Ras proteins regulate cell growth and differentiation by cycling between an inactive, GDP-bound conformation and an active, GTP-bound form that stimulate downstream targets such as Raf-1. Ras is often mutated in different cancer types, and mutated Ras proteins are locked in the active GTP-bound state, thereby stimulating growth autonomously *(33)*. When Ras is activated, effector molecules such as Raf, MEKK, and PI-3K bind to Ras and become activated. Ras must go through several posttranslational modifications to obtain full biological activity. These modifications include farnesylation by the enzyme farnesyl transferase (FTase). This posttranslational modification, which is required for Ras activity, has emerged as a major target for the development of novel anticancer agents *(34,35)*. FTase recognizes and farnesylates the CAAX tetrapeptides with similar affinity to the full-length Ras proteins. Based upon this observation, several competitive inhibitors of FTase were designed and some of them have undergone clinical evaluation *(34,35)*. One of the lead compounds currently in clinical development is R115777 and SCH55335 *(36)*. R115777 was evaluated in patients with advanced solid tumors and in patients with refractory acute leukaemia, and some encouraging results were obtained. FTase inhibitors have been shown to have very little effect on the proliferation of normal cells. Thus, the antitumor activity and lack of toxicity of FTase inhibitors suggest that a farnesylated protein or proteins are critical to tumor survival and oncogenesis. In addition to FT inhibitors, GGT inhibitors were also developed.

Several new methods such as antisense, aptamers, ribozymes, and RNA interference have been developed to assign functions to a large numbers of genes. It should be noted that RNAi is now the leading technique in target validation (*see* Chapters 9–12). Despite the technical difficulties (e.g., delivery, stability), several antisense oligomers are being subjected to phase II and phase III clinical trials *(37)*. ISIS 2503 is a 20-mer phosphorothioate oligonucleotide complementary to the translation initiation site of the human Ha-Ras mRNA. It specifically inhibits Ha-Ras expression and displayed activity against a range of different tumor types *(38)*.

4. Anticancer Drugs Targeting MAP Kinase Kinase (Raf, MEK)

The MAP kinase (MAPK) has emerged as the crucial link between membrane-bound Ras and the nucleus. This pathway involves the activation of three key kinases namely Raf, MEK (MAP kinase kinase), and ERK (MAPK), which represent novel therapeutic targets. Ras interacts with and activates the serine/threonine kinase Raf-1 in a GTP-dependent manner. Impaired Raf-1 expression has been observed in a variety of cancers including breast cancer *(39)* and small-cell lung carcinomas *(40)*. Moreover, Raf mutations have been identified in a range of human tumors *(6)*. Mutated Raf-1 is constitutively active and possesses in vitro transforming potential. Independent of mutations, Raf-1 is also activated in tumors with constitutive active TKR receptors or Ras proteins *(41)*. Once activated, Raf-1 kinase phosphorylates MEK1 and MEK2 which in turn activate ERK1 and ERK2 (ERK1/2). The potential for Raf-1 to play a broad role in tumorigenesis is evidenced by its ability to become activated by other cellular kinases such protein kinase Cα in a Ras-independent manner *(42)*. Because of its important role in cell signaling, several inhibitors for Raf activity were developed (**Table 3**). One of these inhibitors ZM336372 exhibited in vivo activity *(36)*. A search for specific pharmacological inhibitors of Raf kinase has also resulted in the identification of the bis-aryl ureas as lead active compounds *(42)*. The bis-aryl urea BAY 43-9006 has been selected as a candidate for clinical development, and has reached phase II-III studies. Similar to Ras proteins, Raf kinases were also targeted by antisense oligonucleotides and DNAzymes (*see* Chapter 7). In this respect, we recently found that depletion of Raf-1 protein with a DNAzyme induced substantial inhibition of JMML cell colony formation *(44)*. Moreover, when immunodeficient mice engrafted with JMML cells were treated continuously with the DNAzyme via a peritoneal osmotic minipump for 4 wk, a profound reduction in the JMML cell numbers in the recipient murine bone marrows was found, and their survival increased *(44)*. These results indicated that cleaving Raf-1 mRNA by nucleic acid enzymes might hold promise as new therapeutic strategy in several diseases where this kinase is activated. ISIS 5132 is a 20-mer-phosphorothioate oligonucleotide targeting a site in the 3' untranslated region showed antiproliferative and antitumor activity against various tumor cell lines in vitro and in vivo *(45)*. ISIS 5132 has been tested in phase I-II studies.

Activated Raf-1 phosphorylates and activates MEK, which in turn phosphorylates and activates ERK-1 and ERK-2. MEK therefore represents an attractive

Table 3
Anticancer Agents Targeting Raf, MEK

Drug	Type	Target	Malignancies	Development phase
ZM336372	Raf inhibitor	Raf, competitive with ATP	Neuroendocrine tumors	Preclinical
PD184352 (CI-1040)	MEK inhibitor	MEK, inhibits phosphory-lation	Colon, pancreas, breast	I-II
BAY 43-9006	Raf inhibitor (bis-aryl ureas)	Raf	Colorectal, breast, hepatocellular carcinoma, NSCLC, leukemia, renal cell cancers	II-III
ISIS5132	Antisense	Raf	Prostate, colon, ovarian	I-II

target for pharmacological intervention in cancer. MEK is a crucial intracellular kinase for many mitogene-signaling pathways activated by oncogenes *(46)*. Although MEK is not identified as an oncogene, its constitutive activation can result in cellular transformation *(46)*. In this respect, small molecular compounds that inhibit the activity of MEK have been developed *(46)*. PD09059 is a synthetic inhibitor, which inhibits the activation of MEK1 and in lesser extent MEK2 *(47)*. PD184352 is a second inhibitor of MEK and is shown to inhibit tumor growth in mice with colon cancer in approx 80% of the cases *(48)*. Clinical phase I studies of this inhibitor are started *(46)*.

5. Anticancer Drugs Targeting the MAPK Pathways (ERK)

At least five MAPK cascades have been characterized in mammalian cells, including the extracellular-regulated kinases, ERK1 and ERK2, the c-Jun NH_2-terminal kinase, also known as stress-activated MAP kinase, and the p38 kinase pathway *(49)*. A protein kinase cascade activates each of these groups. ERK-1 and -2 are proline-directed protein kinases that phosphorylate Ser/Thr-Pro motifs in the consensus sequence Pro-X_{1-2}-Ser/Thr-Pro, where X is any amino acid *(50)*. Because of their high degree of similarity, ERK1/2 are usually considered to be functionally redundant and have been implicated in the signaling cascades induced by a broad range of receptors, in virtually all cell types. In addition to their activity in the cytoplasm, they translocate into the nucleus and regulate gene expression through phosphorylation of nuclear transcription factors *(50)*. However, neither ERK1/2 contains nuclear localization sequences or nuclear export signals. ERK activation has been found to be required for transformation of certain cells. In this respect, constitutive activation of ERK was found to be necessary for Ras-induced transformation of fibrosarcoma cells *(51)* and for EWS/FLI-1 transformation of NIH3T3 cells *(52)*. Activated MEK phosphorylates and activates ERK. Despite their important role in cell signaling, no selective inhibitor of ERK has been described. However, ERK- and MEK-inhibitors could be expected to have the same effect because ERK only is activated by MEK *(46)*.

6. Anticancer Drugs Targeting STAT Pathways

STAT proteins are a family of cytoplasmic proteins involved in signal transduction pathways used by many growth factors and cytokines, and are activated by phosphorylation of tyrosine and serine residues by upstream JAKs and Src kinase (**Fig. 2**). Notably, Src kinase has been shown to alter the expression or activity of several gene products. JAKs are crucial signal transducers for a variety of cytokines, growth factors, and interferons *(53–55)*. JAKs relay on the signals initiated by extracellular stimuli via corresponding receptors. Either the receptor and/or JAKs can alternatively recruit the STATs proteins via recognition of the SH2 domain near the phosphorylated sites *(56)*. The phosphorylation of the STAT tyrosine residue is essential not only for dimerization, but also for the concomitant translocation of the dimmers into the nucleus. In normal cells, the signaling by STAT proteins is under tight regulation, so that the signal delivered to the cell is transient. However, abnormal activity of certain STAT family members, particularly STAT-3 and -5, has been noted in many tumors, including hematologic, breast, head and neck, and prostate cancers *(9,57–61)*. Constitutively active STAT-3 mutant alone induces transformation, and cells transformed by this active STAT-3 mutant form tumors in vivo. Using in vivo tumor models murine B16 melanoma tumors regress on inhibition of STAT-3. Aberrant STAT-3 signaling is obligatory for growth and survival of various tumors, including multiple myelomas, breast carcinomas, and head and neck squamous cell carcinomas *(9)*. The cancer-causing activity of constitutively activated STAT-3 protein and evidence of potential clinical benefits of blocking constitutive STAT-3 made this kinase an important molecular target for the development of new anticancer treatments.

Tyrosine phosphorylation of STATs constitutes an early event in the activation of these transcription factors that is required for their dimerization and DNA binding activity. Thus, one method of direct regulation of the action of STAT proteins involves the inhibition of dimerization, which is essential for nuclear translocation and transcriptional activity *(56)*. Dimerization inhibition can be brought about by the use of artificial compounds, which have high affinity for the STAT monomer, to generate compounds that are more stable than STAT-STAT homodimers *(57)*. Recently, small phosphotyrosyl-peptides have been used; these bind at the STAT3- SH2 domain, leading to its phosphorylation, dimerization, DNA-binding, and gene activation. Importantly, they inhibited v-Src cell transformation *(61)*. STAT coactivators play an extremely important role in guaranteeing DNA binding and the transcriptional activation carried out by the STATs. Therefore, the use of pseudoactivators with high STAT affinity might block STAT natural function *(59)*.

Following dimerization, STATs translocate into the nucleus and bind to specific regulatory sequences of responsive genes to induce gene transcription. Although the mechanisms of STAT translocation are not fully understood, small-molecule mimics of the translocation machinery might block STAT nuclear translocation *(60)*. The transcriptional activity of STATs requires that they physically interact with the promoter sequences. Knowledge of the crystal structure of STAT bound to its cognate DNA sequence should be important for rational design of artificial competitors. In this respect, phosphotyrosyl peptides inhibited STAT-3 interaction with DNA and therefore cell transformation *(61)*.

Another possible therapeutic approach is the use of antisense oligonucleotides, which block the expression of specific STAT mRNA transcripts, and the use of negative-dominant STAT proteins. Recently, we have found that STAT and Src signaling pathways are extremely important in breast cancer. Inactivation of STAT-3 with a siRNA-inhibited cell proliferation in vitro and in vivo, providing evidence for a functional role of STAT-3 in human cancers.

7. Anticancer Drugs Targeting PKCs

PKCα is a member of the PKC family of serine/threonine kinases, which are activated by many extracellular signals, and are central to many signaling pathways regulating cell growth and differentiation *(62)*. This family of serine/threonine kinases consists of at least 12 isoenzymes, which have been subdivided into three groups *(14)*. The potential role of PKC in carcinogenesis was first suggested by the observation that PKC represents the primary cellular target for tumor-promoting phorbol esters *(63,64)*. Situated at the crossroads of many signal transduction pathways, PKCs are also crucial to the link of a large diversity of signals from the cytoplasm to the nucleus.

PKCs are reversibly activated by upstream signaling elements such as growth factor receptors. Once activated, they can transmit signals to the nucleus via one or more MAPK cascades, which may incorporate Raf-1, MEKs, and ERKs. Overexpressed or hyperactive PKC is among the most distinguished characteristics of malignant brain tumors, in particular gliomas *(65)*. These findings led to the hypothesis that inhibition of PKC could represent a potential therapeutic strategy against high-grade brain malignancies. Reduction of PKC activity in cultured glioma cells using nonspecific PKC inhibitors such as staurosporine, tamoxifen, and calphostin C-inhibited glioma cell growth *(65)*.

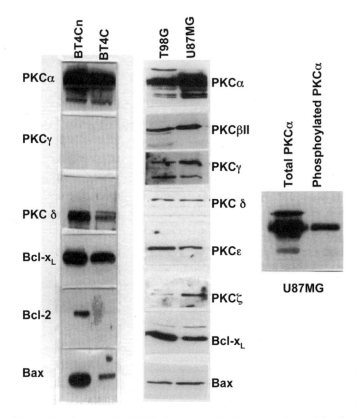

Fig. 4. Expression levels of PKC isoforms and Bcl-2-related proteins in rat (BT4C and BT4Cn) and human (T98MG and U87MG) glioma cell lines. Cytoplasmic protein extracts from each of the cell lines were analyzed by Western blotting using specific antibodies.

Although the overall PKC activity has been shown to be increased in some tumors, the precise role of each isoenzyme upon malignant cell growth is not known. To elucidate the specific role of PKC in cell survival and tumor promotion, we have used the nucleic acid enzyme strategy. Given the specificity of Watson-Crick base pairing, this strategy has the capacity to inhibit individual genes that are structurally related, such as isoenzymes. **Figure 4** shows the expression levels of several PKC isoenzyme and Bcl-2-related proteins. As shown, both human and rat glioma cells upregulated the expression of PCKα as compared to other PKC isoenzymes. In addition, a high percentage of PKCα was in vivo-activated. Specific targeting of PKCα by either a nuclease resistant ribozyme or a DNAzyme-induced apoptosis in glioma cells and inhibited tumor growth in vivo *(66–68)*. In addition, to gliomas, we have investigated the role of PKC-α in breast cancer proliferation and survival. **Figure 5** shows the

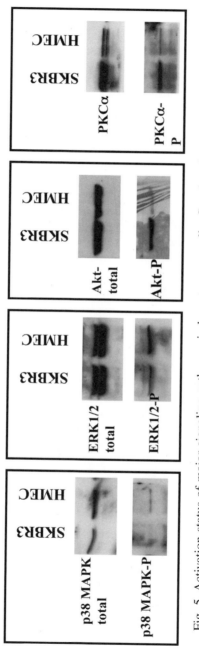

Fig. 5. Activation status of major signaling pathways in breast cancer cells. Cyoplasmic protein extracts were prepared from the breast cancer cell line SKBR3 or normal human mammary epithelial cells and then analyzed by Western blotting. Both total and phosphorylated kinases were detected using commercially available specific antibodies.

17

Table 4
Anticancer Agents Targeting PKC and Bcl-2

Drug	Type	Target	Malignancies	Development phase
ISIS3521	Antisense	PKCα	NSCLC, solid tumors	I-III
G3139	Antisense	Bcl-2	Melanoma, MM, CLL, NSCLC	III

activation status of the four main signaling proteins, p38, ERK, PKCα, and AKT in SKBR3 breast cancer cell line and human mammary epithelial cells. Both AKT and PKCα are constitutively activated in SKBR3 cells when compared to human mammary epithelial cells. By specifically targeting PKCα, Akt, or PI3K with either ribozymes or siRNAs, we have found that PKCα and PI3K are involved in malignant breast cancer cell survival and proliferation. Additionally, we have found that Akt can be phosphorylated by PKCα in vitro. Thus, PKCα might hold promise as a new therapeutic target in breast cancer. Recently, an antisense oligonucleotide targeting PKCα (ISIS 5132) exhibited in vitro and in vivo antitumor activity, and has reached phase I-II clinical trials (*[69]*; **Table 4**).

8. Anticancer Drugs Targeting Bcl-2 (Apoptosis)

Apoptosis is the prevalent form of programmed cell death that, when altered, contributes to a number of human diseases, including cancer. Bcl-2 and related proteins are a growing family of proteins that regulate apoptosis *(16)*. This family includes both death antagonists such Bcl-2, Bcl-x$_L$, Bcl-w, Mcl-1, and A1, and death agonists such as Bax, Bak, Bcl-x$_S$, Bad, Bid, Bik, Bim, Hrk, and Bok, which promote cell death *(70)*. The ratio of death antagonists compared to agonists influences the susceptibility of cells to apoptosis *(71)*. In general apoptosis can be divided into at least three different phases: initiation, effector, and degradation phases. During the initiation phase the cell receives apoptosis-triggering stimuli, which include ligation of certain receptors and cell stresses. The decision to die is made in the effector phase that involves the activation of the Bcl-2 proteins. The degradation phase occurs through the activation of the caspase cascade, which involves transactivation of procaspase-9 to active caspase-9, which in turn cleaves and activates downstream executioner caspases. The Fas-pathway involves the transactivation of procaspase-8 to active caspase-8.

Dysregulation of genes involved in apoptosis can contribute to cancer and resistance of cancer cells to conventional therapies. Proteins in the Bcl-2 family are crucial regulators of programmed cell death, and members that inhibit apoptosis, such as Bcl-X_L, A1, Bcl-2, are overexpressed in many cancers and contribute to tumor initiation and progression *(70)*. Moreover, overexpression of Bcl-2 and Bcl-X_L blocked apoptosis induced by a number of stimuli including anticancer drugs, contributing to resistance to therapy seen in patients *(18,19)*. It is therefore essential to determine whether downregulation of these proteins would benefit cancer patients.

The three-dimensional structure of human Bcl-X_L, a close homolog of Bcl-2 has provided a structural basis for the design and discovery of Bcl-2 binding small molecules *(72)*. Peptides containing the BH3 domain blocked protein interactions involving Bcl-2 and Bcl-X_L. Some of the developed peptide triggered apoptosis via caspase activation. Two natural products antagonized with the antiapoptotic function of Bcl-2 or Bcl-X_L. In addition, low molecular weight organic compound, HA14-1, effectively induced apoptosis in HL60 cells overexpressing Bcl-2 protein. Recently, a high-throughput nuclear magnetic resonance-based method for lead compound discovery was used to screen a chemical library to identify small molecule inhibitors. A small inhibitor ABT-737 was identified. ABT-737 induced apoptosis of cells from lymphoma and small-cell carcinoma lines, as well as primary patient-derived cells. Moreover, it exhibited in vivo antitumor activity *(73)*. Clinical studies of this new agent are under way. This example, illustrate the importance of analyzing protein targets by three-dimensional structure for specific binding sites to evaluate their druggability for small pharmacological components. In principle, this should be done for all protein targets to minimize failures and increase specificity.

In addition to small molecules, antisense oligonucleotides targeting either Bcl-2 or Bcl-X_L induced apoptosis in cells derived from solid tumors and sensitized tumor cells to cancer therapies *(75)*. An 18-mer phosphorothioate antisense targeting the first six codons of the Bcl-2 open reading frame (G3139) has reached phase III studie **(Table 4)**. Although Bcl-X_L is similar to Bcl-2 in function, these two molecules protect cells from apoptosis nonredundantly. Antisense oligonucleotides targeting the Bcl-X_L induced apoptosis in various cancer types including NSCLC, breast cancer and prostate cancer in vitro and in vivo, and sensitize tumor cells to chemotherapy *(74)*. Moreover, a bispecific antisense oligonucleotide targeting both Bcl-2 and Bcl-X_L sensitized breast carcinoma cells to doxorubicin, paclitaxel, and cyclophosphoamide *(76; see* Chapter 7).

9. Conclusion and Perspectives

As illustrated in this review, several signaling proteins have emerged as novel therapeutic targets. A new class of cancer therapies that targets this pathological constitutive activated pathway is currently under development. Notably, the most dramatic therapeutic advances in cancer during the last decade have come from agents targeted against signaling proteins encoded by mutated genes. These include Herpetin (anti-ErbB-2), imatinib (anti-ABL-CBL), and gefitinib (anti-EGRR). Though none of these advances have resulted in cures of many patients with advanced disease, they can substantially improve and prolong lives. Several target genes are now identified (e.g., β-catenin, STAT-3, Bcl-2, PKC-α), and high-throughput analysis of drug discovery should lead to the identification of new generation of drugs.

It is worth noting that solid tumors are composed of two compartments, one consisting of neoplastic epithelial cells and other of stromal cells *(77)*. On the host side, the stromal cells together with extracellular matrix components provide the microenvironment that is important for cancer cell growth, invasion, and metastasis. In general, stroma compartment contain a variety of cell types, including immune cells, muscle and fibroblast cells, and vascular cells. These cells are modifying the phenotype of tumor cells by direct cell-to-cell contacts, via soluble factors or by modification of extracellular matrix. Thus, stromal therapy might become essential therapy in cancer prevention and intervention. By targeting either the expression of CSF-1 or its receptor *c-fms* by siRNAs, we have demonstrated that tumor growth can be inhibited in mice, through blockage of tumor-associated macrophage recruitment with concomitant reduction in local production of VEGF *(78)*.

References

1. Shawver, L. K., Slamon, D., and Ullrich, A. (2002) Smart drugs: tyrosine kinase inhibitors in cancer therapy. *Cancer Cell* **1**, 117–123.
2. Levitzki, A. (1994) Signal-transduction therapy. *Eur. J. Biochem.* **226**, 1–13.
3. Dhanasekaran, N. (1998) Cell signaling: an overview. *Oncogene* **17**, 1329–1330.
4. Schlessinger, J. (2000) Cell signaling by receptor tyrosine kinases. *Cell* **103**, 211–225.
5. Mendelsohn, J. and Baselga, J. (2000) The EGF receptor family as targets for cancer therapy. *Oncogene* **19**, 6550–6565.
6. Campbell, L., Khosravi-Far, R., Rossmann, K. L., Clark, G. J., and Der, C. J. (1998) Increasing complexity of Ras signaling. *Oncogene* **17**, 1395–1413.
7. Manning, G., Whyte, D. B., Martinez, R., Hunter, T., and Sudarsanam, S. (2002) The protein kinase complement of the human genome. *Science* **298**, 1912–1934.
8. Roskoski, R. (2004) The ErbB/HER receptor protein-tyrosine kinases and cancer. *Bioch. Biophys. Res. Commun.* **319**, 1–11.
9. Bowman, T., Garcia, R., Turkson, R., and Jove, R. (2000) STATs in oncogenesis. *Oncogene* **19**, 2474–2488.
10. Bromberg, J. F., Horvath, C. M., Besser, D., Lathem, W. W., and Darnell, J. E., Jr. (1998) *Mol. Cell. Biol.* **18**, 2553–2558.
11. Bromberg, J. F., Wrzeszczynska, M. H., Devgan, G., et al. (1999) Stat3 as an oncogene. *Cell* **98**, 295–303.
12. Polakis, P. (2000) Wnt signalling and cancer. *Genes Devel.* **14**, 1837–1851.

13. Kinzler, K. W. and Vogelstein, B. (1996) Lessons from hereditary colorectal cancer. *Cell* **87,** 159–170.

14. Dekker, L. V. and Parker, P. J. (1994) Protein kinase C—a question of specificity. *TIBS* **19,** 73–77.

15. Hug, H. and Sarre, T. F. (1993) Protein kinase C isoenzymes: divergence in signal transduction? *Biochem. J.* **291,** 329–343.

16. Tsujimoto, Y. and Shimizu, S. (2000) Bcl-2 family: life-or-death switch. *FEBS Letters* **466,** 6–10.

17. Simonian, P. L., Grillot, D. A., and Nunez, G. (1997) Bcl-2 and Bcl-xL can differentially block chemotherapy-induced cell death. *Blood* **90,** 1208–1216.

18. Dole, M., Nunez, G., Merchant, A. K., et al. (1994) Bcl-2 inhibits chemotherapy-induced apoptosis in neuroblastoma. *Cancer Res.* **54,** 3253–3259.

19. Arteaga, C. L. (2001) The epidermal growth factor receptor: From mutant oncogene in nonhuman cancers to therapeutic target in human neoplasia. *J. Clin. Oncol.* **19,** S32–S40.

20. Nicholson, R. I., Gee, J. M., and Harper, M. E. (2001) EGFR and cancer prognosis. *Eur. J. Cancer* **37,** 9–15.

21. Cooke, T., Reeves, J., Lannigan, A., and Stanton, P. (2001) The value of the human epidermal growth factor receptor-2 (Her-2) as a prognostic marker. *Eur. J. Cancer.* **37,** 3–10.

22. Chakravarti, A. Dicker, A., and Mehta, M. (2004) The contribution of epidermal growth factor receptor (EGFR) signaling pathway to radioresistance in human gliomas: a review of preclinical and correlative clinical data. *Int. J. Rad. Oncol. Biol. Phys.* **58,** 927–931.

23. Wong, A. J., Ruppert, J. M., Bigner, S. H., et al. (1992) Structural alterations of the epidermal growth factor receptor gene in human gliomas. *Proc. Natl. Acad. Sci. USA* **89,** 2965–2969.

24. Humphrey, P. A., Wong, A. J., Vogelstein, B., et al. (1990) Anti-synthetic peptide antibody reacting at the fusion junction of deletion-mutant epidermal growth factor receptors in human glioblastoma. *Proc. Natl. Acad. Sci. USA* **87,** 4207–4211.

25. Hung, M. -C. and Lau, Y. -K. (1999) Basic science of HER-2/neu: A Review. *Semin. Oncol.* **26,** 51–59.

26. Amundadottir, L. T. and Leder, P. (1998) Signal transduction pathways activated and required for mammary carcinogenesis in response to specific oncogenes. *Oncogene* **16,** 737–746.

27. Vignot, S., Faivre, S., Aguirre, D., and Raymond, E. (2005) mTOR-targeted therapy of cancer with rapamycin derivatives. *Ann. Oncol.* **16,** 525–537.

28. Mass, R. D. (2004) The HER receptor family: a rich target for therapeutic development. *Int. J. Rad. Oncol. Biol. Phys.* **58,** 932–940.

29. Willems, A., Gauger, K., Henrichs, C., and Harbeck, N. (2005) Antibody therapy for breast cancer. *Anticancer Res.* **25,** 1483–1489.

30. Sebti, S. M. and Hamilton, A. D. (2000) Design of growth factor antagonists with antiangiogenic and antitumor properties. *Oncogene* **19,** 6566–6573.

31. Deininger, M., Goldman, J., and Melo, J. (2000) The molecular biology of chronic myeloid leukaemia. *Blood* **96**, 3343–3356.

32. Bartram, C., de Klein, A., and Hagemeijer, A. (1983) Translocation of c-abl oncogene correlates with the presence of the Philadelphia chromosome in chronic myelocytic leukemia. *Nature* **306**, 277–280.

33. Bos, J. L. (1989) Ras oncogenes in human cancer. *Cancer Res.* **49**, 4682–4689.

34. Adjei, A. A. (2001) Blocking oncogenic Ras signaling for cancer therapy. *J. Natl. Cancer Inst.* **93**, 1062–1074.

35. Johnston, S. R. (2001) Farnesyltransferase inhibitors: a novel targeted therapy for cancer. *Lancet Oncol.* **2**, 18–26.

36. De Bono, J. S. and Rowinsky, E. K. (2002) Therapeutics targeting signal transduction for patients with colorectal carcinoma. *Br. Med. Bulletin.* **64**, 227–254.

37. Cowsert, L. M. (1997) In vitro and in vivo activity of antisense inhibitors of ras: potential for clinical development. *Anticancer Drug. Des.* **12**, 359–371.

38. Monia, B. P., Ecker, D. J., Zounes, M. A., Lima, W. F., and Freier, S. M. (1992) Selective inhibition of mutant Ha-Ras mRNA expression by antisense oligonucleotides. *J. Biol. Chem.* **267**, 19,954–19,962.

39. Callans, L. S., Naama, H., Khandelwal, M., Plotkin, R., and Jardines, L. (1995) Raf-1 protein expression in human breast cancer cells. *Ann. Surg. Oncol.* **2**, 38–42.

40. Sithanandam, G., Dean, M., Brennscheidt, U., et al. (1989) Loss of heterozygosity of the c-raf locus in small cell lung carcionoma. *Oncogene* **4**, 451–455.

41. Morrison, D. K. and Cutler, R. E. (1997) The complexity of Raf-1 regulation. *Curr. Opin. Cell. Biol.* **9**, 174–179.

42. Marquardt, B., Frith, D., and Stabel, S. (1994) Signalling from TPA to MAP kinase requires protein kinase C, raf and MEK: reconstitution of the signalling pathway in vitro. *Oncogene* **9**, 3213–3218.

43. Lyons, J. F., Wilhelm, S., Hibner, B., and Bollag, G. (2001) Discovery of a novel Raf kinase inhibitor. *Endocr. Relat. Cancer* **8**, 219–225.

44. Iversen, P. O., Emanuel, P. D., and Sioud, M. (2002) Targeting Raf-1 gene expression by a DNA enzyme inhibits juvenile myelomonocytic leukemia cell growth. *Blood* **99**, 4147–4153.

45. Monia, B. P., Johnston, J. F., Geiger, T., Muller, M., and Fabbro, D. (1996) Antitumor activity of phosphorothioate antisense oligodeoxynucleotide targeted against c-Raf kinase. *Nat. Med.* **2**, 668–675.

46. Sebolt-Leopold, J. S. (2000) Development of anticancer drugs targeting the MAP kinase pathway. *Oncogene* **19**, 6594–6599.

47. Dudley, D. T., Pang, L., Decker, S. J., Bridges, A. J., and Saltiel, A. R. (1995) A synthetic inhibitor of the mitogen-activated protein kinase cascade. *Proc. Natl. Acad. Sci. USA* **92**, 7686–7689.

48. Sebolt-Leopold, J. S., Dudley, D. T., Herrera, R., et al. (1999) Blockade of the MAP kinase pathway suppresses growth of colon tumors in vivo. *Nat. Med.* **5**, 810–816.

49. Schaeffer, H. J. and Weber, M. J. (1999) Mitogen-activated protein kinases: specific messages from ubiquitous messengers. *Mol. Cell. Biol.* **19**, 2435–2444.

50. Boulton, G., Nye, S. H., Robbibs, D. J., et al. (1991) ERKs: a family of protein-serine/threonine kinases that are activated and tyrosine phosphorylated in response to insulin. *Cell* **65**, 663–675.

51. Plattner, R., Gupta, S., Khosravi-Far, R., et al. (1999) Differential contribution of the ERK and JNK mitogen-activated protein kinase cascades to ras transformation of HT1080 fibrosarcoma and DLD-1 colon carcinoma cells. *Oncogene* **18**, 1807–1817.

52. Silvany, R. E., Eliazer, S., Wolff, N. C., and Ilaria, R. L., Jr. (2000) Interference with the constitutive activation of ERK1 and ERK2 impairs EWS/FLI-1-dependent transformation. *Oncogene* **19**, 4523–4530.

53. Silvennoinen, O., Ihle, J. N., Schlessinger, J., and Levy, D. E. (1993) Interferon-induced nuclear signaling by Jak protein tyrosine kinases. *Nature* **366**, 583–585.

54. O'Shea, J. J., Gadina, M., and Schreiber, R. D. (2002) Cytokine signaling in 2002: new surprises in the JAK/STAT pathway. *Cell* **109**, S121–S131.

55. Schindler, C. W. (2002) JAK-STAT signaling in human disease. *J. Clin. Invest.* **109**, 1133–1137.

56. Chen, X., Bhandari, R., Vinkermeier, U., Van Den Akker, F., Darnell, J. E., Jr., and Kuriyan, J. (2003) A reinterpretation of the dimerization interface of the N-terminal domains of STATs. *Protein Sci.* **12**, 361–365.

57. Luo, C. and Laaja, P. (2004) Inhibitors of JAKs/STATs and the kinases: a possible new cluster of drugs. *DDT* **9**, 268–275.

58. Bromberg, J. F., Horvath, C. M., Besser, D., Lathem, W. W., and Darnell, J. E., Jr. (1998) Stat 3 activation is required for cellular transformation by *v-src*. *Mol. Cell. Biol.* **18**, 2553–2558.

59. Turkson, J. and Jove, R. (2000) STAT proteins: novel molecular targets for cancer drug discovery. *Oncogene* **19**, 6613–6626.

60. Calo, V., Migliavacca, M., Bazan, V., et al. (2003) STAT proteins: from normal control of cellular events to tumorigenesis. *J. Cell. Physiol.* **197**, 157–168.

61. Turkson, J., Ryan, D., Kim, J. S., et al. (2001) Phosphotyrosyl peptides block Stat3-mediated DNA-binding activity, gene regulation, and cell transformation. *J. Biol. Chem.* **276**, 45,443–45,455.

62. Nishizuka, Y. (1992) Intracellular signaling by hydrolysis of phospholipids and activation of protein kinase C. *Science* **258**, 607–614.

63. Kikkawa, U., Takai, Y., Tanaka, Y., Miyake, R., and Nishizuka, Y. (1983) Protein kinase C as a possible receptor protein of tumor-promoting phorbol esters. *J. Biol. Chem.* **258**, 11,442–11,445.

64. Blumberg, P. M. (1988) Protein kinase C as the receptor for the phorbol ester tumor promoters: sixth roads memorial award lecture. *Cancer Res.* **48**, 1–8.

65. Rocha, A. B., Mans, D. R. A., Regner, A., and Schwartsmann, G. (2002) Targeting protein kinase C: new terapeutic opportunities against high-grade malignant gliomas. *The Oncologist* **7**, 17–33.

66. Sioud, M. and Sørensen, D. R. (1998) A nuclease-resistant protein kinase C alpha ribozyme blocks glioma cell growth. *Nat. Biotechnol.* **16**, 556–561.

67. Leirdal, M. and Sioud, M. (1999) Ribozyme inhinition of the protein kinase Ca triggers apoptosis in glioma cells. *Br. J. Cancer.* **80**, 1558–1564.

68. Sioud, M. and Leirdal, M. (2000) Design of nuclease resistant protein kinase Ca DNA enzymes with potential therapeutic application. *J. Mol. Biol.* **296**, 937–947.
69. Geiger, T., Muller, M., Dean, N. M., and Fabbro, D. (1998) Antitumor activity of a PKC-alpha antisense oligonucleotide in combination with standard chemotherapeutic agents against various human tumors transplanted into nude mice. *Anticancer Drug Des.* **13**, 35–45.
70. Reed, J. C. (1998) Bcl-2 family proteins. *Oncogene* **17**, 3225–3236.
71. Zamzami, N., Brenner, C., Marzo, I., Susin, S. A., and Kroemer, G. (1998) Subcellular and submitochondrial mode of action of Bcl-2-like oncoproteins. *Oncogene* **16**, 2265–2282.
72. Muchmore, S. W., Sattler, M., Liang, H., et al. (1996) X-ray and NMR structure of human Bcl-xL, an inhibitor of programmed cell death *Nature* **381**, 335–341.
73. Oltersdorf, T., Elmore, S. W., Shoemaker, A. R., et al. (2005) An inhibitor of Bcl-2 family proteins induces regression of solid tumours. *Nature* **435**, 677–681.
74. Ziegler, A., Luedke, G. H., Fabbro, D., Altmann, K. H., Stahel, R. A., and Zangemeister-Wittke, U. (1997) A novel antisense oligonucleotide targeting the coding region of the bcl-2 mRNA is a potent inducer of apoptosis in small cell lung cancer cells. *J. Natl. Cancer Inst.* **89**, 1027–1036.
75. Leech, S. H., Olie, R. A., Gautschi, O., et al. (2000) Induction of apoptosis in lung cancer cells following bcl-xL antisense treatment. *Int. J. Cancer.* **86**, 570–576.
76. Simoes-Wust, A., Schurpf, T., Hall, J., Stahel, R. A., and Zangemeister-wittke, U. (2002) Bcl-2/bcl-xL bispecific antisense treatment sensitizes breast carcinoma cells to doxorubicin, paclitaxel and cyclophosphoamide. *Breast. Cancer. Res. Treat.* **76**, 157–166.
77. Liotta, L. A. and Kohn, E. C. (2001) The microenvironment of the tumour-host interface. *Nature* **411**, 375–379.
78. Aharinejad, S., Paulus, P., Sioud, M., et al. (2004) Colony-stimulating factor-1 blockage by antisense oligonucleotides and small-interfering RNAs suppresses growth of human mammary tumor xenografts in mice. *Caner Res.* **64**, 5378–5384.

2

DNA Methylation and Histone Modifications in Patients With Cancer

Potential Prognostic and Therapeutic Targets

Michel Herranz and Manel Esteller

Summary

Epigenetics, a combination of DNA modifications, chromatin organization, and variations in its associated proteins, configure a new entity that regulates gene expression throughout methylation, acetylation, and chromatin remodeling. In addition to silencing as a result of mutations, loss of heterozygosity, or *classical* genetic events epigenetic modification symbolizes essential early events during carcinogenesis and tumor development. The reversion of these epigenetic processes restoring normal expression of tumor-suppressor genes has consequently become a new therapeutic target in cancer treatment. Aberrant patterns of epigenetic modifications will be, in a near future, crucial parameters in cancer diagnosis and prognosis.

Key Words: Cancer epigenetics; histone modifications; DNA methylation; prognosis; therapy.

1. Introduction

Epigenetics is concerned with the inheritance of information on the basis of differential gene expression, a process separate from genetic inheritance through gene sequence. Epigenetic modifications do not transform the DNA sequence; however, they are heritable and important in gene expression. Different components comprise the safety of the epigenome. Chromatin organization plays an important role in gene-expression regulation by modifying the tertiary structure to an open or accessible (euchromatin) status or to closed and inaccessible configuration (heterochromatin). Nuclear DNA is packaged into nucleosomes, a protein complex around which the DNA helix is wrapped. A nucleosome is a

From: *Methods in Molecular Biology, vol. 361, Target Discovery and Validation Reviews and Protocols*
Volume 2, Emerging Molecular Targets and Treatment Options
Edited by: M. Sioud © Humana Press Inc., Totowa, NJ

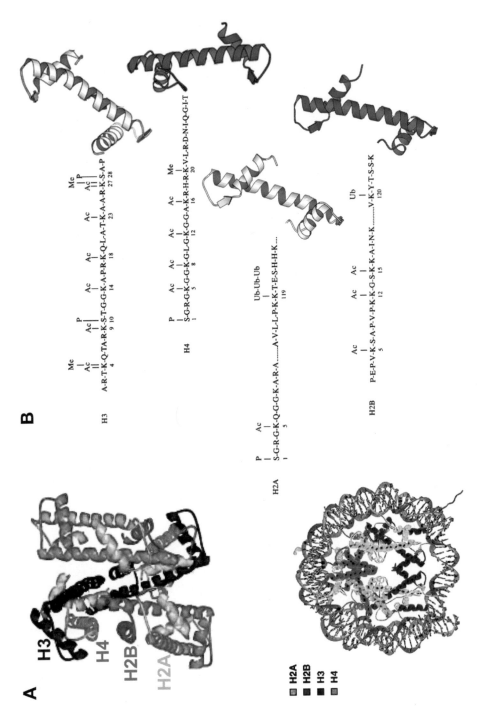

histone octamer core ([H3-H4]$_2$-2[H2A-H2B]). Histone fold domain, present and described in these proteins, is completed by a basic N-terminal and a C-terminal tail *(1)* **(Fig. 1A)**.

Remodeling chromatin can be completed in several and unified ways: (1) covalent modification of histones, (2) intrinsic DNA modification, (3) exchange core histones with mutant or modified histone variants, and (4) disrupting DNA–nucleosome contacts. Histone modifications in the basic N-terminal tails, including acetylation, methylation, ubiquitination, phosporylation, biotinylation, and sumoylation **(Fig. 1B)** *(2–6)*, result in changes in the cell transcriptional state. The best studied of these modifications is histone acetylation; this dynamic posttranslational modification is required for active chromatin configuration. Histone acetylation is a chemical equilibrium state. Acetylation is catalyzed by histone acetyltransferases (HAT), and deacetylation is catalyzed by histone deacetylases (HDAC) using acetyl-CoA as universal acetyl-donor **(Fig. 2)**.

In general, increased levels of histone acetylation (hyperacetylation) are found in euchromatin, a more open conformation of the nuclear chromatin, in which transcription is held in an active state; however, decreased levels of acetylation (hypoacetylation) are found in the tightly compacted chromatin (heterochromatin) associated with transcriptionally silent genomic regions. Another important histone modification in gene expression is histone methylation. Histone methyltransferases direct site-specific methylation of amino acid residues such as lysine (Lys4 and Lys9) and arginine residues. Methylation of Lys4 is important in maintenance of euchromatin structures, where genes are freely accessible and usually active; in contrast, methylation of H3Lys9 is associated with heterochromatin domains, strap, and inactive *(7)*. Lysines can be

---

Fig. 1. *(Opposite page)* The histone octamer assembly in the nucleosome and modifications in histone tails. **(A)** Two molecules of each of the four core histone proteins form the histone octamer via formation of one tetramer of H3 and H4 and two dimers of H2A and H2B. Note that the nucleosome containing the two turns of DNA has the N-terminal tails of the eight-histone protein sticking out from the nucleosome like the legs of a spider. The structure of the portion of these N-terminal tails outside of the DNA is not known, and, more importantly, nor is the 30-nm chromatin fiber. Tetramerization occurs via interactions between the C-terminal halves of two histone molecules and results in a twofold axis of symmetry for the tetramer as shown. **(B)** Histone N-terminal tails are exposed from the nucleosomal interior into the aqueous surroundings. Moreover, these core histone tails have been found to be covalently modified; i.e., they can be methylated, acetylated, phosphorylated, and so on, on a single or on sets of N-terminally located serine and lysine residues. Me, methylated; Ac, acetylated; P, phosphorylated; Ub, ubiquitinated.

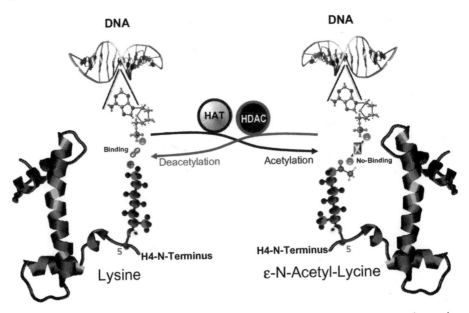

Fig. 2. Equilibrium of steady-state histone acetylation is maintained by opposing activities of histone acetyltransferases and deacetylases. Acetylation is a reversible process, in which histone acetyltransferases (HATs) transfer the acetyl moiety from acetyl coenzyme A to the ε-amino groups of internal, highly conserved lysine residues. This modification neutralizes the positively charged lysine residues of the histone N termini causing a reduction in the affinity of histone–DNA interactions, leading to increased access of transcription factors to the repressed chromatin template. Therefore, in most cases, histone acetylation enhances transcription while histone deacetylation represses transcription. Histone acetylation is catalyzed by HATs and histone deacetylation is catalyzed by histone deacetylases (denoted by HDACs).

mono-, di- or trimethylated, whereas arginines can be mono- or dimethylated, increasing the complexity of histone modifications.

DNA methylation remains the best-studied epigenetic mechanism. Methylation is needed for the normal development of cells because it facilitates static long-term gene silencing and confers genomic stability *(8)*. Abnormal methylation, which confers growth advantages, is tightly connected to cancer development *(9)*. Methylation of cytosines within the CpG dinucleotide (60% of human genes contain a CpG island *[10]*) by transfer of a methyl group from the methyl donor *S*-adenosylmethionine to the carbon 5 position of cytosines (**Fig. 3**) is catalyzed by DNA methyltransferases: DNA methyltransferases 1 (DNMT1; responsible for DNA methylation maintenance during cell division, development, and cancer), DNMT3a, and DNMT3b (responsible for *de novo* methylation during early development) *(11,12)*.

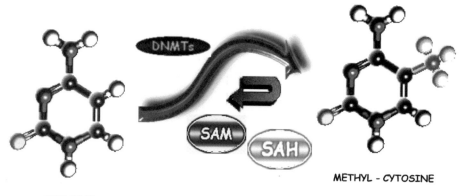

CYTOSINE

METHYL - CYTOSINE

Fig. 3. Epigenetics refers to alterations in gene expression that occur without a change in DNA sequence. The chemistry behind one of these events is simple. It involves the covalent addition of a methyl group to cytosine. Of the four bases that make up DNA—adenine, thymine, cytosine, and guanine—only cytosine has the potential to be methylated in humans and most mammals. The methylation reaction involves flipping the target cytosine out of the intact double helix, so that the transfer of the methyl group from the methyl donor (*S*-adenosylmethionine) can take place. This reaction is catalyzed by the enzyme DNA methyltransferase (DNMTs). Methylation only occurs in cytosines whose 3'-carbon atom is linked by a phosphodiester bond to the 5'-carbon atom of a guanine (CpG dinucleotide). Most CpG dinucleotides are clustered in small stretches of DNA known as CpG islands.

Aberrant methylation patterns associated with cancer appear to be tumor-type specific *(13,14)*.

It is well established that there is a good correlation between methylation state and histone modification. Genes that are methylated are usually related to deacetylated and inactive chromatin, whereas unmethylated promoters and active genes are associated with an open hypoacetylated euchromatin *(15)*. This relationship was, at the beginning, unidirectional; DNA methylation determines histone acetylation status. The molecular event that validates this theory was the MeCP2 discovery. MeCP2 is a methylated DNA-binding protein (MBD) that recruits histone methyltransferase and histone deacetylase activity to the promoter regions of methylation-regulated genes (Jones 1998). However, now it seems to be a bidirectional control, chromatin inactivation recruits DNA methyltransferases to regulatory regions of genes *(16,17)*.

On the basis of our current knowledge, the role of epigenetic events in cancer development, prognosis, and diagnosis is considered to be minor compared with those genetic events. However, nowadays new approaches to cancer therapy

Table 1
Epigenetic Diseases: Symptoms and Etiology[a]

Disease	Symptom	Aetiology
ATR-X syndrome	Intellectual disabilities, α-thalassaemia	Mutations in *ATRX* gene, hypomethylation of certain repeat and satellite sequences
Fragile X syndrome	Chromosome instability, intellectual disabilities	Expansion and methylation of CGG repeat in *FMR1* 5′ UTR, promoter methylation
ICF syndrome	Chromosome instability, immunodeficiency	*DNMT3b* mutations, DNA hypomethylation
Angelman's syndrome	Intellectual disabilities	Deregulation of one or more imprinted genes at 15q11–13 (maternal)
Prader-Willi syndrome	Obesity, intellectual disabilities	Deregulation of one or more imprinted genes at 15q11–13 (paternal)
BWS	Organ overgrowth	Deregulation of one or more imprinted genes at 11p15.5 (e.g. *IGF2*)
Rett syndrome	Intellectual disabilities	*MeCP2* mutations
α-Thalassaemia (one case)	Anaemia	Methylation of α2-globin CpG island, deletion of *HBA1* and *HBQ1*
Rubinstein–Taybi syndrome	Intellectual disabilities	Mutation in CREB-binding protein (histone acetylation)
Coffin–Lowry syndrome	Intellectual disabilities	Mutation in *Rsk-2* (histone phosphorylation)

[a]Neurological diseases related with deregulation of imprinted genes, mutations in MBDs (methylation-binding domain proteins), HATs (histone acetyltransferases), or DNMTs (DNA methyl-transferases).

ATR-X syndrome, α-thalassaemia, mental retardation syndrome; BWS, Beckwith-Wiedemann syndrome; CREB, cAMP-response-element-binding-protien; ICF, immunodeficiency, centromeric region instability, and facial anomalies syndrome; UTR, untranslated region; DNMT, DNA methyl transferase; FMR1, Fragile X mental retardation 1; HBA1, hemoglobin alpha 1; HBQ1, hemoglobin theta 1.

based on epigenetic therapies are emerging, demethylatings agents and histone deacetylases inhibitors predominantly.

2. Epigenetic Diseases: The Neurological Achilles' Heel

Mutations in genes that affect epigenetic profiles are inheritable or somatic acquired. Hereditable mutations in methyltransferases (DNMTs) or MBDs genes, are the phenomenon behind some human syndrome as ICF syndrome (DNMT3b mutation) or Rett syndrome (MeCP2 mutation). Curiously many of this disease results in mental retardation, chromosomal instability, and learning disabilities (**Table 1**). These new platforms of human disease could be considered as epigenetic diseases.

There are syndromes that result in deregulation of imprinted in cluster of same chromosomal location-genes as Angelman's syndrome (AS), a disorder that can be difficult to diagnose, particularly in the first few years of life. Approximately 70% of cases of AS have a deletion of 15q11-q13 in the maternally contributed chromosome. Main characteristics are developmental delay, functionally severe speech impairment, none or minimal use of words, receptive and nonverbal communication skills higher than verbal skills, movement or balance disorder (usually ataxia of gait and/or tremulous movement of limbs), behavioral uniqueness (any combination of frequent laughter/smiling), apparent happy demeanor, easily excitable personality (often with hand flapping movements), hypermotoric behavior, and short attention span.

With the same epigenetic root, but a clinically distinct disorder, is the Prader-Willi syndrome (PWS), a complex disorder, which diagnosis may be difficult to establish on clinical grounds and whose genetic basis is heterogeneous. Approximately 28% of cases of PWS are a result of maternal uniparental disomy. A disorder of chromosome 15 with a prevalence of 1:12,000–15,000 (both sexes, all races). The major characteristics of PWS are hypotonia, hypogonadism, hyperphagia, cognitive impairment, and difficult behaviors.

Finally in these examples, Beckwith-Wiedemann syndrome, and an overgrowth disorder. Wiedemann first recognized it in 1963, and in 1964 by Bruce Beckwith, a pediatric pathologist. Both doctors noted similar characteristics in their patients that were not traceable to other disorders, thereby identifying a new syndrome. The syndrome is usually sporadic, but may be inherited. These children are at risk for developing hypoglycemia and various types of tumors. The clinical picture of this syndrome can vary from mildly to greatly affected. The incidence of BWS has been reported as approx 1:15,000 births. However, exact figures of these kinds of syndromes are impossible to estimate, because so many mildly affected cases are not diagnosed.

Different collections of diseases are related to DNA methyltransferases mutations as ICF syndrome (immunodeficiency-centromeric instability-facial

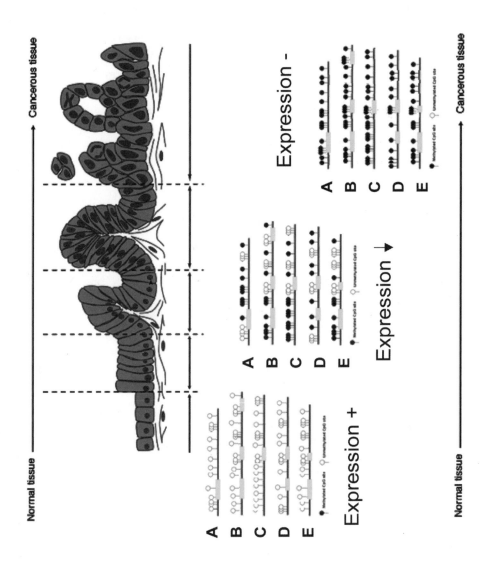

anomalies) is transmitted as an autosomal recessive trait. It is characterized by immune deficiency in association with unstable paracentromeric heterochromatin instability (extensively related with hypomethylated genomic regions) and facial dysmorphism. Patients are affected by recurrent respiratory infections beginning in childhood. The syndrome directly results from mutations in the gene encoding for DNA-methyltransferase 3B. This may explain the hypomethylation in the pericentromeric repeats observed in the chromosomes of patients.

3. Cancer as Epigenetic Disease

A set of human cancers are developed by *de novo* methylations in genes, mainly tumor-suppressor genes, where promoter methylation diminishes or inhibits normal cell expression and thus confers a growth advantage to the tumor cell (**Fig. 4**). Huge expectations have been raised by the large amount of genetic information relating to cancer biology that has been assembled in the past two decades. CpG island hypermethylation of tumor-suppressor genes may be a valuable tool in the essential transfer of research from the "bench" to the "bedside." The detection of hypermethylation is a "positive" signal that can be accomplished in the context of normal cells, whereas certain genetic changes such as LOH or homozygous deletions are not going to be detected in a background of normal DNA.

In recent years, several groups have extensively mapped from most classes of human neoplasia an increasing number of gene CpG islands aberrantly hypermethylated in cancer (**Table 2;** *[9]*).

Epigenetics can offer two components to the treatment of caner: prognostic and predictive factors. Prognostic factors will give us information about the virulence of the tumors. For example, p16INK4a hypermethylation has been linked to tumor virulence in lung and colorectal cancer patients *(18)*. The second component is the group of factors that predict response to therapy. For example, the response to cisplatin and derivatives may be a direct function of the methylation state of the CpG island of hMLH1 *(19)*. Nevertheless, the most compelling evidence is provided by the methylation-associated silencing of the DNA repair methyltransferase (MGMT) in gliomas and lymphomas, which indicates patients who will be sensitive to chemotherapy with carmustine (BCNU)

Fig. 4. *(Opposite page)* Epigenetic events in tumor progression, from normal epithelium (normal tissue) to dysplasia and carcinoma (cancerous tissue). Five methylation-controled-genes (A–E) represented in their promoter regions: ●, methylated CpG; ○, unmethylated CpG. Normal tissue is represented by normal gene expression and an unmethylated state in tumor-suppressor gene promoters; during progression, expression decreases and hypermethylation in promoters increases. Finally, in a cancerous tissue, promoters are extensively methylated and expression is completely inhibited.

Table 2
Examples of Genes Exhibiting Aberrant Methylation in Cancer

Evasion of apoptosis	APAF-1
	DAPK
	DLC-1
	p14ARF
	p53
	p73
	SHP1
	TMS1
	TRAIL-R1
	XAF1
Insensitivity to	CyclinD2
anti-growth signals	ERα
	LOT1
	p15INK4b
	p16INK4a
	p27KIP1
	p57KIP2
	Pax5
	PTEN
	RARα
	RASSF1A
Limitless replicative	pRb
potential	CDX1
	GATA-4 and -5
	Myf-3
	SOCS-3
Angiogenesis	THBS1
	THBS2
	VHL
Intercellular adhesion	ADAM23
and tissue invasion	E-Cadherin
	H-Cadherin
	CLCA2
	CLDN-7
	laminin-5
	Maspin
	OPCML
	TIMP3
	SLIT2
DNA repair	MLH1
	MGMT
	BRCA1

(Continued)

(20) or cyclofosfamide *(21)*. Three major clinical areas can benefit from hypermethylation-based markers: detection, tumor behavior, and treatment.

3.1. DNA Methylation

Epigenetic modifications of DNA do not alter the sequence but are hereditable and involved in gene regulation and transcription. DNA methylation is a very dynamic processes but the regulation behind this mechanism is very tight. Aberrant methylation in the CpG island-containing-promoters of genes is usually correlated with gene silencing, however in some cases abnormal methylation patterns could be related to gene activation *(22)*. Global DNA hypomethylation has been reported in several human diseases *(13,20)*. Such global hypomethylations occur mainly in repetitive elements around pericentromeric areas. In cancer, global genome hypomethylation is a common finding but, generally, is associated with specific promoter hypermethylation *(23,24)*. In normal mammalian cells, CpG islands in the regulatory regions of certain genes are not methylated, whereas CpG in the remaining genes are methylated by DNMT1. In cancer cells, global DNA hypomethylation and specific promoter hypermethylation occurs (**Fig. 4**) *(25)*.

Aberrant patterns of DNA methylation appear to be affected in several pathways: *p53* is the most frequently mutated gene in human cancers, however. *p53* can also become inactivated through methylation-mediated silencing of the tumor-suppressor gene *p14ARF* *(26–28)*, which normally inhibits MDM2, an oncogenic protein that induces p53 degradation. Moreover, *p73*, a *p53* homolog, has been shown to be hypermethylated in leukemia *(29)*. Hypermethylation of the cell-cycle inhibitor p16INK4a, a feature common to many tumors, enables cancer cells to escape senescence and begin to proliferate *(30–32)*. The retinoblastoma gene *(RB)* and the cell-cycle inhibitor p15INK4b can also occasionally undergo aberrant methylation *(33,34)*. DNA methylation has a major role in many repair pathways. The consequences of aberrant methylation of repair

Table 2   *(Opposite page)*

BRCA1, breast cancer 1; DAPK, death-associated protein kinase; E-cadherin, epithelial cadherin; GSTP1, glutathione *S*-transferase p1; MLH1, mutL homolog 1; MGMT, O(6)-methylguanine-DNA methyltransferase; pRb, retinoblastoma; RASSF1a, ras-association domain family 1A; VHL, von Hippel-Lindau; APAF-1, apoptotic protease activating factor 1; DLC1, phosphodynein on microtubules; SHP1, SH2 domain-containing tyrosine phosphatase; TMS1, target of methylation-induced silencing; TRAIL, type II integral membrane protein; XAF1, XIAP-associated factor 1 (XIAP, the X-linked inhibitor of apoptosis); ER, estrogen receptor; PLAGL1/LOT1/ZAC, pleomorphic adenoma of the salivary gland gene like 1; CDX1, homeobox protein CDX-1 (caudal-type-homeobox protein 1); SOCS3, suppressor of cytokine signaling 3; THBS1, thrombospondin 1 precursor; THBS2, thrombospondin 2 precursor; ADAM23; disintegrin and metalloproteinase domain 23; CAV1, caveolin 1; CLCA2, chloride channel, calcium activated, family member 2; CLDN7, claudin 7; OPCML, opioid-binding cell adhesion molecule; TIMP3, tissue inhibitor of metalloproteinase 3; RFC, reduced folate carrier.

pathways include microsatellite instability in sporadic colorectal *(35,36)*, endometrial *(37,38)*, and gastric *(39)* tumors, owing to silencing of the DNA mismatch repair gene *hMLH1*; mutations in *K-RAS* and *p53* caused by hypermethylation of the O6-methylguanine-DNA methyltransferase promoter *(40)*; the prevention of the removal of methyl groups at the O6 position of guanine *(41,42)*; hypermethylation of the mitotic checkpoint gene CHFR *(43)*; and inactivation of *BRCA1* in breast and ovarian tumors *(44)*, which prevents the repair of DNA double-strand breaks and causing global gene-expression changes similar to those present in carriers of *BRCA1* germline mutations *(45)*. Other targets of aberrant methylation, the aberrant methylation of androgen receptors occurs in breast and uterus tumors, may render cancer cells unresponsive to treatment with steroid hormones. Some of the other genes that are affected by DNA methylation are the proapoptotic death-associated protein kinase (DAPK), a target of methylation-induced silencing gene; the von Hippel-Lindau gene in kidney tumors and hemangioblastomas; *LKB1/STK11* (a serine-threonine kinase) in hamartomatous neoplasms, the RAS-related gene, *RASSF1*; thrombospondin 1 (an antiangiogenic factor); cyclo-oxygenase 2; *TPEF*, which comprises epidermal growth-factor domains; and glutathione-*S*-transferase P1 (an electrophilic detoxifier) in tumors of the prostate, breast, and kidney (**Table 2**).

3.2. Histone Acetylation

Chromatin remodeling also plays an important role in the regulation of expression of certain genes. The basic unit of chromatin is the nucleosome, which consists of 146 bp of DNA wrapped around a histone octomer. Modification of the N-terminal group of lysine in histones by acetylation or deacetylation changes the configuration of nucleosomes. The positive charge on unacetylated lysines in the histones is attracted to the negatively charged DNA producing a compact chromatin state that is repressive for transcription. On the other hand, acetylation of the lysines by histone acetylase removes their positive charge and results in an open chromatin structure, which facilitates gene transcription. HDAC removes the acetyl groups from lysine, which reverses this process and silences gene expression (**Fig. 2**). Aberrant deacetylation of histones in nucleosomes is probably a result of a dysregulation of the specificity of HDAC and may be associated with neoplastic transformation. For example, gene translocations in some types of leukemia can generate fusion proteins that recruit HDAC and bind to promoters to silence genes involved in differentiation *(46)*.

For many years, epigenetic research focused on DNA methylation; now, a critical role in epigenetic gene control is assigned to histone modifications. Histone tails are targets for covalent posttranslational modifications, such as acetylation, methylation, and phosphorylation *(47)*. Hypoacetylation of histone-3 and –4 are usually associated with transcriptionally inactive genome regions

inside a global structure called heterochromatin. Acetylation levels and acetylation states are regulated by equilibrium of HAT and HDAC *(48,49)*.

3.3. Histone Methylation

In addition to acetylation of H3 and H4 tails, methylation in lysine residues
(Lys4 and Lys9) of histone 3 has been described **(Fig. 1B)**. The methylation of
lysine in histones by specific histone methylases is also implicated in changes in
chromatin structure and gene regulation. The methylation of lysine-4 in histone-3
is associated with an open chromatin configuration and gene expression. On the
other hand, the methylation of lysine-9 in histone-3 is associated with condensed
and repressive chromatin. This histone modification and the acetylation/deacety-
lation of histones to influence gene expression are called the histone code *(47)*. A
hypermethylated promoter is surrounded by methylated lysine-9 in histone-3,
whereas an unmethylated promoter is surrounded by methylated lysine-4
in histone-3 *(50)*. Treatment of tumor cells with 5-AZA reduces the level of
methylated lysine-9 in histone-3 and increases the level of methylated lysine-
4 in histone-3 in the promoter region of genes silenced by aberrant DNA
methylation *(51)*.

As an example of cooperativity between chromatin modifications, it is interesting to note that Lys9 in histone-3 is acetylated in euchromatin (active state for
gene transcription) but appears to be methylated in regions of gene-expression
silencing *(52)*. Methylated K4 and K79 and acetylated K9 and K14 of H3 are
associated with transcriptionally active regions. H4 methylated at K20 is present
in heterochromatin regions *(53)*. Histone methylation is catalyzed by histone
methyltransferases, a family of proteins with affinity for lysines and arginines.
Recent studies demonstrate that peptidyl arginine deiminase 4 (PADI4) specifically deiminates arginine residues R2, R8, R17, and R26 in the H3 tail. This
deimination by PADI4 prevents arginine methylation by CARM1. These results
define deimination as a novel mechanism for antagonizing the transcriptional
induction mediated by arginine methylation. *(54)*. Histone methylation could be
involved in the replacement of histones during transcription core dislodging *(55)*.
Some histone methyltransferases important in cancer are EZH2 (H3K27 histone
methyltransferase), overexpressed in prostate and breast cancer *(56)*, and SMYD3
(H3K4 histone methyltransferase) overexpressed in colorectal and hepatocellular
carcinomas *(57)*. Notably, there is a dynamic relationship between DNA methylation and histone modifications. Low levels of histone acetylation and H3K9
methylation recruit DNMT1 and DNA methylation to regulatory regions.

4. Epigenetic Therapy of Cancer

Tumorigenesis is known to be a multistep process in which defects in various
cancer genes accumulate *(58,59)*. It is now clear that genetic alterations in
human cancers will not provide a complete answer of genomic alterations

behind tumor development, progression, or metastasis. Epigenetic factors cause changes in mechanisms contributing to the malignant phenotype (**Fig. 4**). Epigenetic causes of human diseases, especially of cancer, has given impetus to the development of new therapies for reversing the processes involved. Inhibitors of DNA methylation were the first molecules to appear on the market. To date, several compounds that inhibit DNA methylation are being used in both in vitro and in vivo studies. Clinical trials have shown an incredible decrease in global methylation and specifically demethylation of tumor-suppressor-promoter-CpG-island cancer cells, recovery of the normal expression levels of these genes, and restoration of the normal phenotype. In this field, compounds such as 5-azacytidine, 5-aza-2'-deoxycytidine, zebularine, procainamide, and so on are emerging as powerful and nontoxic tools for cancer therapy.

Knowledge of CpG-island hypermethylation of tumor-suppressor genes may be an important tool in the essential transfer of research from laboratory to clinical practice. In contrast to genetic markers, in which mutations occur in various sites and can be of very different types, promoter hypermethylation occurs only within CpG islands. Furthermore, hypermethylation is a positive signal that can be observed at background levels in normal cells, whereas particular genetic changes, such as loss of heterozygosity and homozygous deletions, cannot be detected so easily. The impetus for DNA methylation studies in cancer has come from two sources. The first is the identification of well-recognized tumor-suppressor genes that undergo methylation-mediated silencing in human cancer, e.g., *BRCA1*, *hMLH1*, *p16INK4a*, *VHL* (**Table 3**) (*60,61*). The second is the emergence of a new technology to study DNA methylation, one based on bisulphite modification coupled with PCR techniques (*62*).

The study of pigenetic silencing in the last years has been on histone modifications, acetylation, methylation, and phosphorylation of histone tails, but it has already begun a shift to new transcription regulation mechanisms, those catalyzed by two groups of proteins HATs and HDACs. As a result, inhibitors of HDACs are growing as a promising therapeutic compound; inhibition of deacetylation as "word play" increases acetylation levels and maintains or remodels the chromatin to an open or gene-activation state. Some of these newly activated-genes are tumor-suppressor genes and cancer-negative-selected genes. HDAC inhibitors reduce cell growth and induce differentiation and apoptosis. Some of the classic and commonly used compounds in this field are butyric acid, valproic acid, suberoylanilide hydroxamic acid (SAHA), depsipeptide, and so on.

Links between DNA methylation and histone acetylation necessarily favor dual therapies, combining DNA methylation inhibitors with HDAC inhibitors. This synergy was profoundly studied in combinations of 5-AZA-CdR and trichostatin A (TSA) (*63–65*). Four major clinical areas can potentially benefit from hypermethylation-based markers: neoplasm detection, studies of tumor

Table 3
Hypermethylated Genes in Cancer, Role in Tumor Development and Tumor Type

SITE	GENE: role in tumor development
Brain	*MGMT:* DNA repair and drug resistance
Breast	*APC:* cytoskeletal reorganization
	BRCA1: DNA repair
	E-Cadherin: proliferation, invasion and metastasis
	ER: hormone response
	GSTP1: detoxification
	RASSF1A: control of cell proliferation
Colon	*hMLH1:* DNA mistmach repair
Endometrium	*hMLH1:* DNA mistmach repair
Esophageal	*APC:* cytoskeletal reorganization
Gastric	*E-Cadherin:* proliferation, invasion and metastasis
	hMLH1: DNA mistmach repair
Head and Neck	*p16:* cyclin dependent kinase inhibitor
Kidney	*RASSF1A:* control of cell proliferation
Leukemia	*p15:* activation of cell proliferation
Lymphoma	*p15:* activation of cell proliferation
Lung	*APC:* cytoskeletal reorganization
	p16: cyclin dependent kinase inhibitor
	*DAPK1:*Suppression of apoptosis.
	MGMT: DNA repair and drug resistance
	RASSF1A: control of cell proliferation
Nasopharyngeal	*RASSF1A:* control of cell proliferation
NHL	*p16:* cyclin dependent kinase inhibitor
Oligodendroglioma	*Rb:* DNA replication and cell division
Ovarian	*BRCA1:* DNA repair
	hMLH1: DNA mistmach repair
	RASSF1A: control of cell proliferation
Prostate	*ER:* hormone response
	GSTP1: detoxification
Retinoblastoma	*Rb:* DNA replication and cell division
Renal	*GSTP1:* detoxification
	VHL: RNA stability
Squamous cell carcinoma	*p15:* activation of cell proliferation
Thyroid	*E-Cadherin:* proliferation, invasion and metastasis

APC, adenomatous polyposis coli; BRCA1, breast cancer 1; CDKN2A/p16, cyclin-dependent kinase 2A; DAPK1, death-associated protein kinase 1; ER, estrogen receptor; GSTP1, glutathione *S*-transferase Pi 1; hMLH1, mut L homolog 1; MGMT, 0-6 methylguanine-DNA methyltransferase; RASSF1, ras-association domain family member; Rb, retinoblastoma; VHL, von Hippel-Lindau; GIT, gastrointestinal tract; NHL, non-Hodgkin's lymphoma.

Substances that reduce DNMTs expression : antisense DNMTs cDNA oligonucleotides and constructs

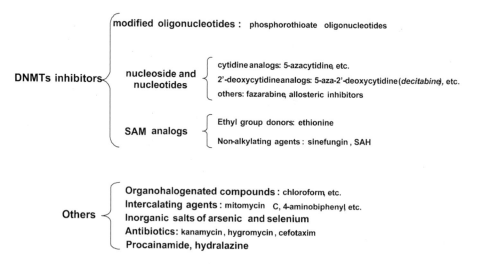

Fig. 5. DNA methylation inhibitors may be used in cancer therapy to modulate hypermethylation of genes and to reactivate antiproliferative, apoptotic, and differentiation-inducing genes in cancer cells. Although some compounds have been proposed for use as DNA methylation inhibitors, these compounds are chemically instable, have weak potency, and can generate toxic metabolites, thus preventing their use as therapeutic agents. Compounds are divided in three categories; substances that directly reduce DNMTs (DNA methyl-transferases), expression, and inhibitors of DNMT activity and others.

behavior, prediction of treatment response, and the development of therapies that target methylated tumor-suppressor genes.

4.1. DNA Methylation in Cancer Therapy

Epigenetic modifications are reversible, whereas genetic modifications are not. This feature makes epigenetic modifications a target for new human therapies. Demethylating agents are "on the crest of the wave" in pharmaceutical development of portfolio molecules (**Fig. 5**).

For several years we have been able to reactivate hypermethylated genes in vitro. One obstacle to the transfer of this technique to human primary cancers is the lack of specificity of the drugs used. Since demethylating agents such as 5-azacytidine or 5-aza-2-deoxicytidine (decitabine) (*66*) inhibit DNMTs and cause global hypomethylation, we cannot reactivate only the particular gene we are targeting. New chemical inhibitors of DNA methylation are being introduced, such as zebularine, and provide us with more hope, but the nonspecificity problem persists. If we consider that only tumor-suppressor genes are hypermethylated, this would not be a great problem. However, we do not know if we have disrupted some essential methylation at certain sites, and global hypomethylation may be associated with even greater chromosomal instability *(67)*. Another drawback is the toxicity to normal cells, a phenomenon that was in fact observed with the initial higher doses. However, these compounds and their derivatives have been used in the clinic with some therapeutic benefit, especially in hematopoietic malignancies *(68,69)*.

Methylation-associated silencing affects many genes in all existing cellular pathways *(13,61)*. As examples of DNA methylation markers of poor prognosis, we can mention that the death-associated protein kinase, p16INK4a hypermethylation, has been linked to tumor virulence in lung and colorectal cancer patients *(61)*. Not all hypermethylation events are bad: in neuroblastoma, the CpG island hypermethylation of *HOXA9* is associated with poor survival, but the hypermethylation of *RARB2* is an excellent marker of good outcome *(70)*.

However, one of the most attractive possibilities is the establishment of clusters of CpG island hypermethylation in human tumors with prognostic value *(70)*. Studying more than 150 neuroblastomas and using an unsupervised hierarchical cluster analysis of all tumors based on methylation of 10 genes, we separated the three clinically relevant groups of tumors *(70)*. CpG island hypermethylation has been used as a tool to detect cancer cells in broncoalveolar lavage *(71)*, lymph nodes *(72)*, sputum *(73)*, urine *(74)*, semen *(75)*, ductal lavage *(76)*, and saliva *(77)*. Thus, we have shown its versatility across multiple tumor types and environments (**Table 4**).

It was possible to screen for hypermethylated promoter loci in serum DNA from lung cancer patients *(78)* , as well as from a broad spectrum of tumor types *(79,80)*, some screening even using semiquantitative and automated methodologies. The detection of DNA hypermethylation in serum or biological fluids of cancer patients (and even patients at risk of cancer) should encourage academic, governmental, and private agencies to create consortiums of different institutions (and even countries) to develop comprehensive studies to validate the use of these markers in the clinical environment. CpG island hypermethylation could be used as a predictor of response to treatment. The methylation-associated silencing of the DNA repair MGMT in human cancer provides the most compelling evidence. The MGMT protein (O6-methylguanine DNA methyltransferase) is directly responsible for repairing the addition of alkyl groups to the guanine base of the DNA *(81)*. MGMT-promoter hypermethylation predicts a good response to chemotherapy, greater overall survival, and longer time to progression in glioma patients treated with BCNU *(20)*. The potential of MGMT methylation to predict the chemoresponse of human tumors to alkylating agents is not limited to BCNU-like alkylating agents; it also extends to other drugs such as cyclophosphamide *(21)*. This has been demonstrated in diffuse large

Table 4
Detection of Cancer in Body Fluids Using DNA Methylation as Marker[a]

SPECIMEN	TUMOR TYPE	GENE	METH. (%)
Serum/plasma	Prostate	GSTP1	72
	NSCL	APC	47
		p16	73
		DAPK	73
		MGMT	73
		GSTP1	73
	Breast	p16	23
	Colorectal	p16	38
	Esophageal	APC	27
	Liver	p15	81
	Head and neck	p16	42
		DAPK	42
		MGMT	42
		GSTP1	42
Urine	Prostate	GSTP1	36
Ejaculates	Prostate	GSTP1	50
Sputum	NSCL	CDKN2A	50
Ductal lavage	Breast	Cyclin D2	85
		RAR-β	85

[a]Tumor type, gene involved, specimen of fluid, and percentage of methylation.

Meth., methylation; GSTP1, glutathione *S*-transferase Pi 1; APC, adenomatous polyposis coli; CDKN2A/p16, cyclin-dependent kinase 2A; DAPK1, death-associated protein kinase 1; MGMT, O-6 methylguanine-DNA methyltransferase.

cell lymphomas treated with cyclophosphamide, where MGMT hypermethylation was the strongest predictor of overall survival and time to progression, and was far superior to classic clinical factors such as the international prognostic index *(21)*.

Finally, gene inactivation by promoter hypermethylation may be the key to understanding the loss of hormone response of many tumors. The inefficacy of the antisteroids estrogen–progesterone–androgen-related compounds such as tamoxifen, raloxifene, or flutemide, in certain breast, endometrial, and prostate cancer cases may be a direct consequence of the methylation-mediated silencing of their respective cellular receptors (*ER*, *PR*, and *AR* genes) *(61,82)*.

Reactivating genes with DNA demethylating agents is an encouraging discovery with respect to avoiding toxic effects. However, it is important to note that the hypermethylation of CpG islands occurs in conjunction with the action of methyl-binding proteins, histone hypoacetylation, and histone methylation, which all contribute to formation of a closed chromatin state and transcriptional silencing *(83)*. Several clinical trials to study these and other mechanisms in patients with cancer are underway in United States and Europe. In such studies, it is essential that the clinical and molecular parameters of response are well defined. Quantitative measurement of 5-methylcytosine DNA after treatment, by use of high-performance capillary electrophoresis *(84,85)*, is an excellent surrogate marker to validate efficacy, as well as demethylation of CpG islands in tumor-suppressor genes, such as p15INK4b *(86)*.

4.2. DNA Methylation Inhibitors as Therapy

Demethylating agents such as 5-aza-cytidine or 5-aza-2-deoxycytidine inhibit DNA methyltransferases and cause global hypomethylation *(87)*. Furthermore, the demethylating effect of 5-aza-2-deoxycytidine seems to be universal, affecting all human cancer cell lines *(68)*. New inhibitors of DNA methylation are being introduced, e.g., procainamide, but the issue of nonspecificity still persists **(Fig. 5)**. Another problem is that at high doses, these agents seem to have toxic effects on normal cells. But despite their drawbacks, these compounds and their derivatives have achieved some therapeutic success in the clinic, especially in hemopoietic disorders such as myelodysplastic syndrome and acute myeloid leukemia *(68,69)*.

One of the most promising clinical scenarios for the use of demethylating drugs is acute promyelocytic leukemia(APL), which is largely caused by transcriptional disruption induced by the PML-RARa translocation. Combined treatment with inhibitors of histone deacetylases, inhibitors of DNA methylation, and differentiating factors (arsenic trioxide may have all three functions) has achieved moderate success in several patients with APL *(88)*. 5-Aza-2'-deoxycytidine alone can also induce the reexpression of silenced, but not hypermethylated, tumor-suppressor genes, such as the proapoptotic gene *APAF1* *(89)*. Although the mechanisms underlying this effect are not fully understood, this drug is known to have additional cytoxic effects, other than those resulting from demethylation, which potentiate the killing capabilities of demethylating compounds, and thus increase their effectiveness in cancer treatment.

The discovery that lower doses of 5-azacytidine associated with inhibitors of HDACs may also reactivate tumor-suppressor genes was encouraging *(63)*. Several phase I trials to test this strategy in human cancer patients are underway. 5-Aza-2'-deoxycytidine alone can even induce reexpression of certain silenced tumor-suppressor genes that do not have an apparent CpG island hypermethylation, such as *APAF-1 (89)*. These new findings have proved very attractive to several pharmacological and biotech companies, and they are now studying how to accomplish demethylation of cancer cells using novel approaches such as antisense constructs or ribozymes against the DNMTs.

4.3. Histone Acetylation Platform for Cancer Therapy

The core histones are N-terminal tails covalently modified by acetylation, methylation, phosporylation, ubiquitination, sumoylation, and biotinylation *(3,90,91)*. Modifications of specific histone residues (Lys, Arg, Ser) are essential for specific proteins interactions important in gene regulation, chromatin condensation, and remodeling and structure *(92)*. Chromatin-modifying enzymes are necessary to generate an open chromatin conformation that permits transcription factors and cofactors positive accessibility to target sequences. Modification of the highly charged lysisne or arginine residues in the N-terminal histone tails is one mechanism of remodeling control (**Figs. 1** and **2**). These residues are susceptible to modifications by acetylation and/or methylation *(47)*. This phenomenon appears to be controlled by a set of new emerging enzyme termed as HDACs, together with the ongoing family of HATs.

4.3.1. HDACs as Therapeutic Targets

HDACs modify chromatin by removing acetyl groups from N-terminal tail of histones and from other proteins such as p53 or tubulin *(93,94)*. The HDAC family is divided in Zn-dependent (class I and II) and Zn-independent (class III) enzymes. Class I and II are the most extensively studies inside the HDAC family proteins. Expression profile of each member is tissue dependent and disease-dependent, critical aim in the development of new therapeutic strategies. Abnormal expression of HDACs is frequent in hematological malignancies. RAR-PML, for instance, could recruit HDACs and cause transcriptional repression and no differentiation *(95)*.

4.3.2. HDACs as Therapeutic Molecules

The importance of histone modifications in cancer is illustrated by the marked antitumor activity of different inhibitors of HDAC, both in animal models and in preliminary clinical trials *(46,96)*. The molecular mechanism of action of HDAC inhibitors is related to their activation of a subset of genes that can produce cell cycle arrest and induce differentiation or apoptosis in tumor cells *(46,96)*.

Inhibition of HDAC includes natural and synthetic molecules. The naturally occurring antifungal antibiotic TSA was one of the first HDAC inhibitor compounds identified as having antiproliferative activity. Agents identified as HDAC inhibitors can be divided into different structural categories: hydroxamates (such as SAHA and TSA), short-chain fatty acids (such as valproic acid), cyclic peptides (such as depsipeptide), and benzamides (MS-275). HDAC inhibitors cause differentiation, cell-cycle arrest in G1 and/or G2 and apoptosis in cultured transformed cells and tumors in animals that arise from both hematological and solid tumors. The mechanisms of genetic silencing by HDACs are associated with activation of selected genes *(97)*. Activation of these silenced genes by inhibition of HDACs contribute to repression of tumor cell growth. In practice, the results of treatment with HDAC inhibitors differ by cell type in having both activate and repressive effects *(98,99)*. However new hypotheses about the mechanism of HDAC inhibitors involvement in cancer are emerging; for example, in HepG2 cells, HDACs increased p21WAF1/CIP1 expression not through changes in chromatin structure or by enhancing promoter activity, but by mRNA stabilization *(100)*. All these findings together indicate that HDAC inhibitor treatment results in changes in chromatin structure and an increase of susceptibility to transcription factors, RNA polymerase, or topoisomerases and mRNA stabilization.

Naturally occurring and synthetic HDAC inhibitors are now of interest to pharmaceutical companies because of their great potential use against cancer and other human pathologies. These compounds can be classified according to their chemical nature and mechanism of inhibition as follows (**Fig. 6**):

4.3.2.1. HYDROXAMIC ACIDS

This is probably the broadest set of HDAC inhibitors. Most of the chemicals in this group are very potent but reversible inhibitors of class I/II HDACs. Among these compounds we find TSA, which was one of the first HDAC inhibitors to be described *(101)* and is widely used as a reference in research in this field. However, its toxicity to patients and lack of specificity for certain HDACs has motivated the search for other substances. The design of many synthetic drugs has been inspired by TSA structure: from the simplicity of SAHA to the latest drugs including NVP-LAQ-824 *(102,103)* and PXD-101 *(104)*.

4.3.2.2. CARBOXYLIC ACIDS

There are few drugs in this group: butanoic *(105)*, valproic *(106,107)*, and 4-phenylbutanoic *(108)*. Despite being much less potent than the hydroxamic acids and their pleiotropic effects, these are currently among the best studied HDAC inhibitors: valproic acid and phenylbutyrate have already been approved for use in treating epilepsy and some cancers, respectively, whereas butanoic acid is undergoing clinical trials *(109,110)*.

4.3.2.3. BENZAMIDES

MS-275 and some of its derivatives inhibit HDACs in vitro at micromolar concentrations, but the mechanism is not clearly understood. MS-275 and *N*-acetyldinaline are undergoing clinical trials *(111–113)*.

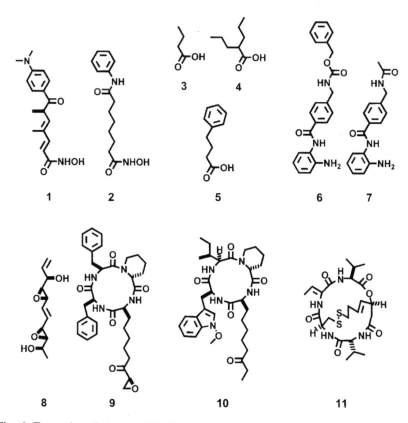

Fig. 6. Examples of chemicals included in the different HDAC inhibitor groups (*see* text). (1) TSA, (2) SAHA, (3) butanoic acid, (4) valproic acid, (5) 4-phenyobutanoic acid, (6) MS-275, (7) N-acetyldinaline, (8) depeudecin, (9) trapoxin A, (10) apicidin, and (11) depsipeptide FK228.

4.3.2.4. Epoxides

The only HDAC inhibitors in this set of compounds are a number of natural products with significant in vitro activity, such as depeudecin, trapoxin A *(114)*.

4.3.2.5. Others

Depsipeptide FK228 (a fungal metabolite) is also undergoing clinical trials, but the mechanism by which it inhibits classical HDACs in vitro remains unknown. Apicidin A is another fungal metabolite that is able to inhibit HDACs in many organisms, from protozoa to humans, at micromolar concentrations. Apicidins B and C (also natural products) have the same structure, differing from apicidin A by a single residue. Trapoxins are also cyclic tetrapeptides that are closely related to apicidins. However, the main difference between the two

Table 5
Mammalian HATs and HDACs[a]

HDAC	HAT
Class I	**GNAT family**
HDAC1	PCAF
HDAC2	GCN5L2
HDAC3	**CREBBP family**
HDAC8	CREBBP
Class II	EP300
HDAC4	**MYST family**
HDAC5	HTATIP
HDAC6	ZNF220
HDAC7	HB01
Sirtuins	MORF
SIRT1	MYST1
SIRT2	**TAFII 250 family**
SIRT3	TAFII 250
SIRT4	**SRC family**
SIRT5	ACTR
SIRT6	SRC1
SIRT7	SRC3
	NCOA2
	Other HATs
	TCF2
	GTF3C1

[a]HATs are divided into six different families (GNAT, CREBBP, MYST, TAFII, SRC, and others) and HDAC in three classes (class I, class II, and sirtuins).

ACTR, activin receptor; CREBBP, CREB-binding protein; EP300, e1a-binding protein p300; GCN5L2, general control of amino-acid synthesis 5-like 2; GNAT, GCN5-related acetyltransferase; GTF3C1, general transcription factor 3c, polypeptide 1; HAT, histone acetyltransferase; HBO, histone acetyltransferase binding to ORC; HDAC, histone deacetylase; HTATIP, HIV tat interactive protein; HIV tat, human immunodeficiency virus type I transacting transcription factor; MORF, MOZ-related factor; MOZ, monocytic leukemia zinc finger protein; MYST, MOZ, YBF2/SAS3, SAS2, TIP60 protein family; NCOA2, nuclear receptor coactivator 2; ORC, original recognition complex; PCAF, EP300/CREBBP-associated factor; SIRT, sirtuin; SRC, steroid receptor coactivators; TAF, TATA box-associated factors; TCF2, transcription factor 2; ZNF220, zinc finger protein 220.

groups of substances is that the former bears epoxyketone functionality rather than an alkylketone functionality, which makes the compound much less stable under physiological conditions *(115–118)*.

4.3.3. HATs as Therapeutic Targets

The addition of acetyl groups from universal donor acetyl-CoA on lysine residues placed on histone tails is catalyzed by HATs **(Table 5)**. Thus, histone tails acetylation is the best-characterized of histone modifications, demonstrating a positive association between acetylation levels and gene expression profiles. In addition, acetylated histones mean actively transcribed regions of chromatin *(119)*. HATs represent an active group of proteins important in replication, apoptosis, repair, and cell cycle. This crucial function in several cellular mechanisms makes HAT damage an important step in human diseases. In cancer, hematological malignancies with chromosomal translocation express chimeric HAT proteins that gain functions *(120)*. In such solid tumors as breast, colon, and gastric cancers, mutation in HAT genes have also been reported *(119)*. Nonfunctional CBP is the main cause of the Rubinstein-Taybi syndrome *(121)* and is in the clinical etiology of neurological disorders such as Huntington disease, Alzheimer's disease, and muscular atrophy *(119,122)*.

HATs specific inhibitors or activators remain on portfolio molecules although much is known about substrates and mechanisms. To date, few molecules have been identified without clinic applicability (Lysyl.CoA, H3-CoA-20, and anacardic acid *[120]*).

5. Epigenetic Diagnosis

Such mapping of DNA methylation has highlighted the existence of a unique profile of hypermethylated CpG islands that defines each tumor type (**Table 2**) *(60,61)*. Several groups are currently attempting to define the DNA methylation signature (methylotype) of each type of human cancer. Only methylation markers that are always unmethylated in normal cells can be used for methylation profiling, but by combining three or four methylation markers, we can extract the greatest possible amount of useful information, because hypermethylation events at different loci are unrelated *(60)*.

For epigenetic markers to be clinically useful, ways of detecting hypermethylation in the CpG islands of tumor-suppressor genes that are quick, non-radioactive, and sensitive are required, such as methylation-specific PCR *(123)*. Methylation-specific primers should be developed in stringent conditions with the inclusion of positive and negative controls to avoid false-positive results. CpG island hypermethylation has been used as a tool to detect cancer cells in several types of biological fluids and biopsy samples. It was possible to screen for hypermethylated promoter loci in DNA from the serum of patients with lung cancer *(78)*. Thus, DNA hypermethylation has proved its applicability in the detection of wide range of tumor types.

The promoter hypermethylation of CpG islands in tumor-suppressor genes occurs early in tumorigenesis. But the presence of aberrant CpG island methylation alone does not necessarily indicate an invasive cancer because premalignant or precursor lesions can also carry this epigenetic marker. This finding has implications for early detection of cancer, especially in people with a high inherited risk, because patterns of CpG island hypermethylation are the same between familial and sporadic cancers *(124)*. Aberrant DNA methylation has been found up to 3 yr before diagnosis of lung cancer in individuals, such as uranium miners and smokers, who have been exposed to large amounts of carcinogens *(73)*.

Standardization and validation of techniques for detecting changes in methylation are vital. Detection of DNA hypermethylation in the biological fluids of patients with cancer and those at risk of cancer should lead to comprehensive studies to justify the use of these markers in the clinic, through the establishment of multidisciplinary consortiums **(Table 4)**.

One of the most important steps for conferring on CpG island hypermethylation a critical role in the origin and progression of a tumor is the demonstration of biological consequences of the inactivation of that particular gene. A good example is provided by the DNA repair genes *hMLH1*, *MGMT*, and *BRCA1*, in which methylation-associated inactivation may change the entire genetic environment of the cell. In the first case, there is a lack of mutations in the mismatch repair genes in sporadic tumors, and the main cause of the presence of microsatellite instability in the sporadic cases of colorectal, endometrial, and gastric cancer is the transcriptional inactivation of hMLH1 by promoter hypermethylation *(125,126)*. In the second case, the DNA repair gene O6-methylguanine DNA MGMT removes the promutagenic O6-methylguanine from the DNA. However, the DNA repair gene MGMT can be transcriptionally silenced by promoter hypermethylation in primary human tumors *(127)*. Most importantly, these MGMT-methylated tumors accumulate a considerable number of G-to-A transition mutations, some of them affecting key genes such as *K-ras* and *p53* *(81)*. Finally, in the case of *BRCA1*, its hypermethylation-associated inactivation *(44)* produces the same profound disruption of expression profiles as do the *BRCA1* germline mutations *(128)*.

One of the most critical steps in giving CpG island methylation of a particular gene its true value is the fact that it should occur in the absence of gene mutations. Both events (genetic and epigenetic) abolish normal gene function and their coincidence in the same allele would be redundant. There are multiple examples but three are worth mentioning. First, the cell cycle inhibitor p16INK4a in one allele of a few colon and bladder cancer cell lines has a genetic mutation while the other is wild-type: p16INK4a hypermethylation occurs only on the wild-type allele, whereas the mutated allele is kept unmethylated *(129,130)*. A second example is that of APC, the gatekeeper of colorectal cancer, which is mutated in the vast majority of colon tumors. When APC methylation occurs in that type, it is clustered in the APC wild-type cases *(131)*. Finally, in tumors from families that harbor a germline mutation in tumor-suppressor genes, only those tumors that still retain one wild-type allele undergo CpG island hypermethylation *(124)*.

6. Epigenetic Prognosis

The most compelling evidence for predicting treatment response is provided by the methylation-associated silencing of O6-methylguanine-DNA methyltransferase. This protein is responsible for the removal of alkyl groups from guanine, which is the preferred point of DNA attack of several alkylating agents used in cancer treatment, such as carmustine, nimustine, procarbazine, streptozotocin, and temozolamide. Thus, tumors that lack function of O6-methylguanine-DNA methyltransferase owing to hypermethylation *(40)* are more sensitive to the action of alkylating agents, because there is no pathway to repair the damage these drugs cause.

In a study of patients with glioma who were treated with carmustine, we found that hypermethylation of the O6-methylguanine-DNA methyltransferase promoter was indicative of a good response to chemotherapy, greater overall survival, and longer time to progression *(20)*. The potential of O6-methylguanine-DNA methyltransferase for predicting the response of tumors to chemotherapy is not limited to carmustine-like alkylating agents, but also extends to drugs such as cyclophosphamide *(61)*. This capability has been shown for diffuse large-cell lymphomas treated with cyclophosphamide, where hypermethylation of O6-methylguanine-DNA methyltransferase was the strongest predictor of overall survival and time to progression, and was far better than classic clinical factors such as the international prognostic index *(121)*. More studies are needed to clarify this issue as the findings may have a direct effect on treatment of cancer.

Gene inactivation by promoter hypermethylation may be a crucial step in the loss of hormone responsiveness of many tumors. The lack of effectiveness of antisteroidal drugs, such as tamoxifen, raloxifene, and flutemide, in some patients with breast, endometrial, and prostate cancer may be a direct consequence of methylation-mediated silencing of their respective cellular receptors. A similar explanation can be applied to the lack of success with preventive retinoid treatment. It may be that premalignant lesions become insensitive to retinoids because of epigenetic silencing of genes that are crucial to the retinoid response, particularly the retinoic acid receptor 2 (RAR 2) *(132,133)*, and the cellular retinol-binding protein I (CRBPI) *(134)*. We have shown that supplementation of dietary retinoids prevents the aberrant methylation of RAR 2 and CRBPI in colorectal tumorigenesis *(134)*; DNA demethylating drugs can be given, if necessary, to improve treatment.

7. Clinical Applications

Most current DNA-demethylating agents **(Fig. 5)** block the action of DNMTs *(135)*. The cytidine and 2-deoxycytidine analogs of cytosine are the most extensively studied drugs. The first analog tested to determine whether it was an inhibitor of DNA methylation was 5-azacytidine. The second analog reported was 5-aza-2-deoxycitidine (decitabine), one of the most commonly used demethylating drugs in assays with cultured cells. All of these compounds only inhibit DNMTs when incorporated into double-strand DNA *(135)*. Zebularine (1-[beta-D-ribofuranosyl]-1,2-dihydropyrimidin-2-one) is another cytidine analog that has recently been developed *(136,137)*. Perhaps the most interesting feature of this DNA-demethylating agent, compared with 5-azacytidine and 5-aza-2-deoxycytidine, is that it is chemically stable and of low toxicity, being the first drug in its class that can be given orally *(136,137)*. The use of the nucleoside analogs in clinical trials has been limited by their side effects, such as thrombocytopenia and neutropenia, which are probably a result of cytotoxic effects associated with the drug's incorporation into the DNA independently of their DNA-hypomethylation value. This has encouraged the search for inhibitors of DNA methylation that are not incorporated into DNA. In this category, the drugs procainamide and procaine, approved by the FDA for the treatment of cardiac arrhythmias and as a local anesthetic, respectively, also act as nonnucleoside inhibitors of DNA methylation *(138,139)*. The demethylating effect of 5-aza-2-deoxycytidine seems to be universal, affecting all human cancer cell lines *(85)*. This is the conclusion that may be drawn from cancer-cell-line and mouse-tumor models, although we really do not know the molecular and cellular responses of cancer patients in their entirety.

Two phases in the clinical use of DNA-demethylating agents can be outlined. The first was during the 1970s and 1980s when high, and frequently significantly toxic, doses of 5-azacytidine and 5-aza-2-deoxycytidine were used to treat leukemia. At this time, their hypomethylating properties had not been fully recognized. The second period is marked by the acceptance of the idea that low doses of these drugs will induce cell differentiation and stop the growth of cancer cells by restoring the expression of silent tumor-suppressor genes.

Several phase I/II trials have been developed for solid tumors. However, it is in the field of hematological malignancies where DNA-demethylating agents have had their greatest success so far. Studies have found overall response rates of 40–54%, with 23–29% complete responses using 5-aza-2-deoxycytidine (decitabine) in myelodysplastic syndrome *(68,69,140)*. For 5-azacytidine, a similar scenario can be drawn with a significant number of complete and partial remissions in myelodysplastic syndrome patients *(141,142)*. The definitive support for an epigenetic treatment of hematological malignancies was provided in 2004, with the approval by the FDA of the use of 5-azacytidine (Vidaza) for the treatment of all myelodysplastic syndrome subtypes (http://www.fda.gov/bbs/topics/news/2004/NEW01069.html).

Table 6
Histone Deacetylase Inhibitors in Preclinical and Clinical Development[a]

Clinical Trials	HDAC Inhibitor	Family
+	Acid bishydroxamic	Hydroxamic acid
+	Acid (CBAH)	Hydroxamic acid
	Oxamflatin	Hydroxamic acid
+	Suberoylamilide	Hydroxamic acid
	SAHA	Hydroxamic acid
+	Trichostatin a (TSA)	Hydroxamic acid
+	Butyrate	Short-Chain-Fatty-Acid
+	Valproic acid	Short-Chain-Fatty-Acid
	Phenylacetate	Short-Chain-Fatty-Acid
	Apicidin	Cyclic Tetrapeptide
	Trapoxin A	Cyclic Tetrapeptide
+	Depsipeptide	Tetrapeptide
	Depudecin	Epoxide
+	MS275	Benzamide
+	LAQ824	

[a]Histone acetylation and deacetylation is modulated by the interplay between histone acetyl-transferases (HATs) and histone deacetylases (HDACs), and imbalances of this process cause multisystem diseases and cancers. Biochemical structures are indicated. "+" Denotes a phase I or II clinical trials.

It is clear from in vitro and preclinical studies that HDACs have great potential as anticancer drugs, but their value will be established by the ongoing clinical trials **(Table 6)**.

Multiple phase I and phase II clinical trials with many HDACs have now been completed, and others are being initiated. A phase I trial for depsipeptide in patients with postthymic lymphoma unresponsive to chemotherapeutic regimens showed partial and complete clinical responses with minimal side effects *(143)*. Another phase I trial of depsipeptide in patients with refractory neoplasms yielded biologically active serum concentrations of the drug and provided a recommended dose for the phase II trials *(144)*. Clinical trials of valproic acid (Mount Sinai School of Medicine), MS-275 (National Cancer Institute), and SAHA (Memorial Sloan-Kettering Cancer Center) are currently in their final stages. In the case of SAHA, a phase I trial has shown that is well tolerated, induces histone acetylation and has antitumor activity in solid and hematological tumors *(145)*.

Clinical trials have also been undertaken to examine the combination of HDAC inhibitors with DNA-demethylating agents, such as decitabine (5-azacytidine). A treatment scheme for acute myelogenous leukemia (AML) patients entailing subcutnaeous injections of 5-azacytidine for seven consecutive days followed by 5 d of iv phenylbutyrate was well tolerated, and a reduction in bone marrow blasts and increased myeloid maturation were observed *(146)*. A similar study initiated at the Johns Hopkins University of patients with myelodysplastic syndrome and AML also indicated good tolerance, and significant hematopoietic improvements were observed in several patients.

8. Future Directions

The main goal in biomedical cancer research is to find therapies that can reverse silencing in human diseases. Epigenetic therapy places new drug discovery in a critical role. Here, it is important to remember that epigenetic diseases are developed by abnormal hypermethylation of CpG island-containing-promoters that seem to be particularly frequent in cancer cells, so DNA demethylating agents or histone deacetylating inhibitor compounds specifically targets cancer cells and certain kind of cancers. Now is just the beginning of our understanding of epigenetic causes of human diseases but is at the same time the beginning of new families of antitumoral compounds. There is much to learn about enzymes involved in the epigenetic pathways and the tight regulation of their activities, but this question will provide new opportunities for cancer therapy. The list of all possible histone modifications is not yet complete. In the future, the manipulation of the epigenetic landscape may indeed prove to be a key element of cancer therapy.

References

1. Luger, K., Mader, A. W., Richmond, R. K., Sargent, D. F., and Richmond, T. J. (1997) Crystal structure of the nucleosome core particle at 2.8 A resolution. *Nature* **389**, 251–260.
2. Strahl, B. D. and Allis, C. D. (2000) The language of covalent histone modifications. *Nature* **403**, 41–45.
3. Davie, J. K. and Dent, S. Y. (2004) Histone modifications in corepressor functions. *Curr. Top. Dev. Biol.* **59**, 145–163.
4. Pickart, C. M. (2001) Ubiquitin enters the new millennium. *Mol. Cell.* **8**, 499–504.
5. Kondo, Y., Shen, L., and Issa, J. P. (2003) Critical role of histone methylation in tumor suppressor gene silencing in colorectal cancer. *Mol. Cell. Biol.* **23**, 206–215.
6. Shiio, Y. and Eisenman, R. N. (2003) Histone sumoylation is associated with transcriptional repression. *Proc. Natl. Acad. Sci. USA* **100**, 13,225–13,230.

7. Rice, J. C. and Allis, C. D. (2001) Code of silence. *Nature* **414**, 258–261.
8. Yoder, J. A., Soman, N. S., Verdine, G. L., and Bestor, T. H. (1997) DNA (cytosine-5)-methyltransferases in mouse cells and tissues. Studies with a mechanism-based probe. *J. Mol. Biol.* **270**, 385–395.
9. Esteller, M., Fraga, M. F., Guo, M., et al. (2001) DNA methylation patterns in hereditary human cancers mimic sporadic tumorigenesis. *Hum. Mol. Genet.* **10**, 3001–3007.
10. Antequera, F. and Bird, A. (1993) Number of CpG islands and genes in human and mouse. *Proc. Natl. Acad. Sci. USA* **90**, 11,995–11,999.
11. Bestor, T. H. (2000) The DNA methyltransferases of mammals. *Hum. Mol. Genet.* **9**, 2395–2402.
12. Bird, A. P. and Wolffe, A. P. (1999) Methylation-induced repression—belts, braces, and chromatin. *Cell* **99**, 451–454.
13. Esteller, M., Corn, P. G., Baylin, S. B., and Herman, J. G. (2001) A gene hypermethylation profile of human cancer. *Cancer. Res.* **61**, 3225–3229.
14. Paz, M. F., Wei, S., Cigudosa, J. C., et al. (2003) Genetic unmasking of epigenetically silenced tumor suppressor genes in colon cancer cells deficient in DNA methyltransferases. *Hum. Mol. Genet.* **12**, 2209–2219.
15. Razin, A. (1998) CpG methylation, chromatin structure and gene silencing-a three-way connection. *Embo. J.* **17**, 4905–4908.
16. Cervoni, N. and Szyf, M. (2001) Demethylase activity is directed by histone acetylation. *J. Biol. Chem.* **276**, 40,778–40,787.
17. Cervoni, N., Detich, N., Seo, S. B., Chakravarti, D., and Szyf, M. (2002) The oncoprotein Set/TAF-1beta, an inhibitor of histone acetyltransferase, inhibits active demethylation of DNA, integrating DNA methylation and transcriptional silencing. *J. Biol. Chem.* **277**, 25,026–25,031.
18. Esteller, M., Cordon-Cardo, C., Corn, P. G., et al. (2001) p14ARF silencing by promoter hypermethylation mediates abnormal intracellular localization of MDM2. *Cancer Res.* **61**, 2816–2821.
19. Plumb, J. A., Strathdee, G., Sludden, J., Kaye, S. B., and Brown, R. (2000) Reversal of drug resistance in human tumor xenografts by 2'-deoxy-5-azacytidine-induced demethylation of the hMLH1 gene promoter. *Cancer Res.* **60**, 6039–6044.
20. Esteller, M., Garcia-Foncillas, J., Andion, E., et al. (2000) Inactivation of the DNA-repair gene MGMT and the clinical response of gliomas to alkylating agents. *N. Engl. J. Med.* **343**, 1350–1354.
21. Esteller, M., Gaidano, G., Goodman, S. N., et al. (2002) Hypermethylation of the DNA repair gene O(6)-methylguanine DNA methyltransferase and survival of patients with diffuse large B-cell lymphoma. *J. Natl. Cancer Inst.* **94**, 26–32.
22. Plass, C., Shibata, H., Kalcheva, I., et al. (1996) Identification of Grf1 on mouse chromosome 9 as an imprinted gene by RLGS-M. *Nat. Genet.* **14**, 106–109.
23. Herman, J. G., Jen, J., Merlo, A., and Baylin, S. B. (1996) Hypermethylation-associated inactivation indicates a tumor suppressor role for p15INK4B. *Cancer Res.* **56**, 722–727.

24. Jones, P. A. and Baylin, S. B. (2002) The fundamental role of epigenetic events in cancer. *Nat. Rev. Genet.* **3**, 415–428.

25. Robertson, K. D. and Jones, P. A. (2000) DNA methylation: past, present and future directions. *Carcinogenesis* **21**, 461–467.

26. Robertson K. D. and Jones, P. A. (1999) The human ARF cell cycle regulatory gene promoter is a CpG island which can be silenced by DNA methylation and down-regulated by wild-type p53. *Mol. Cell. Biol.* **18**, 6457–6473.

27. Esteller, M., Tortola, S., Toyota, M., et al. (2000) Hypermethylation-associated inactivation of p14(ARF) is independent of p16(INK4a) methylation and p53 mutational status. *Cancer Res.* **60**, 129–133.

28. Esteller, M., Cordon-Cardo, C., Corn, P. G., et al. (2001) P14ARF silencing by promoter hypermethylation mediated abnormal intracellular localization of MDM2. *Cancer Res.* **61**, 2816–2821.

29. Corn, P. G., Kuerbitz, S. J., Van Noesel, M. M., et al. (1999) Transcriptional silencing of the p73 gene in acute lymphoblastic leukemia and Burkitt's lymphoma is associated with 5′ CpG island methylation. *Cancer Res.* **59**, 3352–3356.

30. Herman, J. G., Merlo, A., Mao, L. et al. (1995) Inactivation of the CDKN2/p16/MTS1 gene is frequently associated with aberrant DNA methylation in all common human cancers. *Cancer Res.* **55**, 4525–4530.

31. Merlo, A., Herman, J. G., Mao, L., et al. (1995) 5′ CpG island methylation is associated with transcriptional silencing of the tumour suppressor p16/CDKN2/MTS1 in human cancers. *Nat. Med.* **1**, 686–692.

32. Gonzalez-Zulueta, M., Bender, C. M., Yang, A. S., et al. (1995) Methylation of the 5′ CpG island of the p16/CDKN2 tumor suppressor gene in normal and transformed human tissues correlates with gene silencing. *Cancer Res.* **55**, 4531–4535.

33. Greger, V., Passarge, E., Hopping, W., Messmer, E., and Horsthemke, B. (1989) Epigenetic changes may contribute to the formation and spontaneous regression of retinoblastoma. *Hum. Genet.* **83**, 155–158.

34. Herman, J. G., Jen, J., Merlo, A., and Baylin, S. B. (1996) Hypermethylation-associated inactivation indicates a tumor suppressor role for p15INK4B. *Cancer Res.* **56**, 722–727.

35. Kane, M. F., Loda, M., Gaida, G. M., et al. (1997) Methylation of the hMLH1 promoter correlates with lack of expression of hMLH1 in sporadic colon tumors and mismatch repair-defective human tumor cell lines. *Cancer Res.* **57**, 808–811.

36. Herman, J. G., Umar, A., Polyak, K., et al. (1998) Incidence and functional consequences of hMLH1 promoter hypermethylation in colorectal carcinoma. *Proc. Natl. Acad. Sci. USA* **95**, 6870–6875.

37. Esteller, M., Levine, R., Hedrick, L., Ellenson, L. H., and Herman, J. G. (1998) MLH1 promoter hypermethylation is associated with the microsatellite instability phenotype in sporadic endometrial carcinoma. *Oncogene* **17**, 2413–2417.

38. Esteller, M., Lluis, C., Matias-Guiu, X., et al. (1999) HMLH1 promoter hypermethylation is an early event in endometrial tumorigenesis. *Am. J. Pathol.* **155**, 1767–1772.

39. Fleisher, A. S., Esteller, M., Wang, S., et al. (1999) Hypermethylation of the hMLH1 gene promoter in human gastric cancers with microsatellite instability. _Cancer Res._ **59,** 1090–1095.

40. Esteller, M., Hamilton, S. R., Burger, P. C., et al. (1999) Inactivation of the DNA repair gene O-methylguanine-DNA methyltransferase by promoter hypermethylation is a common event in primary human neoplasia. _Cancer Res._ **59,** 793–797.

41. Esteller, M., Toyota, M., Sanchez-Cespedes, M., et al. (2000) Inactivation of the DNA repair gene O6-methylguanine-DNA methyltransferase by promoter hypermethylation is associated with G to A mutations in K-ras in colorectal tumorigenesis. _Cancer Res._ **60,** 2368–2371.

42. Esteller, M., Risques, R. A., Toyota, M., et al. (2001) Promoter hypermethylation of the DNA repair gene O-Methylguanine-DNA methyltransferase is associated with the presence of G:C to A:T transition mutations in p53 in human colorectal tumorigenesis, _Cancer Res._ **61,** 4689–4692.

43. Mizuno, K., Osada, H., Konishi, H., et al. (2002) Aberrant hypermethylation of the CHFR prophase checkpoint gene in human lung cancers. _Oncogene_ **21,** 2328–2333.

44. Esteller, M., Silva, J. M., Dominguez, G., et al. (2000) Promoter hypermethylation is a cause of BRCA1 inactivation in sporadic breast and ovarian tumors. _J. Natl. Cancer Inst._ **92,** 564–569.

45. Hedelfank, I., Duggan, D., Chen, Y., et al. (2001) Gene-expression profiles in hereditary breast cancer. _N. Engl. J. Med._ **343,** 539–548.

46. Johnstone, R. W. (2002) Histone-deacetylase inhibitors: novel drugs for the treatment of cancer. _Nat. Rev. Drug Discov._ **1,** 287–299.

47. Jenuwein, T. and Allis, C. D. (2001) Translating the histone code. _Science_ **293,** 1074–1080.

48. Winston, F. and Allis, C. D. (1999) The bromodomain: a chromatin-targeting module? _Nat. Struct. Biol._ **6,** 601–604.

49. Dhalluin, C., Carlson, J. E., Zeng, L., He, C., Aggarwal, A. K., and Zhou, M. M. (1999) Structure and ligand of a histone acetyltransferase bromodomain. _Nature_ **399,** 491–496.

50. Fahrner, J. A., Eguchi, S., Herman, J. G., and Baylin, S. B. (2002) Dependence of histone modifications and gene expression on DNA hypermethylation in cancer. _Cancer Res._ **62,** 7213–7218.

51. Nguyen, C. T., Weisenberger, D. J., Velicescu, M., et al. (2002) Histone H3-lysine 9 methylation is associated with aberrant gene silencing in cancer cells and is rapidly reversed by 5-aza-2'-deoxycytidine. _Cancer Res._ **62,** 6456–6461.

52. Strahl, B. D., Ohba, R., Cook, R. G., and Allis, C. D. (1999) Methylation of histone H3 at lysine 4 is highly conserved and correlates with transcriptionally active nuclei in Tetrahymena, _Proc. Natl. Acad. Sci. USA_ **96,** 14,967–14,972.

53. Schubeler, D., MacAlpine, D. M., Scalzo, D., et al. (2004) The histone modification pattern of active genes revealed through genome-wide chromatin analysis of a higher eukaryote. _Genes Dev._ **18,** 1263–1271.

54. Cuthbert, G. L., Daujat, S., Snowden, A. W., et al. (2004). Histone deimination antagonizes arginine methylation. *Cell* **118**, 545–553.
55. Workman, J. L. and Abmayr, S. M. (2004) Histone H3 variants and modifications on transcribed genes. *Proc. Natl. Acad. Sci. USA* **101**, 1429–1430.
56. Cao, R. and Zhang, Y. (2004) SUZ12 is required for both the histone methyltransferase activity and the silencing function of the EED-EZH2 complex. *Mol. Cell* **15**, 57–67.
57. Hamamoto, R., Furukawa, Y., Morita, M., et al. (2004) SMYD3 encodes a histone methyltransferase involved in the proliferation of cancer cells. *Nat. Cell Biol.* **6**, 731–740.
58. Fearon, E. R. and Vogelstein, B. (1990) A genetic model for colorectal tumorigenesis. *Cell* **61**, 759–767.
59. Vogelstein, B. (1990) Cancer. A deadly inheritance. *Nature* **348**, 681–682.
60. Esteller, M., Corn, P. G., Baylin, S. B., and Herman, J. G. (2001) A gene hypermethylation profile of human cancer. *Cancer Res.* **61**, 3225–3229.
61. Esteller, M. (2002) CpG island hypermethylation and tumor suppressor genes: a booming present, a brighter future. *Oncogene* **21**, 5427–5440.
62. Fraga, M. F. and Esteller, M. (2002) DNA methylation: a profile of methods and applications. *BioTechniques* **33**, 632–649.
63. Cameron, E. E., Bachman, K. E., Myohanen, S., Herman, J. G., and Baylin, S. B. (1999) Synergy of demethylation and histone deacetylase inhibition in the re-expression of genes silenced in cancer. *Nat. Genet.* **21**, 103–107.
64. Suzuki, H., Gabrielson, E., Chen, W., et al. (2002) A genomic screen for genes upregulated by demethylation and histone deacetylase inhibition in human colorectal cancer. *Nat. Genet.* **31**, 141–149.
65. Yamashita, K., Upadhyay, S., Osada, M., et al. (2002) Pharmacologic unmasking of epigenetically silenced tumor suppressor genes in esophageal squamous cell carcinoma. *Cancer Cell* **2**, 485–495.
66. Baylin, S. B. and Herman, J. G. (2001) Promoter hypermethylation—can this change alone ever designate true tumor suppressor gene function? *J. Natl. Cancer Inst.* **93**, 664–665.
67. Chen, R. Z., Pettersson, U., Beard, C., Jackson-Grusby, L., and Jaenisch, R. (1998) DNA hypomethylation leads to elevated mutation rates. *Nature* **395**, 89–93.
68. Wijermans, P. W., Krulder, J. W., Huijgens, P. C., and Neve, P. (1997) Continuous infusion of low-dose 5-Aza-2'-deoxycytidine in elderly patients with high-risk myelodysplastic syndrome. *Leukemia* **11**, 1–5.
69. Schwartsmann, G., Fernandes, M. S., Schaan, M. D., et al. (1997) Decitabine (5-Aza-2'-deoxycytidine; DAC) plus daunorubicin as a first line treatment in patients with acute myeloid leukemia: preliminary observations. *Leukemia* **11**, S28–S31.
70. Alaminos, M., Davalos, V., Cheung, N. K., Gerald, W. L., and Esteller, M. (2004) Clustering of gene hypermethylation associated with clinical risk groups in neuroblastoma. *J. Natl. Cancer Inst.* **96**, 1208–1219.

71. Ahrendt, S. A., Chow, J. T., Xu, L. H., et al. (1999) Molecular detection of tumor cells in bronchoalveolar lavage fluid from patients with early stage lung cancer. *J. Natl. Cancer Inst.* **91,** 332–339.

72. Sanchez-Cespedes, M., Esteller, M., Hibi, K., et al. (1999) Molecular detection of neoplastic cells in lymph nodes of metastatic colorectal cancer patients predicts recurrence. *Clin. Cancer Res.* **5,** 2450–2454.

73. Palmisano, W. A., Divine, K. K., Saccomanno, G., et al. (2000) Predicting lung cancer by detecting aberrant promoter methylation in sputum. *Cancer Res.* **60,** 5954–5958.

74. Cairns, P., Esteller, M., Herman, J. G., et al. (2001) Molecular detection of prostate cancer in urine by GSTP1 hypermethylation. *Clin. Cancer Res.* **7,** 2727–2730.

75. Goessl, C., Muller, M., and Miller, K. (2000) Methylation-specific PCR (MSP) for detection of tumour DNA in the blood plasma and serum of patients with prostate cancer. *Prostate Cancer Prostatic Dis.* **3,** S17.

76. Evron, E., Dooley, W. C., Umbricht, C. B., et al. (2001) Detection of breast cancer cells in ductal lavage fluid by methylation-specific PCR. *Lancet* **357,** 1335–1336.

77. Rosas, S. L., Koch, W., da Costa Carvalho, M. G., et al. (2001) Promoter hypermethylation patterns of p16, O6-methylguanine-DNA-methyltransferase, and death-associated protein kinase in tumors and saliva of head and neck cancer patients. *Cancer Res.* **61,** 939–942.

78. Esteller, M., Sanchez-Cespedes, M., Rosell, R., Sidransky, D., Baylin, S. B., and Herman, J. G. (1999) Detection of aberrant promoter hypermethylation of tumor suppressor genes in serum DNA from non-small cell lung cancer patients. *Cancer Res.* **59,** 67–70.

79. Kawakami, K., Brabender, J., Lord, R. V., et al. (2000) Hypermethylated APC DNA in plasma and prognosis of patients with esophageal adenocarcinoma. *J. Natl. Cancer Inst.* **92,** 1805–1811.

80. Grady, W. M., Rajput, A., Lutterbaugh, J. D., and Markowitz, S. D. (2001) Detection of aberrantly methylated hMLH1 promoter DNA in the serum of patients with microsatellite unstable colon cancer. *Cancer Res.* **61,** 900–902.

81. Esteller, M. and Herman, J. G. (2004) Generating mutations but providing chemosensitivity: the role of O6-methylguanine DNA methyltransferase in human cancer. *Oncogene* **23,** 1–8.

82. Ottaviano, Y. L., Issa, J. P., Parl, F. F., Smith, H. S., Baylin, S. B., and Davidson, N. E. (1994) Methylation of the estrogen receptor gene CpG island marks loss of estrogen receptor expression in human breast cancer cells. *Cancer Res.* **54,** 2552–2555.

83. Ballestar, E. and Esteller, M. (2002) The impact of chromatin in human cancer: linking DNA methylation to gene silencing. *Carcinogenesis* **23,** 1103–1109.

84. Fraga, M. F., Uriol, E., and Diego, L. B., et al. (2002) High performance capillary electrophoretic method for the quantification of 5-methyl 2'-deoxycytidine in genomic DNA: application to plant, animal and human cancer tissues. *Electrophoresis* **23,** 1677–1681.

85. Paz, M. F., Fraga, M. F., Avila, S., et al. (2003) A systematic profile of DNA methylation in human cancer cell lines. *Cancer Res.* **63**, 1114–1121.
86. Daskalakis, M., Nguyen, T. T., Nguyen, C., et al. (2002) Demethylation of a hypermethylated P15/INK4B gene in patients with myelodysplastic syndrome by 5-Aza-2'-deoxycytidine (decitabine) treatment. *Blood* **100**, 2957–2964.
87. Christman, J. K. (2002) 5-Azacytidine and 5-aza-2'-deoxycytidine as inhibitors of DNA methylation: mechanistic studies and their implications for cancer therapy. *Oncogene* **21**, 5483–5495.
88. Lo Coco, F., Zelent, A., Kimchi, A., et al. (2002) Progress in differentiation induction as a treatment for acute promyelocytic leukemia and beyond. *Cancer Res.* **62**, 5618–5621.
89. Soengas, M. S., Capodieci, P., Polsky, D., et al. (2001) Inactivation of the apoptosis effector Apaf-1 in melanoma. *Nature* **409**, 207–211.
90. Spotswood, H. T. and Turner, B. M. (2002) An increasingly complex code. *J. Clin. Invest.* **110**, 577–582.
91. Peterson, C. L. and Laniel, M. A. (2004) Histones and histone modifications. *Curr. Biol.* **14**, R546–R551.
92. Hake, S. B., Xiao, A., and Allis, C. D. (2004) Linking the epigenetic 'language' of covalent histone modifications to cancer. *Br. J. Cancer* **90**, 761–769.
93. Hubbert, C., Guardiola, A., Shao, R., et al. (2002) HDAC6 is a microtubule-associated deacetylase. *Nature* **417**, 455–458.
94. Marks, P. A., Miller, T., and Richon, V. M. (2003) Histone deacetylases. *Curr. Opin. Pharmacol.* **3**, 344–351.
95. de Ruijter, A. J., van Gennip, A. H., Caron, H. N., Kemp, S., and van Kuilenburg, A. B. (2003) Histone deacetylases (HDACs): characterization of the classical HDAC family. *Biochem. J.* **370**, 737–749.
96. Marks, P., Rifkind, R. A., Richon, V. M., Breslow, R., Miller, T., and Kelly, W. K. (2001) Histone deacetylases and cancer: causes and therapies. *Nat. Rev. Cancer* **1**, 194–202.
97. Deckert, J. and Struhl, K. (2001) Histone acetylation at promoters is differentially affected by specific activators and repressors. *Mol. Cell. Biol.* **21**, 2726–2735.
98. Butler, L. M., Zhou, X., Xu, W. S., et al. (2002) The histone deacetylase inhibitor SAHA arrests cancer cell growth, up-regulates thioredoxin-binding protein-2, and down-regulates thioredoxin. *Proc. Natl. Acad. Sci. USA* **99**, 11,700–11,705.
99. Dehm, S. M., Hilton, T. L., Wang, E. H., and Bonham, K. (2004) SRC proximal and core promoter elements dictate TAF1 dependence and transcriptional repression by histone deacetylase inhibitors. *Mol. Cell. Biol.* **24**, 2296–2307.
100. Hirsch, C. L. and Bonham, K. (2004) Histone deacetylase inhibitors regulate p21WAF1 gene expression at the post-transcriptional level in HepG2 cells. *FEBS Lett.* **570**, 37–40.
101. Yoshida, M., Kijima, M., Akita, M., and Beppu, T. (1990) Potent and specific inhibition of mammalian histone deacetylase both in vivo and in vitro by trichostatin A. *J. Biol. Chem.* **265**, 17,174–17,179.

102. Remiszewski, S. W., Sambucetti, L. C., Bair, K. W., et al. (2003) N-Hydroxy-3-phenyl-2-propenamides as novel inhibitors of human histone deacetylase with in vivo antitumor activity: discovery of (2E)-N-hydroxy-3-[4-[[(2-hydroxyethyl)[2-(1H-indol-3-yl)ethyl]amino]methyl]phenyl]-2-propenamide (NVP-LAQ824). *J. Med. Chem.* **46,** 4609–4624.

103. Atadja, P., Gao, L., Kwon, P., et al. (2004) Selective growth inhibition of tumor cells by a novel histone deacetylase inhibitor, NVP-LAQ824. *Cancer Res.* **64,** 689–695.

104. Plumb, J. A., Finn, P. W., Williams, R. J., et al. (2003) Pharmacodynamic response and inhibition of growth of human tumor xenografts by the novel histone deacetylase inhibitor PXD101. *Mol. Cancer Ther.* **2,** 721–728.

105. Sealy, L. and Chalkley, R. (1978) The effect of sodium butyrate on histone modification. *Cell* **14,** 115–121.

106. Phiel, C. J., Zhang, F., Huang, E. Y., Guenther, M. G., Lazar, M. A., and Klein, P. S. (2001) Histone deacetylase is a direct target of valproic acid, a potent anticonvulsant, mood stabilizer, and teratogen. *J. Biol. Chem.* **276,** 36,734–36,741.

107. Gottlicher, M., Minucci, S., Zhu, P., et al. (2001) Valproic acid defines a novel class of HDAC inhibitors inducing differentiation of transformed cells. *EMBO J.* **20,** 6969–6978.

108. Lea, M. A. and Tulsyan, N. (1995) Discordant effects of butyrate analogues on erythroleukemia cell proliferation, differentiation and histone deacetylase. *Anticancer Res.* **15,** 879–883.

109. Gore, S. D., Weng, L. J., Figg, W. D., et al. (2002) Impact of prolonged infusions of the putative differentiating agent sodium phenylbutyrate on myelodysplastic syndromes and acute myeloid leukemia. *Clin. Cancer Res.* **8,** 963–970.

110. Patnaik, A., Rowinsky, E. K., Villalona, M. A., et al. (2002) A phase I study of pivaloyloxymethyl butyrate, a prodrug of the differentiating agent butyric acid, in patients with advanced solid malignancies. *Clin. Cancer Res.* **8,** 2142–2148.

111. Saito, A., Yamashita, T., Mariko, Y., et al. (1999) A synthetic inhibitor of histone deacetylase, MS-27-275, with marked in vivo antitumor activity against human tumors. *Proc. Natl. Acad. Sci. USA* **96,** 4592–4597.

112. Fournel, M., Trachy-Bourget, M. C., Yan, P. T., et al. (2002) Sulfonamide anilides, a novel class of histone deacetylase inhibitors, are antiproliferative against human tumors. *Cancer Res.* **62,** 4325–4330.

113. Kraker, A. J., Mizzen, C. A., Hartl, B. G., Miin, J., Allis, C. D., and Merriman, R. L. (2003) Modulation of histone acetylation by [4-(acetylamino)-N-(2-aminophenyl)benzamide] in HCT-8 colon carcinoma. *Mol. Cancer Ther.* **2,** 401–408.

114. Furumai, R., Komatsu, Y., Nishino, N., Khochbin, S., Yoshida, M., and Horinouchi, S. (2001) Potent histone deacetylase inhibitors built from trichostatin A and cyclic tetrapeptide antibiotics including trapoxin. *Proc. Natl. Acad. Sci. USA* **98,** 87–92.

115. Darkin-Rattray, S. J., Gurnett, A. M., Myers, R. W., et al. (1996) Apicidin: a novel antiprotozoal agent that inhibits parasite histone deacetylase. *Proc. Natl. Acad. Sci. USA* **93,** 13,143–13,147.

116. Murphy, J. P., McAleer, J. P., Uglialoro, A., et al. (2000) Histone deacetylase inhibitors and cell proliferation in pea root meristems. *Phytochemistry* **55,** 11–18.
117. Murray, P. J., Kranz, M., Ladlow, M., et al. (2001) The synthesis of cyclic tetrapeptoid analogues of the antiprotozoal natural product apicidin. Bioorg. *Med. Chem. Lett.* **11,** 773–776.
118. Hong, J., Ishihara, K., Yamaki, K., et al. (2003) Apicidin, a histone deacetylase inhibitor, induces differentiation of HL-60 cells. *Cancer Lett.* **189,** 197–206.
119. Mei, S., Ho, A. D., and Mahlknecht, U. (2004) Role of histone deacetylase inhibitors in the treatment of cancer (Review). *Int. J. Oncol.* **25,** 1509–1519.
120. Espino, P. S., Drobic, B., Dunn, K. L., and Davie, J. R. (2005) Histone modifications as a platform for cancer therapy. *J. Cell. Biochem.* **94,** 1088–1102.
121. Guasconi, V. and Ait-Si-Ali, S. (2004) Chromatin dynamics and cancer. *Cancer Biol. Ther.* **3,** 825–830.
122. Rouaux, C., Loeffler, J. P., and Boutillier, A. L. (2004) Targeting CREB-binding protein (CBP) loss of function as a therapeutic strategy in neurological disorders. *Biochem. Pharmacol.* **68,** 1157–1164.
123. Herman, J. G., Graff, J. R., Myohanen, S., Nelkin, B. D., and Baylin, S. B. (1996) Methylation-specific PCR: a novel PCR assay for methylation status of CpG islands. *Proc. Natl. Acad. Sci. USA* **93,** 9821–9826.
124. Esteller, M., Fraga, M. F., Guo, M., et al. (2001) DNA methylation patterns in hereditary human cancer mimics sporadic tumorigenesis. *Hum. Mol. Genet.* **10,** 3001–3007.
125. Herman, J. G., Umar, A., Polyak, K., et al. (1998) Incidence and functional consequences of hMLH1 promoter hypermethylation in colorectal carcinoma. *Proc. Natl. Acad. Sci. USA* **95,** 6870–6875.
126. Esteller, M., Levine, R., Baylin, S. B., Ellenson, L. H., and Herman, J. G. (1998) MLH1 promoter hypermethylation is associated with the microsatellite instability phenotype in sporadic endometrial carcinomas. *Oncogene* **17,** 2413–2417.
127. Esteller, M., Hamilton, S. R., Burger, P. C., Baylin, S. B., and Herman, J. G. (1999) Inactivation of the DNA repair gene O6-methylguanine-DNA methyltransferase by promoter hypermethylation is a common event in primary human neoplasia. *Cancer Res.* **59,** 793–797.
128. Hedenfalk, I., Duggan, D., Chen, Y., et al. (2001) Gene-expression profiles in hereditary breast cancer. *N. Engl. J. Med.* **344,** 539–548.
129. Myohanen, S. K., Baylin, S. B., and Herman, J. G. (1998) Hypermethylation can selectively silence individual p16ink4A alleles in neoplasia. *Cancer Res.* **58,** 591–593.
130. Yeager, T. R., DeVries, S., Jarrard, D. F., et al. (1998) Overcoming cellular senescence in human cancer pathogenesis. *Genes Dev.* **12,** 163–174.
131. Esteller, M., Sparks, A., Toyota, M., et al. (2000) Analysis of adenomatous polyposis coli promoter hypermethylation in human cancer. *Cancer Res.* **60,** 4366–4371.
132. Cote, S. and Momparler, R. L. (1997) Activation of the retinoic acid receptor beta gene by 5-aza-2'-deoxycytidine in human DLD-1 colon carcinoma cells. *Anticancer Drugs* **8,** 56–61.

133. Virmani, A. K., Rathi, A., Zochbauer-Muller, S., et al. (2000) Promoter methylation and silencing of the retinoic acid receptor-beta gene in lung carcinomas. *J. Natl. Cancer Inst.* **92,** 1303–1307.

134. Esteller, M., Guo, M., Moreno, V., et al. (2002) Hypermethylation-associated inactivation of the cellular retinol-binding-protein 1 gene in human cancer. *Cancer Res.* **62,** 5902–5905.

135. Villar-Garea, A. and Esteller, M. (2003) DNA demethylating agents and chromatin-remodelling drugs: which, how and why? *Curr. Drug Metab.* **4,** 11–31.

136. Cheng, J. C., Matsen, C. B., Gonzales, F. A., et al. (2003) Inhibition of DNA methylation and reactivation of silenced genes by zebularine. *J. Natl. Cancer Inst.* **95,** 399–409.

137. Cheng, J. C., Yoo, C. B., Weisenberger, D. J., et al. (2004) Preferential response of cancer cells to zebularine. *Cancer Cell* **6,** 151–158.

138. Lin, X., Asgari, K., Putzi, M. J., et al. (2001) Reversal of GSTP1 CpG island hypermethylation and reactivation of pi-class glutathione S-transferase (GSTP1) expression in human prostate cancer cells by treatment with procainamide. *Cancer Res.* **61,** 8611–8616.

139. Villar-Garea, A., Fraga, M. F., Espada, J., and Esteller, M. (2003) Procaine is a DNA-demethylating agent with growth-inhibitory effects in human cancer cells. *Cancer Res.* **63,** 4984–4989.

140. Pinto, A., Zagonel, V., Attadia, V., et al. (1989) 5-Aza-2-deoxycytidine as a differentiation inducer in acute myeloid leukaemias and myelodysplastic syndromes of the elderly. *Bone Marrow Transplant* **4,** 28–32.

141. Silverman, L. R., Holland, J. F., Weinberg, R. S., et al. (1993) Effects of treatment with 5-azacytidine on the in vivo and in vitro hematopoiesis in patients with myelodysplastic syndromes. *Leukemia* **7,** 21–29.

142. Silverman, L. R., Demakos, E. P., Peterson, B. L., et al. (2002) Randomized controlled trial of azacitidine in patients with the myelodysplastic syndrome: a study of the cancer and leukemia group B. *J. Clin. Oncol.* **20,** 2429–2440.

143. Turner, B. M. (2002) Cellular memory and the histone code. *Cell* **111,** 285–291.

144. Bannister, A. J. and Kouzarides, T. (2004) Histone methylation: recognizing the methyl mark. *Methods Enzymol.* **376,** 269–288.

145. Ng, H. H., Zhang, Y., Hendrich, B., et al. (1999) MBD2 is a transcriptional repressor belonging to the MeCP1 histone deacetylase complex. *Nature Genet.* **23,** 58–61.

146. Wade, P. A., Gegonne, A., Jones, P. L., Ballestar, E., Aubry, F., and Wolffe, A. P. (1999) Mi-2 complex couples DNA methylation to chromatin remodelling and histone deacetylation. *Nature Genet.* **23,** 62–66.

3

Wnt Signaling as a Therapeutic Target for Cancer

Andreas Herbst and Frank Thomas Kolligs

Summary

The Wnt/β-catenin signaling pathway is tightly regulated and has important functions in development, tissue homeostasis, and regeneration. Deregulation of Wnt/β-catenin signaling is frequently found in various human cancers. Eighty percent of colorectal cancers alone reveal activation of this pathway by either inactivation of the tumor-suppressor gene adenomatous polyposis coli or mutation of the proto-oncogene β-catenin. Activation of Wnt/β-catenin signaling has been found to be important for both initiation and progression of cancers of different tissues. Therefore, targeted inhibition of Wnt/β-catenin signaling is a rational and promising new approach for the therapy of cancers of various origins.

Key Words: Wnt signalling; adenomatous polyposis coli; *APC*; β-catenin; Tcf; LEF; targeted therapy; small molecules; antisense; siRNA; RNAi.

1. Introduction

The term "targeted therapy" is commonly defined as a treatment strategy focused on a specific molecular target or biological pathway involved in the genesis of a malignant process that can be detected by diagnostic testing prior to therapy *(1)*. Ideally, the target is crucial for the initiation and/or progression of the malignant process, but not for homeostasis and regeneration of normal tissues. Its inhibition only leads to regression of tumors expressing the target. Several monoclonal antibodies, small molecules, and mRNA-targeting approaches are currently under investigation. In fact, the first targeted anticancer therapies were the development of antihormonal treatments in breast, prostate, and thyroid cancer. The antiestrogen tamoxifen is directed against the estrogen receptor and is used in the treatment of breast cancer and for chemoprevention in high-risk women *(2)*.

From: *Methods in Molecular Biology, vol. 361, Target Discovery and Validation Reviews and Protocols*
Volume 2, Emerging Molecular Targets and Treatment Options
Edited by: M. Sioud © Humana Press Inc., Totowa, NJ

Trastuzumab (Herceptin®) is a humanized monoclonal antibody directed against the HER-2/neu (c-erb-B2) antigene. It is successfully used in the treatment of HER-2/neu-positive advanced breast cancer *(3)*. The chimeric monoclonal antibody cetuximab (Erbitux®) binds to the epidermal growth factor receptor (EGFR), which is frequently over expressed in several human cancers *(4)*. Cetuximab has been approved for advanced colorectal cancer in combination with the cytotoxic chemotherapeutic agent irinotecan (CPT-11). The humanized murine monoclonal antibody bevacizumab (Avastin®) targets the vascular endothelial growth factor (VEGF), which regulates vascular proliferation and survival of newly formed blood vessels *(5,6)*. It has received approval for use in metastatic colorectal cancer. Unlike trastuzumab and cetuximab, which require immunohistochemical proof of expression of the targeted receptor protein in the tumor prior to treatment, cetuximab does not require a diagnostic test. The small molecule inhibitor imatinib (Glivec®, Gleevec®) has received approval for use in chronic myelogenous leukemia (CML) and in gastrointestinal stromal tumors (GIST) *(7,8)*. It is directed against the *bcr-abl* fusion gene product in CML and the tyrosine-kinase receptor c-kit, which is oncogenically activated by mutation and overexpressed in GIST. It leads to complete hematologic and cytogenetic remissions in the early chronic phase of CML and to a strong increase in the 1-yr survival rate of patients with advanced GIST *(9,10)*. Antisense oligonucleotides are single-stranded DNA or chimeric DNA/RNA that specifically hybridize to a targeted mRNA and subsequently prevent translation of the mRNA *(11,12)*. Clinical trials are underway targeting genes deregulated in cancer, including *bcl-2* in malignant melanoma and prostate cancer, *c-myc* in prostate cancer, and protein kinase Cα in ovarian cancer *(13–16)*. These and many more targeted therapies are currently under development and clinical testing. They bear great potential for the revolution of treatment of advanced cancers.

Wnt/β-catenin signaling is an essential pathway in embryological development and tissue homeostasis. Its deregulation has been implicated in human cancers of various tissues and a still growing list of inborn diseases and developmental defects including tetra-amelia, an intersex phenotype, polycystic kidney disease, familial exsudative vitreoretinopathy, tooth agenesis, and colon cancer *(17–22)*. As deregulated Wnt/β-catenin signaling is not only involved in cancer initiation but also in cancer progression *(23–25)* its targeted disruption is a rational and promising new approach with great potential in cancer therapy.

2. Regulation of Wnt Signaling

Wnt is a fused term composed of the names of two orthologs, the *Drosophila* segment polarity gene *Wingless (Wg)* and the mouse proto-oncogene *Int-1 (26)*.

The Wnt signaling pathway, first described in *Drosophila* as *Wingless* pathway, is highly conserved among flies, frogs, and mammals. It has critical functions in embryological development, tissue morphogensis, cell-fate determination, and self-renewal of tissues *(27)*. Physiological signaling is initiated by binding of soluble Wnt ligands to the *Frizzled (Fz)* family of seven-pass transmembrane receptors. This results in the activation of one of three different Wnt-regulated pathways: the canonical *Wnt/β-catenin* pathway and the two noncanonical pathways, the *Wnt/planar cell polarity (Wnt/PCP)* and the *Wnt/calcium (Wnt/Ca^{2+})* pathway. The canonical *Wnt/β-catenin* pathway regulates the stability of the proto-oncogene β-catenin, and its activation leads to β-catenin/Tcf-dependent transcription *(28)*. Its constitutive deregulation can result in the development of various benign and malignant tumors *(29)*. The *Wnt/PCP* pathway acts through activation of the *c-Jun* N-terminal kinase (JNK) pathway, the *Wnt/Ca^{2+}* pathway is activated through a heterotrimeric G protein and results in an increase in intracellular calcium and activation of protein kinase C *(30)*. Interestingly, the transcription factor c-Jun is regulated on different levels by both *Wnt/PCP* and *Wnt/β-catenin*: activation of the JNK pathway results in activation of c-Jun by phosphorylation and, in addition, c-Jun is a transcriptional target of β-catenin/Tcf *(31)*. The JNK pathway functions in the control of cell motility, epithelial morphogenesis, and regulation of apoptosis *(32,33)*. It has both been implicated in oncogenic transformation and tumor cell proliferation as well as in the induction of apoptosis in transformed cells *(34)*. The function of the *Wnt/Ca^{2+}* pathway is so far unknown. In the following, this review will focus on the canonical Wnt/β-catenin signaling pathway **(Fig. 1)** and its therapeutic targeting.

2.1. Initiation of Wnt Signaling at the Cell Membrane

Wnt proteins constitute a large family of at least 19 secreted small glycoproteins, all of which contain 23–24 cysteine residues *(35)*. They bind as ligands to the frizzled family of seven-span transmembrane receptors *(36)*. This receptor family of at least 10 members is also characterized by a cysteine-rich domaine. However, canonical Wnt signaling is only initiated when Wnt is simultaneously complexed with both a frizzled receptor and one of the low-density lipoprotein receptor-related proteins LRP-5 or LRP-6, which act as coreceptors *(37)*. Wnt factors and frizzled receptors can be classified in accordance with the Wnt pathway they preferentially activate. However, these preferences are not rigid as several Wnts can interact with different frizzled receptors *(30)*. Wnt signaling can be antagonized at the membrane level by various secreted proteins which include soluble frizzled-related proteins (sFRPs) *(38)*, Wnt inhibitory factor-1 (WIF-1) *(39)*, and Dickkopf (Dkk) *(40,41)*. The sFRP family consists of five members, which can squelch Wnt before binding to Fz and inhibit canonical

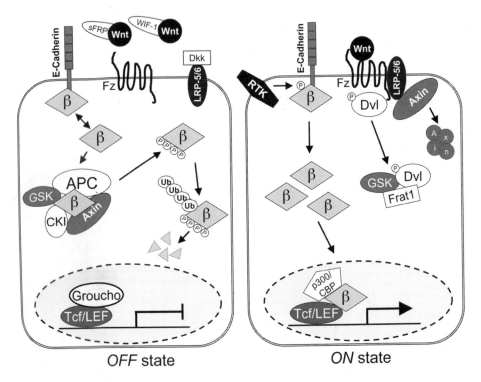

Fig. 1. The main actors of the Wnt/β-catenin signal transduction pathway in the "OFF" and the "ON" state. (Left panel) "OFF" state: β-catenin (β) is found in the cytoplasmic pool and in the E-cadherin bound pool, linking the cell membrane with the actin cytoskeleton. Soluble frizzled related proteins (SFRPs) and Wnt inhibitory factor (WIF)-1 inhibit binding of extracellular Wnt factors to frizzled receptors (Fz), Dkk (Dickkopf) blocks the LRP-5/6 coreceptors. In the absence of Wnt factors binding to Fz the free cytoplasmic pool of the proto-oncogene β-catenin is tightly regulated: the destruction complex composed of the tumor suppressor protein APC (*adenomatous polyposis coli*), the scaffold protein axin, and the kinases glykogen synthase kinase 3β (GSK) and casein kinase I α (CKI) facilitates phosphorylation (P) of 4 serine and threonine residues in the amino-terminus of β-catenin. This is the prerequisite for ubiquitination (Ub) and subsequent proteasomal degradation of β-catenin. In absence of β-catenin in the nucleus the transcriptional repressor Groucho is bound to the Tcf/LEF transcription factors and no target genes are transcribed. (Right panel) "ON" state: upon binding of Wnt ligands to Fz and the LRP-5/6 coreceptors dishevelled (Dvl) is phosphorylated. Phosphorylated Dvl inhibits GSK by forming a complex with GSK and Frat1. Axin is degraded after binding to LRP-5/6. In consequence, the destruction complex can no longer be constituted and β-catenin is stabilized. β-catenin can be liberated from its binding to E-cadherin by phosphorylation of tyrosine residues by receptor tyrosine kinases (RTK). Upon translocation of β-catenin to the nucleus it binds to Tcf/LEF factors and other proteins including p300/CBP and activates the transcription of multiple target genes.

and noncanonical Wnt signaling. Dkk proteins (Dkk-1, -2, -3) block canonical Wnt signaling by binding to LRP-5/6, which inhibits Wnt binding and induces endocytosis of LRP-5/6 *(42,43)*.

2.2. Regulation of β-Catenin in the Cytoplasm

β-catenin is synthesized continuously. The majority of cellular β-catenin is found within the cadherin bound pool at the cell membrane, linking adherens junctions with the cytoskeleton *(44)*. Phosphorylation of tyrosine residues of β-catenin by receptor tyrosine kinases such as c-RON, EGFR, and c-ErbB2 can lead to dissociation of β-catenin from adherens junctions and to its liberation into the cytoplasm *(45–47)*. The free cytoplasmic pool of β-catenin is tightly regulated. This involves three steps: (1) β-catenin phosphorylation of amino-terminal serine and threonine residues, (2) β-catenin ubiquitination, and (3) β-catenin degradation. (1) In the absence of a Wnt signal a multiprotein β-catenin destruction complex is formed in order to facilitate phosphorylation of β-catenin at four serine and threonine residues in its amino terminal destruction box. In addition to β-catenin this complex includes the scaffold protein axin, the tumor suppressor adenomatous polyposis coli (APC), glycogen synthase kinase 3β (GSK3β), casein kinase Iα (CK1α), and the protein phosphatase 2A (PP2A) *(48–52)*. This is the prerequisite for three phosphorylation steps to occur. First, the complex is stabilized by phosphorylation of axin and APC by GSK3β. Second, degradation of β-catenin is initiated by priming phosphorylation of serine residue 45 (S45) by CK 1α *(53,54)*. Third, the three remaining residues threonine T41, S37, and S33 are sequentially phosphorylated by GSK3β *(53)*. (2) Phosphorylated β-catenin is then recognized by β-TrCP, a subunit of an SCF-type E3 ubiquitin ligase complex and ubiquitinated *(55,56)*. (3) This targets β-catenin for degradation by the proteasome system *(57)*.

Degradation of β-catenin is inhibited upon activation of the Wnt signaling cascade. After formation of the Wnt/Fz/LRP-5/6 complex the proteins dishevelled (Dvl) and axin are recruited to the cell membrane. After phosphorylation by casein kinase Iε (CK Iε) *(58)* Dvl forms a complex with Frat1 and GSK3β resulting in the inhibition of GSK3β *(59)*. Of note, Dvl is thought to be the central switch at which the three Wnt signaling pathways branch off. Binding of axin to LRP-5/6 results in its degradation *(60)*. In consequence, the destruction complex is destabilized and β-catenin is no longer phosphorylated. This results in the accumulation of β-catenin in the cytoplasm and its subsequent translocation to the nucleus.

In addition to phosphorylation-dependent ubiquitination β-catenin can also be ubiquitinated by an alternative protein complex requiring the interaction of Siah1, a p53-induced gene, with the carboxy-terminus of APC, and the F-box protein EBI *(61–63)*. However, the significance of this alternative way of β-catenin ubiquitination next to the main phosphorylation-dependent degradation pathway is unknown.

2.3. Execution of β-Catenin/Tcf Signaling in the Nucleus

In the presence of a Wnt signal, free cytoplasmic β-catenin can translocate to the nucleus. As β-catenin cannot bind to DNA itself it must complex with Tcf/LEF factors in order to activate transcription *(64,65)*. Tcf1, Tcf3, Tcf4, and LEF1 constitute the Tcf/LEF family of high mobility group (HMG) proteins. In the absence of nuclear β-catenin they are complexed with the transcriptional repressor Groucho *(66,67)*. Nuclear β-catenin competes with Groucho for Tcf/LEF binding. In the β-catenin/Tcf/LEF complex β-catenin serves as transcriptional activator whereas Tcf/LEF facilitates DNA-binding to the consensus motif (A/T)A/T)CAA(A/T)G *(68)*. The large β-catenin/Tcf/LEF transcriptional complex contains a number of additional proteins including the histone acetyl-transferases p300/CBP, Brg-1, a component of the mammalian SWI/SNF and Rsc chromatin-remodelling complexes, and the TATA-binding protein Pontin52 *(69–73)*. The first β-catenin-regulated target genes identified were c-myc and cyclin D1 *(74–76)*. Other important target genes include the VEGF *(77)*, the matrix metallo-proteinases MMP7, MMP14, and MMP26 *(78–80)*, connexin 43 *(81)*, and the peroxisome proliferator-activated receptor δ (PPARδ) *(82)*. As the list of β-catenin target genes also includes several transcription factors, e.g., c-myc, c-Jun, ITF-2, and Sox9 *(31,74,83,84)* the number of directly and indirectly regulated genes is immense, for a comprehensive overview the reader is referred to the Wnt Homepage (http://www.stanford.edu/~rnusse/wntwindow.html). Together the β-catenin target genes have important functions in the regulation of many cellular processes including cell proliferation, cell cycle progression, apoptosis, differentiation, tissue invasion, and angiogenesis.

3. Wnt Signaling in Cancer

Deregulation of the Wnt signaling pathway can be found in many different human cancers. Changes in expression levels have been described for many components of the Wnt pathway. Overexpression of Wnt factors has been reported in several primary human malignancies including gastric cancer, head and neck squamous cell carcinoma, colon carcinoma, and chronic lymphocytic leukemia *(85–88)*. Several frizzled receptors have been found to be upregulated in esophageal, gastric, and colon cancers as well as in head and neck squamous cell carcinomas *(86,87,89,90)*. The Wnt coreceptor LRP-5 has recently been reported to be overexpressed in osteosarcoma *(91)*. Overexpression of dishevelled has been found in primary breast cancer, cervical squamous cell carcinoma, and mesothelioma *(92–94)*. Also Frat1, which is supposed to be involved in the inhibition of GSK3β, has been described to be overexpressed in several primary human cancers including gastric, esophageal, pancreatic, cervical, and breast *(85,95)*. However, the functional consequences of overexpression of several of these factors remains to be demonstrated.

In addition to upregulation of expression levels of activators of Wnt signaling downregulation of expression has been demonstrated for the secreted inhibitors of Wnt signaling sFRPs and WIF-1. sFRPs have been found to be downregulated in breast, bladder, and colorectal cancers as well as in mesothelioma *(96–99)*. WIF-1 expression has been reported as being repressed in prostate, breast, lung, bladder, and colorectal cancers *(100–102)*. Axin, which serves as the scaffold in the multi-protein complex facilitating phosphorylation of β-catenin, has been found to be biallelically mutated and hereby inactivated in a subset of hepatocellular and colorectal cancers as well as in medulloblastoma *(103–107)*.

Taken together, up to 90% of colorectal cancers harbor inactivating mutations in the *APC* tumor-suppressor gene or activating mutations of the proto-oncogene β-catenin. The tumor-suppressor gene *APC* is inactivated in the hereditary colorectal cancer syndrome familial adenomatous coli (FAP) *(108,109)*. This inherited autosomal-dominant disease inevitably leads to the rise of hundreds to thousands of colorectal adenomas and if no proctocolectomy is performed, to the development of colorectal cancer. Although germline inactivating mutations of APC occur throughout the entire gene, somatic mutations are clustered in exon 15 between codons 1280 and 1500 *(110)*. This results in a frame shift or a premature stop codon and a truncated protein. Mutations close to codon 1300 are mostly associated with allelic loss of the second allele of chromosome 5q, whereas tumors harboring a mutation outside this region tend to have a second truncating mutation *(111,112)*. The APC gene product interacts with multiple proteins including β-catenin, axin, and GSK3β *(51,52,113–116)*. Three different motifs of the APC protein are responsible for the regulation of β-catenin: three 15-amino acid (aa) β-catenin binding repeats, seven 20 aa β-catenin binding and downregulation repeats, and three repeats responsible for axin binding *(113,117–120)*. Loss of one APC allele and truncation of the other results in the incapability to properly bind to axin and β-catenin and to form the multiprotein complex responsible for β-catenin phosphorylation *(119,121)*. APC mutations can be detected in the earliest premalignant lesions of the colon and they are found as frequently in early adenoma as in invasive carcinoma arguing that mutation of APC is a critical step in colorectal carcinogenesis *(122)*. Therefore, the APC tumor suppressor has been named the *gatekeeper* of the colon. Other human tumors that have been found to harbor APC mutations are melanoma, medulloblastoma, and desmoids *(114,123–127)*.

Mutation of one of the four serine or threonine residues in the destruction box or deletion of the whole box in the amino terminus prevents the phosphorylation and subsequent degradation of β-catenin. These molecular changes give rise to the cytoplasmic accumulation of β-catenin and after nuclear translocation, activation of β-catenin/Tcf transcription. β-catenin mutations are present in up to 50% of colorectal cancers with intact APC, adding up to approx 10% of all colorectal cancers harboring β-catenin mutations *(128–132)*. In addition to colorectal cancers, β-catenin mutations have also been described in other gastrointestinal neoplasias including hepatocellular carcinoma and hepatoblastoma, gastric cancer, gastrointestinal carcinoids, and some rare nonductal pancreatic tumors *(103,133–140)*. Other human cancers that have been found to contain β-catenin mutations include ovarian cancer, endometrial cancer, anaplastic thyroid carcinoma, prostate cancer, melanoma, medulloblastoma, and Wilms' tumor *(123,132,141–149)*. For a comprehensive review of β-catenin mutations including mutation frequencies in various tumors *see* Giles et al. *(150)*.

4. Wnt Signaling as a Therapeutic Target in Cancer

Countless in vitro and animal studies have demonstrated the importance of Wnt/β-catenin signaling in human carcinogenesis and presented evidence that this pathway is not only involved in cancer initiation but also in cancer progression *(24,25,150,151)*. Therefore, targeting elements of this cancer pathway is a promising approach for future cancer therapies (**Table 1**). As β-catenin is the central oncogenic switch in the Wnt/β-catenin pathway it is suitable to be the main therapeutic target.

4.1. Targeting the Initiation of Wnt Signaling at the Cell Membrane

Activation of canonical Wnt signaling involves binding of Wnt ligands to frizzled receptors and LRP-5/6 co-receptors. This can be antagonized by the endogenous inhibitors of Wnt signaling sFRPs, WIF-1, and Dkk. Overexpression of Dkk-3 has been demonstrated to inhibit growth of lung cancer cells and invasion and motility of osteosarcoma cells *(152,153)*. The expression of Dkk-1, which is a transcriptional target of p53, has been shown to be induced upon treatment of cancer cells with chemotherapeutic agents, and re-expression of Dkk-1 in cells lacking endogenous Dkk-1 sensitized these to chemotherapy *(154)*. These data suggest a potential of Dkk proteins as adjuvants for chemotherapy.

To directly target Wnt signaling an antibody against Wnt-1 has been utilized *(155)*. This Wnt-1 antibody inhibited β-catenin-mediated signaling, induced apoptosis in human breast and lung cancer cells, sarcoma and mesothelioma cells, and suppressed growth of xenografted tumors in mice. The apoptotic effect was limited to cancer cells expressing high levels of Wnt-1, whereas

Table 1
Overview of Proposed Approaches Targeting the Wnt/β-Catenin Signaling Pathway

Level of action	Target	Method	Evidence	References
Upstream of β-catenin	Wnt-1	Monoclonal antibody, RNA interference	In vitro, xenograft mouse model	*155,156*
	WIF-1	Expression	In vitro	*156*
	sFRPs	Expression	In vitro	*98*
β-catenin mRNA	β-catenin	Antisense oligos	In vitro, xenograft mouse model	*159–163*
	β-catenin	RNA interference	In vitro, xenograft mouse model	*164–167*
β-catenin protein	β-catenin	APC expression	In vitro	*168,169*
	β-catenin	Protein knock-down	In vitro, xenograft mouse model	*170–172*
	β-catenin	Imatinib mesylate	In vitro	*179*
β-catenin dependent transcription	β-catenin	Small molecules	In vitro, xenopus model, xenograft mouse model	*187,188*
	β-catenin	"Death inducing genes"	In vitro, xenograft mouse model	*180,181*
	β-catenin	Oncolytic viruses	In vitro, xenograft mouse model	*182–186*
Downstream effectors of β-catenin	VEGF	Monoclonal antibody	In vivo	*5,6*
	c-Myc	Antisense oligos	In vitro, phase I clinical study	*15*
	Cyclin D1	Cdk inhibitors (R-roscovitine, rapamycin)	In vitro, xenograft mouse model	*190,191*
	c-Jun	Dominant-negative c-Jun	In vitro	*192*
	COX-2	NSAIDs	In vitro, animal studies, regression of colorectal polyps in humans	*198–201*

colon cells lacking Wnt-1 expression were not affected by the antibody treatment. The same group also analyzed the expression of the Wnt antagonist WIF-1 in colorectal cancer cell lines *(156)*. WIF-1 expression was found in normal colon cells, but was missing or downregulated in the cancer cells. The reduced expression of WIF-1 was found to be caused by hypermethylation of the WIF-1 promoter. Restoration of WIF-1 expression, silencing of Wnt-1 by siRNA, or antagonizing Wnt-1 by the anti-Wnt-1 antibody inhibited β-catenin mediated signaling and induced apoptosis in colorectal cancer cell lines already carrying mutations in either β-catenin or APC. The expression of sFRPs has also been found to be downregulated by promoter hypermethylation in colorectal cancers *(98,157,158)*. As was the case with WIF-1, exogenous restoration of sFRP expression in colorectal cancer cell lines already carrying mutations in either β-catenin or APC resulted in suppression of β-catenin-mediated signaling and induction of apoptosis. These findings support the idea that upstream Wnt signaling may be important during the early development of colorectal cancer. In addition, blocking Wnt signaling at the cell membrane may also have a therapeutic potential in the treatment of cancers even if the cancer cells carry mutations in downstream effectors of the Wnt signaling pathway.

4.2. Targeting β-Catenin mRNA

Antisense oligonucleotides specifically hybridize to complimentary mRNAs (*see* Chapter 7). It is thought that the hybrids are recognized and destroyed by RNase H. Alternatively, the RNA hybrids could inhibit the expression of the targeted mRNA by interfering with splicing or blocking translation of the mRNA. Targeting β-catenin mRNA that is continuously transcribed should result in reduced β-catenin protein expression and interruption of Wnt/β-catenin signaling. Accordingly, treatment of APC mutant colon cancer cell lines with antisense oligonucleotides resulted in a reduction of β-catenin mRNA as well as of β-catenin-mediated transcription *(159)*. A reduction of neoplastic growth capabilities of transfected cells, including proliferation, anchorage-independent growth, and cellular invasiveness was observed. Application of the same oligonucleotide in a mouse xenograft model utilizing SW480 colon cancer cells resulted in reduced tumor growth compared to control mice treated with scrambled oligonucleotide *(160)*. Interestingly, transfection of this antisense oligonucleotide into esophageal cancer cell lines that do not commonly reveal mutations of *APC* or β-*catenin* genes *(161,162)* also led to a reduction of β-catenin mRNA levels, β-catenin-mediated transcription, and to reduced growth. Although β-catenin is not expressed in normal peripheral blood T cells it is expressed in tumor cells lines of hematopoietic origin. Transfection of Jurkat T-acute lymphoblastic leukemia cells with β-catenin antisense oligonucleotides reduced β-catenin expression and resulted in the inhibition of cellular adhesion and sensitization to Fas-mediated apoptosis *(163)*.

More recently, RNA interference (RNAi) has been utilized to target β-catenin in colorectal cancer cell lines with deregulated Wnt signaling (*see* Chapters 9–12). Expression of a short-hairpin RNA (shRNA) directed against β-catenin from a plasmid in the colorectal cancer cell line LS174T which contains a mutated β-catenin allele resulted in a reduction of β-catenin-mediated transcription, cellular proliferation, and induction of differentiation *(164)*. Transfection of short-interfering RNAs (siRNA) into the colorectal cancer cell lines SW480 and HCT116, which contain mutant APC and β-catenin alleles, respectively, reduced β-catenin protein expression, β-catenin-mediated transcription, and inhibition of tumor cell growth both in vitro and in a xenograft model *(165)*. However, even though recent improvements in delivering siRNAs to their target cells are likely to give RNAi and its clinical application a boost *(166,167)* studies are needed which demonstrate that downregulation of endogenous β-catenin after systemic application of antisense oligonucleotides or siRNAs does not interfere severely with tissue homeostasis and regeneration of normal tissues.

4.3. Targeting β-Catenin Protein

APC tumor-suppressor function is lost in the majority of colorectal cancers and up to 50% of colorectal cancers with wild-type APC harbor activating β-catenin mutations. In consequence, regulation of β-catenin degradation is severely impaired and β-catenin-mediated signaling is activated. Consistent with the critical function of APC in colorectal carcinogenesis, reexpression of APC in the APC-deficient colorectal cancer cell line HT29 led as a proof of principle to the reduction of β-catenin level, growth arrest, and induction of apoptosis *(168)*. Later studies demonstrated that the central third of the APC protein, which contains the β-catenin binding sites, is sufficient to downregulate β-catenin and to suppress β-catenin-mediated transcription *(169)*. Infection of colorectal cancer cells with an adenovirus expressing this mini-APC fragment resulted in growth inhibition and activation of apoptosis.

Another approach to downregulate β-catenin in cell lines focuses on the ubiquitination and degradation machinery. Phosphorylation is a prerequisite for β-catenin to be recognized by the F-Box protein β-TrCP and subsequent proteasomal degradation. Therefore, bypassing the impaired phosphorylation machinery in cancer cells with deregulated β-catenin would be an intriguing approach targeting deregulated β-catenin expression. To overcome β-catenin from escaping its destruction chimeric F-box proteins have been generated that recognize β-catenin in a phosphorylation-independent manner and promote its proteasomal degradation. One approach engineered a chimeric protein with the β-catenin binding domain of E-cadherin fused to the F-box protein β-TrCP *(170)*. This chimeric protein recruits β-catenin protein to the SCF ubiquitin ligase complex and targets it for degradation by ubiquitination. Expression of the β-TrCP-E-cadherin chimera in DLD-1 colorectal carcinoma cells selectively reduced cytosolic but not E-cadherin-bound β-catenin, resulting in impaired growth and inhibition of colony formation in vitro, as well as loss of tumorigenicity in xenografted mice. Another chimeric protein was constructed to contain multiple copies of a minimal β-catenin-binding element of 15 amino acids derived from the APC protein fused to the F-Box motif of β-TrCP *(171)*. Like the previously mentioned approach, this chimeric protein suppressed the activity of β-catenin-mediated transcription and downregulated the β-catenin target gene *c-myc* by reduction of nuclear and cytosolic β-catenin, but also preserved the membrane-bound pool. Growth of colorectal cancer cells was substantially inhibited in vitro and in vivo. A third chimeric F-box protein, which replaces the WD40 repeat of β-TrCP with the β-catenin-binding domains of Tcf-4 and E-cadherin, has been generated *(172)*. Also this chimera has been shown to downregulate β-catenin independent of phosphorylation. The main advantage of these three approaches is that the cytosolic- and nuclear- but not the membrane-bound pools of β-catenin are reduced. Only the pools responsible for oncogenic signaling but not the membrane-bound pool of β-catenin involved in cell adhesion are targeted. This might be a major advantage when compared to approaches targeting β-catenin mRNA. Discriminating between cytosolic/nuclear and E-cadherin-bound β-catenin might minimize side effects of this therapeutic approach. However, the major drawback of these chimera targeting β-catenin degradation is the delivery of the chimeric proteins to tumors.

Receptor tyrosine kinases have been shown to be involved in the regulation of free cytoplasmic β-catenin *(173–178)*. Phosphorylation of tyrosine residue 654 of β-catenin blocks the E-cadherin/β-catenin interaction and results in an increase of β-catenin/Tcf-regulated transcription. It has been demonstrated that the tyrosine kinase inhibitor imatinib downregulates β-catenin-mediated signaling and suppresses growth of colorectal cancer cells *(179)*. Similar experiments with other tyrosine kinase inhibitors like gefitinib and erlotinib are pending.

4.4. Targeting β-Catenin/Tcf Transcription

Another interesting approach targeting active Wnt/β-catenin signaling is the use of recombinant viruses, which either carry a "death-inducing gene" under the control of a Tcf-dependent promoter or the replication of which is dependent on active β-catenin/Tcf signaling. A recombinant adenovirus containing the apoptosis inducing gene FADD (Fas-associated death domain-containing protein) under the control of a Tcf-dependent promoter has been generated *(180)*. Colorectal cancer cells with activated β-catenin/Tcf signaling were selectively and efficiently killed by the virus, supporting the idea that aberrantly activated β-catenin can be used to selectively target colon cancer cells. In order to maximize the tumor-killing effect in colorectal cancer cells with deregulated Wnt signaling a recombinant adenovirus was generated which carries a herpes simplex virus thymidine kinase gene (HSV-TK) under the control of a Tcf-responsive promoter *(181)*. Treatment of nude mice xenografted with human DLD-1 colon cancer cells with the recombinant adenovirus and ganciclovir significantly suppressed the growth of the tumor cells. Control mice xenografted with a human hepatoma cell line did not respond to this treatment, demonstrating that this approach selectively targets tumor cells with aberrant activation of β-catenin.

Oncolytic viruses selectively lyse malignant cells by cytopathic effects *(182)*. The major advantage of this strategy is the amplification of the virus at the site of the tumor. Brunori and coworkers engineered an oncolytic adenovirus that selectively replicates in cells with aberrantly high β-catenin expression *(183)*. This adenovirus expresses the viral E1B and E2 genes from promoters controlled by b-catenin/Tcf. The Tcf-E1B and Tcf-E2 promoters were found to be active in many cell lines with activated Wnt signaling. Viruses with Tcf-dependent regulation of E2 expression replicated efficiently in SW480 colon cancer cells, but showed a significantly reduced replication in H1299 lung cancer cells and WI38 normal fibroblasts. As a proof of concept, the authors introduced a stable β-catenin mutant into normal WI38 fibroblasts, which rendered these cells permissive for virus replication. Another oncolytic virus with Tcf-binding sites integrated into the promoters of the *E1A, E1B, E2,* and *E4* genes exhibited a strong selectivity for cells with deregulated Wnt signaling *(184)*. This adenovirus preferentially replicated in cells with activated Wnt signaling and resulted in a dramatic increased efficacy in cytopathic assays. Based on a similar idea, Toth and coworkers generated an adenovirus with a synthetic promoter containing five Tcf-consensus binding sites replacing the wild-type E4 promoter *(185)*. The virus preferentially replicated in cells with activated Wnt signaling. In a xenograft model the virus effectively suppressed the growth of SW480 colorectal cancer cells but not of control cells without deregulated Wnt signaling. Instead of using adenoviral vectors Malerba et al. *(186)* modified the minute parvovirus of mice to contain Tcf-binding sites within the P4 promoter. Replication and cytopathic effects of this recombinant virus were also strongly dependent on β-catenin/Tcf activity.

So far, two screens for small molecular compounds targeting active Wnt/β-catenin signaling in cancer have been published. In search for small molecule inhibitors of Wnt signaling, Lepourcelet and coworkers performed a systematic screen of libraries of natural compounds that specifically disrupt the β-catenin/Tcf-4 complex *(187)*. Among 7000 compounds screened, 8 showed dose-dependent inhibition of the β-catenin/Tcf-4 complex. Each of the compounds was able to inhibit β-catenin/Tcf reporter gene activity and transcription of known β-catenin/Tcf target genes. Subsequent analyses revealed that three of the compounds abrogated axis duplication in *Xenopus* embryos, which was induced by injection of β-catenin mRNA. Finally, two compounds of fungal origin were identified as specific inhibitors of the β-catenin/Tcf complex in vitro and in vivo. However, the compounds were also found to inhibit β-catenin binding to APC, which might affect β-catenin phosphorylation by inhibition of its binding to the multiprotein phosphorylation complex. Another screen of 5000 compounds for small-molecule inhibitors of β-catenin-mediated signaling identified a compound, ICG-001, which specifically inhibits the cyclic AMP response element-binding protein, a p300-related coactivator of β-catenin-mediated transcription *(188)*. Treatment of cells with ICG-001 inhibited transcription of a reporter gene and the transcription of β-catenin/Tcf target genes was downregulated. ICG-001 inhibited the proliferation of colorectal cancer cells in vitro and of tumor xenografts in nude mice. These two studies are encouraging as they demonstrate the feasibility of identifying small molecule inhibitors that target protein–protein interactions. However, more studies are needed to exclude toxic side effects and negative effects on tissue homeostasis and regeneration as a compound effective against cancer cells would be expected to also target normal cells that depend on the same pathway, i.e., intestinal epithelium.

4.5. Targeting Downstream Effectors of β-Catenin

β-catenin/Tcf regulate the expression of multiple genes some of which are known to promote tumor growth, including c-Myc, cyclin D1, c-Jun, VEGF, and COX-2. Therefore, targeting these genes in cancers with deregulated Wnt signaling might be a promising alternative to the previously mentioned concepts. The oncogene c-Myc is overexpressed in a variety of human cancers including leukemia, lymphoma, melanoma, breast cancer, and colorectal cancer *(189)*. Being a direct target gene of β-catenin, c-Myc is crucial for the development of cancer and inhibiton of c-Myc is an important step to limit tumor growth. An antisense oligonucleotide targeting c-Myc mRNA was able to significantly reduce the growth and induce apoptosis in prostate cancer cells *(15)*. When tested in a xenograft model, the antisense oligonucleotide caused a dramatic reduction of tumor load. Moreover, antisense oligonucleotides against c-Myc have been shown to limit proliferation in leukemia, lymphoma, melanoma, prostate, breast and liver cancer cells *(15)*. Several approaches have been done to target the cell cycle regulator cyclin D1. The function of cyclin D1 to phosphorylate the tumor suppressor Rb in complex with the cyclin-dependent kinases (CDK) 4 and 6 is inhibited by the CDK inhibitor R-roscovitine (CYC202) and by rapamycin *(190,191)*.

C-Jun and Fos proteins form hetero- and homodimers to constitute the activator protein (AP)-1. To investigate the role of AP-1 in colorectal cancer, a dominant-negative mutant of c (DN)-Jun lacking the transcription activation domain was used *(192)*. Transfection of HT29 colorectal cancer cells with DN-Jun inhibited tumor cell proliferation in vitro and in vivo, suggesting that the β-catenin-regulated gene *c-Jun* might be a useful target in colorectal cancer. VEGF stimulates the vascular permeability and acts a mitogen and survival factor for endothelial cells through interaction with its cognate cell surface receptors. Treatment of HCT116 colorectal cancer cells with β-catenin antisense oligonucleotides led to a reduction of VEGF expression by more than 50% *(193)*. Therefore, targeting VEGF by small molecules or antibodies will indirectly inhibit part of β-catenin function in cancer.

Cyclooxygenase-2 is overexpressed in many tumors and its direct or indirect regulation by Wnt/β-catenin signaling has been demonstrated *(82,194–196,208)*. Its activity can be inhibited by selective cyclooxygenase (COX)-2 inhibitors and nonselective nonsteroidal antiinflammatory drugs *(197)*. Epidemiological and experimental studies have demonstrated that COX-2 inhibitors and nonselective nonsteroidal antiinflammatory drugs can inhibit the development of colorectal cancer *(198–201)*. The COX-2 inhibitor celecoxib has been approved for reduction and regression of colorectal polyps in FAP patients. However, to effectively downregulate Wnt/β-catenin signaling by inhibiting downstream effectors of the pathway more than one β-catenin/Tcf-regulated gene needs to be targeted. This kind of an approach is appealing but specific studies are pending.

5. Conclusions and Future Perspectives

Targeting deregulated Wnt/β-catenin signaling in cancer is a rationale therapeutic approach. Accordingly, many different strategies focusing on different levels of the pathway have been developed. However, none of these has so far reached clinics. It needs to be kept in mind with all new approaches targeting Wnt signaling that the Wnt pathway has vital functions in the maintenance and self-renewal of various pluripotent stem cells and progenitor cells *(202–204,209)*. Interruption of Wnt signaling in the intestinal crypt may lead to depletion of the epithelial stem-cell compartment and consequently to a loss of intestinal regeneration *(205,206)*. Moreover, not every single cancer cell with deregulated Wnt/β-catenin signaling might also be dependent on this pathway for maintenance of the transformed phenotype as has been demonstrated by direct targeting of β-catenin by knock-out of the mutant allele in the colorectal cancer cell line HCT116 *(207)*. The individual genetic background of a tumor might be of great importance for its response to a targeted therapy even if the targeted pathway is indeed deregulated. As our understanding of the Wnt/β-catenin pathway is progressing with new activators, inhibitors, target genes, and cross-connections to other pathways being identified, more therapeutic approaches to target this pathway will appear. In conclusion, as most tumors carry mutations in several genes and reveal various deregulated pathways, the majority of tumors will most likely not be treated successfully by targeting only one single pathway. As multiple pathways in a single cell contribute to the transformed phenotype, only a treatment focusing on more than one target will ultimately be successful in the majority of cases.

Acknowledgments

This work was supported in part by research grants from the German Research Foundation DFG and the Wilhelm Sander-Foundation.

References

1. Ross, J. S., Schenkein, D. P., Pietrusko, R., et al. (2004) Targeted therapies for cancer 2004. *Am. J. Clin. Pathol.* **122**, 598–609.
2. Jordan, V. C. (2003) Tamoxifen: a most unlikely pioneering medicine. *Nat. Rev. Drug Discov.* **2**, 205–213.
3. McKeage, K. and Perry, C. M. (2002) Trastuzumab: a review of its use in the treatment of metastatic breast cancer overexpressing HER2. *Drugs* **62**, 209–243.
4. Reynolds, N. A. and Wagstaff, A. J. (2004) Cetuximab: in the treatment of metastatic colorectal cancer. *Drugs* **64**, 109–121.
5. McCarthy, M. (2003) Antiangiogenesis drug promising for metastatic colorectal cancer. *Lancet* **361**, 1959.
6. Sparano, J. A., Gray, R., Giantonio, B., O'Dwyer, P., and Comis, R. L. (2004) Evaluating antiangiogenesis agents in the clinic: the Eastern Cooperative Oncology Group Portfolio of Clinical Trials. *Clin. Cancer Res.* **10**, 1206–1211.
7. Goldman, J. M. and Melo, J. V. (2003) Chronic myeloid leukemia—advances in biology and new approaches to treatment. *N. Engl. J. Med.* **349**, 1451–1464.
8. von Mehren, M. (2003) Gastrointestinal stromal tumors: a paradigm for molecularly targeted therapy. *Cancer Invest.* **21**, 553–563.
9. Druker, B. J. (2003) Imatinib mesylate in the treatment of chronic myeloid leukaemia. *Expert Opin. Pharmacother.* **4**, 963–971.
10. Verweij, J., van Oosterom, A., Blay, J. Y., et al. (2003) Imatinib mesylate (STI-571 Glivec, Gleevec) is an active agent for gastrointestinal stromal tumours, but does not yield responses in other soft-tissue sarcomas that are unselected for a molecular target. Results from an EORTC Soft Tissue and Bone Sarcoma Group phase II study. *Eur. J. Cancer* **39**, 2006–2011.
11. Dean, N. M. and Bennett, C. F. (2003) Antisense oligonucleotide-based therapeutics for cancer. *Oncogene* **22**, 9087–9096.

12. Wang, H., Prasad, G., Buolamwini, J. K., and Zhang, R. (2001) Antisense anti-cancer oligonucleotide therapeutics. *Curr. Cancer Drug Targets* **1**, 177–196.
13. Jansen, B., Wacheck, V., Heere-Ress, E., et al. (2000) Chemosensitisation of malignant melanoma by BCL2 antisense therapy. *Lancet* **356**, 1728–1733.
14. Chi, K. N., Gleave, M. E., Klasa, R., et al. (2001) A phase I dose-finding study of combined treatment with an antisense Bcl-2 oligonucleotide (Genasense) and mitoxantrone in patients with metastatic hormone-refractory prostate cancer. *Clin. Cancer Res.* **7**, 3920–3927.
15. Iversen, P. L., Arora, V., Acker, A. J., Mason, D. H., and Devi, G. R. (2003) Efficacy of antisense morpholino oligomer targeted to c-myc in prostate cancer xenograft murine model and a Phase I safety study in humans. *Clin. Cancer Res.* **9**, 2510–2519.
16. Advani, R., Peethambaram, P., Lum, B. L., et al. (2004) A Phase II trial of aprinocarsen, an antisense oligonucleotide inhibitor of protein kinase C alpha, administered as a 21-day infusion to patients with advanced ovarian carcinoma. *Cancer* **100**, 321–326.
17. Niemann, S., Zhao, C., Pascu, F., et al. (2004) Homozygous WNT3 mutation causes tetra-amelia in a large consanguineous family. *Am. J. Hum. Genet.* **74**, 558–563.
18. Jordan, B. K., Shen, J. H., Olaso, R., Ingraham, H. A., and Vilain, E. (2003) Wnt4 overexpression disrupts normal testicular vasculature and inhibits testosterone synthesis by repressing steroidogenic factor 1/beta-catenin synergy. *Proc. Natl. Acad. Sci. USA* **100**, 10,866–10,871.
19. Rodova, M., Islam, M. R., Maser, R. L., and Calvet, J. P. (2002) The polycystic kidney disease-1 promoter is a target of the beta-catenin/T-cell factor pathway. *J. Biol. Chem.* **277**, 29,577–29,583.
20. Robitaille, J., MacDonald, M. L., Kaykas, A., et al. (2002) Mutant frizzled-4 disrupts retinal angiogenesis in familial exudative vitreoretinopathy. *Nat. Genet.* **32**, 326–330.
21. Toomes, C., Bottomley, H. M., Jackson, R. M., et al. (2004) Mutations in LRP5 or FZD4 underlie the common familial exudative vitreoretinopathy locus on chromosome 11q. *Am. J. Hum. Genet.* **74**, 721–730.
22. Lammi, L., Arte, S., Somer, M., et al. (2004) Mutations in AXIN2 cause familial tooth agenesis and predispose to colorectal cancer. *Am. J. Hum. Genet.* **74**, 1043–1050.
23. Kim, J. S., Crooks, H., Foxworth, A., and Waldman, T. (2002) Proof-of-principle: oncogenic beta-catenin is a valid molecular target for the development of pharmacological inhibitors. *Mol. Cancer Ther.* **1**, 1355–1359.
24. Gunther, E. J., Moody, S. E., Belka, G .K., et al. (2003) Impact of p53 loss on reversal and recurrence of conditional Wnt-induced tumorigenesis. *Genes Dev.* **17**, 488–501.
25. Derksen, P. W., Tjin, E., Meijer, H. P., et al. (2004) Illegitimate WNT signaling promotes proliferation of multiple myeloma cells. *Proc. Natl. Acad. Sci. USA* **101**, 6122–6127.

26. Rijsewijk, F., Schuermann, M., Wagenaar, E., Parren, P., Weigel, D., and Nusse, R. (1987) The Drosophila homolog of the mouse mammary oncogene int-1 is identical to the segment polarity gene wingless. *Cell* **50,** 649–657.

27. Cadigan, K. M. and Nusse, R. (1997) Wnt signaling: a common theme in animal development. *Genes Dev.* **11,** 3286–3305.

28. Papkoff, J., Rubinfeld, B., Schryver, B., and Polakis, P. (1996) Wnt-1 regulates free pools of catenins and stabilizes APC-catenin complexes. *Mol. Cell. Biol.* **16,** 2128–2134.

29. Polakis, P. (2000) Wnt signaling and cancer. *Genes Dev.* **14,** 1837–1851.

30. Veeman, M. T., Axelrod, J. D., and Moon, R. T. (2003) A second canon. Functions and mechanisms of beta-catenin-independent Wnt signaling. *Dev. Cell.* **5,** 367–377.

31. Mann, B., Gelos, M., Siedow, A., et al. (1999) Target genes of beta-catenin-T cell-factor/lymphoid-enhancer-factor signaling in human colorectal carcinomas. *Proc. Natl. Acad. Sci. USA* **96,** 1603–1608.

32. Xia, Y. and Karin, M. (2004) The control of cell motility and epithelial morphogenesis by Jun kinases. *Trends Cell Biol.* **14,** 94–101.

33. Wada, T. and Penninger, J. M. (2004) Mitogen-activated protein kinases in apoptosis regulation. *Oncogene* **23,** 2838–2849.

34. Kennedy, N. J. and Davis, R. J. (2003) Role of JNK in tumor development. *Cell Cycle* **2,** 199–201.

35. Miller, J. R. (2002) The Wnts. *Genome Biol* **3,** REVIEWS3001.

36. Huang, H. C. and Klein, P. S. (2004) The Frizzled family: receptors for multiple signal transduction pathways. *Genome Biol.* **5,** 234.

37. Tamai, K., Semenov, M., Kato, Y., et al. (2000) LDL-receptor-related proteins in Wnt signal transduction. *Nature* **407,** 530–535.

38. Jones, S. E. and Jomary, C. (2002) Secreted Frizzled-related proteins: searching for relationships and patterns. *Bioessays* **24,** 811–820.

39. Hsieh, J. C., Kodjabachian, L., Rebbert, M. L., et al. (1999) A new secreted protein that binds to Wnt proteins and inhibits their activities. *Nature* **398,** 431–436.

40. Brott, B. K. and Sokol, S. Y. (2002) Regulation of Wnt/LRP signaling by distinct domains of Dickkopf proteins. *Mol. Cell. Biol.* **22,** 6100–6110.

41. Fedi, P., Bafico, A., Nieto Soria, A., et al. (1999) Isolation and biochemical characterization of the human Dkk-1 homologue, a novel inhibitor of mammalian Wnt signaling. *J. Biol. Chem.* **274,** 19,465–19,472.

42. Mao, B., Wu, W., Li, Y., et al. (2001) LDL-receptor-related protein 6 is a receptor for Dickkopf proteins. *Nature* **411,** 321–325.

43. Mao, B., Wu, W., Davidson, G., et al. (2002) Kremen proteins are Dickkopf receptors that regulate Wnt/beta-catenin signalling. *Nature* **417,** 664–667.

44. Barth, A. I., Nathke, I. S., and Nelson, W. J. (1997) Cadherins, catenins and APC protein: interplay between cytoskeletal complexes and signaling pathways. *Curr. Opin. Cell. Biol.* **9,** 683–690.

45. Graham, N. A. and Asthagiri, A. R. (2004) Epidermal growth factor-mediated T-cell factor/lymphoid enhancer factor transcriptional activity is essential but

not sufficient for cell cycle progression in nontransformed mammary epithelial cells. *J. Biol. Chem.* **279,** 23,517–23,524.

46. Danilkovitch-Miagkova, A., Miagkov, A., Skeel, A., Nakaigawa, N., Zbar, B., and Leonard, E. J. (2001) Oncogenic mutants of RON and MET receptor tyrosine kinases cause activation of the beta-catenin pathway. *Mol. Cell. Biol.* **21,** 5857–5868.

47. Bonvini, P., An, W. G., Rosolen, A., et al. (2001) Geldanamycin abrogates ErbB2 association with proteasome-resistant beta-catenin in melanoma cells, increases beta-catenin-E-cadherin association, and decreases beta-catenin-sensitive transcription. *Cancer Res.* **61,** 1671–1677.

48. Hinoi, T., Yamamoto, H., Kishida, M., Takada, S., Kishida, S., and Kikuchi, A. (2000) Complex formation of adenomatous polyposis coli gene product and axin facilitates glycogen synthase kinase-3 beta-dependent phosphorylation of beta-catenin and down-regulates beta-catenin. *J. Biol. Chem.* **275,** 34,399–34,406.

49. Ikeda, S., Kishida, M., Matsuura, Y., Usui, H., and Kikuchi, A. (2000) GSK-3beta-dependent phosphorylation of adenomatous polyposis coli gene product can be modulated by beta-catenin and protein phosphatase 2A complexed with Axin. *Oncogene* **19,** 537–545.

50. Yamamoto, H., Kishida, S., Kishida, M., Ikeda, S., Takada, S., and Kikuchi, A. (1999) Phosphorylation of axin, a Wnt signal negative regulator, by glycogen synthase kinase-3beta regulates its stability. *J. Biol. Chem.* **274,** 10,681–10,684.

51. Kishida, S., Yamamoto, H., Ikeda, S., et al. (1998) Axin, a negative regulator of the wnt signaling pathway, directly interacts with adenomatous polyposis coli and regulates the stabilization of beta-catenin. *J. Biol. Chem.* **273,** 10,823–10,826.

52. Ikeda, S., Kishida, S., Yamamoto, H., Murai, H., Koyama, S., and Kikuchi, A. (1998) Axin, a negative regulator of the Wnt signaling pathway, forms a complex with GSK-3beta and beta-catenin and promotes GSK-3beta-dependent phosphorylation of beta-catenin. *Embo. J.* **17,** 1371–1384.

53. Liu, C., Li, Y., Semenov, M., Han, C., et al. (2002) Control of beta-catenin phosphorylation/degradation by a dual-kinase mechanism. *Cell* **108,** 837–847.

54. Amit, S., Hatzubai, A., Birman, Y., et al. (2002) Axin-mediated CKI phosphorylation of beta-catenin at Ser 45: a molecular switch for the Wnt pathway. *Genes Dev.* **16,** 1066–1076.

55. Latres, E., Chiaur, D. S., and Pagano, M. (1999) The human F box protein beta-Trcp associates with the Cul1/Skp1 complex and regulates the stability of beta-catenin. *Oncogene* **18,** 849–854.

56. Hart, M., Concordet, J. P., Lassot, I., et al. (1999) The F-box protein beta-TrCP associates with phosphorylated beta-catenin and regulates its activity in the cell. *Curr. Biol.* **9,** 207–210.

57. Aberle, H., Bauer, A., Stappert, J., Kispert, A., and Kemler, R. (1997) beta-catenin is a target for the ubiquitin-proteasome pathway. *Embo J.* **16,** 3797–3804.

58. Kishida, M., Hino, S., Michiue, T., et al. (2001) Synergistic activation of the Wnt signaling pathway by Dvl and casein kinase Iepsilon. *J. Biol. Chem.* **276,** 33,147–33,155.

59. Lee, E., Salic, A., and Kirschner, M. W. (2001) Physiological regulation of [beta]-catenin stability by Tcf3 and CK1epsilon. *J. Cell. Biol.* **154**, 983–993.
60. Mao, J., Wang, J., Liu, B., et al. (2001) Low-density lipoprotein receptor-related protein-5 binds to Axin and regulates the canonical Wnt signaling pathway. *Mol. Cell.* **7**, 801–809.
61. Matsuzawa, S. I. and Reed, J. C. (2001) Siah-1, SIP, and Ebi collaborate in a novel pathway for beta-catenin degradation linked to p53 responses. *Mol. Cell.* **7**, 915–926.
62. Liu, J., Stevens, J., Rote, C. A., et al. (2001) Siah-1 mediates a novel beta-catenin degradation pathway linking p53 to the adenomatous polyposis coli protein. *Mol. Cell.* **7**, 927–936.
63. Sadot, E., Geiger, B., Oren, M., and Ben-Ze'ev, A. (2001) Down-regulation of beta-catenin by activated p53. *Mol. Cell. Biol.* **21**, 6768–6781.
64. Behrens, J., von Kries, J. P., Kuhl, M., et al. (1996) Functional interaction of beta-catenin with the transcription factor LEF-1. *Nature* **382**, 638–642.
65. Molenaar, M., van de Wetering, M., Oosterwegel, M., et al. (1996) XTcf-3 transcription factor mediates beta-catenin-induced axis formation in Xenopus embryos. *Cell* **86**, 391–399.
66. Cavallo, R. A., Cox, R. T., Moline, M. M., et al. (1998) Drosophila Tcf and Groucho interact to repress Wingless signalling activity. *Nature* **395**, 604–608.
67. Roose, J., Molenaar, M., Peterson, J., et al. (1998) The Xenopus Wnt effector XTcf-3 interacts with Groucho-related transcriptional repressors. *Nature* **395**, 608–612.
68. Brantjes, H., Barker, N., van Es, J., and Clevers, H. (2002) TCF: Lady Justice casting the final verdict on the outcome of Wnt signalling. *Biol. Chem.* **383**, 255–261.
69. Hecht, A., Vleminckx, K., Stemmler, M. P., van Roy, F., and Kemler, R. (2000) The p300/CBP acetyltransferases function as transcriptional coactivators of beta-catenin in vertebrates. *Embo. J.* **19**, 1839–1850.
70. Sun, Y., Kolligs, F. T., Hottiger, M. O., Mosavin, R., Fearon, E. R., and Nabel, G. J. (2000) Regulation of beta-catenin transformation by the p300 transcriptional coactivator. *Proc. Natl. Acad. Sci. USA* **97**, 12,613–12,618.
71. Takemaru, K. I. and Moon, R. T. (2000) The transcriptional coactivator CBP interacts with beta-catenin to activate gene expression. *J. Cell. Biol.* **149**, 249–254.
72. Barker, N., Hurlstone, A., Musisi, H., Miles, A., Bienz, M., and Clevers, H. (2001) The chromatin remodelling factor Brg-1 interacts with beta-catenin to promote target gene activation. *Embo. J.* **20**, 4935–4943.
73. Bauer, A., Huber, O., and Kemler, R. (1998) Pontin52, an interaction partner of beta-catenin, binds to the TATA box binding protein. *Proc. Natl. Acad. Sci. USA* **95**, 14,787–14,792.
74. He, T. C., Sparks, A. B., Rago, C., et al. (1998) Identification of c-MYC as a target of the APC pathway. *Science* **281**, 1509–1512.
75. Shtutman, M., Zhurinsky, J., Simcha, I., et al. (1999) The cyclin D1 gene is a target of the beta-catenin/LEF-1 pathway. *Proc. Natl. Acad. Sci. USA* **96**, 5522–5527.

76. Tetsu, O. and McCormick, F. (1999) Beta-catenin regulates expression of cyclin D1 in colon carcinoma cells. *Nature* **398,** 422–426.
77. Zhang, X., Gaspard, J. P., and Chung, D. C. (2001) Regulation of vascular endothelial growth factor by the Wnt and K-ras pathways in colonic neoplasia. *Cancer Res.* **61,** 6050–6054.
78. Brabletz, T., Jung, A., Dag, S., Hlubek, F., and Kirchner, T. (1999) beta-catenin regulates the expression of the matrix metalloproteinase-7 in human colorectal cancer. *Am. J. Pathol.* **155,** 1033–1038.
79. Takahashi, M., Tsunoda, T., Seiki, M., Nakamura, Y., and Furukawa, Y. (2002) Identification of membrane-type matrix metalloproteinase-1 as a target of the beta-catenin/Tcf4 complex in human colorectal cancers. *Oncogene* **21,** 5861–5867.
80. Marchenko, N. D., Marchenko, G. N., Weinreb, R. N., et al. (2004) Beta-catenin regulates the gene of MMP-26, a novel metalloproteinase expressed both in carcinomas and normal epithelial cells. *Int. J. Biochem. Cell. Biol.* **36,** 942–956.
81. van der Heyden, M. A., Rook, M. B., Hermans, M. M., et al. (1998) Identification of connexin43 as a functional target for Wnt signalling. *J. Cell. Sci.* **111,** 1741–1749.
82. He, T. C., Chan, T. A., Vogelstein, B., and Kinzler, K. W. (1999) PPARdelta is an APC-regulated target of nonsteroidal anti-inflammatory drugs. *Cell* **99,** 335–345.
83. Kolligs, F. T., Nieman, M. T., Winer, I., et al. (2002) ITF-2, a downstream target of the Wnt/TCF pathway, is activated in human cancers with beta-catenin defects and promotes neoplastic transformation. *Cancer Cell.* **1,** 145–155.
84. Blache, P., van de Wetering, M., Duluc, I., et al. (2004) SOX9 is an intestine crypt transcription factor, is regulated by the Wnt pathway, and represses the CDX2 and MUC2 genes. *J. Cell. Biol.* **166,** 37–47.
85. Saitoh, T., Mine, T., and Katoh, M. (2002) Frequent up-regulation of WNT5A mRNA in primary gastric cancer. *Int. J. Mol. Med.* **9,** 515–519.
86. Rhee, C. S., Sen, M., Lu, D., et al. (2002) Wnt and frizzled receptors as potential targets for immunotherapy in head and neck squamous cell carcinomas. *Oncogene* **21,** 6598–6605.
87. Holcombe, R. F., Marsh, J. L., Waterman, M. L., Lin, F., Milovanovic, T., and Truong, T. (2002) Expression of Wnt ligands and Frizzled receptors in colonic mucosa and in colon carcinoma. *Mol. Pathol.* **55,** 220–226.
88. Lu, D., Zhao, Y., Tawatao, R., et al. (2004) Activation of the Wnt signaling pathway in chronic lymphocytic leukemia. *Proc. Natl. Acad. Sci. USA* **101,** 3118–3123.
89. Tanaka, S., Akiyoshi, T., Mori, M., Wands, J. R., and Sugimachi, K. (1998) A novel frizzled gene identified in human esophageal carcinoma mediates APC/beta-catenin signals. *Proc. Natl. Acad. Sci. USA* **95,** 10,164–10,169.
90. Kirikoshi, H., Sekihara, H., and Katoh, M. (2001) Up-regulation of Frizzled-7 (FZD7) in human gastric cancer. *Int. J. Oncol.* **19,** 111–115.
91. Hoang, B. H., Kubo, T., Healey, J. H., et al. (2004) Expression of LDL receptor-related protein 5 (LRP5) as a novel marker for disease progression in high-grade osteosarcoma. *Int. J. Cancer* **109,** 106–111.

92. Nagahata, T., Shimada, T., Harada, A., et al. (2003) Amplification, up-regulation and over-expression of DVL-1, the human counterpart of the Drosophila disheveled gene, in primary breast cancers. *Cancer Sci.* **94**, 515–518.

93. Okino, K., Nagai, H., Hatta, M., et al. (2003) Up-regulation and overproduction of DVL-1, the human counterpart of the Drosophila dishevelled gene, in cervical squamous cell carcinoma. *Oncol. Rep.* **10**, 1219–1223.

94. Uematsu, K., Kanazawa, S., You, L., et al. (2003) Wnt pathway activation in mesothelioma: evidence of Dishevelled overexpression and transcriptional activity of beta-catenin. *Cancer Res.* **63**, 4547–4551.

95. Saitoh, T. and Katoh, M. (2001) FRAT1 and FRAT2, clustered in human chromosome 10q24.1 region, are up-regulated in gastric cancer. *Int. J. Oncol.* **19**, 311–315.

96. Ugolini, F., Charafe-Jauffret, E., Bardou, V. J., et al. (2001) WNT pathway and mammary carcinogenesis: loss of expression of candidate tumor suppressor gene SFRP1 in most invasive carcinomas except of the medullary type. *Oncogene* **20**, 5810–5817.

97. Stoehr, R., Wissmann, C., Suzuki, H., et al. (2004) Deletions of chromosome 8p and loss of sFRP1 expression are progression markers of papillary bladder cancer. *Lab. Invest.* **84**, 465–478.

98. Suzuki, H., Watkins, D. N., Jair, K. W., et al. (2004) Epigenetic inactivation of SFRP genes allows constitutive WNT signaling in colorectal cancer. *Nat. Genet.* **36**, 417–422.

99. Lee, A. Y., He, B., You, L., et al. (2004) Expression of the secreted frizzled-related protein gene family is downregulated in human mesothelioma. *Oncogene* **23**, 6672–6676.

100. Wissmann, C., Wild, P. J., Kaiser, S., et al. (2003) WIF1, a component of the Wnt pathway, is down-regulated in prostate, breast, lung, and bladder cancer. *J. Pathol.* **201**, 204–212.

101. Mazieres, J., He, B., You, L., et al. (2004) Wnt inhibitory factor-1 is silenced by promoter hypermethylation in human lung cancer. *Cancer Res.* **64**, 4717–4720.

102. He, B., Lee, A. Y., Dadfarmay, S., et al. (2005) Secreted frizzled-related protein 4 is silenced by hypermethylation and induces apoptosis in beta-catenin-deficient human mesothelioma cells. *Cancer Res.* **65**, 743–748.

103. Satoh, S., Daigo, Y., Furukawa, Y., et al. (2000) AXIN1 mutations in hepatocellular carcinomas, and growth suppression in cancer cells by virus-mediated transfer of AXIN1. *Nat. Genet.* **24**, 245–250.

104. Taniguchi, K., Roberts, L. R., Aderca, I. N., et al. (2002) Mutational spectrum of beta-catenin, AXIN1, and AXIN2 in hepatocellular carcinomas and hepatoblastomas. *Oncogene* **21**, 4863–4871.

105. Liu, W., Dong, X., Mai, M., et al. (2000) Mutations in AXIN2 cause colorectal cancer with defective mismatch repair by activating beta-catenin/TCF signalling. *Nat. Genet.* **26**, 146–147.

106. Dahmen, R. P., Koch, A., Denkhaus, D., et al. (2001) Deletions of AXIN1, a component of the WNT/wingless pathway, in sporadic medulloblastomas. *Cancer Res.* **61**, 7039–7043.

107. Yokota, N., Nishizawa, S., Ohta, S., et al. (2002) Role of Wnt pathway in medulloblastoma oncogenesis. *Int. J. Cancer* **101,** 198–201.
108. Groden, J., Thliveris, A., Samowitz, W., et al. (1991) Identification and characterization of the familial adenomatous polyposis coli gene. *Cell* **66,** 589–600.
109. Nishisho, I., Nakamura, Y., Miyoshi, Y., et al. (1991) Mutations of chromosome 5q21 genes in FAP and colorectal cancer patients. *Science* **253,** 665–669.
110. Miyoshi, Y., Nagase, H., Ando, H., et al. (1992) Somatic mutations of the APC gene in colorectal tumors: mutation cluster region in the APC gene. *Hum. Mol. Genet.* **1,** 229–233.
111. Lamlum, H., Ilyas, M., Rowan, A., et al. (1999) The type of somatic mutation at APC in familial adenomatous polyposis is determined by the site of the germline mutation: a new facet to Knudson's 'two-hit' hypothesis. *Nat. Med.* **5,** 1071–1075.
112. Rowan, A. J., Lamlum, H., Ilyas, M., et al. (2000) APC mutations in sporadic colorectal tumors: A mutational "hotspot" and interdependence of the "two hits." *Proc. Natl. Acad. Sci. USA* **97,** 3352–3357.
113. Su, L. K., Vogelstein, B., and Kinzler, K. W. (1993) Association of the APC tumor suppressor protein with catenins. *Science* **262,** 1734–1737.
114. Rubinfeld, B., Albert, I., Porfiri, E., Munemitsu, S., and Polakis, P. (1997) Loss of beta-catenin regulation by the APC tumor suppressor protein correlates with loss of structure due to common somatic mutations of the gene. *Cancer Res.* **57,** 4624–4630.
115. Hart, M. J., de los Santos, R., Albert, I. N., Rubinfeld, B., and Polakis, P. (1998) Downregulation of beta-catenin by human Axin and its association with the APC tumor suppressor, beta-catenin and GSK3 beta. *Curr. Biol.* **8,** 573–581.
116. Rubinfeld, B., Albert, I., Porfiri, E., Fiol, C., Munemitsu, S., and Polakis, P. (1996) Binding of GSK3beta to the APC-beta-catenin complex and regulation of complex assembly. *Science* **272,** 1023–1026.
117. Rubinfeld, B., Souza, B., Albert, I., et al. (1993) Association of the APC gene product with beta-catenin. *Science* **262,** 1731–1734.
118. Munemitsu, S., Albert, I., Souza, B., Rubinfeld, B., and Polakis, P. (1995) Regulation of intracellular beta-catenin levels by the adenomatous polyposis coli (APC) tumor-suppressor protein. *Proc. Natl. Acad. Sci. USA* **92,** 3046–3050.
119. Behrens, J., Jerchow, B. A., Wurtele, M., et al. (1998) Functional interaction of an axin homolog, conductin, with beta-catenin, APC, and GSK3beta. *Science* **280,** 596–599.
120. Peifer, M., Pai, L. M., and Casey, M. (1994) Phosphorylation of the Drosophila adherens junction protein Armadillo: roles for wingless signal and zeste-white 3 kinase. *Dev. Biol.* **166,** 543–556.
121. Kawahara, K., Morishita, T., Nakamura, T., Hamada, F., Toyoshima, K., and Akiyama, T. (2000) Down-regulation of beta-catenin by the colorectal tumor suppressor APC requires association with Axin and beta-catenin. *J. Biol. Chem.* **275,** 8369–8374.
122. Kinzler, K. W. and Vogelstein, B. (1996) Lessons from hereditary colorectal cancer. *Cell* **87,** 159–170.

123. Reifenberger, J., Knobbe, C. B., Wolter, M., et al. (2002) Molecular genetic analysis of malignant melanomas for aberrations of the WNT signaling pathway genes CTNNB1, APC, ICAT and BTRC. *Int. J. Cancer* **100,** 549–556.

124. Koch, A., Waha, A., Tonn, J. C., et al. (2001) Somatic mutations of WNT/wingless signaling pathway components in primitive neuroectodermal tumors. *Int. J. Cancer* **93,** 445–449.

125. Huang, H., Mahler-Araujo, B. M., Sankila, A., et al. (2000) APC mutations in sporadic medulloblastomas. *Am. J. Pathol.* **156,** 433–437.

126. Tejpar, S., Nollet, F., Li, C., et al. (1999) Predominance of beta-catenin mutations and beta-catenin dysregulation in sporadic aggressive fibromatosis (desmoid tumor). *Oncogene* **18,** 6615–6620.

127. Alman, B. A., Li, C., Pajerski, M. E., Diaz-Cano, S., and Wolfe, H. J. (1997) Increased beta-catenin protein and somatic APC mutations in sporadic aggressive fibromatoses (desmoid tumors). *Am. J. Pathol.* **151,** 329–334.

128. Sparks, A. B., Morin, P. J., Vogelstein, B., and Kinzler, K. W. (1998) Mutational analysis of the APC/beta-catenin/Tcf pathway in colorectal cancer. *Cancer Res.* **58,** 1130–1134.

129. Morin, P. J., Sparks, A. B., Korinek, V., et al. (1997) Activation of beta-catenin-Tcf signaling in colon cancer by mutations in beta-catenin or APC. *Science* **275,** 1787–1790.

130. Kitaeva, M. N., Grogan, L., Williams, J. P., et al. (1997) Mutations in beta-catenin are uncommon in colorectal cancer occurring in occasional replication error-positive tumors. *Cancer Res.* **57,** 4478–4481.

131. Iwao, K., Nakamori, S., Kameyama, M., et al. (1998) Activation of the beta-catenin gene by interstitial deletions involving exon 3 in primary colorectal carcinomas without adenomatous polyposis coli mutations. *Cancer Res.* **58,** 1021–1026.

132. Mirabelli-Primdahl, L., Gryfe, R., Kim, H., et al. (1999) Beta-catenin mutations are specific for colorectal carcinomas with microsatellite instability but occur in endometrial carcinomas irrespective of mutator pathway. *Cancer Res.* **59,** 3346–3351.

133. Wong, C. M., Fan, S. T., and Ng, I. O. (2001) beta-Catenin mutation and overexpression in hepatocellular carcinoma: clinicopathologic and prognostic significance. *Cancer* **92,** 136–145.

134. Koch, A., Denkhaus, D., Albrecht, S., Leuschner, I., von Schweinitz, D., and Pietsch, T. (1999) Childhood hepatoblastomas frequently carry a mutated degradation targeting box of the beta-catenin gene. *Cancer Res.* **59,** 269–273.

135. Park, W. S., Oh, R. R., Park, J. Y., et al. (1999) Frequent somatic mutations of the beta-catenin gene in intestinal-type gastric cancer. *Cancer Res.* **59,** 4257–4260.

136. Clements, W. M., Wang, J., Sarnaik, A., et al. (2002) beta-Catenin mutation is a frequent cause of Wnt pathway activation in gastric cancer. *Cancer Res.* **62,** 3503–3506.

137. Fujimori, M., Ikeda, S., Shimizu, Y., Okajima, M., and Asahara, T. (2001) Accumulation of beta-catenin protein and mutations in exon 3 of beta-catenin gene in gastrointestinal carcinoid tumor. *Cancer Res.* **61,** 6656–6659.

138. Abraham, S. C., Nobukawa, B., Giardiello, F. M., Hamilton, S. R., and Wu, T. T. (2001) Sporadic fundic gland polyps: common gastric polyps arising through activating mutations in the beta-catenin gene. *Am. J. Pathol.* **158,** 1005–1010.

139. Abraham, S. C., Wu, T. T., Hruban, R. H., et al. (2002) Genetic and immunohistochemical analysis of pancreatic acinar cell carcinoma: frequent allelic loss on chromosome 11p and alterations in the APC/beta-catenin pathway. *Am. J. Pathol.* **160,** 953–962.

140. Abraham, S. C., Klimstra, D. S., Wilentz, R. E., et al. (2002) Solid-pseudopapillary tumors of the pancreas are genetically distinct from pancreatic ductal adenocarcinomas and almost always harbor beta-catenin mutations. *Am. J. Pathol.* **160,** 1361–1369.

141. Gamallo, C., Palacios, J., Moreno, G., Calvo de Mora, J., Suarez, A., and Armas, A. (1999) beta-catenin expression pattern in stage I and II ovarian carcinomas: relationship with beta-catenin gene mutations, clinicopathological features, and clinical outcome. *Am. J. Pathol.* **155,** 527–536.

142. Wu, R., Zhai, Y., Fearon, E. R., and Cho, K. R. (2001) Diverse mechanisms of beta-catenin deregulation in ovarian endometrioid adenocarcinomas. *Cancer Res.* **61,** 8247–8255.

143. Fukuchi, T., Sakamoto, M., Tsuda, H., Maruyama, K., Nozawa, S., and Hirohashi, S. (1998) Beta-catenin mutation in carcinoma of the uterine endometrium. *Cancer Res.* **58,** 3526–3528.

144. Kobayashi, K., Sagae, S., Nishioka, Y., Tokino, T., and Kudo, R. (1999) Mutations of the beta-catenin gene in endometrial carcinomas. *Jpn. J. Cancer Res.* **90,** 55–59.

145. Garcia-Rostan, G., Camp, R. L., Herrero, A., Carcangiu, M. L., Rimm, D. L., and Tallini, G. (2001) Beta-catenin dysregulation in thyroid neoplasms: down-regulation, aberrant nuclear expression, and CTNNB1 exon 3 mutations are markers for aggressive tumor phenotypes and poor prognosis. *Am. J. Pathol.* **158,** 987–996.

146. Voeller, H. J., Truica, C. I., and Gelmann, E. P. (1998) Beta-catenin mutations in human prostate cancer. *Cancer Res.* **58,** 2520–2523.

147. Chesire, D. R., Ewing, C. M., Sauvageot, J., Bova, G. S., and Isaacs, W. B. (2000) Detection and analysis of beta-catenin mutations in prostate cancer. *Prostate* **45,** 323–334.

148. Zurawel, R. H., Chiappa, S. A., Allen, C., and Raffel, C. (1998) Sporadic medulloblastomas contain oncogenic beta-catenin mutations. *Cancer Res.* **58,** 896–899.

149. Koesters, R., Niggli, F., von Knebel Doeberitz, M., and Stallmach, T. (2003) Nuclear accumulation of beta-catenin protein in Wilms' tumours. *J. Pathol.* **199,** 68–76.

150. Giles, R. H., van Es, J. H., and Clevers, H. (2003) Caught up in a Wnt storm: Wnt signaling in cancer. *Biochim. Biophys. Acta* **1653,** 1–24.

151. Kim, J. S., Crooks, H., Foxworth, A., and Waldman, T. (2002) Proof-of-principle: oncogenic beta-catenin is a valid molecular target for the development of pharmacological inhibitors. *Mol. Cancer Ther.* **1,** 1355–1359.

152. Tsuji, T., Nozaki, I., Miyazaki, M., et al. (2001) Antiproliferative activity of REIC/Dkk-3 and its significant down-regulation in non-small-cell lung carcinomas. *Biochem. Biophys. Res. Commun.* **289,** 257–263.

153. Hoang, B. H., Kubo, T., Healey, J. H., et al. (2004) Dickkopf 3 inhibits invasion and motility of Saos-2 osteosarcoma cells by modulating the Wnt-beta-catenin pathway. *Cancer Res.* **64,** 2734–2739.

154. Shou, J., Ali-Osman, F., Multani, A. S., Pathak, S., Fedi, P., and Srivenugopal, K. S. (2002) Human Dkk-1, a gene encoding a Wnt antagonist, responds to DNA damage and its overexpression sensitizes brain tumor cells to apoptosis following alkylation damage of DNA. *Oncogene* **21,** 878–889.

155. He, B., You, L., Uematsu, K., et al. (2004) A monoclonal antibody against Wnt-1 induces apoptosis in human cancer cells. *Neoplasia* **6,** 7–14.

156. He, B., Reguart, N., You, L., et al. (2005) Blockade of Wnt-1 signaling induces apoptosis in human colorectal cancer cells containing downstream mutations. *Oncogene* **24,** 3054–3058.

157. Suzuki, H., Gabrielson, E., Chen, W., et al. (2002) A genomic screen for genes upregulated by demethylation and histone deacetylase inhibition in human colorectal cancer. *Nat. Genet.* **31,** 141–149.

158. Caldwell, G. M., Jones, C., Gensberg, K., et al. (2004) The Wnt antagonist sFRP1 in colorectal tumorigenesis. *Cancer Res.* **64,** 883–888.

159. Roh, H., Green, D. W., Boswell, C. B., Pippin, J. A., and Drebin, J. A. (2001) Suppression of beta-catenin inhibits the neoplastic growth of APC-mutant colon cancer cells. *Cancer Res.* **61,** 6563–6568.

160. Green, D. W., Roh, H., Pippin, J. A., and Drebin, J. A. (2001) Beta-catenin antisense treatment decreases beta-catenin expression and tumor growth rate in colon carcinoma xenografts. *J. Surg. Res.* **101,** 16–20.

161. Choi, Y. W., Heath, E. I., Heitmiller, R., Forastiere, A. A., and Wu, T. T. (2000) Mutations in beta-catenin and APC genes are uncommon in esophageal and esophagogastric junction adenocarcinomas. *Mod. Pathol.* **13,** 1055–1059.

162. Wijnhoven, B. P., Dinjens, W. N., and Pignatelli, M. (2000) E-cadherin-catenin cell-cell adhesion complex and human cancer. *Br. J. Surg.* **87,** 992–1005.

163. Chung, E. J., Hwang, S. G., Nguyen, P., et al. (2002) Regulation of leukemic cell adhesion, proliferation, and survival by beta-catenin. *Blood* **100,** 982–990.

164. van de Wetering, M., Oving, I., Muncan, V., et al. (2003) Specific inhibition of gene expression using a stably integrated, inducible small-interfering-RNA vector. *EMBO Rep.* **4,** 609–615.

165. Verma, U. N., Surabhi, R. M., Schmaltieg, A., Becerra, C., and Gaynor, R. B. (2003) Small interfering RNAs directed against beta-catenin inhibit the in vitro and in vivo growth of colon cancer cells. *Clin. Cancer Res.* **9,** 1291–1300.

166. Soutschek, J., Akinc, A., Bramlage, B., et al. (2004) Therapeutic silencing of an endogenous gene by systemic administration of modified siRNAs. *Nature* **432,** 173–178.

167. Rossi, J. J. (2004) Medicine: a cholesterol connection in RNAi. *Nature* **432,** 155–156.

168. Morin, P. J., Vogelstein, B., and Kinzler, K. W. (1996) Apoptosis and APC in colorectal tumorigenesis. *Proc. Natl. Acad. Sci. USA* **93,** 7950–7954.

169. Shih, I. M., Yu, J., He, T. C., Vogelstein, B., and Kinzler, K. W. (2000) The beta-catenin binding domain of adenomatous polyposis coli is sufficient for tumor suppression. *Cancer Res.* **60,** 1671–1676.

170. Cong, F., Schweizer, L., Chamorro, M., and Varmus, H. (2003) Requirement for a nuclear function of beta-catenin in Wnt signaling. *Mol. Cell. Biol.* **23,** 8462–8470.
171. Su, Y., Ishikawa, S., Kojima, M., and Liu, B. (2003) Eradication of pathogenic beta-catenin by Skp1/Cullin/F box ubiquitylation machinery. *Proc. Natl. Acad. Sci. USA* **100,** 12,729–12,734.
172. Liu, J., Stevens, J., Matsunami, N., and White, R. L. (2004) Targeted degradation of beta-catenin by chimeric F-box fusion proteins. *Biochem. Biophys. Res. Commun.* **313,** 1023–1029.
173. Papkoff, J. and Aikawa, M. (1998) WNT-1 and HGF regulate GSK3 beta activity and beta-catenin signaling in mammary epithelial cells. *Biochem. Biophys. Res. Commun.* **247,** 851–858.
174. Playford, M. P., Bicknell, D., Bodmer, W. F., and Macaulay, V. M. (2000) Insulin-like growth factor 1 regulates the location, stability, and transcriptional activity of beta-catenin. *Proc. Natl. Acad. Sci. USA* **97,** 12,103–12,108.
175. Piedra, J., Martinez, D., Castano, J., Miravet, S., Dunach, M., and de Herreros, A. G. (2001) Regulation of beta-catenin structure and activity by tyrosine phosphorylation. *J. Biol. Chem.* **276,** 20,436–20,443.
176. Vlahovic, G. and Crawford, J. (2003) Activation of tyrosine kinases in cancer. *Oncologist* **8,** 531–538.
177. Lu, Z., Ghosh, S., Wang, Z., and Hunter, T. (2003) Downregulation of caveolin-1 function by EGF leads to the loss of E-cadherin, increased transcriptional activity of beta-catenin, and enhanced tumor cell invasion. *Cancer Cell.* **4,** 499–515.
178. Lu, Z. and Hunter, T. (2004) Wnt-independent beta-catenin transactivation in tumor development. *Cell Cycle* **3,** 571–573.
179. Zhou, L., An, N., Haydon, R. C., et al. (2003) Tyrosine kinase inhibitor STI-571/Gleevec down-regulates the beta-catenin signaling activity. *Cancer Lett.* **193,** 161–170.
180. Chen, R. H. and McCormick, F. (2001) Selective targeting to the hyperactive beta-catenin/T-cell factor pathway in colon cancer cells. *Cancer Res.* **61,** 4445–4449.
181. Kwong, K. Y., Zou, Y., Day, C. P., and Hung, M. C. (2002) The suppression of colon cancer cell growth in nude mice by targeting beta-catenin/TCF pathway. *Oncogene* **21,** 8340–8346.
182. Ring, C. J. (2002) Cytolytic viruses as potential anti-cancer agents. *J. Gen. Virol.* **83,** 491–502.
183. Brunori, M., Malerba, M., Kashiwazaki, H., and Iggo, R. (2001) Replicating adenoviruses that target tumors with constitutive activation of the wnt signaling pathway. *J. Virol.* **75,** 2857–2865.
184. Fuerer, C. and Iggo, R. (2002) Adenoviruses with Tcf binding sites in multiple early promoters show enhanced selectivity for tumour cells with constitutive activation of the wnt signalling pathway. *Gene Ther.* **9,** 270–281.
185. Toth, K., Djeha, H., Ying, B., et al. (2004) An oncolytic adenovirus vector combining enhanced cell-to-cell spreading, mediated by the ADP cytolytic protein, with selective replication in cancer cells with deregulated wnt signaling. *Cancer Res.* **64,** 3638–3644.

186. Malerba, M., Daeffler, L., Rommelaere, J., and Iggo, R. D. (2003) Replicating parvoviruses that target colon cancer cells. *J. Virol.* **77,** 6683–6691.
187. Lepourcelet, M., Chen, Y. N., France, D. S., et al. (2004) Small-molecule antagonists of the oncogenic Tcf/beta-catenin protein complex. *Cancer Cell* **5,** 91–102.
188. Emami, K. H., Nguyen, C., Ma, H., et al. (2004) A small molecule inhibitor of beta-catenin/CREB-binding protein transcription [corrected]. *Proc. Natl. Acad. Sci. USA* **101,** 12,682–12,687.
189. Dang, C. V. (1999) c-Myc target genes involved in cell growth, apoptosis, and metabolism. *Mol. Cell. Biol.* **19,** 1–11.
190. Whittaker, S. R., Walton, M. I., Garrett, M. D., and Workman, P. (2004) The Cyclin-dependent kinase inhibitor CYC202 (R-roscovitine) inhibits retinoblastoma protein phosphorylation, causes loss of Cyclin D1, and activates the mitogen-activated protein kinase pathway. *Cancer Res.* **64,** 262–272.
191. Hidalgo, M. and Rowinsky, E. K. (2000) The rapamycin-sensitive signal transduction pathway as a target for cancer therapy. *Oncogene* **19,** 6680–6686.
192. Suto, R., Tominaga, K., Mizuguchi, H., et al. (2004) Dominant-negative mutant of c-Jun gene transfer: a novel therapeutic strategy for colorectal cancer. *Gene Ther.* **11,** 187–193.
193. Easwaran, V., Lee, S. H., Inge, L., et al. (2003) beta-Catenin regulates vascular endothelial growth factor expression in colon cancer. *Cancer Res.* **63,** 3145–3153.
194. Gupta, R. A. and DuBois, R. N. (2000) Translational studies on Cox-2 inhibitors in the prevention and treatment of colon cancer. *Ann. NY Acad. Sci.* **910,** 196–204.
195. Araki, Y., Okamura, S., Hussain, S. P., et al. (2003) Regulation of cyclooxygenase-2 expression by the Wnt and ras pathways. *Cancer Res.* **63,** 728–734.
196. Dimberg, J., Hugander, A., Sirsjo, A., and Soderkvist, P. (2001) Enhanced expression of cyclooxygenase-2 and nuclear beta-catenin are related to mutations in the APC gene in human colorectal cancer. *Anticancer Res.* **21,** 911–915.
197. Thun, M. J., Henley, S. J., and Patrono, C. (2002) Nonsteroidal anti-inflammatory drugs as anticancer agents: mechanistic, pharmacologic, and clinical issues. *J. Natl. Cancer Inst.* **94,** 252–266.
198. Koehne, C. H. and Dubois, R. N. (2004) COX-2 inhibition and colorectal cancer. *Semin. Oncol.* **31,** 12–21.
199. Oshima, M. and Taketo, M. M. (2002) COX selectivity and animal models for colon cancer. *Curr. Pharm. Des.* **8,** 1021–1034.
200. Ricchi, P., Palma, A. D., Matola, T. D., et al. (2003) Aspirin protects Caco-2 cells from apoptosis after serum deprivation through the activation of a phosphatidylinositol 3-kinase/AKT/p21Cip/WAF1pathway. *Mol. Pharmacol.* **64,** 407–414.
201. Lew, J. I., Guo, Y., Kim, R. K., Vargish, L., Michelassi, F., and Arenas, R. B. (2002) Reduction of intestinal neoplasia with adenomatous polyposis coli gene replacement and COX-2 inhibition is additive. *J. Gastrointest. Surg.* **6,** 563–568.
202. Kielman, M. F., Rindapaa, M., Gaspar, C., et al. (2002) Apc modulates embryonic stem-cell differentiation by controlling the dosage of beta-catenin signaling. *Nat. Genet.* **32,** 594–605.

203. Reya, T., Duncan, A. W., Ailles, L., et al. (2003) A role for Wnt signalling in self-renewal of haematopoietic stem cells. *Nature* **423,** 409–414.

204. Sato, N., Meijer, L., Skaltsounis, L., Greengard, P., and Brivanlou, A. H. (2004) Maintenance of pluripotency in human and mouse embryonic stem cells through activation of Wnt signaling by a pharmacological GSK-3-specific inhibitor. *Nat. Med.* **10,** 55–63.

205. Korinek, V., Barker, N., Moerer, P., et al. (1998) Depletion of epithelial stem-cell compartments in the small intestine of mice lacking Tcf-4. *Nat. Genet.* **19,** 379–383.

206. van de Wetering, M., Sancho, E., Verweij, C., et al. (2002) The beta-catenin/TCF-4 complex imposes a crypt progenitor phenotype on colorectal cancer cells. *Cell* **111,** 241–250.

207. Chan, T. A., Wang, Z., Dang, L. H., Vogelstein, B., and Kinzler, K. W. (2002) Targeted inactivation of CTNNB1 reveals unexpected effects of beta-catenin mutation. *Proc. Natl. Acad. Sci. USA* **99,** 8265–8270.

208. Kim, S. J., Im, D. S., Kim, S. H., et al. (2002) Beta-catenin regulates expression of cyclooxygenase-2 in articular chondrocytes. *Biochem. Biophys. Res. Commun.* **296,** 221–226.

209. Willert, K., Brown, J. D., Danenberg, E., et al. (2003) Wnt proteins are lipid-modified and can act as stem cell growth factors. *Nature* **423,** 448–452.

4

NG2/HMP Proteoglycan as a Cancer Therapeutic Target

Martha Chekenya and Heike Immervoll

Summary

Neuroepithelial cells of the central nervous system constitute neuroglia (astrocytes, oligodendrocytes, and microglia), ependyma, and neurons, which make up the stromal cells of the brain. The stromal tissue organization of the brain is tightly regulated, but occasionally the signals that define the normal contexts become disrupted and result in cancer. Malignant progression is then maintained by cross-talks between the tumor and its stroma, where the activated stroma nurtures the proliferative and invasive neoplastic cells, by providing neovasculature, extracelluar matrix components, and stimulatory growth factors. The NG2/HMP plays a major role in tumor–stroma activation through alterations in cellular adhesion, migration, proliferation, and vascular morphogenesis. Therapeutic strategies specifically targeting NG2/HMP may be useful in normalizing the tumor stroma and may reduce the toxic side effects when used in combination with conventional treatments.

Key Words: NG2; siRNA; immunotherapy; glioma; melanoma.

1. Introduction

1.1. The Brain Stroma as the Glioma Backdrop

The human brain is made up of numerous cell types that interact physically through cell–cell, and cell–extracellular matrix (ECM) contacts, and biochemically via soluble and insoluble signaling molecules. Neuroepithelial cells of the central nervous system (CNS) constitute neuroglia (astrocytes, oligodendrocytes, and microglia) and neurons, which are derived from the neuroectoderm. These cells produce the ECM, an important feature of the normal stroma, which provides structural scaffolding as well as contextual information to the cells. However, with the exception of the vascular basement membrane and the *glia limitans externa*, the adult CNS is poorly endowed with the classical ECM

From: *Methods in Molecular Biology, vol. 361, Target Discovery and Validation Reviews and Protocols*
Volume 2, Emerging Molecular Targets and Treatment Options
Edited by: M. Sioud © Humana Press Inc., Totowa, NJ

components, such as collagens, laminin, tenascin, vitronectin, elastin, and fibronectin *(1)*. These glycoproteins contain an Arg-Gly-Asp (RGD)-peptide adhesion domain that is recognized by members of the integrin family of *(2,3)* adhesion receptors. The brain ECM is composed of several proteoglycans, including chondroitin sulphate proteoglycans (CSPG) *(1)*. These macromolecules, with core proteins covalently linked to glycosaminoglycan chains are believed to mediate multiple cellular functions, such as the regulation of ECM structural organization, proliferation, trophic-factor binding, cellular adhesion, and motility *(4,5)*. The vascular and perivascular cells of the endothelium interact with the basement membrane, a specialized form of ECM that provides structural support to cells. The vascular system provides nutrients, oxygen, and circulating immune cells that combat pathogens and remove apoptotic cell debris. The normal brain is considered an "immune-privileged site" because of the lack of resident immune-competent cells (T cells and B cells). This stromal tissue organization of the brain is tightly regulated, but occasionally the signals that define the normal contexts become disrupted in cancer. Malignant progression is thus maintained by cross-talks between the tumor and its stroma, where the activated stroma nurtures the proliferative and invasive neoplastic cells, by providing neovasculature, ECM components, and stimulatory growth factors **(Fig. 1)**.

1.2. NG2 at the Tumor–Stroma Interface

NG2 is a 300-kDa membrane spanning CSPG that was originally identified as a surface epitope on a subset of tumor cell lines derived from rat embryos after ethylnitrosourea administration *(6)*. The cell lines were characterized by the presence of Na^+ and K^+ ion channels, but an inability to generate full-fledged action potentials, features characteristic of neural precursor cells. NG2 positive neural precursors can differentiate into either neuroglia or neurons, hence the designation nerve/glial antigen 2 (NG2) *(6)*. Structurally, NG2 is composed of an extensive extracellular domain, which is further segregated into three functionally distinct subunits (designated domains 1–3) **(Fig. 2)**. Domain 1 comprises two globular "dumb-bell" structures stabilized by intramolecular disulphide bonds *(2,3)*. Domain 2 contains one chondroitin sulfate chain at serine –999 *(7)*, and an α-helical site for collagen V and VI binding *(2,3)*. Domain 3 is the globular juxtamembrane site for proteolysis of NG2 that leads to its cleavage and release from the cell surface *(8)*. Although four internal repeats resembling the Ca^{2+}-binding motifs of cadherins are scattered throughout the ectodomain, no homology is found between NG2 and other proteoglycans, e.g., syndecans, aggrecans, glypicans, and so on *(9,10)*. NG2/HMP has single transmembrane domain, and a short cytoplasmic tail. The extreme C terminus of the cytoplasmic tail contains a QYWV motif responsible for PDZ-binding *(11)* and

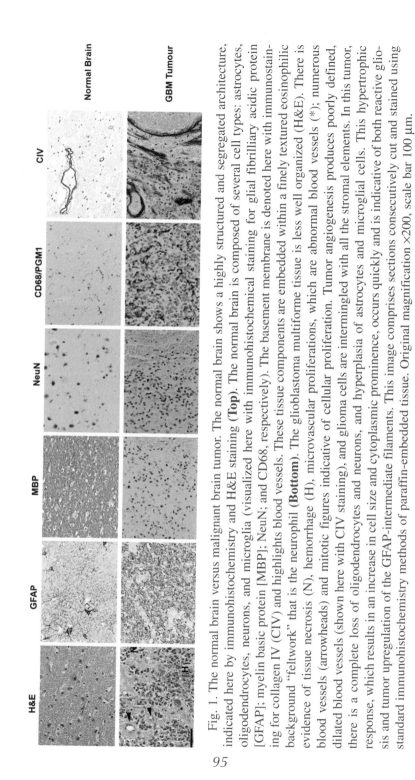

Fig. 1. The normal brain versus malignant brain tumor. The normal brain shows a highly structured and segregated architecture, indicated here by immunohistochemistry and H&E staining (**Top**). The normal brain is composed of several cell types: astrocytes, oligodendrocytes, neurons, and microglia (visualized here with immunohistochemical staining for glial fibrillary acidic protein [GFAP]; myelin basic protein [MBP]; NeuN; and CD68, respectively). The basement membrane is denoted here with immunostaining for collagen IV (CIV) and highlights blood vessels. These tissue components are embedded within a finely textured eosinophilic background "feltwork" that is the neuropil (**Bottom**). The glioblastoma multiforme tissue is less well organized (H&E). There is evidence of tissue necrosis (N), microvascular proliferations, which are abnormal blood vessels (*); numerous blood vessels (arrowheads) and mitotic figures indicative of cellular proliferation. Tumor angiogenesis produces poorly defined, dilated blood vessels (shown here with CIV staining), and glioma cells are intermingled with all the stromal elements. In this tumor, there is a complete loss of oligodendrocytes and neurons, and hyperplasia of astrocytes and microglial cells. This hypertrophic response, which results in an increase in cell size and cytoplasmic prominence, occurs quickly and is indicative of both reactive gliosis and tumor upregulation of the GFAP-intermediate filaments. This image comprises sections consecutively cut and stained using standard immunohistochemistry methods of paraffin-embedded tissue. Original magnification ×200, scale bar 100 µm.

95

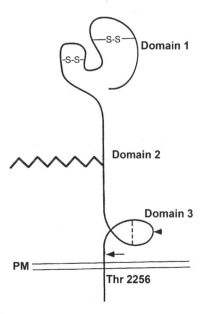

Fig. 2. The schematic structure of NG2. Domain 1 comprises the ligand binding globular head that is stabilized by disulphide bonds. Domain 2 contains type VI collagen binding sites and a single chondroitin sulfate chain (jagged line). Domain 3 is the site for proteolytic cleavage (arrowheads). The cytoplasmic tail contains PDZ-binding motifs and proline-rich regions and several sites for phosphorylation, including threonine 2256, which has been shown to be phosphorylated by PKCα, *(156)*.

may be the site for NG2 interaction with MUPP1, a multi-PDZ domain-containing cytoplasmic scaffolding protein *(12)*. The NG2 cytoplasmic domain also contains phospho-threonine residues, four of which are candidates for phoshorylation *(13)*. Recently, the threonine residue 2256 has been identified as a primary phosphorylation site for PKCα. Finally, although a classical PXXP SH3-binding motif is lacking *(14)*, the C terminal half of the cytoplasmic tail is rich in prolines, the significance of which remains to be elucidated *(6)*.

NG2 shares high-sequence homology with the high-molecular-weight melanoma-associated antigen (HMW-MAA) or human melanoma proteoglycan (HMP) *(15–18)*, where 18 residues of the NG2 amino-terminus are identical to the HMP, identifying it as the human homolog, and shall hereon be denoted NG2/HMP. In contrast, HMP contains three nucleotides in the juxtamembrane domain that are absent from the NG2 sequence *(13)*. The mouse NG2 homolog, designated AN2, has also been identified *(19,20)* indicating that it is evolution-ary conserved. NG2/HMP is a well-established marker for glial progenitor cells in the CNS *(21–26)*. Although differentiation of NG2/HMP-positive progeni-tors into oligodendrocytes in vivo has been demonstrated, derivation of astrocytes

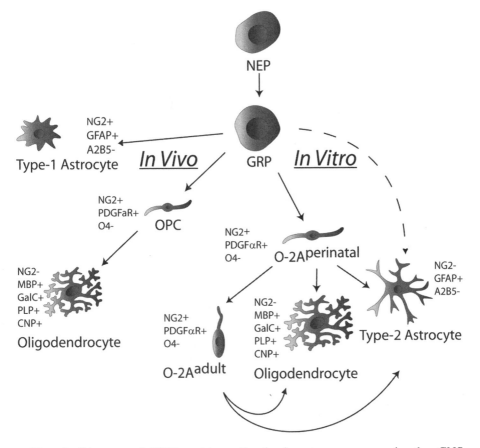

Fig. 3. Lineage of NG2-positive oligodendrocyte precursors in the CNS. Neuroepithelial stem cells (NEP) become lineage restricted to give glial-restricted precursors (GRP), which are tri-potent, giving rise to oligodendrocytes and two astrocytes: type 1 and type 2 astrocytes (O-2A cells). This lineage has only been demonstrated in vitro. The generation of oligodendrocytes in vivo has been demonstrated from oligodendrocyte precursors (OPC), which are lineage restricted from GRP. Type 1 astrocytes have also been demonstrated in vivo to be derived from GRP cells.

from the same lineage has been elusive *(21–23,25,27–30)* (**Fig. 3**). NG2/HMP expression by oligodendrocyte progenitor cells is preceded by expression of the PDGFα receptor, which is critical for progenitor development and provides another stringency marker for this population *(31–33)*. Oligodendrocyte progenitors expressing both NG2/HMP and PDGFα receptor in the rodent CNS are present as early as embryonic day 16–17 *(24)* in the ventral spinal cord. Their distribution expands with time to the first postnatal week, when they are located throughout both the gray and white matter in the CNS. Oligodendrocyte progenitor cells have a characteristic unipolar or bipolar morphology in vitro and small cell bodies (10- to 15-µm in diameter) that give rise to multiple stellate branches in vivo *(34,35)*. The processes have a radial orientation in the gray matter, but are more longitudinal in the white matter *(35)*.

2. The Role of NG2/HMP in Tumor–Stroma Activation

2.1. Reactive Response to Injury

NG2/HMP positive cells undergo morphological changes in response to a variety of injuries *(36–41)*, characterized by (1) upregulation of NG2/HMP expression *(42)*, (2) an increased density and change in morphology to become shorter and thicker *(34,35,39,40)*, and (3) appearance of fine filopodia on their cell bodies and processes *(39)*. The onset is rapid (within hours of injury) and may persist for several weeks, indicating that these dynamic cells *(39,40)* can be involved in stromal activation.

2.1.1. Cell Adhesion and Migration

Cell adhesion and migration on ECM components are promoted by a number of membrane receptors, of which, integrins represent a major class *(43)*. Several lines of evidence indicate that NG2/HMP is also capable of modulating both cell–ECM and cell–cell adhesion. For example, NG2/HMP is localized on microspikes in melanoma cells where it participates in cellular adhesion *(44)*. Furthermore, the human 9.2.27 monoclonal antibody (mAb), which recognizes the NG2/HMP human homolog, HMW-MAA, inhibits melanoma cell migration on ECM proteins *(45)*. The extracellular domain of NG2 can be proteolytically cleaved from the cell surface both in vitro and in vivo *(8,42)* and is then deposited at the interface between the substrata and the migrating tumor *(46)*, and endothelial cells *(47)*. Although brain CSPGs can promote transient adhesion of neuronal cells, they generally inhibit stable cell adhesion and neurite outgrowth *(48)*. NG2/HMP negatively modulates adhesion of melanoma cells via cluster of differentiation 44 (CD44), hyaluronic acid (HA), fibronectin, and $\alpha 4\beta 1$ integrin *(49)*. CD44 is ubiquitously expressed in several tumors *(50)*, including gliomas *(51)*, where it mediates tumor cell adhesion and migration *(52,53)*.

NG2/HMP may indirectly regulate cell–ECM interactions by serving as a co-receptor for $\alpha 4\beta 1$ integrin, which it communicates with by outside–in and inside–out signaling mechanisms *(54,55)* during adhesion and migration *(55)*. NG2/HMP also interacts with the $\beta 1$ integrin-subunit, where it modulates adhesion to type II and VI collagen *(54,56)*. NG2/HMP is best characterized as a cell surface receptor for type VI collagen *(2,57–59)*, which is a major component of the basement membrane in some types of vasculature *(60,61)*. The normal brain stroma is composed of very little classical ECM, but glioma cells and activated stromal astrocytes can synthesize tenascin, HA, and collagen *de novo* during invasion and migration *(62,63)*. The fact that NG2/HMP interacts with these ECM components *(2,3,58,59)*, and it is highly expressed on some gliomas, suggests that NG2/HMP may modulate neoplastic cell adhesion to various ECM components. Indeed, we previously reported that NG2/HMP expressing glioma cells failed to migrate on laminin, vitronectin, and fibronectin substrates, and only migrated efficiently on collagen IV-coated substrates in vitro *(64)*. Others have shown that NG2/HMP-expressing glioma cells migrate most efficiently on type VI collagen *(3)*, and that this can be inhibited by NG2/HMP blocking antibodies or by mutations in NG2/HMP's collagen-binding domain. We have also compared the NG2/HMP spatial distribution in neoplastic tissue that originated from the tumor main mass with that obtained from the interface between the tumor and the infiltrated brain. The results indicated that the NG2/HMP expression was confined to the tumor main mass but was markedly reduced in the infiltrative edge *(65)*. It has been reported that NG2/HMP poses a barrier to cell migration and axonal growth on laminin substrates *(66–70)* through Gi protein receptor signaling *(70)*. Because laminin is abundantly deposited in the border zones between the tumor tissue and the brain parenchyma in vivo *(71,72)*, we speculated whether NG2/HMP expressing cells may be restricted to the tumor main mass owing to the inhibition of cell adhesion and migration on certain ECM components *(65)*.

NG2/HMP-positive oligodendrocyte progenitor cells produced in the germinative neuroepithelium during embryogenesis migrate to the optic nerve and chiasma *(73)* by guidance of the repulsive sematophorins, Netrin1 and Sema3a, which are secreted from the optic chiasma *(74)*. However, the mechanisms by which NG2/HMP induces tumor cell motility involve modification of the cytoskeletal dynamics *(75)*, because NG2/HMP localizes to radial actin spikes associated with filopodia in migrating cells. This indicates a role for NG2/HMP in cell migration through Rho-dependent mechanisms *(7,75,76)*.

2.1.2. Cell Proliferation and Tumor Growth

Fibroblast growth factor (FGF)-2 and PDGF AA are critical mitogens and chemoattractants, which alter the differentiation of cultured oligodendrocyte progenitor cells *(77,78)*, and are upregulated during pathological conditions *(79)*. Both NG2/HMP and PDGF receptors are coexpressed on oligodendrocyte progenitor cells *(24)*, and on the surface of vascular pericytes and smooth muscle cells *(23,24,80,81)*. NG2/HMP binds and activates both PDGF-AA and FGF-2, modulating their pleiotropic effects on the signaling receptors. Moreover, antibodies against NG2/HMP block the mitogenic effects of PDGF-AA on both oligodendrocyte progenitor and aortic smooth muscle cells. The PDGFα receptor is unresponsive to PDGF-AA in aortic smooth muscle cells derived from NG2/HMP knockout mice *(23,63,80,81)*, indicating that NG2/HMP is important for both the proliferative and migratory responses to the PDGF-AA/PDGFα receptor pathway.

Using Ki67 (MIB-1) immunolabeling, which recognizes proliferation associated nuclear proteins expressed during G1 to M phases of the cell cycle, we showed that NG2/HMP expressing glioblastoma cells were more proliferative than their NG2/HMP negative counterparts *(65,82)*, and similar observations have been reported for melanoma cells, where NG2/HMP expression increased their proliferation rates in vitro, tumorigenicity, and their metastatic potential in vivo *(49)*. Using magnetic resonance imaging (MRI) we showed that NG2/HMP expressing xenografts grew faster and exhibited greater spread within the brain compared to NG2/HMP negative control tumors *(82,83)*. NG2/HMP's binding and activation of the PDGF-AA/PDGFαR pathway is one putative mechanism for enhancing the growth of neoplastic cells. The *PDGFαR* gene on chromosome 4q11-p12 is amplified in some glioblastomas *(84)* and is over expressed in most astrocytomas *(85,86)* and this may lead to both autocrine and paracrine growth factor stimulation. In addition, NG2/HMP–collagen interactions may also potentiate mitogen-driven proliferative and migratory responses, because the collagen types are capable of binding PDGF. These findings might indicate that NG2/HMP expressing cancer cells generate a supportive microenvironment by producing stroma-modulating growth factors. These disrupt normal homeostasis and act in paracrine manner to induce stromal reactions such as angiogenesis *(87)*, inflammatory responses, as well as activating other surrounding stromal cells, such as microglia and macrophages, resulting in secretion of additional growth factors and proteases.

2.1.3. Vascular Morphogenesis and Tumor Angiogenesis

NG2/HMP is widely expressed during both normal and pathological angiogenesis *(65,82,83,88,89)* by the mural cell component of the neovasculature. NG2/HMP is expressed by pericytes on immature brain capillaries as early as embryonic day 10–12 (E10–12) in the rat and continues throughout the period of rapid expansion of the brain vasculature *(23,80,88,90)*. Microvascular pericytes are characterized by their coexpression of NG2/HMP and PDGF β-receptor, which is just as important to their development *(91,92)* as the PDGFα receptor is to oligodendrocyte progenitors. However, as the brain matures and CNS capillaries become quiescent, NG2/HMP expression decreases *(90)*. Outside the CNS, the earliest and most prominent expression of NG2/HMP is in the heart, on cardiomyocytes *(80,89)* and smooth-muscle cells in the dorsal aorta from E10 to 14 *(89)*. NG2/HMP expression is primarily confined to perivascular cells along arterioles and capillaries, and continuous expression is not observed along venules and never beyond the immediate postcapillary vessels *(93)*. During tumor angiogenesis and wound healing, NG2/HMP expressing mural cells respond to environmental cues by migrating to sites where vessel growth and repair are occurring *(94–96)*. The close apposition of pericytes to endothelial cells also indicates a seminal role during angiogenesis *(97)*. NG2/HMP is proteolytically cleaved into a soluble form *(8,98)*, which is highly angiogenic, stimulating endothelial and pericytic tube formation both in vitro and in vivo *(47)*.

Furthermore, NG2/HMP binds specifically and saturably to plasminogen, which can be proteolytically cleaved to release the endogenous angiogenesis inhibitors, angiostatin consisting of kringle domains (K1–4) and miniplasminogen (K5) *(99)*. In agreement with these findings, we have shown that overexpression of NG2/HMP in human glioblastoma cells directly increased tumor angiogenesis *(83)*, by binding and sequestration of angiostatin. Furthermore, we have recently demonstrated that the tumor vasculature in NG2/HMP-positive tumors is structurally and functionally defected compared to that in NG2/HMP-negative tumors *(82)*. As a cell surface component of mural cells, NG2/HMP is adequately positioned to sequester angiostatin, which otherwise would be available to inhibit proliferation and migration of endothelial cells *(83,99)*.

3. Normalizing the Stroma Through Targeting NG2/HMP

3.1. mAb-Directed Therapy

Antibody-based immunotherapy has been greatly investigated as a therapeutic strategy against NG2/HMP-expressing melanomas. This method utilizes a molecular vehicle, mAb, to selectively deliver radionuclides or toxins to tumor cells *(100)*. Several studies have used various mAbs that recognize the NG2/HMP because the majority of melanomas extensively express it. There is limited intra- and intertumor heterogeneity, where it has been detected on >90% of melanoma cells *(49,101,102)*. Furthermore, because it is expressed on both tumor cells and the associated vasculature, it offers several advantages over therapies that are strictly tumor-directed. Therapies that target only tumor cells, are limited by both the heterogeneous expression of the NG2/HMP within the tumor, as well as by the high rate of tumor cell mutation *(103,104)*. In contrast, the host activated-stromal vascular cells are relatively homogenous and lack the problems associated with drug resistance *(103,105–107)*. Other than the tumor-associated vascular cells, and oligodendrocyte precursors in the brain, the NG2/HMP has a restricted distribution in normal tissues *(108,109)*.

The 9.2.27 mAb has been most frequently chosen as the drug-targeting device because it effectively targets and has a high affinity for melanoma cells *(108–110)*. The antibody does not cause antigen modulation in vivo and expression of the NG2/HMP antigen it recognizes is not cell cycle dependent *(111)*. Although it is not clear at this point whether NG2/HMP antigen is internalised, other mechanisms can still mediate the clinical benefits of mA3-directed therapy. These mechanisms involve both immunological and nonimmunological effector functions **(Fig. 4)**.

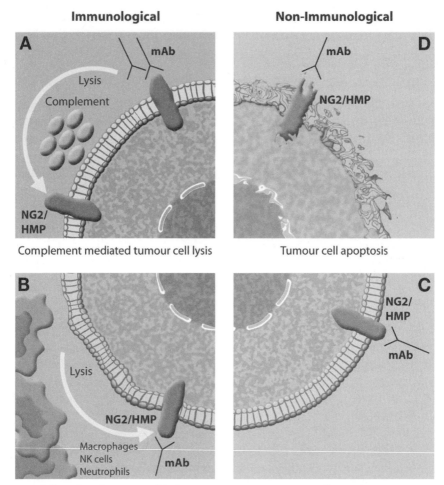

Fig. 4. Mechanisms underlying antibody-based immunotherapy. Immunological mechanisms include **(A)** complement dependent, where membrane-bound tumor-associated antigens (e.g., NG2/HMP) bound to mAb are recognized and destroyed by complement membrane attack complexes. Alternatively, **(B)** lysis of tumor cells is initiated by macrophages bearing Fcγ III receptors, natural killer cells, and neutrophils. Nonimmunological mechanisms include **(C)**, tumor cell growth arrest, and **(D)**, tumor cell apoptosis induced by mAb-specific antibody binding to the antigens that trigger signal transduction events in the tumor cells. Models are proposed from the literature *(157–159)*.

The methods of preperation for mAbs and antibody fragments include hybridoma technology *(112)*, antibody phage display *(113)*, ribosome display *(114)*, and iterative colony filter screening *(115)*. The dissociation constants for mAbs are in micromolar to picomolar range but might require further affinity maturation procedures *(116)*. Antibody formats include single-chain variable fragments, Fab fragments, miniantibodies, or immunoglobulins, which all show different pharmacokinetics and tumor-targeting properties *(117)*.

Although this treatment strategy is highly attractive, the therapeutic efficacy of antibody-directed immunotherapy has been limited by several shortcomings *(118)* including (1) the loss or downregulation of antigenic epitopes on tumor cells; (2) lack of tumor-specific antigens; (3) antibody toxicity; (4) failure of the large antibody complexes to cross the blood brain barrier *(119)*; (5) high interstitial pressure leading to poor diffusion of antibodies into all parts of the tumor *(120)*; (6) dehalogenation or removal of radioactive label from mAb; (7) enzymatic removal of mAb from tumors; and (8) lack of mAb humanization. Nonetheless, several preclinical experimental studies and clinical trials targeting the tumor- and vessel-associated NG2/HMP have been developed (*see* **Table 1**).

3.2. Targeting Peptides

In order to circumvent the problems associated with antibody-directed immunotherapeutic strategies, an alternative approach can involve using small peptides. Phage display of random peptide libraries has previously enabled isolation of peptides that successfully bind to integrin receptors *(121–124)*, growth factor receptors *(125)*, and other tumor-associated proteins *(126,127)*. NG2/HMP-binding decapeptides that home directly to the angiogenic neovasculature of melanoma xenografts in mice have been developed *(128)*. The localization and accessibility of NG2/HMP on pericytes suggested a potential use of these vessel homing sequences for targeted delivery of therapeutic agents to tumors. Several reports have suggested that pericytes play an important role in controlling endothelial cell proliferation and vessel stabilization during angiogenesis *(91,129–131)*. Thus, anticancer strategies targeting pericytes in the angiogenic vasculature may complement approaches targeting endothelial cells. Because NG2/HMP is also expressed on tumor cells *(132–134)*, the peptides could deliver therapeutic agents both to the tumor cells and their vasculature. The small peptides may prove superior to antibodies in terms of penetration into tumors.

Methods of preparation for peptides include phage display of random peptide libraries *(135,136)*, including in vivo panning *(137)* and solid phase parallel synthesis *(138)*. Typical dissociation constants are in micromolar range, although avidity can be improved by multimerisation *(139)*. The in vivo stability may differ greatly among peptides.

3.3. siRNA Targeted Therapy

RNA interference (RNAi) is a process whereby small, noncoding double stranded RNAs posttranscriptionally silence specific genes (*see* Chapters 9, 11,

Table 1
Monoclonal Antibody-Mediated Immunotherapeutic Strategies
For Targeting NG2/HMP in Tumor Stroma

Monoclonal antibody	IgG class	Conjugate	Tumor type	Reference
9.2.27 mAb	γ2a	^{125}I	Human melanoma xenografts in athymic mice	*(148)*
9.2.27 mAb	γ2a	Diphtheria toxin A chain	Human melanoma xenografts in athymic mice	*(17)*
9.2.27 mAb	γ2a	Doxorubicin via cis-acotinic anhydride	Human melanoma xenografts in athymic mice	*(149,150)*
Me1–14 F(ab')$_2$	IgG2a	^{131}I-labeled	D54 MG human glioblastoma xenografts in athymic mice	*(151,152)*
Me1–14	IgG2a	^{131}I-labeled	Human glioblastoma patients	*(153)*
Me1–14 F(ab')$_2$	IgG2a	^{131}I-labeled	Phase I trial of a patient with neoplastic meningitis secondary to melanoma	*(154)*
Me1–14 F(ab')$_2$	IgG2a	(^{211}At)	Human glioblastoma and melanoma cells in vitro	*(155)*

and 12). RNAi is a highly conserved mechanism *(140)* that was first recognized as an antiviral immune response in plants to protect against random transposable elements. Double stranded RNAs are processed into short interfering RNAs (siRNA), about 22 nucleotides in length, by the RNA enzyme Dicer. These siRNAs are then incorporated into RNA-induced silencing complexes (RISC), which identify and silence complementary messenger RNAs (**Fig. 4**).

RNAi has produced a paradigm shift in the process of drug discovery. Its strong appeal in therapeutics is the potency and specificity with which gene expression can be silenced. However, two key challenges to the use of RNAi in therapeutics are avoiding off-target effects and ensuring efficient delivery. The potential risk for side effects stems from the inherent use of host cellular machinery for directing the sequence specific silencing. The use of RNAi to target specific cellular transcripts essentially hijacks the endogenous RNAi pathway, which can potentially be saturated. The issue of delivery has been the greatest hindrance to the successful treatment of gliomas. Because siRNAs are double-stranded molecules, delivery and cellular uptake is more of a challenge than for single stranded antisense agents, which are taken up by binding to serum proteins *(141)*. It is feasible to modify the backbone of synthetic siRNAs in order to enable resistance to serum nucleases and increase their half-life in vivo *(142)*. Nevertheless achieving intracellular delivery at therapeutically effective concentrations is a still major challenge. The alternative approach is viral-vector mediated delivery, but there are several safety concerns and systemic delivery of viral vectors is still a major hurdle.

The presence of a blood brain barrier precludes passage of macromolecules with molecular weights more than 100,000 Da, including mAbs, liposomes, and gene therapy vectors, which are generally excluded from more than 95% of the tumor tissue *(143,144)*. Once present in the tumor microvasculature the siRNA must be transported across the capillary walls, and penetrate the ECM to reach the tumor cells. Transport through the ECM involves both diffusion and convection owing to the absence of osmotic or pressure gradients in solid tumors. These are relatively slow processes, because the time required to move some distance by diffusion is proportional to the square of that distance *(145)*. During these processes the siRNA might further miss its target because of nonspecific binding to proteins or other tissue components. Moreover, because the siRNA must travel through the vasculature to reach its target, a functional and well distributed vascular network facilitating the tumor blood flow is necessary for efficient drug delivery *(146,147)*. From a clinical point of view this represents a therapeutic quagmire, because tumor blood flow also improves tumor growth. The tumor interstitium is characterized by elevated levels of interstitial fluid pressure, which reduces fluid filtration and consequently impedes the influx of therapeutic agents *(120)*. One strategy used to circumvent these barriers is to administer large enough doses of the drug to achieve therapeutic concentrations to the brain. However, this often results in significant systemic toxicity. Furthermore, because all perivascular cells along arterioles express NG2, therapeutic strategies targeting it in brain tumors must involve local delivery. Nevertheless some of the delivery issues previously discussed need to be taken into account to ensure an adequate biodistribution within the tumor bed. However, should the delivery be optimized and the highest intracellular concentration of the siRNA is achieved, gene silencing may be limited by their transient effects and restricted by the rate of cell division. Mammalian cells do not have mechanisms to amplify and propagate RNAi-like *C. elegans* and plants.

We have recently uncovered a novel role of NG2/HMP in glioma cell death resistance and confirmed it using RNAi. We demonstrated that the expression of NG2/HMP results in significant resistance to death induced by tumor necrosis factor (TNF)-α, daunorubicin, or etoposide. NG2/HMP expression in various glioma cells was transiently inhibited by siRNAs, which resulted in their increased sensitivity to apoptotic stimuli such as TNF-α. Furthermore, stable downregulation of NG2/HMP in glioblastoma tumors in vivo led to marked reduction of tumor growth rates and volumes, identifying it as an antitumor target. The growth of these tumors in vivo was considerably retarded after TNF-α treatment indicating that the glioma sensitivity to cell death mediators can be restored by siRNA gene silencing (unpublished data).

4. Conclusion and Future Directions

Agents that target the tumor microenvironment represent an important strategy in cancer therapy. Just as the normal brain exists in dynamic equilibrium to maintain normal tissue function, likewise, the tumor adopts many mechanisms to maintain its functional disorder and to evade anticancer therapies. By expressing NG2, the tumor can interact with growth factors to modulate proliferation and angiogenesis; can interact with integrin receptors and ECM components to mediate cellular motility, as well as stimulate signal transduction pathways to avoid apoptosis. Several questions remain to be answered. Can the therapeutic effects of anti-NG2/HMP mAb-mediated immunotherapy be enhanced to overcome the hurdles to efficient delivery and penetrance? Can the administration of small molecule inhibitors of the NG2/HMP or the different signal transduction pathways mediated by the NG2/HMP be targeted? With the use of RNAi in whole animals increasing, its growing implementation in experimental therapy is anticipated. Despite considerable hurdles to overcome, it seems likely that RNAi might find a place alongside conventional approaches in brain tumor treatment, although it is unclear how long it will be before the first RNAi-based drug.

Acknowledgments

The authors are grateful to Dr. Per Øyvind Enger for technical assistance.

References

1. Rutka, J. T., Apodaca, G., Stern, R., and Rosenblum, M. (1988) The extracellular matrix of the central and peripheral nervous systems: structure and function. *J. Neurosurg.* **69,** 155–170.
2. Tillet, E., Ruggiero, F., Nishiyama, A., and Stallcup, W. B. (1997) The membrane-spanning proteoglycan NG2 binds to collagens V and VI through the central nonglobular domain of its core protein. *J. Biol. Chem.* **272,** 10,769–10,776.
3. Burg, M. A., Nishiyama, A., and Stallcup, W. B. (1997) A central segment of the NG2 proteoglycan is critical for the ability of glioma cells to bind and migrate toward type VI collagen. *Exp. Cell Res.,* **235,** 254–264.

4. Schlessinger, J., Lax, I., and Lemmon, M. (1995) Regulation of growth factor activation by proteoglycans: what is the role of the low affinity receptors? *Cell,* **83,** 357–360.
5. David, G. (1993) Integral membrane heparan sulfate proteoglycans. *FASEB J.* **7,** 1023–1030.
6. Stallcup, W. B. (2002) The NG2 proteoglycan: past insights and future prospects. *J. Neurocytol.* **31,** 423–435.
7. Stallcup, W. B., and Dahlin-Huppe, K. (2001) Chondroitin sulfate and cytoplasmic domain-dependent membrane targeting of the NG2 proteoglycan promotes retraction fiber formation and cell polarization. *J. Cell Sci.* **114,** 2315–2325.
8. Nishiyama, A., Lin, X. H., and Stallcup, W. B. (1995) Generation of truncated forms of the NG2 proteoglycan by cell surface proteolysis. *Mol. Biol. Cell* **6,** 1819–1832.
9. Yamaguchi, Y. (2000) *Chondroitin sulfate proteoglycans in the nervous system.* Marcel Dekker, Inc., New York.
10. Yamaguchi, Y. (2001) Heparin sulfate proteoglycans in the nervous system: Their diverse roles in neurogenesis,axon guidance, and synaptogenesis. *Sem. Cell Dev. Biol.* **12,** 96–106.
11. Songyang, Z., Fanning, A. S., Fu, C., et al. (1997) Recognition of unique carboxyl-terminal motifs by distinct PDZ domains. *Science* **275,** 73–77.
12. Barritt, D. S., Pearn, M. T., Zisch, A. H., et al. (2000) The multi-PDZ domain protein MUPP1 is a cytoplasmic ligand for the membrane-spanning proteoglycan NG2. *J. Cell Biochem.* **79,** 213–224.
13. Nishiyama, A., Dahlin, K. J., Prince, J. T., Johnstone, S. R., and Stallcup, W. B. (1991) The primary structure of NG2, a novel membrane-spanning proteoglycan. *J. Cell Biol.* **114,** 359–371.
14. Yu, H., Chen, J. K., Feng, S., Dalgarno, D. C., Brauer, A. W., and Schreiber, S. L. (1994) Structural basis for the binding of proline-rich peptides to SH3 domains. *Cell* **76,** 933–945.
15. Stallcup, W. B., Beasley, L. and Levine, J. (1983) Cell-surface molecules that characterize different stages in the development of cerebellar interneurons. *Cold Spring Harb Symp. Quant. Biol.* **48 Pt 2,** 761–774.
16. Houghton, A. N., Eisinger, M., Albino, A. P., Cairncross, J. G., and Old, L. J. (1982) Surface antigens of melanocytes and melanomas. Markers of melanocyte differentiation and melanoma subsets. *J. Exp. Med.,* **156,** 1755–1766.
17. Bumol, T. F., Walker, L. E., and Reisfeld, R. A. (1984) Biosynthetic studies of proteoglycans in human melanoma cells with a monoclonal antibody to a core glycoprotein of chondroitin sulfate proteoglycans. *J. Biol. Chem.,* **259,** 12,733–12,741.
18. Bumol, T. F. and Reisfeld, R. A. (1982) Unique glycoprotein-proteoglycan complex defined by monoclonal antibody on human melanoma cells. *Proc. Natl. Acad. Sci. USA* **79,** 1245–1249.
19. Schneider, S., Bosse, F., D'Urso, D., et al. (2001) The AN2 protein is a novel marker for the Schwann cell lineage expressed by immature and nonmyelinating Schwann cells. *J. Neurosci.,* **21,** 920–933.

20. Niehaus, A., Stegmuller, J., Diers-Fenger, M., and Trotter, J. (1999) Cell-surface glycoprotein of oligodendrocyte progenitors involved in migration. *J. Neurosci.* **19**, 4948–4961.

21. Trapp, B. D., Nishiyama, A., Cheng, D., and Macklin, W. (1997) Differentiation and death of premyelinating oligodendrocytes in developing rodent brain. *J. Cell Biol.* **137**, 459–468.

22. Reynolds, R. and Hardy, R. (1997) Oligodendroglial progenitors labeled with the O4 antibody persist in the adult rat cerebral cortex in vivo. *J. Neurosci. Res.* **47**, 455–470.

23. Nishiyama, A., Lin, X. H., Giese, N., Heldin, C. H., and Stallcup, W. B. (1996) Interaction between NG2 proteoglycan and PDGF alpha-receptor on O2A progenitor cells is required for optimal response to PDGF. *J. Neurosci. Res.*, **43**, 315–330.

24. Nishiyama, A., Lin, X. H., Giese, N., Heldin, C. H., and Stallcup, W. B. (1996) Co-localization of NG2 proteoglycan and PDGF alpha-receptor on O2A progenitor cells in the developing rat brain. *J. Neurosci. Res.*, **43**, 299–314.

25. Levine, J. M., Stincone, F., and Lee, Y. S. (1993) Development and differentiation of glial precursor cells in the rat cerebellum. *Glia*, **7**, 307–321.

26. Keirstead, H. S., Levine, J. M., and Blakemore, W. F. (1998) Response of the oligodendrocyte progenitor cell population (defined by NG2 labelling) to demyelination of the adult spinal cord. *Glia* **22**, 161–170.

27. Luskin, M. B., Parnavelas, J. G., and Barfield, J. A. (1993) Neurons, astrocytes, and oligodendrocytes of the rat cerebral cortex originate from separate progenitor cells: an ultrastructural analysis of clonally related cells. *J. Neurosci.* **13**, 1730–1750.

28. Levison, S. W., Young, G. M., and Goldman, J. E. (1999) Cycling cells in the adult rat neocortex preferentially generate oligodendroglia. *J. Neurosci. Res.* **57**, 435–446.

29. Levison, S. W. and Goldman, J. E. (1993) Both oligodendrocytes and astrocytes develop from progenitors in the subventricular zone of postnatal rat forebrain. *Neuron* **10**, 201–212.

30. Grove, E. A., Williams, B. P., Li, D. Q., Hajihosseini, M., Friedrich, A. and Price, J. (1993) Multiple restricted lineages in the embryonic rat cerebral cortex. *Development* **117**, 553–561.

31. Richardson, W. D., Pringle, N., Mosley, M. J., Westermark, B., and Dubois-Dalcq, M. (1988) A role for platelet-derived growth factor in normal gliogenesis in the central nervous system. *Cell*, **53**, 309–319.

32. Raff, M. C., Lillien, L. E., Richardson, W. D., Burne, J. F., and Noble, M. D. (1988) Platelet-derived growth factor from astrocytes drives the clock that times oligodendrocyte development in culture. *Nature* **333**, 562–565.

33. Ellison, J. A. and de Vellis, J. (1994) Platelet-derived growth factor receptor is expressed by cells in the early oligodendrocyte lineage. *J. Neurosci. Res.* **37**, 116–128.

34. Tanaka, K., Nogawa, S., Ito, D., et al. (2001) Activation of NG2–positive oligodendrocyte progenitor cells during post-ischemic reperfusion in the rat brain. *Neuroreport* **12**, 2169–2174.

35. Levine, J. M., Reynolds, R., and Fawcett, J. W. (2001) The oligodendrocyte precursor cell in health and disease. *Trends Neurosci.* **24,** 39–47.
36. Shee, W. L., Ong, W. Y., and Lim, T. M. (1998) Distribution of perlecan in mouse hippocampus following intracerebroventricular kainate injections. *Brain Res.* **799,** 292–300.
37. Reynolds, R., Cenci di Bello, I., Dawson, M., and Levine, J. (2001) The response of adult oligodendrocyte progenitors to demyelination in EAE. *Prog. Brain Res.* **132,** 165–174.
38. McTigue, D. M., Wei, P., and Stokes, B. T. (2001) Proliferation of NG2–positive cells and altered oligodendrocyte numbers in the contused rat spinal cord. *J. Neurosci.* **21,** 3392–3400.
39. Levine, J. M., Enquist, L. W., and Card, J. P. (1998) Reactions of oligodendrocyte precursor cells to alpha herpesvirus infection of the central nervous system. *Glia* **23,** 316–328.
40. Levine, J. M. (1994) Increased expression of the NG2 chondroitin-sulfate proteoglycan after brain injury. *J. Neurosci.*, **14,** 4716–4730.
41. Back, S. A., Luo, N. L., Borenstein, N. S., Levine, J. M., Volpe, J. J., and Kinney, H. C. (2001) Late oligodendrocyte progenitors coincide with the developmental window of vulnerability for human perinatal white matter injury. *J. Neurosci.* **21,** 1302–1312.
42. Jones, L. L., Yamaguchi, Y., Stallcup, W. B., and Tuszynski, M. H. (2002) NG2 is a major chondroitin sulfate proteoglycan produced after spinal cord injury and is expressed by macrophages and oligodendrocyte progenitors. *J. Neurosci.* **22,** 2792–2803.
43. Humphries, M. J. (2000) Integrin cell adhesion receptors and the concept of agonism. *Trends Pharmacol. Sci.* **21,** 29–32.
44. Garrigues, H. J., Lark, M. W., Lara, S., Hellstrom, I., Hellstrom, K. E., and Wight, T. N. (1986) The melanoma proteoglycan: restricted expression on microspikes, a specific microdomain of the cell surface. *J. Cell Biol.* **103,** 1699–1710.
45. Harper, J. R., Bumol, T. F., and Reisfeld, R. A. (1984) Characterization of monoclonal antibody 155.8 and partial characterization of its proteoglycan antigen on human melanoma cells. *J. Immunol.* **132,** 2096–2104.
46. de Vries, J. E., Keizer, G. D., te Velde, A. A., et al. (1986) Characterization of melanoma-associated surface antigens involved in the adhesion and motility of human melanoma cells. *Int. J. Cancer* **38,** 465–473.
47. Fukushi, J., Makagiansar, I. T., and Stallcup, W. B. (2004) NG2 proteoglycan promotes endothelial cell motility and angiogenesis via engagement of galectin-3 and alpha3beta1 integrin. *Mol. Biol. Cell* **15,** 3580–3590.
48. Gladson, C. L. (1999) The extracellular matrix of gliomas: modulation of cell function. *J. Neuropathol. Exp. Neurol.* **58,** 1029–1040.
49. Burg, M. A., Grako, K. A., and Stallcup, W. B. (1998) Expression of the NG2 proteoglycan enhances the growth and metastatic properties of melanoma cells. *J. Cell Physiol.* **177,** 299–312.

50. East, J. A., Mitchell, S. D., and Hart, I. R. (1993) Expression and function of the CD44 glycoprotein in melanoma cell lines. *Melanoma Res.* **3,** 341–346.

51. Kuppner, M. C., Van Meir, E., Gauthier, T., Hamou, M. F., and de Tribolet, N. (1992) Differential expression of the CD44 molecule in human brain tumours. *Int., J. Cancer* **50,** 572–577.

52. Merzak, A., Koocheckpour, S., and Pilkington, G. J. (1994) CD44 mediates human glioma cell adhesion and invasion in vitro. *Cancer Res.* **54,** 3988–3992.

53. Akiyama, Y., Jung, S., Salhia, B., et al. (2001) Hyaluronate receptors mediating glioma cell migration and proliferation. *J. Neurooncol.* **53,** 115–127.

54. Midwood, K. S. and Salter, D. M. (2001) NG2/HMPG modulation of human articular chondrocyte adhesion to type VI collagen is lost in osteoarthritis. *J. Pathol.* **195,** 631–635.

55. Iida, J., Meijne, A. M., Spiro, R. C., Roos, E., Furcht, L. T., and McCarthy, J. B. (1995) Spreading and focal contact formation of human melanoma cells in response to the stimulation of both melanoma-associated proteoglycan (NG2) and alpha 4 beta 1 integrin. *Cancer Res.* **55,** 2177–2185.

56. Doane, K. J., Howell, S. J., and Birk, D. E. (1998) Identification and functional characterization of two type VI collagen receptors, alpha 3 beta 1 integrin and NG2, during avian corneal stromal development. *Invest. Ophthalmol. Vis. Sci.* **39,** 263–275.

57. Burg, M. A., Tillet, E., Timpl, R., and Stallcup, W. B. (1996) Binding of the NG2 proteoglycan to type VI collagen and other extracellular matrix molecules. *J. Biol. Chem.* **271,** 26,110–26,116.

58. Nishiyama, A. and Stallcup, W. B. (1993) Expression of NG2 proteoglycan causes retention of type VI collagen on the cell surface. *Mol. Biol. Cell* **4,** 1097–1108.

59. Stallcup, W. B., Dahlin, K., and Healy, P. (1990) Interaction of the NG2 chondroitin sulfate proteoglycan with type VI collagen. *J. Cell Biol.,* **111,** 3177–3188.

60. Kuo, H. J., Maslen, C. L., Keene, D. R., and Glanville, R. W. (1997) Type VI collagen anchors endothelial basement membranes by interacting with type IV collagen. *J. Biol. Chem.* **272,** 26,522–26,529.

61. Rand, J. H., Wu, X. X., Potter, B. J., Uson, R. R., and Gordon, R. E. (1993) Co-localization of von Willebrand factor and type VI collagen in human vascular subendothelium. *Am. J. Pathol.* **142,** 843–850.

62. Chintala, S. K., Sawaya, R., Gokaslan, Z. L., Fuller, G., and Rao, J. S. (1996) Immunohistochemical localization of extracellular matrix proteins in human glioma, both in vivo and in vitro. *Cancer Lett.* **101,** 107–114.

63. Paulus, W., Roggendorf, W., and Schuppan, D. (1988) Immunohistochemical investigation of collagen subtypes in human glioblastomas. *Virchows Arch. A Pathol. Anat. Histopathol.* **413,** 325–332.

64. Chekenya, M., Rooprai, H. K., Davies, D., Levine, J. M., Butt, A. M., and Pilkington, G. J. (1999) The NG2 chondroitin sulfate proteoglycan: role in malignant progression of human brain tumours. *Int J. Dev. Neurosci.* **17,** 421–435.

65. Chekenya, M., Enger, P., Thorsen, F., et al. (2002) The glial precursor proteoglycan, NG2, is expressed on tumour neovasculature by vascular pericytes in human malignant brain tumours. *Neuropathol. Appl. Neurobiol.* **28,** 367–380.

66. Lemmon, V., Farr, K. L., and Lagenaur, C. (1989) L1–mediated axon outgrowth occurs via a homophilic binding mechanism. *Neuron* **2**, 1597–1603.
67. Edgar, D., Timpl, R., and Thoenen, H. (1984) The heparin-binding domain of laminin is responsible for its effects on neurite outgrowth and neuronal survival. *EMBO J.* **3**, 1463–1468.
68. Fidler, P. S., Schuette, K., Asher, R. A., et al. (1999) Comparing astrocytic cell lines that are inhibitory or permissive for axon growth: the major axon-inhibitory proteoglycan is NG2. *J. Neurosci.* **19**, 8778–8788.
69. Fawcett, J. W., and Asher, R. A. (1999) The glial scar and central nervous system repair. *Brain Res. Bull* **49**, 377–391.
70. Dou, C. L., and Levine, J. M. (1994) Inhibition of neurite growth by the NG2 chondroitin sulfate proteoglycan. *J. Neurosci.* **14**, 7616–7628.
71. Pedersen, P. H., Marienhagen, K., Mork, S., and Bjerkvig, R. (1993) Migratory pattern of fetal rat brain cells and human glioma cells in the adult rat brain. *Cancer Res.* **53**, 5158–5165.
72. Giordana, M. T., Germano, I., Giaccone, G., Mauro, A., Migheli, A., and Schiffer, D. (1985) The distribution of laminin in human brain tumors: an immunohisto-chemical study. *Acta. NeuroPathol. (Berl)* **67**, 51–57.
73. Noble, M. -P. (2001) *Glial Restricted Precursors*. Humana Press, Totowa, New Jersey.
74. Sugimoto, Y., Taniguchi, M., Yagi, T., Akagi, Y., Nojyo, Y., and Tamamaki, N. (2001) Guidance of glial precursor cell migration by secreted cues in the developing optic nerve. *Development* **128**, 3321–3330.
75. Fang, X., Burg, M. A., Barritt, D., Dahlin-Huppe, K., Nishiyama, A., and Stallcup, W. B. (1999) Cytoskeletal reorganization induced by engagement of the NG2 proteoglycan leads to cell spreading and migration. *Mol. Biol. Cell* **10**, 3373–3387.
76. Lin, X. H., Dahlin-Huppe, K., and Stallcup, W. B. (1996) Interaction of the NG2 proteoglycan with the actin cytoskeleton. *J. Cell Biochem.* **63**, 463–477.
77. Bogler, O., Wren, D., Barnett, S. C., Land, H., and Noble, M. (1990) Cooperation between two growth factors promotes extended self-renewal and inhibits differentiation of oligodendrocyte-type-2 astrocyte (O-2A) progenitor cells. *Proc. Natl. Acad. Sci. USA* **87**, 6368–6372.
78. Baron, W., Metz, B., Bansal, R., Hoekstra, D., and de Vries, H. (2000) PDGF and FGF-2 signaling in oligodendrocyte progenitor cells: regulation of proliferation and differentiation by multiple intracellular signaling pathways. *Mol. Cell Neurosci.* **15**, 314–329.
79. Redwine, J. M., Blinder, K. L., and Armstrong, R. C. (1997) In situ expression of fibroblast growth factor receptors by oligodendrocyte progenitors and oligodendrocytes in adult mouse central nervous system. *J. Neurosci. Res.* **50**, 229–237.
80. Grako, K. A., and Stallcup, W. B. (1995) Participation of the NG2 proteoglycan in rat aortic smooth muscle cell responses to platelet-derived growth factor. *Exp. Cell Res.* **221**, 231–240.
81. Goretzki, L., Burg, M. A., Grako, K. A., and Stallcup, W. B. (1999) High-affinity binding of basic fibroblast growth factor and platelet-derived growth factor-AA to the core protein of the NG2 proteoglycan. *J. Biol. Chem.* **274**, 16,831–16,837.

82. Brekke, C., Lundervold, A., Enger, P. Ø., et al. (2006) NG2 expression regulates vascular morphology and function in human brain tumours. *NeuroImage* **29,** 965–976. Epub Oct 25, 2005.

83. Chekenya, M., Hjelstuen, M., Enger, P. O., et al. (2002) NG2 proteoglycan promotes angiogenesis-dependent tumor growth in CNS by sequestering angiostatin. *FASEB J.* **16,** 586–588.

84. Hermanson, M., Funa, K., Koopmann, J., et al. (1996) Association of loss of heterozygosity on chromosome 17p with high platelet-derived growth factor alpha receptor expression in human malignant gliomas. *Cancer Res.* **56,** 164–171.

85. Nister, M., Libermann, T. A., Betsholtz, C., et al. (1988) Expression of messenger RNAs for platelet-derived growth factor and transforming growth factor-alpha and their receptors in human malignant glioma cell lines. *Cancer Res.* **48,** 3910–3918.

86. Fleming, T. P., Saxena, A., Clark, W. C., et al. (1992) Amplification and/or overexpression of platelet-derived growth factor receptors and epidermal growth factor receptor in human glial tumors. *Cancer Res.* **52,** 4550–4553.

87. Bergers, G., and Benjamin, L. E. (2003) Tumorigenesis and the angiogenic switch. *Nat. Rev. Cancer* **3,** 401–410.

88. Ozerdem, U., Monosov, E., and Stallcup, W. B. (2002) NG2 Proteoglycan Expression by Pericytes in Pathological Microvasculature. *Microvasc. Res.* **63,** 129–134.

89. Ozerdem, U., Grako, K. A., Dahlin-Huppe, K., Monosov, E., and Stallcup, W. B. (2001) NG2 proteoglycan is expressed exclusively by mural cells during vascular morphogenesis. *Dev. Dyn* **222,** 218–227.

90. Miller, B., Sheppard, A. M., Bicknese, A. R., and Pearlman, A. L. (1995) Chondroitin sulfate proteoglycans in the developing cerebral cortex: the distribution of neurocan distinguishes forming afferent and efferent axonal pathways. *J. Comp. Neurol.* **355,** 615–628.

91. Lindahl, P., Johansson, B. R., Leveen, P., and Betsholtz, C. (1997) Pericyte loss and microaneurysm formation in PDGF-B-deficient mice. *Science* **277,** 242–245.

92. Hellstrom, M., Kalen, M., Lindahl, P., Abramsson, A., and Betsholtz, C. (1999) Role of PDGF-B and PDGFR-beta in recruitment of vascular smooth muscle cells and pericytes during embryonic blood vessel formation in the mouse. *Development* **126,** 3047–3055.

93. Murfee, W. L., Skalak, T. C., and Peirce, S. M. (2005) Differential arterial/venous expression of NG2 proteoglycan in perivascular cells along microvessels: identifying a venule-specific phenotype. *Microcirculation* **12,** 151–160.

94. Schwartz, S. M., Heimark, R. L., and Majesky, M. W. (1990) Developmental mechanisms underlying pathology of arteries. *Physiol. Rev.* **70,** 1177–1209.

95. Ross. (1993) The pathogenesis of atherosclerosis: a perspective for the 1990s. *Nature* **362,** 801–809.

96. Grako, K. A., Ochiya, T., Barritt, D., Nishiyama, A., and Stallcup, W. B. (1999) PDGF (alpha)-receptor is unresponsive to PDGF-AA in aortic smooth muscle cells from the NG2 knockout mouse. *J. Cell Sci.* **112 (Pt 6),** 905–915.

97. Orlidge, A., and D'Amore, P. A. (1987) Inhibition of capillary endothelial cell growth by pericytes and smooth muscle cells. *J. Cell Biol.* **105,** 1455–1462.

98. Asher, R. A., Morgenstern, D. A., Properzi, F., Nishiyama, A., Levine, J. M., and Fawcett, J. W. (2005) Two separate metalloproteinase activities are responsible for the shedding and processing of the NG2 proteoglycan in vitro. *Mol. Cell Neurosci.* **29,** 82–96.

99. Goretzki, L., Lombardo, C. R., and Stallcup, W. B. (2000) Binding of the NG2 proteoglycan to kringle domains modulates the functional properties of angiostatin and plasmin(ogen). *J. Biol. Chem.* **275,** 28,625–28,633.

100. Ashley, D. M., Batra, S. K., and Bigner, D. D. (1997) Monoclonal antibodies to growth factors and growth factor receptors: their diagnostic and therapeutic potential in brain tumors. *J. Neurooncol.* **35,** 259–273.

101. Harper, J. R., and Reisfeld, R. A. (1983) Inhibition of anchorage-independent growth of human melanoma cells by a monoclonal antibody to a chondroitin sulfate proteoglycan. *J. Natl. Cancer Inst.* **71,** 259–263.

102. Bumol, T. F., Wang, Q. C., Reisfeld, R. A., and Kaplan, N. O. (1983) Monoclonal antibody and an antibody-toxin conjugate to a cell surface proteoglycan of melanoma cells suppress in vivo tumor growth. *Proc. Natl. Acad. Sci. USA* **80,** 529–533.

103. Folkman, J. (1995) Angiogenesis in cancer, vascular, rheumatoid and other disease. *Nat. Med.* **1,** 27–31.

104. Burrows, F. J., and Thorpe, P. E. (1993) Eradication of large solid tumors in mice with an immunotoxin directed against tumor vasculature. *Proc. Natl. Acad. Sci. USA* **90,** 8996–9000.

105. Kerbel, R. S. (1997) A cancer therapy resistant to resistance. *Nature* **390,** 335–336.

106. Kerbel, R. S. (1991) Inhibition of tumor angiogenesis as a strategy to circumvent acquired resistance to anti-cancer therapeutic agents. *Bioessays* **13,** 31–36.

107. Boehm, T., Folkman, J., Browder, T., and O'Reilly, M. S. (1997) Antiangiogenic therapy of experimental cancer does not induce acquired drug resistance. *Nature* **390,** 404–407.

108. Natali, P. G., Imai, K., Wilson, B. S., et al. (1981) Structural properties and tissue distribution of the antigen recognized by the monoclonal antibody 653.40S to human melanoma cells. *J. Natl. Cancer Inst.* **67,** 591–601.

109. Ferrone, S. G. P., Natali, P. G., et al. (1983) A human high molecular weight-melanoma associated antigen (HMWW_MAA) defined by monoclonal antibodies: a useful marker to radioimage tumor lesions in patients with melanoma. Brookhaven National Laboratories. Associated Universities, Inc., Brookhaven, New York.

110. Giacomini, P., Natali, P., and Ferrone, S. (1985) Analysis of the interaction between a human high molecular weight melanoma-associated antigen and the monoclonal antibodies to three distinct antigenic determinants. *J. Immunol.* **135,** 696–702.

111. Lindmo, T., Boven, E., Cuttitta, F., Fedorko, J., and Bunn, P. A., Jr. (1984) Determination of the immunoreactive fraction of radiolabeled monoclonal antibodies

by linear extrapolation to binding at infinite antigen excess. *J. Immunol. Methods* **72,** 77–89.

112. Kohler, G., and Milstein, C. (1975) Continuous cultures of fused cells secreting antibody of predefined specificity. *Nature* **256,** 495–497.

113. Winter, G., Griffiths, A. D., Hawkins, R. E., and Hoogenboom, H. R. (1994) Making antibodies by phage display technology. *Annu. Rev. Immunol.* **12,** 433–455.

114. Schaffitzel, C., Hanes, J., Jermutus, L., and Pluckthun, A. (1999) Ribosome display: an in vitro method for selection and evolution of antibodies from libraries. *J. Immunol. Methods* **231,** 119–135.

115. Giovannoni, L., Viti, F., Zardi, L., and Neri, D. (2001) Isolation of anti-angiogenesis antibodies from a large combinatorial repertoire by colony filter screening. *Nucleic Acids Res.* **29,** E27.

116. Graff, C. P., Chester, K., Begent, R., and Wittrup, K. D. (2004) Directed evolution of an anti-carcinoembryonic antigen scFv with a 4–day monovalent dissociation half-time at 37 degrees C. *Protein Eng. Des. Sel.* **17,** 293–304.

117. Olafsen, T., Tan, G. J., Cheung, C. W., et al. (2004) Characterization of engineered anti-p185HER-2 (scFv-CH3)2 antibody fragments (minibodies) for tumor targeting. *Protein Eng. Des. Sel.* **17,** 315–323.

118. Epenetos, A. A., Snook, D., Durbin, H., Johnson, P. M., and Taylor-Papadimitriou, J. (1986) Limitations of radiolabeled monoclonal antibodies for localization of human neoplasms. *Cancer Res.* **46,** 3183–3191.

119. Neuwelt, E. A., Specht, H. D., Barnett, P. A., et al. (1987) Increased delivery of tumor-specific monoclonal antibodies to brain after osmotic blood-brain barrier modification in patients with melanoma metastatic to the central nervous system. *Neurosurgery* **20,** 885–895.

120. Jain, R. K., and Baxter, L. T. (1988) Mechanisms of heterogeneous distribution of monoclonal antibodies and other macromolecules in tumors: significance of elevated interstitial pressure. *Cancer Res.* **48,** 7022–7032.

121. Murayama, O., Nishida, H., and Sekiguchi, K. (1996) Novel peptide ligands for integrin alpha 6 beta 1 selected from a phage display library. *J. Biochem. (Tokyo)* **120,** 445–451.

122. Koivunen, E., Wang, B., and Ruoslahti, E. (1995) Phage libraries displaying cyclic peptides with different ring sizes: ligand specificities of the RGD-directed integrins. *Biotechnology (NY)* **13,** 265–270.

123. Koivunen, E., Restel, B. H., Rajotte, D., Lahdenranta, J., Hagedorn, M., Arap, W., and Pasqualini, R. (1999) Integrin-binding peptides derived from phage display libraries. *Methods Mol. Biol.* **129,** 3–17.

124. Koivunen, E., Arap, W., Valtanen, H., et al. (1999) Tumor targeting with a selective gelatinase inhibitor. *Nat. Biotechnol.* **17,** 768–774.

125. Yanofsky, S. D., Baldwin, D. N., Butler, J. H., et al. (1996) High affinity type I interleukin 1 receptor antagonists discovered by screening recombinant peptide libraries. *Proc. Natl. Acad. Sci. USA* **93,** 7381–7386.

126. Pennington, M. E., Lam, K. S., and Cress, A. E. (1996) The use of a combinatorial library method to isolate human tumor cell adhesion peptides. *Mol. Divers,* **2,** 19–28.

127. Goodson, R. J., Doyle, M. V., Kaufman, S. E., and Rosenberg, S. (1994) High-affinity urokinase receptor antagonists identified with bacteriophage peptide display. *Proc. Natl. Acad. Sci. USA* **91,** 7129–7133.

128. Burg, M. A., Pasqualini, R., Arap, W., Ruoslahti, E., and Stallcup, W. B. (1999) NG2 proteoglycan-binding peptides target tumor neovasculature. *Cancer Res.* **59,** 2869–2874.

129. Sims, D., Horne, M. M., Creighan, M., and Donald, A. (1994) Heterogeneity of pericyte populations in equine skeletal muscle and dermal microvessels: a quantitative study. *Anat. Histol. Embryol.* **23,** 232–238.

130. Lindahl, P., and Betsholtz, C. (1998) Not all myofibroblasts are alike: revisiting the role of PDGF-A and PDGF-B using PDGF-targeted mice. *Curr. Opin. Nephrol. Hypertens.* **7,** 21–26.

131. Hirschi, K. K., and D'Amore, P. A. (1997) Control of angiogenesis by the pericyte: molecular mechanisms and significance. *Exs.* **79,** 419–428.

132. Schrappe, M., Klier, F. G., Spiro, R. C., Waltz, T. A., Reisfeld, R. A., and Gladson, C. L. (1991) Correlation of chondroitin sulfate proteoglycan expression on proliferating brain capillary endothelial cells with the malignant phenotype of astroglial cells. *Cancer Res.* **51,** 4986–4993.

133. Leger, O., Johnson-Leger, C., Jackson, E., Coles, B., and Dean, C. (1994) The chondroitin sulfate proteoglycan NG2 is a tumour-specific antigen on the chemically induced rat chondrosarcoma HSN. *Int J. Cancer* **58,** 700–705.

134. Behm, F. G., Smith, F. O., Raimondi, S. C., Pui, C. H., and Bernstein, I. D. (1996) Human homologue of the rat chondroitin sulfate proteoglycan, NG2, detected by monoclonal antibody 7.1, identifies childhood acute lymphoblastic leukemias with t(4;11)(q21;q23) or t(11;19)(q23;p13) and MLL gene rearrangements. *Blood* **87,** 1134–1139.

135. Scott, J. K., and Smith, G. P. (1990) Searching for peptide ligands with an epitope library. *Science* **249,** 386–390.

136. Collins, J., Horn, N., Wadenback, J., and Szardenings, M. (2001) Cosmix-plexing: a novel recombinatorial approach for evolutionary selection from combinatorial libraries. *J. Biotechnol.* **74,** 317–338.

137. Pasqualini, R., Koivunen, E., and Ruoslahti, E. (1997) Alpha v integrins as receptors for tumor targeting by circulating ligands. *Nat. Biotechnol.* **15,** 542–546.

138. Pinilla, C., Appel, J. R., Borras, E., and Houghten, R. A. (2003) Advances in the use of synthetic combinatorial chemistry: mixture-based libraries. *Nat. Med.* **9,** 118–122.

139. Wrighton, N. C., Balasubramanian, P., Barbone, F. P., et al. (1997) Increased potency of an erythropoietin peptide mimetic through covalent dimerization. *Nat. Biotechnol.* **15,** 1261–1265.

140. Hannon, G. J. (2002) RNA interference. *Nature* **418,** 244–251.

141. Wang, L., Prakash, R. K., Stein, C. A., Koehn, R. K., and Ruffner, D. E. (2003) Progress in the delivery of therapeutic oligonucleotides: organ/cellular distribution and targeted delivery of oligonucleotides in vivo. *Antisense Nucleic Acid Drug Dev.* **13,** 169–189.

142. Czauderna, F., Fechtner, M., Dames, S., et al. (2003) Structural variations and stabilising modifications of synthetic siRNAs in mammalian cells. *Nucleic Acids Res.* **31**, 2705–2716.

143. Reed, R. K., Lepsoe, S., and Wiig, H. (1989) Interstitial exclusion of albumin in rat dermis and subcutis in over- and dehydration. *Am. J. Physiol.* **257**, H1819–H1827.

144. Krol, A., Maresca, J., Dewhirst, M. W., and Yuan, F. (1999) Available volume fraction of macromolecules in the extravascular space of a fibrosarcoma: implications for drug delivery. *Cancer Res.* **59**, 4136–4141.

145. Jain, R. K. (1997) Delivery of molecular and cellular medicine to solid tumors. *Adv. Drug Deliv. Rev.* **26**, 71–90.

146. Vaupel, P., Kallinowski, F., and Okunieff, P. (1989) Blood flow, oxygen and nutrient supply, and metabolic microenvironment of human tumors: a review. *Cancer Res.* **49**, 6449–6465.

147. Jain, R. K. (1988) Determinants of tumor blood flow: a review. *Cancer Res.* **48**, 2641–2658.

148. Hwang, K. M., Fodstad, O., Oldham, R. K., and Morgan, A. C., Jr. (1985) Radiolocalization of xenografted human malignant melanoma by a monoclonal antibody (9.2.27) to a melanoma-associated antigen in nude mice. *Cancer Res.* **45**, 4150–4155.

149. Yang, H. M., and Reisfeld, R. A. (1988) Doxorubicin conjugated with a monoclonal antibody directed to a human melanoma-associated proteoglycan suppresses the growth of established tumor xenografts in nude mice. *Proc. Natl. Acad. Sci. USA*, **85**, 1189–1193.

150. Yang, H. M., and Reisfeld, R. A. (1988) Pharmacokinetics and mechanism of action of a doxorubicin-monoclonal antibody 9.2.27 conjugate directed to a human melanoma proteoglycan. *J. Natl. Cancer Inst.* **80**, 1154–1159.

151. Colapinto, E. V., Zalutsky, M. R., Archer, G. E., et al. (1990) Radioimmunotherapy of intracerebral human glioma xenografts with 131I-labeled F(ab')2 fragments of monoclonal antibody Mel-14. *Cancer Res.* **50**, 1822–1827.

152. Colapinto, E. V., Humphrey, P. A., Zalutsky, M. R., et al. (1988) Comparative localization of murine monoclonal antibody Mel-14 F(ab')2 fragment and whole IgG2a in human glioma xenografts. *Cancer Res.* **48**, 5701–5707.

153. Bigner, D. D., Brown, M., Coleman, R. E., et al. (1995) Phase I studies of treatment of malignant gliomas and neoplastic meningitis with ^{131}I-radiolabeled monoclonal antibodies anti-tenascin 81C6 and anti-chondroitin proteoglycan sulfate Mel-14 F (ab')2–a preliminary report. *J. Neurooncol.* **24**, 109–122.

154. Cokgor, I., Akabani, G., Friedman, H. S., et al. (2001) Long term response in a patient with neoplastic meningitis secondary to melanoma treated with (131)I-radiolabeled antichondroitin proteoglycan sulfate Mel-14 F(ab')(2): a case study. *Cancer* **91**, 1809–1813.

155. Larsen, R. H., Akabani, G., Welsh, P., and Zalutsky, M. R. (1998) The cytotoxicity and microdosimetry of astatine-211–labeled chimeric monoclonal antibodies in human glioma and melanoma cells in vitro. *Radiat. Res.* **149**, 155–162.

156. Makagiansar, I. T., Williams, S., Dahlin-Huppe, K., Fukushi, J., Mustelin, T., and Stallcup, W. B. (2004) Phosphorylation of NG2 proteoglycan by protein kinase C-alpha regulates polarized membrane distribution and cell motility. *J. Biol. Chem.* **279,** 55,262–55,270.
157. Smith, M. R. (2003) Rituximab (monoclonal anti-CD20 antibody): mechanisms of action and resistance. *Oncogene* **22,** 7359–7368.
158. Lin, C. C., Shen, Y. C., Chuang, C. K., and Liao, S. K. (2001) Analysis of a murine anti-ganglioside GD2 monoclonal antibody expressing both IgG2a and IgG3 isotypes: monoclonality, apoptosis triggering, and activation of cellular cytotoxicity on human melanoma cells. *Adv. Exp. Med. Biol.* **491,** 419–429.
159. Baselga, J., and Albanell, J. (2001) Mechanism of action of anti-HER2 monoclonal antibodies. *Ann. Oncol.* **12 Suppl 1,** S35–S41.

5

Heterotrimeric G Proteins and Disease

Øyvind Melien

Summary

Heterotrimeric G proteins attached to the cell membrane convey signals from G protein-coupled receptors in response to stimulation by a number of hormones, neurotransmitters, chemokines, and pharmacological agents to intracellular signaling cascades. The heterotrimeric G proteins are also located in the cell interior, and receptor-independent mechanisms may elicit their activation. Thus, G proteins may possibly exert cellular functions other than acting as signaling transducers. There is also increasing evidence for roles in different diseases including infections, inflammation, neurological diseases, cardiovascular diseases, cancer, and endocrine disorders. This review describes characteristics of the heterotrimeric G proteins, evidence for their involvement in different diseases, and outlines some of the therapeutic options utilizing G protein targets.

Key Words: Heterotrimeric G proteins; disease; therapy.

1. Introduction

Heterotrimeric guanine nucleotide-binding proteins (G proteins) belong to a superfamily of guanosine triphosphate (GTP)ases acting as key transducing components of cellular signaling cascades (*1–8*). Attached to the plasma membrane they transmit signals from G protein-coupled receptors (GPCR) in response to hormones, neurotransmitters, chemokines as well as a number of pharmacological agents to intracellular pathways, which include adenylyl cyclases (AC), phospholipases, and ion channels (**Fig. 1**).

The G proteins are composed of an α- (39–52 kDa), β- (35 kDa), and γ- (7–8 kDa) subunit. Altogether, 21 different Gα-subunits (from 17 genes) have been described sharing approx 20% conserved amino acids. Based on the amino acid sequence of the α-subunits, the heterotrimeric G proteins are

From: *Methods in Molecular Biology, vol. 361, Target Discovery and Validation Reviews and Protocols*
Volume 2, Emerging Molecular Targets and Treatment Options
Edited by: M. Sioud © Humana Press Inc., Totowa, NJ

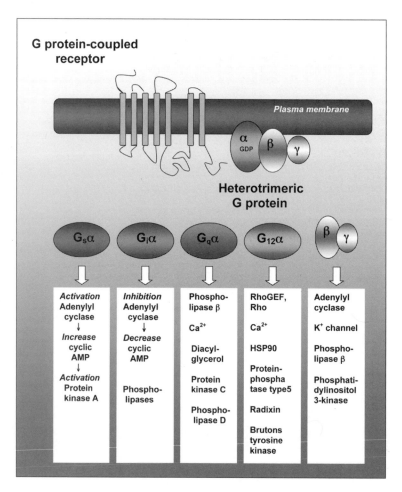

Fig. 1. G protein signaling. Heterotrimeric G proteins are activated in response to stimulation of G protein-coupled receptors by numerous hormones, neurotransmitters, chemokines, pharmacological agents, and other substances. Upon activation, the heterotrimeric G protein dissociates into its α- and βγ-subunits, which transduce signals to various effectors in the cell illustrated here for the different subunit groups.

divided into the four main families G_s, G_i, $G_{q/11}$, and $G_{12/13}$. Six β- and 12 γ-subunits have been identified. The β- and γ-subunits form tightly bound functional dimers that only dissociate after denaturation. Whereas combinations of β- and γ-subunits assembling with specific α-subunits have been defined in various cell types, there is still limited understanding with regard to the biological significance and regulation of G protein heterotrimeric composition.

The GTPase activity of the G proteins is localized within the α-subunit, which also possess a single guanine–nucleotide-binding site. In the resting, inactive state the G protein exists as a heterotrimer with the α-subunit in a GDP-bound form. The activation of G proteins is believed to involve two major events, a guanine–nucleotide-exchange step and dissociation of the α- and βγ-subunits. Upon receptor stimulation by hormones, neurotransmitters, or other agents, the activated receptor interacts with the G protein resulting in release of GDP. Subsequently, a complex is formed between receptor and the G protein in its guanine–nucleotide-deficient ("empty pocket") state before GTP is inserted *(8)*. The binding of GTP to the α-subunit produces conformational changes resulting in decreased affinity of α for the βγ dimer allowing them to separate and signal to various effectors. The G protein deactivation involves hydrolysis of GTP bound to the α-subunit, mediated by the intrinsic GTPase activity, resulting in subunit reassociation and termination of signaling.

In addition to the intrinsic GTPase activity of heterotrimeric G proteins, the group of regulators of G protein signaling (RGS) *(9,10)* act as GTPase-activating proteins (GAP) accelerating the termination of the GTP bound state of Gα, resulting in a shortened timespan of Gα to exert signaling. In addition, the RGS proteins may counteract the interaction between Gα and its effector molecules. Thus, the RGS proteins, presently counting over 30 members, add to the mechanisms of a temporal fine-tuning of signal transduction mediated through heterotrimeric G proteins.

It has been claimed that the dissociation of the α- and βγ-subunits during G protein activation may imply reassociation in an accidental, unregulated manner possibly affecting the signaling outputs that are generated through successive cycles of G protein activation *(11)*. An alternative model to activation through subunit dissociation would be conformational changes of α and βγ within the frame of a heterotrimeric structure still allowing subunit access to effector molecules. This mechanism is supported by observations indicating that G proteins retain their heterotrimeric state during signaling *(11–14)*.

Although the activation of heterotrimeric G proteins mainly results from stimulation of GPCRs *(15)*, receptor-independent mechanisms involving activators of G protein signaling (AGS) have also been identified *(16,17)*. These discoveries, as well as the observations of several intracellular locations for G proteins, such as in the Golgi apparatus or the nucleus *(18–24)* suggest additional roles for G proteins beyond acting as signal transducers. Furthermore, the knowledge of G protein interactions with AGS, RGS, and other accessory proteins *(17)*, which may also function as scaffolding proteins, as well as with particular cellular microdomains, like caveolae and the Golgi apparatus, suggests additional mechanisms for the achievement of signaling specificity and effects.

2. Heterotrimeric G Proteins Families

2.1. G_s

G_s proteins (44–52 kDa) were the first heterotrimeric G proteins to be discovered *(25–27)*. G_s stimulates AC directly, through the α- or $\beta\gamma$-subunit, to produce cyclic adenosine monophosphate (AMP), which is a central signaling molecule for a range of hormones. The increase in cyclic AMP levels activates protein kinase A, resulting in phosphorylation of several enzymes, ion channels, and transcription factors thereby regulating various metabolic and growth-related processes. G_s proteins may also regulate ion channels independent of AC activation *(18)*. In HEK293 cells, β_2-adrenoceptors switched their coupling from G_s proteins to G_i to convey signals that stimulated extracellular signal-regulated kinase (ERK)1/2 *(28)*. Notably, β-adrenoceptor regulation of ERK1/2 in COS-7 cells was conveyed through G_s proteins in a bimodal manner, i.e., the $\beta\gamma$-subunit-mediated activation, whereas the α_s-subunit exerted inhibition *(29)*. Moreover, in PC12 cells, G_s is involved in stimulation of ERK1/2 through protein kinase A-dependent activation of the small G protein Rap1 and B-Raf *(30)*.

Evidence for active signaling role(s) of G proteins in their heterotrimeric state is obtained for G_s *(11,31)*. Furthermore, a notable observation is the ability of EGF to activate AC in cardiac cells *(32)* involving the $G_s\alpha$-subunit. This supports data from other cells suggesting the existence of signaling interactions between receptor tyrosine kinases and heterotrimeric G proteins *(33)*.

The G_s proteins occur in several splice variants, also within a single cell type. In addition, observations in pituitary cells have provided evidence for the presence of biologically active $G_s\alpha$ variants resulting from limited proteolytic cleavage by calpain *(34)*. The $G_s\alpha$ proteins share the susceptibility to be adenosine diphosphate (ADP)-ribosylated at a highly conserved arginine residue in the N-terminal end of the α-subunit by cholera toxin (CTX), an enterotoxin from *Vibrio cholerae* *(35)*. This modification constitutively activates G_s, by inactivating intrinsic GTPase function, as well as inhibiting the interaction between $G_s\alpha$ and $G\beta\gamma$, resulting in marked elevation of cyclic AMP. Notably, $G\alpha$-subunits belonging to other G protein families also contain the CTX-sensitive arginine residue, and members of the G_i family may be ADP-ribosylated by CTX under certain conditions.

G_{olf} is a member of the G_s family distributed in olfactory epithelium capable of stimulating AC and susceptible to ADP-ribosylation by CTX.

2.2. Gi

G_i proteins (40–41 kDa) include several subtypes. G_{i1}, G_{i2}, G_{i3}, G_o, and G_z inhibit AC, thereby decreasing cyclic AMP production, whereas the retinal subtypes G_{t1} and G_{t2} activate cyclic guanosine monophosphate (cGMP)-specific phosphodiesterase *(18)*. All members of the G_i family except G_z are sensitive to pertussis toxin (PTX) *(36)* produced by the bacteria *Bordetella pertussis*. Using nicotinamide adenine dinucleotide as a substrate, PTX ADP-ribosylates the α-subunit of G_i at a cystein residue four positions from the C-terminal end, thereby inactivating the G_i protein. It has been observed in various cell types that G_i proteins are more abundant than other members of the G protein family, and $G_o\alpha$ constitutes up to 1–2% of membrane protein in brain.

G_i proteins are involved in regulation of ion channels for K^+, Ca^{2+}, Na^+, or Cl^- *(37)*. The regulation of the cardiac K^+ channel is conceivably mediated by G_i in a direct manner. Activation of PLCβ enzymes may involve G_i proteins, conceivably their βγ-subunits *(38)*, and also phosphoinositide 3 (PI 3) kinases are reported to be activated by G_i proteins, through both α and βγ-subunits *(37)*. The G_i-mediated activation of ERK is promoted through various signaling pathways. In some cells activation of ERK1/2 through G_i proteins involves the βγ-subunit in Ras-dependent and protein kinase C (PKC)-independent pathways *(39)*. There is also evidence that G_i proteins mediate activation of ERK1/2 in a βγ-independent manner; i.e., suggesting a role for α_i, and as well independent of Ras *(40)*. In CHO cells a G_i-dependent pathway to ERK1/2 was identified which bypassed Ras and Raf, but involved PI 3-kinase γ and atypical PKC-ζ *(41)*. A complex formed of a 100-kDa tyrosine-phosphorylated protein (p100) and Grb2, but not Src kinases or Shc, was found to be critical for G_i-mediated ERK activation in Rat-1 fibroblasts and COS cells *(42)*.

There are also observations suggesting that certain receptor tyrosine kinases activate ERK in part involving G_i-dependent mechanisms *(43)*. A role for heterotrimeric G proteins in signaling pathways from receptor tyrosine kinases *(33)* has support from observations in different experimental models. In hematopoietic cells both colony-stimulating factor 1 and erythropoietin activate mechanisms that conceivably involve G_i proteins *(44–45)*. In breast cancer cells, epidermal growth factor (EGF) activation was found to implicate G_i proteins *(46)*. A direct interaction between the EGF receptor and G_i protein was suggested in rat hepatocytes *(47)* and similar interactions were reported for the insulin receptor and G_i in hepatoma cells *(48)*. Furthermore, a recent report suggests that Gβγ-subunits are needed in EGF-induced formation of complexes between EGF receptor and G protein-coupled receptor kinase 2 (GRK2) *(49)*. These and other data suggest that the function of heterotrimeric G proteins is not confined to signaling from seven transmembrane receptors, although the molecular basis for this interplay is rather elusive.

Observations in different cell types support role(s) of G_i proteins, especially G_{i3}, in functions of the Golgi apparatus *(18,50–52)*. Data suggest that Gβγ-subunits may mediate several of these Golgi regulatory functions through direct pleckstrin homology domain interactions with protein kinase D, a subtype of PKC *(53)*. Furthermore, G_i has also been implicated in nuclear import of proteins, although the mechanism for this is unclear *(19,54)*, and $G_{12}\alpha$ is believed to play a role in the biogenesis of tight junctions *(55)*.

The major roles of G_0 proteins have not been clearly determined. As they are both relatively weak inhibitors of AC and highly abundant in certain tissues, other functions have been sought. It may be that G_0 proteins are involved in regulation of various ion channels. Furthermore, G_0 is implicated in activation of ERK *(39)* conceivably through a particular mechanism depending on the GTPase activating protein Rap1GAP *(56)*. G_0 is involved in pathways that activate the signal transducer and activator of transcription 3 (STAT3) *(57)*, and it appears that the protein GAP43 exerts a regulatory control of G_0 *(58)*.

G_z is primarily distributed in brain, adrenal medulla, and platelets. Whereas the understanding of the biological role of G_z are still only partially understood, it is believed that G_z is involved in functions of the nervous system and in platelets and recently it has been reported a role for G_z in the pancreatic islet β cells *(59)*. In addition to its inhibitory effect on AC, it is reported that βγ dimers from G_z mediate regulation of G protein-activated K^+ channels from muscarinic m2 receptors *(60)*, and in a previous report a role for G_z in production of tumor necrosis factor-α was suggested *(61)*. A well described effector for G_z is Rap1GAP, which is a GAP for the Ras family protein Rap1 *(62)*. Activated $G\alpha_z$ recruit Rap1GAP from cytosol to the cell membrane, thus resulting in downregulation of Rap1-signaling *(63)*. $G\alpha_z$ also interacts with a specific regulator of G protein signaling, RGSZ1 as well as the transcriptional cofactor Eya2 *(64)*.

2.3. $G_{q/11}$

Members of the phospholipase(PLC)β family are main substrates for the $G_{q/11}$ proteins (40–41 kDa) *(38,65)*. This activation is mediated through the α-subunit and results in generation of inositol (1,4,5)-trisphosphate (IP_3) from phosphatidyl-inositol 4,5-bisphosphate together with diacylglycerol, which activates PKC. Also Bruton's tyrosine kinase is reported to be substrate for G_q *(66)*, and $G_{q/11}$ proteins are as well involved in ERK activation *(39)* and growth regulation *(67)*. The G_q-mediated activation of ERK is reported to involve PKC in Ras-independent pathways *(39)*, or may converge with pathways from βγ of G_i that involve Ras *(68)*. G_q is activated by pasteurella multocida toxin *(69)* causing athrophic rhinitis in pigs.

G_{14}, G_{15}, and G_{16}, which are members of the $G_{q/11}$ family, also activate the β forms of PLC. The distribution of G_{14} is mainly restricted to spleen, kidney, lung, testis, bone marrow, and early myeloid and progenitor B cells, whereas G_{15} and G_{16} are expressed in hematopoietic cells. $G_{14}\alpha$ is reported to stimulate c-Jun N-terminal kinases (JNK), ERK, and STAT3 *(70,71)*. G_{16} has also been found to be involved in activation of mitogen-activated protein (MAP) kinases as well as STAT3. Thus, melatonin stimulates JNK involving G_{16} *(72)*, and constitutive active $G_{16}\alpha$ is reported to stimulate STAT3 involving c-Src/Janus kinase and ERK *(73)*. Moreover, G_{16} appears to couple a wide range of different GPCRs, and has attained interest as a tool to compare agonist properties *(74)*.

2.4. $G_{12/13}$

The widely distributed G_{12} and G_{13} proteins (42–43 kDa) constitute the most recently discovered class of heterotrimeric G proteins *(65,75,76)*. Although G_{12} and G_{13} are insensitive to PTX, novel observations suggest that pasteurella multocida toxin activates these proteins *(77)*, in addition to its effect on G_q. G_{12} and G_{13} exhibit 67% amino acid identity and couple thrombin, thromboxan A_2 and lysophosphatidic acid receptors. Actin polymerization, phospholipase A_2 activity, and activation of Na^+/H^+ exchanger are reported to implicate $G_{12/13}$. On the other hand, $G_{12/13}$ proteins do not stimulate IP_3 generation *(76)*, but may elicit increases in intracellular Ca^{2+} levels *(78)*. Several of the effects mediated by $G_{12/13}$ such as the stimulation of JNK and activation of the cyclooxygenase-2 promoter involve small G proteins like Rho, Rac, or Ras *(79,80)*. $G_{13}\alpha$ activate Rho through direct stimulation of guanine nucleotide exchange factor RhoGEF *(81)* and $G_{12}\alpha$ is reported to directly stimulate Brutons tyrosine kinase and a Ras GTPase-activating protein *(82)*. In COS-7 cells, ERK was reported to be inhibited by $G_{12/13}$ *(83)*. Moreover, there is evidence that G_{12} interacts with the heat shock protein 90 and that G_{13} interacts with radixin whereas both G proteins interact with protein phosphatase type 5 *(84)*. Despite intensive research the understanding of the roles and signaling mediated by G_{12} and G_{13} proteins is still limited, in part as a result of a lack of identified effector systems *(85)*.

3. G Proteins in Disease

The heterotrimeric G proteins are involved in various diseases through mechanisms involving modifications of $G\alpha$-subunits, genetic changes and conceivably by acting as transducers of signals implicated in pathogenetic processes, which, in some cases, may involve quantitative changes in certain subgroups of G proteins. However, it is difficult to define how tight the observed alterations in G protein levels are connected to the disease mechanisms; i.e., whether they only reflect secondary changes or if they are integrated in significant pathogenetic steps. The disease groups covered here, that could have been even more extended, represent main clinical areas wherere there is evidence, although to a variable extent, for an involvement of G proteins.

3.1. Infections

Bacteria, viruses as well as parasites may utilize G protein-dependent pathways in disease mechanisms. One of the early recognized G protein diseases was cholera involving modification of the $G\alpha$-subunit. The watery diarrhea induced by *V. cholerae* is a result of the actions mediated by CTX, which ADP-ribosylates $G_s\alpha$ *(35)*. This modification strongly activates AC leading to an increase in intracellular cyclic AMP levels in intestinal cells and, finally, secretion of salt and water. In whooping cough or pertussis, caused by the bacteria *B. pertussis*, the main secreted toxin, PTX, inactivates $G_i\alpha$ *(36)*. The precise role of this particular molecular mechanism in the pathogenesis of pertussis is, however, still not fully understood. Furthermore, it is reported that nontypeable *Haemophilus influenza* invades host cells in a G_i-dependent manner *(86)*.

Disease states induced by several viruses involve GPCRs through different mechanisms *(87)*. Herpesviruses and poxviruses encode GPCRs that are homologues to chemokine receptors and may act in a constitutive manner. For example, there is evidence that the human herpesvirus 8 or Kaposi's sarcoma-associated virus encodes a chemokine GPCR, which promotes the development of Kaposi's sarcomas *(88,89)*. Also the Epstein–Barr virus, which is involved in diseases like infectious mononucleosis and Burkitt's lymphoma, encode a GPCR acting through G_i-dependent mechanisms *(90)*. On the other hand, the molecular pathways utilized by HIV involve chemokine receptors representing coreceptors for virus cell entry, primarily the CXC-chemokine receptor-4 and the chemokine-receptor-5 *(87)*. The receptors, which couple to heterotrimeric G proteins, may be affected by genetic defects, and thus it was previously reported that homozygous loss of function in such coreceptors provides resistance to HIV-1 cell entry *(91)*.

The *GNB3* C825T polymorphism, affecting the G-protein β3-subunit, is reported to be associated with increased function of immune cells in humans *(92)*. On the other hand, recent findings in patients with hepatitis C who carry the *GNB3* 825 CC genotype, showed an association to a lack of treatment effect in response to the combination of interferon-α and ribavirin *(93)*. The *GNB3* 825 CC genotype has recently also been found to be associated with sudden infant death as a result of infection *(94)*. Thus, it appears that the *GNB3* 825 CC genotype somehow is unfavorable in relation to certain infectious states.

Also parasite infections have been reported to involve heterotrimeric G proteins, as it was detected that the β_2-adrenergic receptor with its cognate $G_s\alpha$ protein regulates the entry of *Plasmodium falciparum* into erythrocytes *(95)*.

3.2. Inflammation

Several observations indicate a role for heterotrimeric G proteins in inflammatory responses. Mice deficient of $G_{12}\alpha$ develop a lethal diffuse colitis, which is related to ulcerative colitis *(96)*, and the development of the colitis was preceded by activation of the immune system in the intestine *(97)*. Recent findings have shown that long-term treatment with anti-α4-integrin antibodies aggravated the colitis in these animals, whereas short-term treatments performed in earlier studies counteracted the inflammation *(98)*.

In other experimental models, it has been shown that lysophospholipids produced from activated platelets and acting as wound-healing factors in the endothelium involve G_i-dependendent mechanisms *(99)*. A role for $G_{12}\alpha$ has also recently been reported in a model of pulmonary immune complex inflammation *(100)*. Based on studies in $G_{12}\alpha$-deficient mice, it is suggested that the $G_{13}\alpha$ protein may be involved in homing of T cells. Also G_{12} and G_{13} proteins are believed to be implicated in B- and T-cell functions, including homing and motility. Lsc, which is the murine homolog to the human guanine exchange factor RhoGEF, is activated by $G_{13}\alpha$ and plays an important role in actin polymerization in both B and T cells, marginal zone B-cell homeostasis and immune responses *(101)*.

Furthermore, previous experiments in a human lymphoblastic B-cell line also indicated a role for heterotrimeric Gβγ-proteins in the assembly of terminal complement complexes (C5b-7, C5b-8, and C5b-9) in inflammatory reactions *(102)*. On the other hand, G_s signaling in response to stimulation of the A2A adenosine receptor attenuates proinflammatoric transcription and appears to play an important role in regulating overactive immune cells *(103)*.

3.3. Neurological Diseases

Certain data suggest that G protein pathways may play a role in neurological diseases including epilepsy and Alzheimer's disease. Various experimental models used in studies of epilepsy shed light on mechanisms involving GPCRs and their heterotrimeric G proteins. In mice it was found that the neuropeptide Y receptor, Y5R, mediated antiepileptic actions of neuropeptide Y regulating limbic seizures *(104)*. Limbic status epilepticus in a rat model was also recently reported to be counteracted by galanin through the GPCRs, GalR1, and GalR2, whereas inhibition with PTX increased the severity of the epileptic state *(105)*. In rats with genetic absence epilepsy from Strasbourg (GAERS), injections with PTX decreased seizures suggesting a role for G_i-dependent mechanisms *(106)*.

In a rat-kindling model of epilepsy, where epileptogenesis is induced in response to electric stimulation, increases in mRNA levels in brain for both $G_s\alpha$ (bilaterally) and $G_{12}\alpha$ (only on stimulated side) were detected *(107)*. In accordance with a possible role for $G_s\alpha$, it was earlier demonstrated that intrahippocampal administration of CTX into rats resulted in epileptic seizures *(108)*. Interestingly, recent observations have also demonstrated that γ-subunits of

G proteins may play a role in epilepsy, as mice deficient of the γ_3-subunit are more susceptible to seizures *(109)*.

In Alzheimer's disease, which involves dysfynctional cholinergic signaling observed at early stages, there is evidence of a decreased coupling of muscarinic M_1-receptors to heterotrimeric G proteins assessed in postmortem neocortex of Alzheimer patients *(110)*. This is in accordance with earlier observations suggesting an uncoupling between receptors and G proteins in Alzheimer's disease *(111)*. In familial Alzheimer's disease, a majority of the patients have a mutation in genes for presenilin. Presenilin is a membrane protein localized in the endoplasmatic reticulum as well as in other areas, and it has been reported that presenilin-1 interacts with the G_o protein and thereby possibly regulating the G protein activity *(112)*.

Also the G_q group of G proteins may play a role in the pathogenesis of neurological disease as it has been described ataxia and dysregulation of motor coordination in $G_q\alpha$-deficient mice *(113)*.

3.4. Cardiovascular Diseases

Different disease states in the cardiovascular system appear to implicate components of G protein pathways. Thus, G protein-dependent mechanisms have been reported with relation to hypertension, cardiac hypertrophy, heart failure, as well as atrial fibrillation (AF).

G proteins may influence hypertension both with regard to the control mediated by the autonomic nervous system and the peripheral vasoregulatory control exerted by opposing actions of vasodilators and vasoconstrictors acting on GPCRs. One of the mechanisms characterized in hypertensive patients is an impaired vasodilator response *(114)*. Thus, it was observed early that there was a decreased β-adrenergic response in lymphocytes of hypertensive patients *(115)*. The explanation for this might relate to a weakened interaction between the GPCR and its G protein, an interaction that is modulated, in part, by the phosphorylation state of the receptor. Phosphorylation of the GPCRs are mediated by GPCR kinase family members (GRK) as well as other kinases, and it has been shown in various hypertensive models that the GRKs are overexpressed *(114)*. These findings thus suggest a role for components exerting a regulatory control of G protein pathways in the disease mechanism. This is also the case in a recent study indicating a role for regulator of G protein signaling 2 (RGS2) in hypertension *(116)*. In this study of hypertensive patients, two single-nucleotide polymorphisms were found to be associated with the hypertensive phenotype *(116)*. These observations are of particular interest with regard to the regulatory role of RGS2 proteins toward G protein signaling. RGS2 acts selectively toward the G protein subunit $G_q\alpha$, which is a main signal transducer for vasoconstrictory agents. Thus, an intact RGS2 function with the ability to attenuate $G_q\alpha$ activity is presumably an important mechanism to counteract the effect of vasoconstrictors and thereby regulate bloodpressure. In concert with this is the recent reported finding that RGS2 acts as an effector of the nitric oxide-cyclic GMP pathway, which itself is a principal counteractor of vasoconstriction *(117)*.

Other G protein mechanisms may also play a role in hypertension. Thus, it has been found that expression of the $G_{12}\alpha$ protein was significantly higher in fibroblasts from hypertensive individuals compared to controls *(118)*, and the *GNB3* C825T polymorphism, affecting the G protein β3-subunit *(119)*, has been found associated with hypertension. Recent findings also suggest a role for G_s proteins in hypertension as an association was found to a GNAS1 gene variant *(120)*.

GPCRs, G proteins and their downstream effectors are involved in normal and pathological regulation of the mammalian myocardium. Cardiac hypertrophy, which is an independent risk factor for heart failure and death, may result from a number of different physiological and pathological conditions. A G protein-dependent pathway, which is believed to play an important role in the development of hypertrophy, involves enhanced $G_{\alpha q}$ signaling *(121,122)*. Agonists such as angiotensin II, α-adrenergic agents and endothelin-1 stimulate through their membrane receptors $G_q\alpha$ signaling and have also been linked to hypertrophic responses. Furthermore, a recent report also describes an association of the *GNB3* C825T polymorphism with left-ventricular hypertrophy *(123)*.

The underlying molecular mechanisms in heart failure are reported to involve an impaired β-adrenergic receptor function in heart that affects both receptor density as well as sensitivity *(124)*. The amount of β-adrenergic receptors of the β1-subtype decreases, whereas the sensitivity both in β-1- and β-2-adrenergic receptors is lowered through desensitization, which in part is mediated by GRK, denoted β-adrenergic receptor kinases (βARK). There are typical changes in βARK function in heart failure involving increases in the level of βARK-subtype 1 appearing even before the disease is precipitated *(124)*. Thus, inhibition of βARK function is a potential treatment strategy in heart failure *(124)*. In heart failure models it has also been detected changes in the levels of G proteins including increases of $G_q\alpha$ and $G_i\alpha$ *(122,125)*.

The *GNB3* C825T polymorphism has recently been linked also to the risk for AF *(126)*. In a study of 292 patients with AF compared to an equal control group the prevalence of GNB3 TT genotype was 5.8% in the group of AF-patients and 12.0% in the controls. Thus, homozygous carriers of the T allele had a 54% lower risk for AF. However, this risk reduction did not apply to the heterozygous T-allele carriers. The explanation for the observed risk reduction in the homozygous T-allele carriers is not clear. Findings of increased activity in atrial inward rectifier potassium currents in homozygous T-allele carriers might be of relevance *(127)*. The *GNB3* C825T polymorphism presumably results in an increased signal transduction possibly mediated through G_i proteins *(119)*, which in some way may be favorable with regard to the risk of AF. Of note are novel findings using a gene therapeutic strategy by overexpression of the $G_{i2}\alpha$ protein in porcine atrioventricular node resulting in improved heart rate control in a model of persistent AF *(128)*.

3.5. Cancer

Heterotrimeric G proteins are involved in cell growth and proliferation through their integration with intracellular cascades and networks *(129–131)*. However, the more direct evidence for their transforming potentials are derived primarily from studies of mutant forms of their G protein α-subunits.

Several data support a role of G_i proteins in regulation of gene expression *(132)* and cell growth *(133–135)*, and in hepatocellular carcinoma increased levels of G_i proteins have been detected *(136)*. The mutated $G_{i2}\alpha$ protein *gip2* has been found in ovarian sex chord tumors and adrenal cortical tumors and transforms Rat1a fibroblasts *(137–140)*. The constitutive active Q205L $G_o\alpha$ protein is also reported to transform NIH3T3 cells, murine fibroblasts, through activation of STAT3 *(141)*.

$G_{q/11}$ proteins are involved in ERK activation *(39)* as well as growth regulation *(67)*, but mutant forms of these proteins have so far not been identified in any tumors *(131)*. Expression of the GTPase-deficient $G_q\alpha$ mutant, $G_{\alpha q}$Q209L was observed to cause either cell death *(142)* or transformation *(143)*. In addition, certain data suggest that $G_{q/11}$ proteins may somehow be involved in development of hepatocellular carcinoma *(144)*.

$G_{12/13}$ proteins are involved in growth regulation and exhibit marked transforming properties in fibroblasts *(145–147)*, but no mutations have been detected so far in human cancers. However, overexpression of the native $G_{12/13}$ proteins has been detected in prostate, breast, and colon adenocarcinoma cells *(131)*, but the precise role of these changes are not clear. Recent studies in NIH3T3 murine fibroblasts stimulating protease-activated receptor-1 with thrombin, suggest a more concerted action by different G proteins in the processes of cellular transformation *(148)*. Although $G_i\alpha$ was found to be involved in ERK activation, also $G_q\alpha$ and/or $G_{13}\alpha$ were needed to achieve cellular transformation.

GTPase-deficient mutants of $G_s\alpha$, initially discovered in various endocrine tumors, activate the cyclic AMP/protein kinase A pathways constitutively *(140)*. Although expression of these mutated G proteins do not result in transformation of Swiss 3T3 cells *(149)*, and suppressed Ras-induced transformation of NIH 3T3 cells *(150)*, findings in prostate cancer cells support a role for

$G_s\alpha$-induced pathways in tumor progression and metastatic capability *(151)*. Furthermore, recent data indicate that a polymorphism in the $G_s\alpha$ protein, GNAS1 T393C is a marker for survival in colorectal cancer stages I and II *(152)*. The GNB3 C825T polymorphism has also recently been reported to influence disease progression in bladder cancer *(153)*.

3.6. Endocrine Disorders

Defects in G protein-signaling have been detected in certain endocrine disorders caused by mutations in the $G_s\alpha$ gene, *GNAS1*, and are thoroughly reviewed *(154,155)*. To date, no mutations resulting in monogenic diseases in humans have been detected in the genes for the β- or γ-subunits. In principle, the mutations in the $G_s\alpha$ gene are either gain-of-function mutations resulting in increased signal transduction owing to a constitutive G protein activity thereby mimicking states of endocrine hyperfunction, or loss-of-function mutations causing hormonal resistance and endocrine hypofunction. An example is the McCune-Albright syndrome involving a somatic gain-of-function mutation in the $G_s\alpha$ gene causing polyostotic fibrous dysplasia, café-au-lait skin hyperpigmentation, and autonome hyperfunction of endocrine organs. This syndrome is not believed to be inherited, although possible exceptions may have been discovered, and presents a variable clinical picture presumably dependent on the time in embryogenesis for the occurrence of the mutation.

Albright's hereditary osteodystrophy is caused by a heterozygous loss-of-function mutation in the $G_s\alpha$ gene resulting in a clinical picture with presentation of short stature, short fingers and toes, obesity, mild mental retardation, as well as other components. However, clinical presentations may vary. Furthermore, it has become evident that the phenomena of genetic imprinting, affects $G_s\alpha$. Thus, patients who receive $G_s\alpha$ mutations maternally develop hormonal resistance (pseudohypoparathyroidism type Ia) in addition to the Albright's hereditary osteodystrophy, because the maternal defect allele tends to be expressed in various organs under hormonal control. On the other hand, the paternally derived defect $G_s\alpha$ alleles are silenced owing to genetic imprinting, and thus the phenotype will be limited to Albright's hereditary osteodystrophy.

Several observations suggest that heterotrimeric G proteins can be linked to actions and regulation of insulin. G_i proteins have been implicated in mediating insulin signaling as well as in the development of insulin resistance, and also G_q might play a role for insulin action. *(48,118,156)*. Furthermore, recent observations support a physiological role of the G_z protein in the pancreatic β-cell function *(59)*. Somatostatin, prostaglandin E_1, and other agents have the ability to reduce the insulin secretion from β cells in response to glucose. The recent findings demonstrated that $G_z\alpha$ is necessary for the prostaglandin E_1-induced inhibition of the glucose-stimulated insulin secretion in these cells.

The data also show that the components of the specific $G_z\alpha$ axis, i.e., $G_z\alpha$, Rap1GAP, and Rap1, are functionally active in the β cells. These observations thus implicate G proteins in the regulatory control of pancreatic islet β-cell function.

A recently discovered polymorphism affecting a β-subunit of G proteins, the so called *GNB3* C825T polymorphism is reported to be associated with diabetes type 2 and obesity *(119,157)*. This polymorphism, affecting the $G\beta_3$ gene, results in a truncated splice variant of the $G\beta_3$ protein, denoted $G\beta_{3s}$, lacking 41 amino acids compared to the native protein. The expression of the $G\beta_{3s}$-splice variant is reported to enhance G protein activation, preferentially through G_i proteins.

4. Concluding Remarks and Potentials for Therapeutic Options

Heterotrimeric G proteins transduce signals in response to a number of hormones and neurotransmitters. Furthermore, about 50% of all drugs used in therapy act through GPCRs, thus emphasizing the importance of GPCR/G protein signaling pathways in medical treatment. In addition to the role of G proteins in signaling mechanisms, the identification of their localization also intracellularly as well as the discovery of novel receptor-independent mechanisms for their activation, suggest that G proteins may have other important cellular functions than acting as signal transducers. In light of this, the growing body of evidence that connects heterotrimeric G proteins to various diseases, is not surprising. Added to the initial discoveries that toxin-mediated modifications of G proteins may cause infectious disease as well as the delineation of $G_s\alpha$ mutations as the cause of certain endocrine disorders, is an emerging understanding of a more complex role for G proteins in disease mechanisms. Thus, it is conceivable that G proteins may contribute as transducers or components within more integrated signaling networks in diseases of multigenic/multifactorial origin. For example, the recently discovered *GNB3* C825T polymorphism has been associated with various diseases such as hypertension, diabetes type 2, AF, disease progression in bladder cancer, and response to a certain treatment of hepatitis C. Presently, it is not known how this particular single-nucleotide polymorphism may affect disease development in these different clinical settings. However, it is possible that the *GNB3* C825T polymorphism provides a mechanism, possibly enhanced G_i protein signaling, which somehow might facilitate or act in a permissive manner related to different pathogenetic processes. In any case, this example of a potential G protein-dependent pathogenetic mechanism challenges the approach of understanding more complex disease states.

The possibility that heterotrimeric G proteins may become candidates for medical treatment will depend on several conditions, first, the identification of significant and clinically relevant targets as well as the development of efficient and selective molecular strategies. Of the numerous possible G protein targets, both the Gβγ dimer and the G_i protein have been explored in experimental models with relevance for cardiovascular diseases. A molecular strategy for targeting the Gβγ dimer utilizes an inhibitor of the enzyme β-adrenergic receptor kinase, βARK1, denoted βARKct, which is a peptide consisting of the last 194 amino acids of βARK1 *(158)*. This sequence also contains a specific Gβγ-binding domain, and the βARK1ct can thus be used to counteract Gβγ-mediated signaling, which, in turn, also blocks the Gβγ-dependent translocation of βARK1 to the membrane. This translocation is necessary for the activation of βARK1. These inhibitory actions of βARK1ct have been studied in various models. Thus, inhibition of the Gβγ-subunit in arterial vascular smooth muscle through adenovirus-mediated gene transfer of βARKct was shown to dramatically reduce intima hyperplasia and thereby may reveal a novel strategy to treat restenosis after percutaneous transluminal coronary angioplasty *(158)*. Furthermore, as increased expression and function of the βARK1 is believed to be implicated in heart failure by mediating downregulation of β-adrenergic receptors, the use of βARKct may represent a potential treatment strategy *(124)*. Recent studies with gene transfer of βARKct in a rabbit model for cardiac dysfunction showed increased right-ventricular afterload owing to pulmonary artery banding (inducing early right ventricular hypertrophy and dilatation), also resulted in improvement of ventricular performance *(159)*.

Other models have explored direct manipulation of the levels of G proteins. Notably, in studies of persistent AF the overexpression of G_i-protein resulted in improved heart rate control *(128)*. The further characterization of possible strategies to target G proteins in various disease-related systems may also take advantage of tools such as ribozymes and RNA interference *(160)*.

The increasing knowledge of the mechanisms in G protein signaling including the discovery of a number of accessory G protein partners, may uncover novel targets for drug treatment. In this regard, both AGS as well as regulators of G protein signaling (RGS) might be candidates. The RGS2 protein, which appears to be implicated in hypertension *(116)*, mediating actions of nitric oxide, is one possible target.

Finally, an important issue concering the potential of targeting intracellular signaling components in medical therapy, such as G proteins, is the risk level for unwanted effects. As outlined in the first part of this review, G proteins are key elements in numerous signaling pathways, and may exert other important cellular functions. Therefore, the possibility of provoking serious side effects, by targeting key signaling molecules, must obviously be carefully evaluated. This circumstance is an essential condition, which needs to be addressed in terms of demands for a high degree of cell and target selectivity, if a further development of G protein therapeutic strategies shall succeed.

References

1. Rodbell, M. (1980) The role of hormone receptors and GTP-regulatory proteins in membrane transduction. *Nature* **284,** 17–22.
2. Rodbell, M. (1995) Signal transduction: evolution of an idea. *Biosci. Rep.* **15,** 117–133.
3. Rodbell, M. (1997) The complex regulation of receptor-coupled G-proteins. *Adv. Enzyme Reg.* **37,** 427–435.
4. Gilman, A. (1995) G proteins and regulation of adenylyl cyclase. *Biosci. Rep.* **15,** 65–97.
5. Neer, E. J. (1995) Heterotrimeric G proteins: organizers of transmembrane signals. *Cell* **80,** 249–257.
6. Birnbaumer, L. and Birnbaumer, M. (1995) Signal transduction by G proteins: 1994 edition. *J. Recept. Signal. Transduct. Res.* **15,** 213–252.
7. Birnbaumer, M. (1995) Mutations and diseases of G protein-coupled receptors. *J. Recept. Signal Transduct. Res.* **15,** 131–160.
8. Hamm, H. E. (1998) The many faces of G protein signaling. *J. Biol. Chem.* **273,** 669–672.
9. Berman, D. M. and Gilman, A. G. (1998) Mammalian RGS proteins: barbarians at the gate. *J. Biol. Chem.* **273,** 1269–1272.
10. Hepler, J. R. (1999) Emerging roles for RGS proteins in cell signalling. *Trends Pharmacol. Sci.* **20,** 376–382.
11. Rebois, R. V., Warner, D. R., and Basi, N. S. (1997) Does subunit dissociation necessarily accompany the activation of all heterotrimeric G proteins? *Cell. Signal.* **9,** 141–151.
12. Basi, N. S., Okuya, S., and Rebois, R. V. (1996) GTP binding to G$_s$ does not promote subunit dissociation. *Cell Signal.* **8,** 209–215.
13. Chidiac, P. (1998) Rethinking receptor-G protein-effector interactions. *Biochem. Pharmacol.* **55,** 549–556.
14. Klein, S., Reuveni, H., and Levitzki, A. (2000) Signal transduction by a nondissociable heterotrimeric yeast G protein. *Proc. Acad. Nat. Sci. USA* **97,** 3219–3223.
15. Gutkind, J. S. (1998) Cell growth control by G protein-coupled receptors: from signal transduction to signal integration. *Oncogene* **17,** 1331–1342.
16. Takesono, A., Cismowski, M. J., Ribas, C., et al. (1999) Receptor-independent activators of heterotrimeric G-protein signaling pathways. *J. Biol. Chem.* **274,** 33,202–33,205.
17. Sato, M., Blumer, J. B., Simon, V., and Lanier S. M. (2005) Accessory proteins for G proteins: partners in signaling. *Ann. Rev. Pharmacol.* **46,** 151–187.
18. Hepler, J. R. and Gilman, A. G. (1992) G proteins. *Trends Biochem. Sci.* **17,** 383–387.

19. Takei, Y., Kurosu, H., Takahashi, K., and Katada, T. (1992) A GTP-binding protein in rat liver nuclei serving as the specific substrate of pertussis toxin-catalyzed ADP-ribosylation. *J. Biol. Chem.* **267**, 5085–5089.

20. Cadrin, M., McFarlane-Anderson, N., Harper, M. E., Gaffield, J., and Begin-Heick, N. (1996) Comparison of the subcellular distribution of G-proteins in hepatocytes in situ and in primary cultures. *J. Cell. Biochem.* **62**, 334–341.

21. Crouch, M. F. and Simson, L. (1997) The G-protein G_i regulates mitosis but not DNA synthesis in growth factor-activated fibroblasts: a role for the nuclear translocation of G_i. *FASEB J.* **11**, 189–198.

22. Khan, Z. U. and Gutierrez, A. (2004) Distribution of C-terminal splice variant of $G_{\alpha i2}$ in rat and monkey brain. *Neuroscience* **127**, 833–843.

23. Simonds, W. F., Woodard G. E., and Zhang, J. -H. (2004) Assays of nuclear localization of R7/$G\beta_5$ compelxes. *Meth. Enzymol.* **390**, 210–223.

24. Kino, T., Tiulpakov, A., Ichijo, T., Chheng, L., Kozasa, T., and Chrousos, G. P. (2005) G protein β interacts with the glucocorticoid receptor and suppresses its transcriptional activity in the nucleus. *J. Cell Biol.* **169**, 885–896.

25. Rodbell, M., Birnbaumer, L., Pohl, S. L., and Krans, H. M. J. (1971) The glucagon-sensitive adenylyl cyclase system in plasma membranes of rat liver. V. An obligatory role of guanyl nucleotides in glucagon action. *J. Biol. Chem.* **246**, 1877–1882.

26. Pfeuffer, T. and Helmreich, E. J. M. (1975) Activation of pigeon erythrocyte membrane adenylate cyclase by guanyl nucleotide analogues and separation of nucleotide-binding protein. *J. Biol. Chem.* **250**, 867–876.

27. Ross, E. M., and Gilman, A. G. (1977) Resolution of some components of adenylate cyclase necessary for catalytic activity. *J. Biol. Chem.* **252**, 6966–6969.

28. Daaka, Y., Luttrell. L. M., and Lefkowitz, R. J. (1997) Switching of the coupling of the β_2-adrenergic receptor to different G proteins by protein kinase A. *Nature* **390**, 88–91.

29. Crespo, P., Cachero, T. G., Xu, N., and Gutkind, J. S. (1995) Dual effect of β-adrenergic receptors on mitogen-activated protein kinase. Evidence for a βγ-dependent activation and a $G\alpha_s$- cAMP-mediated inhibition. *J. Biol. Chem.* **270**, 25,259–25,265.

30. Grewal, S. S., Horgan, A. M., York, R. D., Withers, G. S., Banker, G. A., and Stork. P. J. S. (2000) Neuronal calcium activates a Rap1 and a B-Raf signaling pathway via the cyclic adenosine monophosphate-dependent protein kinase. *J. Biol. Chem.* **275**, 3722–3728.

31. Ganpat, M. M., Nishimura, M., Toyoshige, M., Okuya, S., Pointer, R. H. and Rebois, R. V. (1999) Evidence for stimulation of adenylyl cyclase by an activated G(s) heterotrimer in cell membranes: an experimental method for controlling the G(s) subunit composition of cell membranes. *Cell Signal.* **12**, 113–122.

32. Nair, B. G., Parikh, B., Milligan, G., and Patel, T. B. (1990) Gs alpha mediates epidermal growth factor-elicited stimulation of rat cardiac adenylate cyclase. *J. Biol. Chem.* **265**, 21,317–21,322.

33. Ramirez, I., Tebar, F., Grau, M., and Soley, M. (1995) Role of heterotrimeric G-proteins in epidermal growth factor signalling. *Cell. Signal.* **7**, 303–311.
34. Sato-Kubasata, K., Yajima, Y., and Kawashima, S. (2000) Persistent activation of $G_s\alpha$ through limited proteolysis by calpain. *Biochem. J.* **347**, 733–740.
35. Moss, J. and Vaughan, M. (1979) Activation of adenylate cyclase by choleragen. *Ann. Rev. Biochem.* **48**, 581–600.
36. Murayama, T. and Ui, M. (1983) Loss of the inhibitory function of the guanine nucleotide regulatory component of adenylate cyclase due to its ADP ribosylation by islet-activating protein, pertussis toxin, in adipocyte membranes. *J. Biol. Chem.* **258**, 3319–3326.
37. Morris, A. J. and Malbon, C. C. (1999) Physiological regulation of G protein-linked signaling. *Physiol. Rev.* **79**, 1373–1430.
38. Exton, J. H. (1997) Cell signalling through guanine-nucleotide-binding regulatory proteins (G proteins) and phospholipases. *Eur. J. Biochem.* **243**, 10–20.
39. van Biesen, T., Luttrell, L. M., Hawes, B. E., and Lefkowitz, R. J. (1996) Mitogenic signaling via G protein-coupled receptors. *Endocr. Rev.* **17**, 698–714.
40. Hedin, K. E., Bell, M. P., Huntoon, C. J., Karnitz, L. M., and McKean, D. J. (1999) G_i proteins use a novel $\beta\gamma$- and Ras-independent pathway to activate extracellular signal-regulated kinase and mobilize AP-1 transcription factors in Jurkat T lymphocytes. *J. Biol. Chem.* **274**, 19,992–20,001.
41. Takeda, H., Matozaki, T., Takada, T., et al. (1999) PI 3-kinase γ and protein kinase C-ζ mediate RAS-independent activation of MAP kinase by a G_i protein-coupled receptor. *EMBO J.* **18**, 386–395.
42. Kranenburg, O., Verlaan, I., Hordijk, P. L., and Molenaar, W. H. (1997) G_i-mediated activation of the Ras/MAP kinase pathway involves a 100 kDa tyrosine-phosphorylated Grb2 SH3 binding protein, but not Src nor Shc. *EMBO J.* **16**, 3097–3105.
43. Melien, Ø., Thoresen, G. H., Sandnes, D., Østby, E., and Christoffersen, T. (1998) Activation of p42/p44 mitogen-activated protein kinase by angiotensin II, vasopressin, norepinephrine, and prostaglandin $F_{2\alpha}$ in hepatocytes is sustained, and like the effect of epidermal growth factor, mediated through pertussis toxin-sensitive mechanisms. *J. Cell. Physiol.* **175**, 348–358.
44. Corre, I. and Hermouet, S. (1995) Regulation of colony-stimulating factor 1-induced proliferation by heterotrimeric G_{i2} proteins. *Blood* **86**, 1776–1783.
45. Miller, B. A., Bell, L., Hansen, C. A., Robishaw, J. D., Linder, M. E., and Cheung, J. Y. (1996) G-protein α subunit Giα2 mediates erythropoietin signal transduction in human erythroid precursors. *J. Clin. Invest.* **98**, 1728–1736.
46. Church, J. G. and Buick, R. N. (1988) G-protein-mediated epidermal growth factor signal transduction in a human breast cancer cell line. Evidence for two intracellular pathways distinguishable by pertussis toxin. *J. Biol. Chem.* **263**, 4242–4246.
47. Liang, M. and Garrison, J. C. (1991) The epidermal growth factor receptor is coupled to a pertussis toxin-sensitive guanine nucleotide regulatory protein in rat hepatocytes. *J. Biol. Chem.* **266**, 13,342–13,349.

48. Sanchez-Margalet, V., Gonzalez-Yanes, C., Santos-Alvarez, J., and Najib, S. (1999) Insulin activates $G\alpha_{i1,2}$ protein in rat hepatoma (HTC) cell membranes. *Cell. Mol. Life. Sci.* **55**, 142–147.

49. Gao, J., Li, J., Chen, Y., and Ma, L. (2005) Activation of tyrosine kinase of EGFR induces Gβγ-dependent GRK-EGFR complex formation. *FEBS Lett.* **579**, 122–126.

50. Stow, J. L., de Almeida, J. B., Narula, N., Holtzman, E. J., Ercolani, L., and Ausiello, D. A. (1991) A heterotrimeric G protein, G alpha i-3, on Golgi membranes regulates the secretion of a heparan sulfate proteoglycan in LLC-PK$_1$ epithelial cells. *J. Cell. Biol.* **114**, 1113–1124.

51. Nürnberg, B. and Ahnert-Hilger, G. (1996) Potential roles of heterotrimeric G proteins of the endomembrane system. *FEBS Lett.* **389**, 61–65.

52. Yamaguchi, T., Yamamoto, A., Furuno, A., et al. (1997) Possible involvement of heterotrimeric G proteins in the organization of the Golgi apparatus. *J. Biol. Chem.* **272**, 25,260–25,266.

53. Jamora, C., Yamanouye, N., Van Lint, J., et al. (1999) Gβγ-mediated regulation of Golgi organization is through the direct activation of protein kinase D. *Cell* **98**, 59–68.

54. Takei, Y., Takahashi, K., Kanaho, Y., and Katada, T. (1994) Possible involvement of a pertussis toxin-sensitive GTP-binding protein in protein transport into nuclei isolated from rat liver. *J. Biochem. (Tokyo)* **115**, 578–583.

55. Saha, C., Nigam, S. K., and Denker, B. M. (1996) Involvement of $G\alpha_{i2}$ in the maintenance and biogenesis of epithelial cell tight junctions. *J. Biol. Chem.* **273**, 21,629–21,633.

56. Jordan, J. D., Carey, K. D., Stork, P. J. S., and Iyengar, R. (1999) Modulation of Rap Activity by direct interaction of $G\alpha_o$ with Rap1 GTPase-activating protein. *J. Biol. Chem.* **274**, 21,507–21,510.

57. Ram, P. T., Horvath, C. M., and Iyengar, R. (2000) Stat3-mediated transformation of NIH-3T3 cells by the constitutively active Q205L $G\alpha_o$ protein. *Science* **287**, 142–144.

58. Strittmatter, S. M., Valenzuela, D., Kennedy, T. E., Neer, E. J., and Fishman, M. C. (1990) G_o is a major growth cone protein subject to regulation by GAP-43. *Nature* **344**, 836–841.

59. Kimple, M. E., Nixon, A. B., Kelly, P., et al. (2005) A role for G_z in pancreatic islet β-cell biology. *J. Biol. Chem.* **280**, 31,708–31,713.

60. Vorobiov, D., Bera, A. K., Keren-Raifman, T., Barzilai, R., and Dascal, N. (2000) Coupling of the muscarinic m2 receptor to G protein-activated K$^+$ channels via $G\alpha_z$ and a receptor-$G\alpha_z$ fusion protein. *J. Biol. Chem.* **275**, 4166–4170.

61. Baumgartner, R. A., Hirasawa, N., Ozawa, K., Gusovsky, F., and Beaven, M. A. (1996) Enhancement of TNF-alpha synthesis by overexpression of G alpha z in a mast cell line. *J. Immunol.* **157**, 1625–1629.

62. Meng, J., Glick, J. L. Polakis, P., and Casey, P. J. (1999) Functional interaction between $G\alpha_z$ and Rap1GAP suggest a novel form of cellular cross-talk. *J. Biol. Chem.* **274**, 36,663–36,669.

63. Meng, J. and Casey, P. J. (2002) Activation of G_z attenuates Rap-1mediated differentiation of PC12 cells. *J. Biol. Chem.* **277**, 43,417–43,424.
64. Fan, X., Brass, L. F., Poncz, M., Spitz, F., Maire, P., and Manning, D. R. (2000). The α subunits of G_z and G_i interact with the eyes absent transcription cofactor Eya2, preventing its interaction with the six class of homeodomain-containing proteins. *J. Biol. Chem.* **275**, 32,129–32,134.
65. Fields, T. A. and Casey, P. J. (1997) Signalling functions and biochemical properties of pertussis toxin-resistant G-proteins. *Biochem. J.* **321**, 561–571.
66. Bence, K., Ma, W., Kozasa, T., and Huang, X. (1997) Direct stimulation of Bruton's tyrosine kinase by G(q)-protein α-subunit. *Nature* **389**, 296–299.
67. LaMorte, V. J., Harootunian, A. T., Spiegel, A. M., Tsien, R. Y., and Feramisco, J. R. (1993) Mediation of growth factor induced DNA synthesis and calcium mobilization by G_q and G_{12}. *J. Cell. Biol.* **121**, 91–99.
68. Della Rocca, G. J., van Biesen, T., Daaka, Y., Luttrell, D. K., Luttrell, L. M., and Lefkowitz, R. J. (1997) Ras-dependent mitogen-activated protein kinase activation by G protein- coupled receptors. Convergence of G_i- and G_q-mediated pathways on calcium/calmodulin, Pyk2, and Src kinase. *J. Biol. Chem.* **272**, 19,125–19,132.
69. Wilson, B., Zhu, X., Ho, M., and Lu, L. (1997) *Pasteurella multocida* toxin activates the inositol triphosphate signaling pathway in *Xenopus* oocytes via $G_q\alpha$-coupled phospholipase C-β1. *J. Biol. Chem.* **272**, 1268–1275.
70. Chan, A. S. and Wong, Y. H. (2000) Regulation of c-Jun N-terminal kinase by the ORL(1) receptor through multiple G proteins. *J. Pharmacol. Exp. Ther.* **295**, 1094–1100.
71. Lo, R. K. H. and Wong Y. H. (2004) Signal transducer and activator of transcription 3 activation by the δ-opioid receptor via $G\alpha_{14}$ involves multiple intermediates. *Mol. Pharmacol.* **65**, 1427–1439.
72. Chan, A. S., Lai, F. P., Lo, R. K., Voyno-Yasenetskaya, T. A., Stanbridge, E. J., and Wong, Y. H (2002) Melatonin mt1 and MT2 receptors stimulate c-Jun N-terminal kinase via pertussis toxin-sensitive and –insensitive G proteins. *Cell Signal.* **14**, 249–257.
73. Lo, R. K. H., Cheung, H., and Wong, Y. H. (2003) Constitutively active $G\alpha_{16}$ stimulates STAT3 via a c-Src/JAK- and ERK-dependent mechanism. *J. Biol. Chem.* **278**, 52,154–52,165.
74. Milligan, G., Marshall, F., and Rees, S. (1996) G_{16} as a universal G protein adapter: implications for agonist screening strategies. *Trends Pharm. Sci.* **17**, 235–237.
75. Offermanns, S. and Schultz, G. (1994) What are the functions of the pertussis toxin-insensitive G proteins G_{12}, G_{13}, G_z? *Mol. Cell. Endocrinol.* **100**, 71–74.
76. Dhanasekaran, N. and Dermott, J. M. (1996) Signaling by the G_{12} class of G proteins. *Cell Signal.* **8**, 235–245.
77. Orth, J. H. C., Lang, S., Taniguchi, M., and Aktories, K. (2005) *Pasteurella multocida*-induced activation of RhoA is mediated via two Gα proteins Gα_q and G$\alpha_{12/13}$. *J. Biol. Chem.* **280**, 36,701–36,707.

78. Macrez, N., Morel, J. -L., Kalkbrenner, F., Viard, P., and Schultz, G. (1997) A βγ dimer derived from G_{13} transduces the angiotensin AT_1 receptor signal to stimulation of Ca^{2+} channels in rat portal vein myocytes. *J. Biol. Chem.* **272,** 23,180–23,185.

79. Collins, L. R., Minden, A., Karin, M., and Brown, J. H. (1996) Galpha12 stimulates c-Jun NH2-terminal kinase through the small G proteins Ras and Rac. *J. Biol. Chem.* **271,** 17,349–17,353.

80. Slice, L. W., Walsh, J. H., and Rozengurt, E. (1999) Galpha(13) stimulates Rho-dependent activation of the cyclooxygenase-2 promoter. *J. Biol. Chem.* **274,** 27,562–27,566.

81. Hart, M. J., Jiang, X., Kozasa, T., et al. (1998) Direct stimulation of the guanine nucleotide exchange activity of p115 RhoGEF by $G\alpha_{13}$. *Science* **280,** 2112–2114.

82. Jiang, Y., Ma, W., Wan, Y., Kozasa, T., Hattori, S., and Huang, X. -Y. (1998) The G protein Gα12 stimulates Bruton's tyrosine kinase and rasGAP through a conserved PH/BM domain. *Nature* **395,** 808–813.

83. Voyno-Yasenetskaya, T. A., Faure, M. P., Ahn, N. G., and Bourne, H. R. (1996) Gα12 and Gα13 regulate extracellular signal-regulated kinase and c-Jun kinase pathways by different mechanisms in COS-7 cells. *J. Biol. Chem.* **271,** 21,081–21,087.

84. Kurose, H. (2003) Gα12 and Gα13 as key regulatory mediater in signal transduction. *Life Sci.* **74,** 155–161.

85. Riobo, N. A. and Manning, D. R. (2005) Receptors coupled to heterotrimeric G proteins of the G_{12} family. *Trends Pharmacol. Sci.* **26,** 146–154.

86. Swords, W. E., Ketterer, M. R., Shao, J., Campbell, C. A., Weiser, J. N., and Apicella, M. A. (2001) Binding of the non-typeable *Haemophilus influenzae* lipooligosaccharide to the PAF receptor initiates host cell signalling. *Cell Microbiol.* **3,** 525–536.

87. Sodhi, A., Montaner, S., and Gutkind, J. S. (2004) Viral hijacking of G-protein-coupled-receptor signalling networks. *Nature Mol. Cell. Biol.* **5,** 998–1012.

88. Arvantakis, L., Geras-Raaka, E., Varma, A., Gershengorn, M. C., and Cesarman, E. (1997) Human herpesvirus KSHV encodes a constitutively active G-proetin-coupled receptor linked to cell proliferation. *Nature* **385,** 347–350.

89. Yang, T. -Y., Chen, S. -C., Leach, M. W., et al. (2000) Transgenic expression of the chemokine receptor encoded by Human Herpesvirus 8 indices angioproliferative disease resembling Kaposi's sarcoma. *J. Exp. Med.* **191,** 445–453.

90. Beisser, P. S., Verzijl, D., Gruijthuijsen, Y. K., et al. (2005) The Epstein-Barr vis-rud BILF1 gene encodes a G protein-coupled receptor that inhibits phosphorylation of RNA-dependent protein kinase. *J. Virol.* **79,** 441–449.

91. Liu, R., Paxton, W. A., Choe, S., et al. (1996) Homozygous defect in HIV-1 coreceptor accounts for resistance of some multiply exposed individuals to HIV-1 infection. *Cell* **86,** 367–377.

92. Virchow, S., Ansorge, N., Rubben, H., Siffert, G., and Siffert, W. (1998) Enhanced fMLP-stimulated chemotaxis in human neutrophils from individuals carrying the G protein beta3 subunit 825 T-allele. *FEBS Lett.* **436,** 155–158.

93. Sarrazin, C., Berg, T., Weich, V., et al. (2005) *GNB* C825T polymorphism and response to interferon-alfa/ribavirin treatment in patients with hepatitis C virus genotype 1 (HCV-1) infection. *J. Hepatol.* **43,** 388–393.

94. Opdal, S., Melien, Ø., Rootwelt, H., Vege, Å., Arnestad, M., and Rognum, T. O. *(in press)* The G protein β3 subunit 825C allele is associated with sudden infant death due to infection. *Aeta PQDae.*

95. Harrison, T., Samuel, B. U., Akompong, T., et al. (2003) Erythrocyte G protein-coupled receptor signaling in malarial infection. *Science* **301,** 1734–1736.

96. Rudolph, U., Finegold, M. J., Rich, S. S., et al. (1995) Ulcerative colitis and adenocarcinoma of the colon in αG_{i2}-deficient mice. *Nature Gen.* **10,** 143–150.

97. Öhman, L., Franzén, L., Rudolph, U., Harriman, G. R., and Hörnquist Hultgren, E. (2000) Immune activation in the intestinal mucosa before the onset of colitis in $G\alpha_{i2}$-deficient mice. *Scand. J. Immunol.* **52,** 80–90.

98. Bjursten, M., Bland, P. W., Willén, R., and Hultgren Hörnquist, E. (2005) Long-term treatment with anti-α4 integrin antibodies aggravates colitis in $G\alpha_{i2}$-deficient mice. *Eur. J. Immunol.* **35,** 2274–2283.

99. Lee, H., Chi, L. I., Liao, J. -J., et al. (2004) Lysophospholipids increase ICAM-1 expression in HUVEC through a G_i– and NF-κB-dependent mechanism. *Am. J. Physiol. Cell. Physiol.* **287,** C1657–C1666.

100. Skokowa, J., Syed, A. R., Felda, O., et al. (2005) Macrophages induce the inflammatory response in the pulmonary Arthus reaction through $G\alpha_{i2}$ activation that controls C5aR and Fc receptor cooperation. *J. Immunol.* **174,** 3041–3050.

101. Girkontainte, I., Karine, M., Sakk, V., et al. (2001) Lsc is required for marginal zone B cells, regulation of lymphocyte motility and immune responses. *Nature Immunol.* **2,** 855–862.

102. Niculescu, F., Rus, H., van Biesen, T., and Shin, M. L. (1997) Activation of Ras and mitogen-activated proetin kinase pathways by terminal complement compelxes is G protein dependent. *J. Immunol.* **158,** 4405–4412.

103. Lukashev, D., Ohta, A., Apasov, S., Chen, J. -F., and Sitkovsky, M. (2004) Cutting edge: physiologic attenuation of proinflammatory transcription by the G_s protein-coipled A2A adenosine receptor in vivo. *J. Immunol.* **173,** 21–24.

104. Marsh, D. J., Baraban, S. C., Hollopeter, G., and Palmiter, R. D. (1999) Role of the Y5 neuropeptide Y receptor in limbic seizures. *Proc. Natl. Acad. Sci.* **96,** 13,518–13,523.

105. Mazarati, A. and Lu, X. (2005) Regulation of limbic status epilepticus by hippocampal galanin type 1 and type 2 receptors. *Neuropeptides* **39,** 277–280.

106. Bowery, N. G., Parry, K., Boehrer, A., Mathivet, P., Marescaux, C., and Bernasconi, R. (1999) Pertussis toxin decreases absence seizures and $GABA_B$ receptor binding in thalamus of a genetically prone rat (GAERS). *Neuropharmacol.* **38,** 1691–1697.

107. Iwasa, H., Kikuchi, S., Miyagishima, H., Mine, S., Koseki, K., and Hasegawa, S. (1999) Altered expression levels of G protein subclass mRNAs in various seizure stages of the kindling model. *Brain Res.* **818**, 570–574.

108. Williams, S. F., Colling, S. B., Whittinton, M. A., and Jeffreys, J. G. (1993) Epileptic focus induced by intrahippocampal cholera toxin in rat: time course and properties in vivo and in vitro. *Epilepsy Res.* **16**, 137–146.

109. Schwindlinger, W. F., Giger, K. E., Betz, K. S., et al. (2004) Mice with deficiency of G protein γ_3 are lean and have seizures. *Mol. Cell. Biol.* **24**, 7758–7768.

110. Tsang, S. W. Y., Lai, M. K. P., Kirvell, S., et al. (2005) Impaired coupling of muscarinic M_1 receptors to G-proteins in the neocortex is associated with severity of dementia in Alzheimer's disease. *Neurobiol. Aging* Epub ahead of print.

111. Wang, H. Y. and Friedman, E. (1994) Receptor-mediated activation of G proteins is reduced in postmortem brains from Alzheimer's disease patients. *Neurosci. Lett.* **23**, 37–39.

112. Smine, A., Xu, X., Nishiyama, K., et al. (1998) Regulation of brain G-protein G_o by Alzheimer's disease gene presenilin-1. *J. Biol. Chem.* **273**, 16,281–16,288.

113. Offermanns, S., Hashimoto, K., Watanabe, M., et al. (1997) Impaired motor coordination and presistent multiple climbing fiber innervation of cerebellar Purkinje cells in mice lacking Gαq. *Proc. Nat. Acad. Sci.* **94**, 14,089–14,094.

114. Feldmann, R. D. (2002) Deactivation of vasodilator responses by GRK2 overexpression: a mechanism or *the* mechanism for hypertension? *Mol. Pharmacol.* **61**, 707–709.

115. Feldman, R. D. (1990) Defective venous beta-adrenergic response in borderline hypertensive subjects is corrected by a low sodium diet. *J. Clin. Invest.* **85**, 647–652.

116. Yang, J., Kamide, K., Kokubo, Y., et al. (2005) Genetic variations of regulator of G-protein signaling 2 in hypertensive patients and in the general population. *J. Hypertension* **23**, 1497–1505.

117. Sun, X., Kaltenbronn, K. M., Steinberg, T. H., and Blumer, K. J. (2005) RGS2 is a mediator of nitric oxide action on blood pressure and vasoconstrictor signaling. *Mol. Pharmacol.* **67**, 631–639.

118. Baritono, E., Ceolotto, G., Papparella, I., et al. (2003) Abnormal regulation of G protein α_{i2} subunit in skin fibroblasts from insulin-resistant hypertensive individuals. *J. Hypertension* **22**, 783–792.

119. Siffert, W. (2005) G protein polymorphisms in hypertension, atherosclerosis, and diabetes. *Annu. Rev. Med.* **56**, 17–28.

120. Yamamoto, M., Abe, M., Jin, J. J., et al. (2004) Association of a GNAS1 Gene variant with hypertension and diabetes mellitus. *Hypertens. Res.* **27**, 919–924.

121. Knowlton, K. U., Michel, M. C., Itani, M., et al. (1993) The alpha 1A-adrenergic receptor subtype mediates biochemical, molecular, and morphological features of cultured myocardial cell hypertrophy. *J. Biol. Chem.* **268**, 15,374–15,380.

122. Adams, J. W., Sakata, Y., Davis, M. G., et al. (1998) Enhanced Gαq signaling: a common pathway mediates cardiac hypertrophy and apoptotic heart failure. *Proc. Nat. Acad. Sci.* **95**, 10,140–10,145.

123. Mahmood, M. S., Mian, Z. S., and Afzal, A. (2005) G-protein beta-3 subunit gene 825C>T dimorphism is associated with left ventricular hypertrophy but not essential hypertension. *Med. Sci. Monit.* **11**, CR6–CR9.

124. Hata, J. A., Williams, M. L., and Koch, W. J. (2004) Genetic manipulation of myocardial β-adrenergic receptor activation and desensitization. *J. Mol. Cell. Cardiol.* **37**, 11–21.

125. El-Armouche, A., Zolk, O., Rau, T., and Eschenhagen, T. (2003) Inhibitory G-proteins and their role in desensitization of the adenylyl cyclase pathways in heart failure. *Cardiovasc. Res.* **60**, 478–487.

126. Schreieck, J., Dostal, S., von Beckerath, N., et al. (2004) C825T polymorphism of the G-protein β3 subunit gene and atrial fibrillation: association of the TT genotype with a reduced risk for atrial fibrillation. *Am. Heart. J.* **148**, 545–550.

127. Dobrev, D., Wettwer, E., Himmel, H. M., et al. (2000) G-protein β3 subunit 825T allele is associated with enhanced human atrial inward rectifier potassium currents. *Circulation* **102**, 692–697.

128. Bauer, A., McDonald, A. D., Nasir, K., et al. (2004) Inhibitory G protein overexpression provides physiologically relevant heart rate control in persistent atrial fibrillation. *Circulation* **110**, 3115–3120.

129. Dhanasekaran, N. and Prasad, M. V. (1998) G protein subunits and cell proliferation. *Biol. Signals. Recept.* **7**, 109–117.

130. Christoffersen, T., Thoresen, G. H., Dajani, O. F., et al. (2000) Mechanisms of hepatocyte growth regulation by hormones and growth factors, in *The Hepatocyte Review*, (Berry M. N., Edwards, A. M. eds.), Kluwer Academic Publishers, Dordrecht/ Boston/London pp. 209–246.

131. Marinissen, M. J. and Gutkind, J. S. (2001) G protein-coupled receptors and signaling networks: emerging paradigms. *Trends Pharmacol. Sci.* **22**, 368–376.

132. Chuprun, J. K., Raymond, J. R., and Blackshear, P. J. (1997) The heterotrimeric G protein $G_{\alpha i2}$ mediates lysophosphatidic acid-stimulated induction of the c-*fos* gene in mouse fibroblasts. *J. Biol. Chem.* **272**, 773–781.

133. Harbers, M., Borowski, P., Fanick, W., et al. (1992) Epigenetic activation of Gi-2 protein, the product of a putative protooncogene, mediates tumor promotion in vitro. *Carcinogenesis* **13**, 2403–2406.

134. LaMorte, V. J., Goldsmith, P. K., Spiegel, A. M., Meinkoth, J. L., and Feramisco, J. R. (1992) Inhibition of DNA synthesis in living cells by microinjection of G_{i2} antibodies. *J. Biol. Chem.* **267**, 691–694.

135. Johnson, G. L., Gardner, A. M., Lange-Carter, C., Qian, N. X., Russell, M., and Winitz, S. (1994) How does the G protein, Gi2, transduce mitogenic signals? *J. Cell. Biochem.* **54**, 415–422.

136. McKillop, I. H., Wu, Y., Cahill, P. A., and Sitzmann, J. V. (1998) Altered expression of inhibitory guanine nucleotide regulatory proteins (Gi-proteins) in experimental hepatocellular carcinoma. *J. Cell. Physiol.* **175**, 295–304.

137. Gupta, S. K., Gallego, C., Johnson, G. L., and Heasley, L. E. (1992) MAP kinase is constitutively activated in *gip2* and Src-transformed Rat 1a fibroblasts. *J. Biol. Chem.* **267**, 7987–7990.

138. Vallar, L. (1996) Oncogenic role of heterotrimeric G proteins. *Cancer Surv.* **27**, 325–338.
139. Edamatsu, H., Kaziro, Y., and Itoh, H. (1998) Expression of an oncogenic mutant Gαi2 activates Ras in Rat-1 fibroblast cells. *FEBS Lett.* **440**, 231–234.
140. Dhanasekaran, N., Tsim, S. T., Dermott, J. M., and Onesime, D. (1998) Regulation of cell proliferation by G proteins. *Oncogene* **17**, 1383–1394.
141. Ram, P. T., Horvath, C. M., and Iyengar, R. (2000) Stat3-mediated transformation of NIH-3T3 cells by the constitutively active Q205L Gα$_o$ protein. *Science* **287**, 142–144.
142. Wu, D., Lee, C. H., Rhee, S. G., and Simon, M. I. (1992) Activation of phospholipase C by the α subunits of G$_q$ and G$_{11}$ proteins in transfected Cos-7 cells. *J. Biol. Chem.* **267**, 1811–1817.
143. Kalinec, G., Nazarali, A. J., Hermouet, S., Xu, N., and Gutkind, J. S. (1992) Mutated alpha subunit of the Gq protein induces malignant transformation in NIH 3T3 cells. *Mol. Cell. Biol.* **12**, 4687–4693.
144. McKillop, I. H., Schmidt, C. M., Cahill, P. A., and Sitzmann, J. V. (1999) Altered Gq/G11 guanine nucleotide regulatory protein expression in a rat model of hepatocellular carcinoma: role in mitogenesis. *Hepatology* **29**, 371–378.
145. Xu, N., Voyno-Yasenetskaya, T., and Gutkind, J. S. (1994) Potent transforming activity of the G13 alpha subunit defines a novel family of oncogenes. *Biochem. Biophys. Res. Commun.* **201**, 603–609.
146. Voyno-Yasenetskaya, T. A., Pace, A. M., and Bourne, H. R. (1994) Mutant α subunits of G12 and G13 proteins induce neoplastic transformation of Rat-1 fibroblasts. *Oncogene* **9**, 2559–2565.
147. Dermott, J. M., Reddy, M. V. R., Onesime, D., Reddy, E. P., and Dhanasekaran, N. (1999) Oncogenic mutant of Gα$_{12}$ stimulates cell proliferation through cycloxygenase-2 signaling pathway. *Oncogene* **18**, 7185–7189.
148. Marinissen, M. J., Servitja, J. -M., Offermanns, S., Simon, M. I., and Gutkind, J. S. (2003) Thrombin protease-activated receptor-1 signals through G$_q$- and G$_{13}$- initiated MAPK cascades regulating c-Jun expression to induce cell transformation. *J. Biol. Chem.* **278**, 46,814–46,825.
149. Zachary, I., Masters, S. B., and Bourne, H. R. (1990) Increased mitogenic responsiveness of Swiss 3T3 cells expressing constitutively active Gsα. *Biochem. Biophys. Res. Commun.* **168**, 1184–1193.
150. Chen, J. and Iyengar, R. (1994) Suppression of Ras-induced transformation of NIH 3T3 cells by activated Gα$_s$. *Science* **263**, 1278–1281.
151. Chien, J., Wong, E., Nikes, E., Noble, M. J., Pantazis, C. G., and Shah, G. V. (1999) Constitutive activation of stimulatory guanine nucleotide binding protein (G$_s$αQL)-mediated signaling increases invasiveness and tumorigenicity of PC-3M prostate cancer cells. *Oncogene* **18**, 3376–3382.
152. Frey, U. H., Alakhus, H., Wohlschlaeger, J., et al. (2005) *GNAS1* T393C polymorphism and survival in patients with sporadic colorectal cancer. *Clin. Cancer. Res.* **11**, 5071–5077.

153. Eisenhardt, A., Siffert, W., Rosskopf, D., et al. (2005) Association study of the G-protein beta3 subunit C825T polymorphism with disease progression in patients with bladder cancer. *World J. Urol.* **25,** 1–8.

154. Spiegel, A. M. and Weinstein, L. S. (2004) Inherited disease involving G proteins and G protein-coupled receptors. *Annu. Rev. Med.* **55,** 27–39.

155. Lania, A., Mantovani, G., and Spada, A. (2001) G protein mutations in endocrine diseases. *Eur. J. Endocrinol.* **145,** 543–559.

156. Dalle, S., Ricketts, W., Imamura, T., Vollenweider, P., and Olefsky, J. M. (2001). Insulin and insulin-like growth factor I receptors utilize different G protein signalling components. *J. Biol. Chem.* **276,** 15,688–15,695.

157. Kiani, J. G., Saeed, M., Parvez, S. H., and Frossard, P. M. (2005) Association of G-protein beta-3 subunit gene (GNB3) T825 allele with type II diabetes. *Neuro. Endocrinol. Lett.* **26,** 87–88.

158. Iaccarino, G., Smithwick, L. A., Lefkowitz, R. J., and Koch, W. J. (1999) Targeting $G_{\beta\gamma}$ signalling in arterial vascular smooth muscle proliferation: A novel strategy to limit restenosis. *Proc. Nat. Acad. Sci.* **96,** 3945–3950.

159. Emani, S. M., Shah, A. S., Bowman, M. K., et al. (2004). Right ventricular targeted gene transfer of a β-adrenergic receptor kinase inhibitor improves ventricular performance after pulmonary artery banding. *J. Thorac. Cardiovasc. Surg.* **127,** 787–793.

160. Robishaw, J. D., Guo, Z. P., and Wang, Q. (2004) Ribozymes as tools for suppression of G protein gamma subunits. *Methods. Mol. Biol.* **237,** 169–180.

6

High-Mobility Group Box-1 Isoforms as Potential Therapeutic Targets in Sepsis

William Parrish and Luis Ulloa

Summary

High-mobility group box-1 (HMGB1) protein was originally described as a nuclear DNA-binding protein that functions as a structural cofactor critical for proper transcriptional regulation and gene expression. Recent studies indicate that damaged, necrotic cells liberate HMGB1 into the extracellular milieu where it functions as a proinflammatory cytokine. Indeed, HMGB1 represents a novel family of inflammatory cytokines composed of intracellular proteins that can be recognized by the innate immune system as a signal of tissue damage. Posttranslational modifications of HMGB1 determine its interactions with other proteins and modulate its biological activity. However, very little is known about how these posttranslational modifications of HMGB1 affect its extracellular inflammatory activity and pathological potential. These studies can provide more efficient therapeutic strategies directed against specific HMGB1 isoforms. Therapeutic strategies against these specific HMGB1 isoforms can serve as models for more efficient therapeutic strategies against rheumatoid arthritis or sepsis. This article reviews the recent studies on HMGB1 regulation and their impact on the inflammatory activity and pathological contribution of HMGB1 to infectious and inflammatory disorders.

Key Words: HMGB1; proinflammatory cytokines; sepsis; posttranslational modifications.

1. Introduction

High-mobility group box-1 (HMGB1) was originally identified as a nuclear DNA-binding protein that participates in the assembly of transcriptional complexes in somatic cells *(1,2)*. Recent studies indicate that damaged necrotic cells or activated leukocytes can liberate HMGB1 into the extracellular milieu where it functions as a proinflammatory cytokine *(1–6)*. Thus, HMGB1 represents an intracellular protein that when present in the extracellular milieu is recognized by the innate immune system as a signal of tissue damage. In this context, extracellular

From: *Methods in Molecular Biology, vol. 361, Target Discovery and Validation Reviews and Protocols*
Volume 2, Emerging Molecular Targets and Treatment Options
Edited by: M. Sioud © Humana Press Inc., Totowa, NJ

HMGB1 appears to be a sufficient mediator of systemic inflammation because administration of exogenous HMGB1 causes a constellation of symptoms similar to that found in clinical trauma or severe sepsis *(4–7)*. HMGB1 is a powerful chemotactic and activating signal for inflammation-mediating immune cells such as neutrophils, monocytes, and macrophages *(8–10)*. HMGB1 also acts as a chemotactic and mitogenic signal for smooth muscle cells *(11)*, and specific types of tissue stem cells such as mesoangioblasts, which can differentiate into most mesoderm-derived cell types, including endothelium and muscle *(12,13)*. Collectively, these results suggest that HMGB1 represents a comprehensive cytokine that is able to orchestrate the regulation of both inflammation and tissue regeneration to promote wound healing.

There are two basic mechanisms for cells to liberate HMGB1 into the extracellular milieu **(Fig. 1)**. The first mechanism is a "passive release" of HMGB1 from damaged or necrotic cells. In this context, the extracellular HMGB1 released during necrosis acts as an immune-stimulatory signal that indicates the extent of tissue injury *(7)*. The second mechanism is by "active secretion" of HMGB1 from immune cells. During an immunological challenge, extracellular HMGB1 secreted by immune cells acts as a conventional proinflammatory cytokine *(14,15)*. Both mechanisms result in significant levels of extracellular HMGB1 that can trigger a systemic inflammatory response to ischemia, trauma, burn, infection, or sepsis. Active secretion of HMGB1 requires the execution of a cellular program in activated cells of the innate immune system, especially macrophages and monocytes *(15)*. Although the molecular details of HMGB1 secretion remain unknown, an obligate event in this process is the accumulation of HMGB1 in the cytosol *(14,15)*. Normally, HMGB1 protein is translocated from the cytosol into the nucleus where it binds to DNA and regulates transcription. Nuclear translocation of HMGB1 is controlled by at least two nuclear localization signals (NLS): NLS1 is composed of amino acids 28–44, and NLS2, amino acids 180–185 *(14)*. However, during an immunological challenge, macrophages are activated and HMGB1 becomes acetylated on groups of lysine residues within the NLS **(Fig. 2)**. Extensive acetylation of these domains is thought to inhibit nuclear HMGB1 translocation, and, therefore, hyperacetylated forms of HMGB1 accumulate in the cytosol where they are packaged through an unknown mechanism into specialized secretory lysosomes *(14,15)*. The fusion of these secretory lysosomes with the plasma membrane liberates HMGB1 into the extracellular environment. Consequently, immune cells secrete hyperacetylated isoforms of HMGB1, which are molecularly different from the predominantly hypoacetylated forms released from necrotic cells **(Fig. 1)**.

Although the functional consequences of the mode of HMGB1 release are currently unknown, acetylation modulates HMGB1 interactions with other

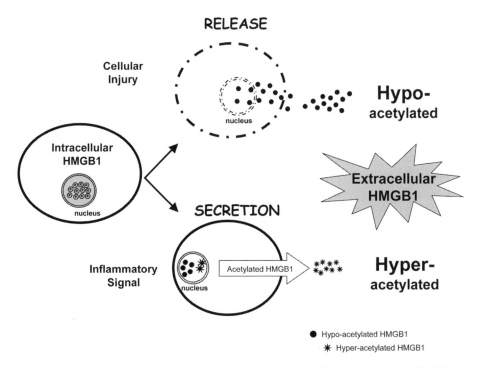

Fig. 1. "Passive release" of hypoacetylated high-mobility group box-1 (HMGB1) isoforms from necrotic cells vs "active secretion" of hyperacetylated HMGB1 isoforms from activated immune cells. Somatic cells contain large amounts of hypoacetylated nuclear HMGB1 that is passively released into the environment following cell membrane perturbation during necrotic death. Alternatively, macrophages, monocytes, and dendritic cells have a specialized regulated secretory mechanism that leads to the active secretion of HMGB1 in response to proinflammatory stimuli. Activated immune cells hyperacetylate nuclear HMGB1 on several lysine residues, which presumably blocks the function of nuclear localization signals and promotes the cytoplasmic accumulation of these HMGB1 isoforms. These hyperacetylated HMGB1 isoforms are then sequestered into specialized secretory lysosomes, which will fuse with the plasma membrane to release hyperacetylated HMGB1 into the extracellular milieu. Note that actively secreted hyperacetylated HMGB1 isoforms are molecularly different from passively released hypoacetylated isoforms. Posttranslational modifications such as acetylation are important for modulating HMGB1 interaction with other proteins and might determine its ability to bind to and activate cell surface receptors, determining its pathological potential.

nuclear proteins *(16–18)*. Likewise, acetylation can impact HMGB1 interactions with specific cell surface receptors and modulate its cytokine and inflammatory activity. The extent to which acetylation or other posttranslational modifications determine extracellular HMGB1-inflammatory activity and

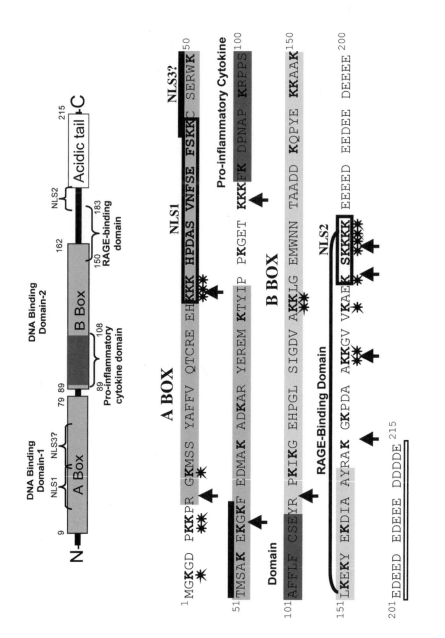

pathological contribution to infectious and immunoinflammatory disorders is presently unknown. Currently, there is a great deal of interest in the characterization of HMGB1 isoforms and their relative contributions to infectious and inflammatory disorders *(4,6)*. This renewed interest in the inflammatory activity of HMGB1 has fueled the need for precise methods to purify contaminant-free HMGB1 that retains biological activity. Different methods for the purification and characterization of functionally active HMGB1 are under current development.

2. HMGB1 Purification

There are several recent reports describing refined methods for the purification of biologically active HMGB1 from either prokaryotic (recombinant) or eukaryotic (endogenous or transfected) sources *(19,20)*. These methods represent a major advance in the ability to purify significant amount of HMGB1 and study its cytokine activity and pathological potential under diverse conditions. As the methods employed in these studies are very detailed in the respective publications, the purpose here is to discuss differences in the procedures that affect the levels of contaminants, and the biological activity of the purified HMGB1 protein.

HMGB1 purification from prokaryotic sources. HMGB1 is a proinflammatory cytokine that activates the innate immune system. A major potential problem with expression and purification of HMGB1 from microbial sources is that contamination with bacterial cellular debris, including endotoxin (LPS), can also activate the innate immune system and evoke very similar responses as HMGB1. Complicating purification is the fact that HMGB1 contains an inordinately large number of charged residues (43 lysines and 9 arginines in the N-terminal

---

Fig. 2. *(Opposite page)* Structural characteristics of high-mobility group box-1 (HMGB1). Primary amino acid sequence and structural organization scheme of human HMGB1 (PubMed accession no. NP_002119). The acetylation state of bovine HMGB1 lysine residues have been previously studied *(14,58)*. (Note that HMGB1 is extremely well conserved in evolution, and human and bovine HMGB1 differ only at amino acid 206, which is aspartic acid in human and glutamic acid in the cow *[58]*). Lysine residues that were found acetylated are indicated with asterisk. Sequences corresponding to the two DNA-binding A- and B-box are highlighted in light gray. Sequences comprising the minimal proinflammatory cytokine-inducing domain of the B-box are highlighted in dark gray. The two characterized HMGB1 nuclear localization signal (NLS) sequences (amino acids 28–44, and amino acids 180–185) are boxed *(14)*, and sequences that comprise a third potential NLS predicted by PROSITE (amino acids 43–59) are underlined. The RAGE-binding domain (amino acids 150–183) is indicated with a bracket *(41)*. Sites that match preferred plasmin digestion sequences *(42)* are denoted by black arrowheads.

DNA-binding domains, and 36 glutamic acids and 20 aspartic acids in the C-terminal acidic tail) that confer strong dipolar, charged properties to the protein **(Fig. 2)**. This dipolar feature promotes the binding and copurification of contaminating bacterial components, including bacterial CpG DNA and LPS *(19)*. These contaminants induce immune responses similar to that of recombinant HMGB1, and can potentially obscure specific cytokine effects in different immune cells, including macrophages and neutrophils *(21,22)*. Therefore, a critical step in the purification of recombinant HMGB1 is to avoid bacterial contaminants. The different methods described for HMGB1 purification lead to differences in the final concentration of contaminant endotoxin that can range from 6 pg/mL to >50 ng/mL. The highest reported levels of purity can be best attributed to polymyxin B chromatography followed by a further fractionation using triton X-114 phase separation *(19)*. Recombinant HMGB1 purified in this manner elicits a tumor necrosis factor (TNF) response from primary human blood cells similar to that of protein purified by other methods, indicating that multiple procedures result in recombinant HMGB1 that retains a similar level of biological activity *(19,20)*. Future studies are warranted to determine whether differences in the HMGB1 obtained by these methods might affect other immune responses induced in different cell types.

HMGB1 purification from eukaryotic sources. An important limitation of studies using recombinant protein generated in bacteria is that eukaryotic HMGB1 is extensively modified posttranslationally by mechanisms that are lacking in prokaryote. Therefore, modifications that could potentially modulate the cytokine activity of HMGB1 would be missing from bacterially purified protein. For these reasons, it is important to compare the effects of recombinant and eukaryote-derived HMGB1. Eukaryote-derived HMGB1 has been purified from cultures of Chinese hamster ovary (CHO) *(19,20)*. The methods described in these reports include the generation of stably transfected CHO cells expressing rat HMGB1 *(19)* and the isolation of a CHO cell line that naturally secreted large quantities of endogenous hamster HMGB1 *(20)*. These methods differ primarily in the efficacy of purification. Transfected rat HMGB1 was N-terminally tagged with three tandem copies of the FLAG epitope to facilitate purification from the medium, resulting in highly pure (>90%) HMGB1 at about 50 µg/L of conditioned medium with few chromatography steps *(19)*. Hamster HMGB1, naturally secreted in large quantities, was purified from the culture medium using a series of chromatography steps that resulted in a roughly 90% pure preparation at about 500 µg/L of culture supernatant *(20)*. Similar to the bacterially expressed HMGB1, both eukaryotic preparations result in a similar cytokine activity, and both recombinant and native HMGB1 induce TNF production in human blood, murine RAW264.7 and monocytic THP1 cells in a dose-dependent manner. Both recombinant and native HMGB1 also induce similar proliferation of NIH/3T3 fibroblasts. However, bacterial expressed recombinant HMGB1 elicits stronger responses from cultured cells than equivalent doses of HMGB1 purified from eukaryotic sources *(19,20)*. These results suggest that eukaryotic posttranslational modifications are not required for HMGB1 to function as a proinflammatory cytokine on primary human blood cells.

Since recombinant unmodified HMGB1 is more robust at evoking inflammatory responses than secreted HMGB1 purified from culture supernatants, modifications such as acetylation may actually restrict the ability of HMGB1 to activate TNF or other immune responses. These observations might reflect differences in the physiological mode by which HMGB1 is liberated into the extracellular milieu. For example, nuclear hypoacetylated HMGB1 leaked into the environment by damaged or necrotic cells could signify local tissue damage requiring a strong and immediate immune response to protect against further injury or dissemination of infection. On the other hand, hyperacetylated HMGB1, secreted by activated immune cells even hours after the initial immune insult *(23)*, could serve the more limited purpose of prolonging the initial inflammatory response to promote wound healing and the resolution of tissue damage. A major limitation of these studies is that the test of analysis in vitro, are normally performed at very low concentrations of inactivated fetal serum, which may not mimic the stability of HMGB1 in serum. Future studies will determine whether these results can be translated in vivo, and whether specific responses in different cell types are affected by posttranslational modifications of HMGB1.

3. Cellular Responses to Extracellular HMGB1

The cellular responses to extracellular HMGB1 vary considerably depending upon the cell type. As such, cell-type specific responses to HMGB1 stimulation, and their relative contributions to inflammatory responses are addressed specifically (**Fig. 3**).

Immune cells: HMGB1 is a proinflammatory cytokine that acts as a very potent activator of macrophages and monocytes. HMGB1 stimulates the migration and phagocytosis of these cells *(24,25)*, and activates the production and secretion of a battery of proinflammatory cytokines including TNF, interleukin (IL)-1, IL-6, IL-8, macrophage inflammatory protein-1, and HMGB1 *(8,23,24)*. Thus, HMGB1 can stimulate a self-perpetuating, positive-feedback autocrine loop in macrophages that amplifies and sustains inflammatory cascades. Similar to that described for macrophages, HMGB1 also acts as a chemotactic factor to drive the recruitment of neutrophils to sites of inflammation *(24)*. HMGB1-activated neutrophils produce and secrete proinflammatory cytokines such as TNF, IL-1, and IL-8 *(9)*. HMGB1 also stimulates dendritic cell maturation

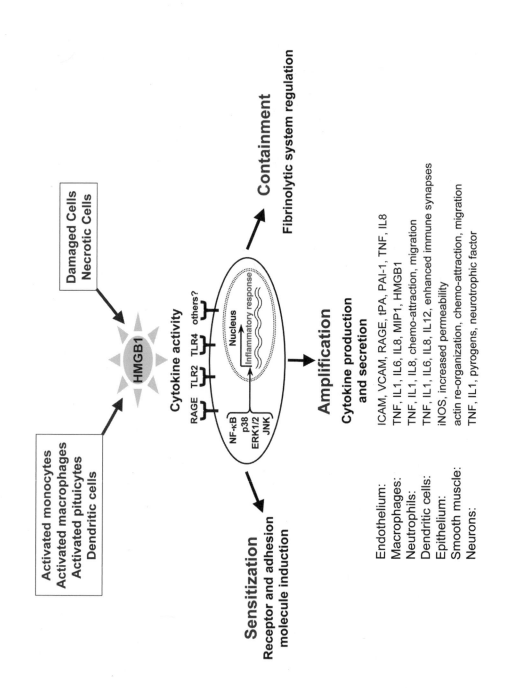

Activated monocytes
Activated macrophages
Activated pituicytes
Dendritic cells

Damaged Cells
Necrotic Cells

HMGB1

Containment

Fibrinolytic system regulation

Cytokine activity

RAGE   TLR2   TLR4   others?

NF-κB
p38
ERK1/2
JNK

Nucleus

Inflammatory response

Sensitization

Receptor and adhesion
molecule induction

Amplification

Cytokine production
and secretion

Endothelium: ICAM, VCAM, RAGE, tPA, PAI-1, TNF, IL8
Macrophages: TNF, IL1, IL6, IL8, MIP1, HMGB1
Neutrophils: TNF, IL1, IL8, chemo-attraction, migration
Dendritic cells: TNF, IL1, IL6, IL8, IL12, enhanced immune synapses
Epithelium: iNOS, increased permeability
Smooth muscle: actin re-organization, chemo-attraction, migration
Neurons: TNF, IL1, pyrogens, neurotrophic factor

and subsequent secretion of TNF, IL-1, IL-6, IL-8, and IL-12, which functions to further enhance immune reactions in other immune cell types *(5,26,27)*.

Endothelium: in response to HMGB1, microvascular endothelial cells upregulate the expression of cellular adhesion molecules like intracellular adhesion molecule (ICAM)-1 and vascular cell adhesion molecule (VCAM)-1, which promote the attachment of different immune cells to the endothelial vessel wall. HMGB1 also disrupts endothelial barrier functions and facilitates the extravasation of immune cells into tissues, but also increases the risk of vascular leakage and edema, which can contribute to tissue damage *(13)*. HMGB1 also stimulates endothelial cells to produce a variety of proinflammatory cytokines including TNF and IL-8, and causes the secretion of tissue-type plasminogen activator as well as plasminogen activator inhibitor, which influence hemostasis *(28)*. Therefore, stimulation of the endothelium by HMGB1 provokes inflammatory responses that are important during injury or infection.

Smooth muscle: HMGB1 acts as a strong chemotactic signal that promotes the reorganization of the actin cytoskeleton, leading to smooth muscle cell migration *(11)*, which is critical to the process of wound healing. The chemotactic induction of smooth muscle cells in response to HMGB1 is also thought to play a role in the pathogenesis of certain vascular diseases such as atherosclerosis and restenosis *(29)*.

Other cell types: HMGB1 can also alter the permeability of cultured enterocytes through the stimulation of a nitric oxide-dependent pathway and impair the intestinal barrier function in mice *(30)*. HMGB1 is also a key neurotrophic factor that plays an important role in directing neurite outgrowth during brain development *(31,32)*. As a ligand for RAGE, HMGB1 has also been implicated in tumor cell metastasis *(33)*. HMGB1 abundance at the invasive front of solid tumors correlates with matrix metalloprotease activation and the depth of tumor invasion and lymph node metastasis *(34)*.

Overall, HMGB1 is nearly ubiquitous, and participates in a large number of molecular processes in a variety of cell types. This feature allows HMGB1 to

---

Fig. 3. *(Opposite page)* Cytokine activity of high-mobility group box-1 (HMGB1). HMGB1 can be secreted by mononuclear leukocytes as a delayed response to activation by inflammatory signals such as endotoxin, tumor necrosis factor, or interleukin-1, as serum levels of HMGB1 are not elevated until 16–20 h postimmunological challenge in animals, and peaks about 24 h after the onset of sepsis *(23)*. Once released, HMGB1 functions as a convential proinflammatory cytokine, exerting its effects through cell surface receptors like advanced glycation end-products, Toll-like receptors-2, and Toll-like receptors-4, which activate a variety of cellular responses that vary depending upon the cell type. Typical responses from cell types that have key roles in the normal and pathophysiological outcomes of HMGB1 signaling are indicated.

orchestrate a plethora of cellular signaling events in diverse cell types to coordinate specific biological process (**Fig. 3**). During infection, trauma, or shock, stimulated macrophages can secrete large amounts of HMGB1 into the extracellular milieu *(35)*. Extracellular HMGB1 promotes macrophage and dendritic cell maturation, and induces the production of other proinflammatory cytokines, which further enhance immune reactions *(5,26)*. HMGB1 can also activate endothelial cells, inducing the expression of cellular adhesion molecules and tissue-type plasminogen activator *(2)*. The expression of these molecules promotes the adhesion of immune cells to the endothelial vessel wall and permits their extravasation into tissues. Although this process is critical for the proper resolution of infection or injury, excessive secretion of HMGB1 may result in the disruption of endothelial barrier functions, leading to vascular leakage similar to that observed in sepsis *(13)*. Likewise, HMGB1 can also alter the permeability of cultured enterocytes and impair the intestinal barrier function in mice *(30)*. Thus, similar to other proinflammatory cytokines, HMGB1 can elicit a beneficial defensive immune response against injury or infection. However, excessive release of HMGB1 can become more dangerous than the original stimuli and thus contribute to the pathogenesis of different inflammatory disorders *(1,2)*.

4. Receptors and Cytokine Activity of HMGB1

HMGB1 is considered a cytokine because it is secreted by activated immune cells, transduces signals through cell surface receptors, and induces conventional inflammatory responses in immune and endothelial cells *(1,2)*. Extracellular HMGB1 binds to the cellular receptor for advanced glycation end-products (RAGE) in a concentration-dependent manner *(36)*. RAGE is a transmembrane protein that belongs to the immunoglobulin super-family, and acts as a receptor for diverse ligands including RAGE, amyloid peptide, members of the S100 family of inflammatory-mediating peptides, and is currently the best characterized cellular receptor for HMGB1 *(37–39)*. RAGE is expressed on the surface of a variety of cell types including endothelium, vascular smooth muscle, neurons, macrophages, and monocytes *(38)*. Stimulation of RAGE results in the activation of multiple intracellular signaling pathways including the small Rho-like GTPases Rac and CDC42, mitogen-activated protein kinases (p38, c-Jun N-terminal kinase, and ERK1/2) and the nuclear factor (NF)-κB pathway *(37)*. It is noteworthy that both RAGE and HMGB1 are NF-κB-responsive genes, and their expression can be dramatically enhanced upon RAGE stimulation in various cell types *(38)*. This self-enhancing property of RAGE signaling could function to further sensitize cells to RAGE ligands such as HMGB1 or S100 proinflammatory peptides, and has important implications for the progression of inflammatory responses. One specific example of this mechanism is the requirement of HMGB1-RAGE signaling for the maturation of plasmacytoid dendritic cells (PDCs) and their contribution to T-cell activation *(27)*. Activated PDCs accumulate HMGB1 in the cytosol in response to bacterial CpG DNA-mediated Toll-like receptor (TLR)-9 signaling, and the subsequent secretion of HMGB1 by these PDCs is crucial to direct their maturation in an autocrine fashion *(27)*. The pools of HMGB1 secreted from activated dendritic cells appears to be essential for the clonal expansion, survival, and functional polarization of naive T cells *(5,26)*, which then drive adaptive immune responses. These observations may in part explain why certain therapies that target HMGB1 can short-circuit the progression of experimental sepsis *(4,6,23,40)*.

Recent studies indicate that specific stimulation of RAGE alone cannot account for the full array of cellular responses induced by HMGB1 *(39)*. First, neutralizing antibodies directed against RAGE only partially inhibit HMGB1-mediated cytokine activity *(10,28,29)*. Second, although the RAGE-binding domain has been mapped to the C-terminus (amino acids 150–183) of HMGB1 *(41)* (**Fig. 2**), structure/function studies of HMGB1 show that the first 20 amino acids of the DNA-binding B-box (corresponding to residues 89–108) are sufficient for stimulating macrophage TNF secretion *(10)*. Also consistent with alternative cellular HMGB1 receptors is the observation that the RAGE-binding domain of HMGB1 contains several preferred plasmin recognition sequences (**Fig. 2**) whose availability for digestion is likely to be controlled by acetylation *(42)*. Therefore, acetylation might play multiple roles in controlling HMGB1–RAGE interactions, not only by potentially modulating receptor affinity through targeting the RAGE-binding domain of HMGB1, but also by potentially protecting it from proteolytic inactivation. Taken together, these observations suggest that the cytokine-inducing activity of HMGB1 might be partially independent of RAGE. Recent studies suggest that in addition to RAGE, TLR-2 and TLR-4 also mediate the cytokine activity of HMGB1. The ability of necrotic cells to maximally stimulate NF-κB activity in macrophages is at least in part dependent on a TLR-mediated signaling pathway *(43)*, and both TLR-2 and TLR-4 have been implicated in the activation of macrophages by HMGB1 *(21)*. The specific contributions of RAGE, TLR-2, and TLR-4 to the cytokine activity of HMGB1 remain unclear in part because these receptors share common downstream effector molecules (especially NF-κB, c-Jun N-terminal kinase, and p38 mitogen-activated protein kinases) that stimulate similar intracellular signaling events *(2,40)*. This sharing of signaling components makes genetic studies using dominant-negative constructs and heterologous expression systems difficult to interpret, and has lead to contradictory conclusions in the literature regarding the roles of RAGE, TLR-2, and TLR-4 in executing the cytokine activity of HMGB1 *(2,21,39)*. The TLR receptors also form homo- and hetero-oligomers that function in signaling, and the oligomeric state of TLRs can dramatically increase the complexity of receptor isoforms *(22,36,44)*. Each oligomeric state might have alternative substrate specificities and different capacities for the recruitment and activation of downstream signaling adaptors in a cell type-specific manner. This phenomenon has been already described for G protein-coupled receptors; the biological significance of G protein-coupled receptors oligomerization has only recently coming to light *(45,46)*, and could potentially explain some apparent discrepancies regarding HMGB1 signal transduction.

HMGB1 has the capacity to act through nonreceptor-mediated mechanisms to facilitate delivery of other molecules across cellular membranes *(47,48)*. Because HMGB1 can effectively transport plasmid DNA into cells for transfection, it might also facilitate the delivery of other biologically active molecules into cells, especially those derived from necrotic cells or invading pathogens. In this respect, HMGB1 has similar properties to proteins like lactoferrin and the HIV-1 Tat protein, which contain protein transduction domains and promote cargo delivery across cell and organelle membranes *(49)*. These protein transduction domains are typically rich in basic amino acids (lysine, arginine, and histidine), and convey the ability to transport other proteins, DNA, and RNA into cells *(50)*. This property of HMGB1 adds another potential dimension to its signaling capabilities, as it could potentially act as a carrier to present unmethylated CpG DNA to TLR-9, an intracellular TLR expressed in dendritic cells and B cells that responds to bacterial or viral DNA *(51)*. This mechanism could be analogous to TLR-4, which requires additional cofactors such as LPS-binding protein, CD14, and MD-2 to respond to LPS. The potential for HMGB1 as an alternative carrier for the presentation of LPS to TLR-4 could represent an interesting mechanism to explain why HMGB1 and LPS can elicit similar responses from macrophages in culture *(21)*. Detailed studies are needed to define the relative contribution of RAGE, TLR-2, and TLR-4 to HMGB1 cytokine activity and to its roles in the pathological progression of infectious and inflammatory disorders *(4,40,52)*.

5. Future Directions

HMGB1 was recently described as a therapeutic target for different infectious and inflammatory disorders *(1,2,4,52)*. However, little is known about the contribution of posttranslational modifications to the extracellular regulation of HMGB1 cytokine activity, or its pathological effects in infectious and inflammatory disorders. Indeed, HMGB1 is a member of a novel family of inflammatory cytokines composed of intracellular proteins that when present in the extracellular milieu, are recognized by the innate immune system as a signal of tissue damage. Posttranslational modifications of HMGB1 modulate its intracellular biological activity by controlling its interactions with other proteins

(14,18). It is now proposed that posttranslational modifications of HMGB1 modulate its cytokine and inflammatory activity by determining its interactions with cell surface receptors.

HMGB1 purified from calf thymus exists in several distinct isoforms including at least 10 acetylated species *(14)*, which may also bear ADP ribose, glycosylation, phosphorylation, and methylation moieties *(1,2)*, each of which may contribute differentially to determine the biological activity of HMGB1. The acetylated isoforms of HMGB1 were described for protein purified from the thymus of healthy animals *(14)*, and thus it is uncertain whether they reflect the acetylation state of HMGB1 secreted during pathological or inflammatory conditions. Thus, it is probable that lysine residues found unmodified in this study could represent important sites to control the inflammatory activity of HMGB1. For instance, several studies indicate that under normal conditions HMGB1 moves and accumulates into the nucleus. During immune challenges, acetylation of lysine residues within NLS (NLS1 and NLS2) is thought to prevent HMGB1 translocation into the nucleus **(Fig. 2)**. However, lysine residues in NLS1 (lysines 28, 29, 30), and in NLS2 (lysines 180, 182, 183, 184, and 185) were acetylated in healthy animals, and a mutant HMGB1 protein compromised for the function of both NLS sequences by substitution of six of these lysines (either to alanine or to glutamine) still showed nuclear localization *(14)*. These results suggest a putative third NLS (NLS3) within HMGB1. Accordingly, a PROSITE scan of HMGB1 reveals a putative NLS3 corresponding to the amino acids 43–59 **(Fig. 2)**. Because none of the lysine residues within this putative NLS were found acetylated, this motif could represent a potential target for preventing HMGB1 nuclear translocation during immune stimulation. Hyperacetylation of HMGB1 on lysines within NLS2 (lysines 180, 182, 183, 184, and 185), which are located inside the RAGE-binding domain **(Fig. 2)**, is thought to promote secretion during immune challenges *(14)*. Therefore, hyperacetylated HMGB1 (in the RAGE-binding domain) might have lower affinity for RAGE and induce a weaker immune response, perhaps mimicking the weaker responses induced by HMGB1 purified from eukaryotic sources in vitro *(19,20)*. However, hypoacetylated nuclear HMGB1 that leaks into the extracellular milieu during injury or necrosis might have higher affinity for RAGE, and induce a stronger immune response, similar to that described for bacterial expressed recombinant HMGB1 *(19,20)*.

Posttranslational modifications can also determine HMGB1 interaction with specific proteases and modulate its extracellular stability. Although there is currently no data regarding the stability of HMGB1 in the extracellular environment, one possibility is that acetylation can provide greater stability to HMGB1 in the extracellular environment. Acetylation in lysine residues during immune active secretion of HMGB1 can block lysine residues that constitute sensitive protease digestion sites for tissue and serum proteases, such as a plasmin. In support of this hypothesis, HMGB1 interacts with tissue-type plasminogen activator and stimulates the conversion of the zymogen plasminogen to plasmin, a highly active lysine-specific endoprotease *(53)*. Because HMGB1 is itself a lysine-rich protein that serves as a plasmin substrate, hypoacetylated extracellular HMGB1 would be more susceptible to degradation, restricting it to a local environment *(42)*. This same mechanism would potentially allow hyperacetylated HMGB1 secreted from macrophages and other immune cells to disseminate into the serum and contribute to systemic inflammation, which appears to be the case in severe sepsis.

In addition to acetylation, HMGB1 has also been found to be methylated, glycosylated, ADP-ribosylated, and phosphorylated *(2)*, all of which can contribute to the regulation its biological functions. Indeed, HMGB1 can be polyADP-ribosylated, which is a common phenotypic change in proteins present in cells with damaged DNA. HMGB1 is also a substrate for protein kinase C (PKC) phosphorylation *(54)*, and the activity of several PKC isoforms is stimulated upon leukocyte activation *(55–57)*. Although the PKC phosphorylation sites on HMGB1 remain uncharacterized, it is noteworthy that there are PKC consensus phosphorylation sites in each of the NLS sequences (NLS1, NLS2, and the putative NLS3), in the proinflammatory cytokine domain of the B-box, and in the RAGE-binding domain **(Fig. 2)**. These potential phosphorylation sites may represent additional mechanisms for regulating HMGB1 cytokine and inflammatory activity. Because of recent methodological advances in the ability to generate large quantities of relatively contaminant-free HMGB1 preparations *(19,20)*, in vivo experimental approaches can now be targeted to determine the relative contribution of these posttranslational modifications of HMGB1 to its proinflammatory cytokine activity and pathological contribution to infectious or inflammatory disorders *(1,2,4,52)*.

References

1. Ulloa, L. and Tracey, K. J. (2005) The "cytokine profile": a code for sepsis. *Trends Mol. Med.* **11,** 56–63.
2. Lotze, M. T. and Tracey, K. J. (2005) High-mobility group box 1 protein (HMGB1): nuclear weapon in the immune arsenal. *Nat. Rev. Immunol.* **5,** 331–342.
3. Ulloa, L. (2005) The vagus nerve and the nicotinic anti-inflammatory pathway. *Nat. Rev. Drug Disc.* **4,** 673–684.
4. Ulloa, L., Ochani, M., Yang, H., et al. (2002) Ethyl pyruvate prevents lethality in mice with established lethal sepsis and systemic inflammation. *PNAS* **99,** 12,351–12,356.
5. Messmer, D., Yang, H., Telusma, G., et al. (2004) High mobility group box protein 1: an endogenous signal for dendritic cell maturation and Th1 polarization. *J. Immunol.* **173,** 307–313.

6. Yang, H., Ochani, M., Li, J., et al. (2004) Reversing established sepsis with antagonists of endogenous high-mobility group box 1. *PNAS* **101,** 296–301.

7. Scaffidi, P., Misteli, T., and Bianchi, M. E. (2002) Release of chromatin protein HMGB1 by necrotic cells triggers inflammation. *Nature* **418,** 191–195.

8. Andersson, U., Wang, H., Palmblad, K., et al. (2000) High mobility group 1 protein (HMG-1) stimulates proinflammatory cytokine synthesis in human monocytes. *J. Exp. Med.* **192,** 565–570.

9. Park, J. S., Arcaroli, J., Yum, H.-K., et al. (2003) Activation of gene expression in human neutrophils by high mobility group box 1 protein. *Am. J. Physiol. Cell. Physiol.* **284,** C870–C879.

10. Li, J., Kokkola, R., Tabibzadeh, S., et al. (2003) Structural basis for the proinflammatory cytokine activity of high mobility group box 1. *Mol. Med.* **9,** 37–45.

11. Degryse, B., Bonaldi, T., Scaffidi, P., et al. (2001) The high mobility group (HMG) boxes of the nuclear protein HMG1 induce chemotaxis and cytoskeleton reorganization in rat smooth muscle cells. *J. Cell Biol.* **152,** 1197–1206.

12. Cossu, G. and Bianco, P. (2003) Mesoangioblasts—vascular progenitors for extravascular mesodermal tissues. *Curr. Opin. Genet. Dev.* **13,** 537–542.

13. Palumbo, R., Sampaolesi, M., De Marchis, F., et al. (2004) Extracellular HMGB1, a signal of tissue damage, induces mesoangioblast migration and proliferation. *J. Cell Biol.* **164,** 441–449.

14. Bonaldi, T., Talamo, F., Scaffidi, P., et al. (2003) Monocytic cells hyperacetylate chromatin protein HMGB1 to redirect it towards secretion. *EMBO* **22,** 5551–5560.

15. Gardella, S., Andrei, C., Ferrera, D., et al. (2002) The nuclear protein HMGB1 is secreted by monocytes via a non-classical, vesicle-mediated secretory pathway. *EMBO Rep.* **3,** 995–1001.

16. Alexandrova, E. A. and Beltchev, B. G. (1988) Acetylated HMG1 protein interacts specifically with homologous DNA polymerase alpha in vitro. *Biochem. Biophys. Res. Commun.* **154,** 91–927.

17. Dimov, S. I., Alexandrova, E. A., and Beltchev, B. G. (1990) Differences between some properties of acetylated and nonacetylated forms of HMG1 protein. *Biochem. Biophys. Res. Commun.* **166,** 819–826.

18. Ugrinova, I., A, P. E., Armengaud, J., and Pashev, I. G. (2001) In vivo acetylation of HMG1 protein enhances its binding affinity to distorted DNA structures. *Biochemistry* **40,** 14,655–14,660.

19. Li, J., Wang, H., Mason, J. M., et al. (2004) Recombinant HMGB1 with cytokine-stimulating activity. *J. Immunol. Methods.* **289,** 211–223.

20. Zimmermann, K., Volkel, D., Pable, S., et al. (2004) Native versus recombinant high-mobility group B1 proteins: functional activity in vitro. *Inflammation* **28,** 221–229.

21. Park, J. S., Svetkauskaite, D., He, Q., et al. (2004) Involvement of Toll-like receptors 2 and 4 in cellular activation by high mobility group box 1 protein. *J. Biol. Chem.* **279,** 7370–7377.

22. Akira, S. and Takeda, K. (2004) Toll-like receptor signalling. *Nat. Rev. Immunol.* **4,** 499–511.

23. Wang, H., Bloom, O., Zhang, M., et al. (1999) HMG-1 as a late mediator of endotoxin lethality in mice. *Science* **285,** 248–251.

24. Abraham, E., Arcaroli, J., Carmody, A., Wang, H., and Tracey, K. J. (2000) Cutting Edge: HMG-1 as a Mediator of Acute Lung Inflammation. *J. Immunol.* **165,** 2950–2954.

25. Pullerits, R., Jonsson, I. M., Verdrengh, M., et al. (2003) High mobility group box chromosomal protein 1, a DNA binding cytokine, induces arthritis. *Arthritis Rheum.* **48,** 1693–1700.

26. Dumitriu, I. E., Baruah, P., Valentinis, B., et al. (2005) Release of high mobility group box 1 by dendritic cells controls T cell activation via the receptor for advanced glycation end products. *J. Immunol.* **174,** 7506–7515.

27. Dumitriu, I. E., Baruah, P., Bianchi, M. E., Manfredi, A. A., and Rovere-Querini, P. (2005) Requirement of HMGB1 and RAGE for the maturation of human plasmacytoid dendritic cells. *Eur. J. Immunol.* **35,** 2184–2190.

28. Fiuza, C., Bustin, M., Talwar, S., et al. (2003) Inflammation-promoting activity of HMGB1 on human microvascular endothelial cells. *Blood* **101,** 2652–2660.

29. Degryse, B. and Virgilio, M. (2003) The nuclear protein HMGB1, a new kind of chemokine? *FEBS Lett.* **553,** 11–17.

30. Sappington, P. L., Yang, R., Yang, H., Tracey, K. J., Delude, R. L. and Fink, M. P. (2002). HMGB1 B box increases the permeability of Caco-2 enterocytic monolayers and impairs intestinal barrier function in mice. *Gastroenterology* **123,** 790–802.

31. Rauvala, H. and Pihlaskari, R. (1987) Isolation and some characteristics of an adhesive factor of brain that enhances neurite outgrowth in central neurons. *J. Biol. Chem.* **262,** 16,625–16,635.

32. Merenmies, J., Pihlaskari, R., Laitinen, J., Wartiovaara, J., and Rauvala, H. (1991) 30-kDa heparin-binding protein of brain (amphoterin) involved in neurite outgrowth. Amino acid sequence and localization in the filopodia of the advancing plasma membrane. *J. Biol. Chem.* **266,** 16,722–16,729.

33. Parkkinen, J., Raulo, E., Merenmies, J., et al. (1993) Amphoterin, the 30-kDa protein in a family of HMG1-type polypeptides. Enhanced expression in transformed cells, leading edge localization, and interactions with plasminogen activation. *J. Biol. Chem.* **268,** 19,726–19,738.

34. Kuniyasu, H., Oue, N., Wakikawa, A., et al. (2002) Expression of receptors for advanced glycation end-products (RAGE) is closely associated with the invasive and metastatic activity of gastric cancer. *J. Pathol.* **196,** 163–170.

35. Yang, H., Wang, H., Czura, C. J., and Tracey, K. J. (2005) The cytokine activity of HMGB1. *J. Leukoc. Biol.* **78,** 1–8.

36. Hori, O., Brett, J., Slattery, T., et al. (1995) The receptor for advanced glycation end products (RAGE) is a cellular binding site for amphoterin. *J. Biol. Chem.* **270,** 25,752–25,761.

37. Huttunen, H. J. and Rauvala, H. (2004) Amphoterin as an extracellular regulator of cell motility: from discovery to disease. *J. Intern. Med.* **255,** 351–366.

38. Schmidt, A. M., Yan, S. D., Yan, S. F., and Stern, D. M. (2001) The multiligand receptor RAGE as a progression factor amplifying immune and inflammatory responses. *J. Clin. Invest.* **108**, 949–955.

39. Kokkola, R., Andersson, A., Mullins, G., et al. (2005) RAGE is the major receptor for the proinflammatory activity of HMGB1 in rodent macrophages. *Scand. J. Immunol.* **61**, 1–9.

40. Wang, H., Liao, H., Ochani, M., et al. (2004) Cholinergic agonists inhibit HMGB1 release and improve survival in experimental sepsis. *Nat. Med.* **10**, 1216–1221.

41. Huttunen, H. J., Fages, C., Kuja-Panula, J., Ridley, A. J., and Rauvala, H. (2002) Receptor for advanced glycation end products-binding COOH-terminal motif of amphoterin inhibits invasive migration and metastasis. *Cancer Res.* **62**, 4805–4811.

42. Hervio, L. S., Coombs, G. S., Bergstrom, R. C., Trivedi, K., Corey, D. R., and Madison, E. L. (2000) Negative selectivity and the evolution of protease cascades: the specificity of plasmin for peptide and protein substrates. *Chem. Biol.* **7**, 443–453.

43. Li, M., Carpio, D. F., Zheng, Y., et al. (2001) An essential role of the NF-κB/Toll-like receptor pathway in induction of inflammatory and tissue-repair gene expression by necrotic cells. *J. Immunol.* **166**, 7128–7135.

44. Dunne, A. and O'Neill, L. A. (2005) Adaptor usage and Toll-like receptor signaling specificity. *FEBS Lett.* **579**, 3330–3335.

45. Rashid, A. J., O'Dowd, B. F., and George, S. R. (2004) Minireview: diversity and complexity of signaling through peptidergic G protein-coupled receptors. *Endocrinology* **145**, 2645–2652.

46. Rios, C. D., Jordan, B. A., Gomes, I., and Devi, L. A. (2001) G-protein-coupled receptor dimerization: modulation of receptor function. *Pharmacol Ther.* **92**, 71–87.

47. Mistry, A. R., Falciola, L., Monaco, L., et al. (1997) Recombinant HMG1 protein produced in Pichia pastoris: a nonviral gene delivery agent. *Biotechniques* **22**, 718–729.

48. Bottger, M., Vogel, F., Platzer, M., Kiessling, U., Grade, K., and Strauss, M. (1988) Condensation of vector DNA by the chromosomal protein HMG1 results in efficient transfection. *Biochim. Biophys. Acta.* **950**, 221–228.

49. Rubartelli, A. and Sitia, R. (1995) Entry of exogenous polypeptides into the nucleus of living cells: facts and speculations. *Trends Cell Biol.* **5**, 409–412.

50. Dietz, G. P. and Bahr, M. (2004) Delivery of bioactive molecules into the cell: the Trojan horse approach. *Mol. Cell. Neurosci.* **27**, 85–131.

51. Krieg, A. M. (2002) CPG Motifs in bacterial DNA and their immune effects. *Ann. Rev. Immunol.* **20**, 709–760.

52. Ulloa, L., Batliwalla, F. M., Andersson, U., Gregersen, P. K., and Tracey, K. J. (2003) High mobility group box chromosomal protein 1 as a nuclear protein, cytokine, and potential therapeutic target in arthritis. *Arthritis Rheum.* **48**, 876–881.

53. Parkkinen, J. and Rauvala, H. (1991) Interactions of plasminogen and tissue plasminogen activator (t-PA) with amphoterin. Enhancement of t-PA-catalyzed plasminogen activation by amphoterin. *J. Biol. Chem.* **266**, 16,730–16,735.

54. Ramachandran, C., Yau, P., Bradbury, E., Shyamala, G., Yasuda, H., and Walsh, D. (1984) Phosphorylation of high-mobility-group proteins by the calcium-phospholipid-dependent protein kinase and the cyclic AMP-dependent protein kinase. *J. Biol. Chem.* **259,** 13,495–13,503.

55. von Knethen, A., Tautenhahn, A., Link, H., Lindemann, D., and Brune, B. (2005) Activation-induced depletion of protein kinase Cα provokes desensitization of monocytes/macrophages in sepsis. *J. Immunol.* **174,** 4960–4965.

56. Chen, L.-Y., Doerner, A., Lehmann, P. F., Huang, S., Zhong, G., and Pan, Z. K. (2005) A novel protein kinase C (PKCε) is required for fMet-Leu-Phe-induced activation of NF-κB in human peripheral blood monocytes. *J. Biol. Chem.* **280,** 22,497–22,501.

57. Aksoy, E., Goldman, M., and Willems, F. (2004) Protein kinase C epsilon: a new target to control inflammation and immune-mediated disorders. *Int. J. Biochem. Cell Biol.* **36,** 183–188.

58. Sterner, R., Vidali, G., and Allfrey, V. G. (1979) Studies of acetylation and deacetylation in high mobility group proteins. Identification of the sites of acetylation in HMG-1. *J. Biol. Chem.* **254,** 11,577–11,583.

7

Antisense Oligonucleotides
Target Validation and Development of Systemically Delivered Therapeutic Nanoparticles

Chuanbo Zhang, Jin Pei, Deepak Kumar, Isamu Sakabe, Howard E. Boudreau, Prafulla C. Gokhale, and Usha N. Kasid

Summary

Antisense oligonucleotides (ASO) against specific molecular targets (e.g., Bcl-2 and Raf-1) are important reagents in cancer biology and therapy. Phosphorothioate modification of the ASO backbone has resulted in an increased stability of ASO in vivo without compromising, in general, their target selectivity. Although the power of antisense technology remains unsurpassed, dose-limiting side effects of modified ASO and inadequate penetration into the tumor tissue have necessitated further improvements in ASO chemistry and delivery systems. Oligonucleotide delivery systems may increase stability of the unmodified or minimally modified ASO in plasma, enhance uptake of ASO by tumor tissue, and offer an improved therapy response. Here, we provide an overview of ASO design and in vivo delivery systems, and focus on preclinical validation of a liposomal nanoparticle containing minimally modified *raf* antisense oligodeoxynucleotide (LErafAON). Intact rafAON (15-mer) is present in plasma and in normal and tumor tissues of athymic mice systemically treated with LErafAON. Raf-1 expression is decreased in normal and tumor tissues of LErafAON-treated mice. Therapeutic benefit of a combination of LErafAON and radiation or an anticancer drug exceeds radiation or drug alone against human prostate, breast, and pancreatic tumors grown in athymic mice. Further improvements in ASO chemistry and nanoparticles are promising avenues in antisense therapy of cancer.

Key Words: Raf-1, antisense oligonucleotides; liposomes; radiation; chemotherapeutic drugs; preclinical validation; cancer therapy.

1. Introduction

Sequence-specific depletion of molecular targets via antisense strategies, including antisense oligonucleotides (ASO) and short-interfering RNA, has enormous potential in cancer biology and therapy (*1,2*; *see* Chapters 9 and 12).

From: *Methods in Molecular Biology, vol. 361, Target Discovery and Validation Reviews and Protocols*
Volume 2, Emerging Molecular Targets and Treatment Options
Edited by: M. Sioud © Humana Press Inc., Totowa, NJ

During the past two decades, considerable progress has been made in the design and application of synthetic ASO *(3–8)*. The applications of ASO in target discovery and validation and in functional genomics have been well established. Further improvements in ASO chemistry and development of safe and effective tumor-targeted ASO nanoparticles are likely to close the gap between ASO drug discovery and clinical practice. This chapter provides an overview of current state-of-the-art ASO technology, and focuses on our efforts to develop and validate a therapeutic nanoparticle containing minimally modified c-*raf* ASO.

2. ASO Design and Validation

Ideally, an antisense therapeutic is expected to fulfill all of the following criteria: (1) nuclease resistance; (2) lack of cytosine–guanine motifs; (3) acceptable pharmacokinetics and bioavailability; (4) nontoxicity in animal models; (5) transport through cell membrane; (6) maximal inhibition of the target protein preferentially in tumor tissues; (7) preclinical efficacy; (8) cost-effective scale-up and production; (9) clinical tolerability; and (10) therapeutic benefit over existing treatment modalities. Various modifications of ASO chemistry and in vitro and in vivo applications of ASO targeted against specific molecules in cancer cells are summarized in **Table 1**. The reader is referred to recent reviews for further details of ASO chemistries and their advantages and disadvantages *(4,7)*. In general, phosphorothioate and chimeric modifications, which include partial or complete modification of the backbone and/or ribose moiety (2'-OH group), have resulted in significant improvements in pharmacokinetics, bioavailability, and target inhibition. As a prototype example, Raf-1 protein expression is inhibited in several human cancer cells exposed, albeit in the presence of lipofectin, to a phosphorothioate ASO targeted to the 3'-untranslated region of c-*raf*-1 mRNA sequence (ISIS 5132) **(Fig. 1)**. Similar effects have been seen using a phosphorothioate ASO targeted to the same region of c-*raf*-1 mRNA and it also has a 2' methoxyethyl group on the sugar moiety (ISIS 13650) **(Fig. 1)**. ISIS 5132, ISIS 13650, and a mismatch phosphorothioate oligo ISIS 10353 were kindly provided by Dr. Brett Monia (ISIS Pharmaceuticals) *(9,10)*. Currents efforts are directed at further improvements in chemistry so that the clinical side effects are minimized and access to the target site and penetration/retention of ASO into tumor cells are maximized. In preclinical studies, as single agents, most ASO exhibit tumor growth arrest properties, consistent with the oncogenic/prosurvival phenotype of their target molecules. The combinatorial antisense approach, whereby disease-specific signaling pathway(s) can be simultaneously disrupted by approaching redundant and multiple targets, and has the potential to enhance therapeutic efficacy of radiation or anticancer drugs against refractory cancers.

Table 1
Antisense Oligonucleotides in Cancer Biology and Therapy[a]

Molecular target	ASO design and application (I.D., size, chemistry, in vitro, in vivo)[b]	Ref.
Bcl-2	G3139, 18-mer, PS, in vitro, and in vivo	*35*
Bcl-xL	ISIS 16009, 20-mer, PS, and 5 nt at the 5'- and 3'-ends with 2'-MOE, in vitro	*36*
Bcl-x pre-mRNA	ISIS 22783, 20-mer, PS with 2'-MOE, in vitro	*37*
Bcl-2/Bcl-XL	4625, 20-mer, PS, and 5 nt at the 5'- and 3'-ends with 2'-MOE, in vitro	*38*
	5005, 20-mer, PS, and LNA modification of 5 nt at the 5'- and 3'-ends, in vitro	*39*
Bcr-Abl	NLS-asPNA, 13-mer, basic peptide (VKRKKKP)-linked PNA, in vitro	*40*
Clusterin	OGX-011, 21-mer, PS, chimeric 2' MOE/2'-deoxynucleotide, in vitro, in vivo	*41*
CRE-transcription factor	CRE-decoy, 24-mer CRE palindrome, PS, in vitro, in vivo	*42*
CSF-1	CSF-1 ODN-196, 15-mer, PS, in vivo	*43*
HER2/ErbB2/Neu	AS HER-2 ODN, PS, 15-mer, in vitro	*44*
	AP7-2, 15-mer, PS, ASO containing dithiodipyridine group at 3'-end and conjugated to a peptide (LTVSPWYC), in vitro	*45*
Mcl-1	ISIS 20408, 20-mer, PS, chimeric 2'-MOE/2'-deoxynucleotide, in vitro, in vivo	*46*
MDM2	AS, 20-mer, PS, MBO, in vitro, in vivo	*47*
	T5-12-Acr, Acr-PNA, in vitro	*48*
c-Myc	INX-6295, 16-mer, PS, in vitro, in vivo	*49*
Translocated c-Myc	PNAE μwt, 18-mer, NLS peptide (PKKKRKV)-linked PNA, in vitro	*50*
PKA (RIα)	GEM 231, 18-mer, PS, MBO, in vitro, in vivo	*51*
PKC-α	ISIS 3521, 20-mer, PS, in vitro, in vivo	*52*
PML/PML-RAR-α	PNA no 1 15-mer, adamantyl(*Ada*)-linked PNA, in vitro	*53*
B-Raf	BRAF-AS, 18-mer, PS, in vitro	*54*
c-Raf	As-raf/rafAON, 15-mer, one base at 5'- and 3'-ends has PS-linkage, in vitro	*30,55*
	ISIS 5132, 20-mer, PS, in vitro, and in vivo	*9*
	ISIS 13650, 20-mer, PS with 2'-MOE, in vitro	*10*

(Continued)

Table 1 *(Continued)*

Molecular target	ASO design and application (I.D., size, chemistry, in vitro, in vivo)[b]	Ref.
Ribonucleotide reductase (R2)	GTI-2040, 20-mer, PS, in vitro, in vivo	**56**
Telomerase	ISIS 24691, 13-mer, PS, 2'-MOE RNA, in vitro	**57**
XIAP	GEM640/AEG 35156, 19-mer, MBO, in vitro	**58**

[a]Selected ASO and their applications are listed. ASO tested using specialized in vivo delivery systems are listed in **Table 2**.

[b]In vitro, cultured cells; in vivo, animal models; PO, phosphodiester; PS, phosphorothioate; PNA, peptide nucleic acid; Acr-PNA, 9-aminoacridine conjugated PNA; LNA, locked nucleic acid; 2' MOE, 2'-*O*-(2-methoxy)ethyl; MBO: modified oligodeoxynucleotide or oligoribonucleotide segment (2'-*O*-methylribonucleoside PS/2'-*O*-methylribonucleoside PO/deoxynucleoside methylphosphonate *(59)*.

3. In Vivo Delivery of Antisense Oligonucleotides

The criteria of a clinically and commercially compatible ASO delivery system include nanoparticle size (<1 µ in diameter), biodegradability, high encapsulation/entrapment efficiency, ASO stability and favorable pharmacokinetics, tumor-specific drug delivery, easy formulation, scalability, and safety profiles in animals and humans. Such an optimal in vivo delivery system offers merits that may complement not only the chemically modified ASO but also natural ASO. First, a suitable vehicle may protect the unmodified/minimally modified ASO from nuclease degradation and alleviate chemistry-related side effects. Second, it may preferentially carry ASO to its desired destination, decreasing the dose required and normal tissue toxicity. Third, it may facilitate ASO transport through the cell membrane and enhance its retention in cytoplasm or transport to the nucleus, effectively blocking translation and/or transcription of the target molecule. Limited studies of ASO in vivo delivery systems have been reported **(Table 2)**. Nontargeted and tumor-targeted cationic liposomes have been shown to deliver minimally modified ASO and modified ASO, respectively **(Figs. 2 and 3; Table 2)**. In addition, several laboratories have reported the use of stabilized antisense lipid particles. Further investigations are necessary to develop validated composition(s) of safe and efficacious ASO nanoparticles. Efforts in our laboratory have been focused on development of liposome-entrapped ASO nanoparticles. One of these formulations, liposomal nanoparticle containing minimally modified *raf* antisense oligodeoxynucleotide (LErafAON), is discussed in the following section.

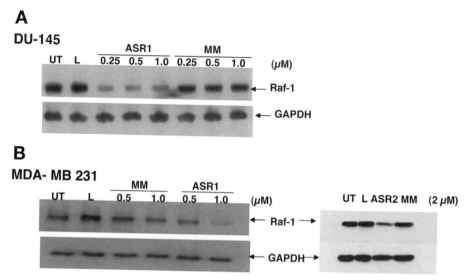

Fig. 1. Inhibition of Raf-1 protein expression in human prostate (DU-145) and breast cancer cells (MDA-MB 231). Tumor cells were treated with indicated concentration of phosphorothioate *c-raf* ASO (ASR1, ISIS 13650; ASR2, ISIS 5132) or a mismatch ASO (MM, ISIS 10353). Cells were grown to 80% confluency in improved minimum essential medium containing 10% fetal bovine serum (FBS) and 2 mM L-glutamine. For ASR1 treatment, on day 1 cells were treated with indicated concentration of ASO or MM for 6 h in the presence of lipofectin (15 µg/mL) in medium containing 1% FBS. Cells were then washed twice with 10% FBS containing medium and maintained overnight in 1% FBS containing medium in the presence of indicated concentration of antisense oligonucleotides (ASO) or MM. On day 2, cells were treated as on day 1. On day 3, Raf-1 expression was detected in cell lysates by Western blotting using monoclonal anti-Raf-1 antibody. The blots were reprobed with polyclonal anti-GAPDH antibody. For ASR2 treatment, cells were washed twice with serum-free medium and then treated with indicated concentration of ASO or MM for 6 h in serum-free medium containing 20 µg/mL lipofectin. Cells were washed twice with 10% FBS containing medium and incubated overnight in 10% FBS containing medium in the presence of indicated concentration of ASO or MM. On day 2, cells were treated as on day 1, followed by cell lysis and Western blotting on day 3. UT, untreated; L, lipofectin control.

4. Liposome-Entrapped raf Antisense Oligonucleotide: A Therapeutic Nanoparticle

4.1. Raf-1 Is a Validated Target in Cancer Therapy

Raf-1 (c-Raf), B-Raf, and A-Raf are members of a family of serine-threonine kinases known to regulate extracellular signal-regulated kinase -mediated mitogenic signal transduction pathways *(11)*. Numerous reports from our laboratory and others have shown that Raf-1 plays a key role in cell proliferation, survival,

Table 2
In Vivo Delivery Systems of Antisense Oligonucleotides[a]

In vivo delivery system	Molecular target	Formulation I.D. and ASO parameters in vivo[b]	Ref.
Cationic liposomes (first generation)	Raf-1	LE-ATG-AS, one base at 5'- and 3'-ends has PS-linkage, 15-mer, IV/IT, PK, TIB, TI	*34*
		LE-5132, PS, 20-mer, IV, PK, TIB, TI, EF	*60*
Cationic liposomes (second generation)	Raf-1	LErafAON, one base at 5'- and 3'-ends has PS-linkage, 15-mer, IV, EntEf, S, TX, PK, TIB, TUB, TI, EF	*26–28*
Cationic liposomes (easy to use)	Raf-1	LErafAON-ETU, one base at 5'- and 3'-ends has PS-linkage, 15-mer, IV, PK, TIB, E	*32,61*
Folate-liposomes	HER2	AS HER-2 ODN, PS, 15-mer, S, IV, TT, TI, EF	*62*
Cationic and immunoliposomes- (scFv against TfR)	HER2	scL-AS HER-2 ODN, PS, 15-mer, IV, TT, TI, EF	*63*, Personal communication
Coated-cationic immunoliposomes (GD2-targeted)	c-Myc	aGD$_2$-CCL-myc-as, PS, 16-mer, IV, TT, PK, TI, EF	*64*
	c-Myb	Targeted liposome-CpG-myb-as, PS, 24-mer, IV, EF	*65*
PIHCA nanoparticles	Mutated Ha-Ras	AS-VAL, unmodified 12-mer, IT, TI, EF	*66*
PACA nanocapsules	EWS-FLi-1	NC AS, PS, 25-mer, IT, EF	*67*
SALP	c-Myc	SALP INX-6295, PS, 16-mer, IV, PK, TUB, TI, EF	*68*

[a]In vivo refers to preclinical studies in animal models. Selected in vivo ASO delivery systems in cancer biology or therapy are listed.

[b]EntEf, ASO entrappment efficiency; S, ASO stability; IV intravenous, IT intratumoral; TT, tumor-targeted; PK, plasma pharmacokinetics; TIB, normal tissue biodistribution; TUB, tumor tissue biodistribution; TX, toxicology; TI, target inhibition; EF, in vivo antitumor efficacy; PIHCA, polyisohexylcyanoacrylate; PACA, polyisobutylcyanoacrylate; TfR, transferrin receptor; GD2, disialoganglioside; SALP, stabilized antisense lipid particles.

damage-induced signal transduction, and metabolism *(12–17)*. Growing evidence also suggests an extracellular signal-regulated kinase-independent role of Raf-1 in cell survival *(5,18,19)*. Using sense and antisense c-*raf*-1 cDNA

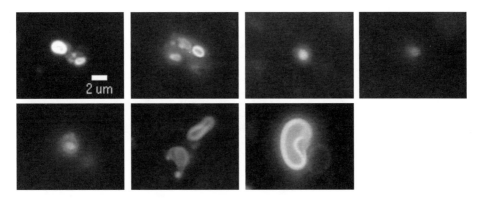

Fig. 2. Fluorescence microscopy showing first generation of liposome-entrapped *raf* antisense oligodeoxynucleotide (LE-ATG-AS *raf* ODN). 5'-Fluorescein-labeled minimally modified rafAON (ATG-AS *raf* ODN) was entrapped in liposomes as described earlier *(34)*.

molecules and Raf short-interfering RNA, expression of Raf-1 has been associated with resistance of human tumors to radiation and chemotherapeutic drugs *(2,20–25)*. A correlation between ASO-specific inhibition of Raf-1 in vivo, tumor growth arrest, and enhanced sensitivity to radiation or chemotherapeutic drugs has also been demonstrated, further establishing Raf-1 as a validated target in cancer drug discovery *(5,9)*. We summarize next our recently reported preclinical and clinical studies of liposome-entrapped *raf* antisense oligonucleotide (LErafAON) as a novel liposomal antisense therapeutic *(26–29)*.

4.2. Preclinical Development and Validation of Liposome-Entrapped raf Antisense Oligonucleotide

A schematic diagram of LErafAON formulation is shown in **Fig. 4A**. The rafAON is a 15-mer ASO with phosphorothioate linkage limited to one base at 5'- and 3'-ends *(30)*. The rafAON sequence is targeted against the translation initiation region of c-*raf*-1 mRNA. The liposome formulation consists of a mixture of a cationic lipid (dimethyldioctadecyl ammonium bromide), egg phosphatidylchloline, and cholesterol in a molar ratio of 1:3.2:1.6. The rafAON to lipid ratio is 1:15 (w/w). The particle size was found to be approx 500 nm and entrapment efficiency was >85%. The LErafAON formulation was stable at room temperature for at least 1 wk as shown by the presence of 15-mer rafAON **(Fig. 4B)**.

In CD2F1 mice, systemic administration (intravenous via tail vein [iv]) of LErafAON produced no morbidity/mortality (35 mg/kg/dose, iv, ×12). Dose-related elevations in liver enzymes (alanine aminotransferase [ALT] and aspartate aminotransferase [AST]) and histopathological changes in liver were noted

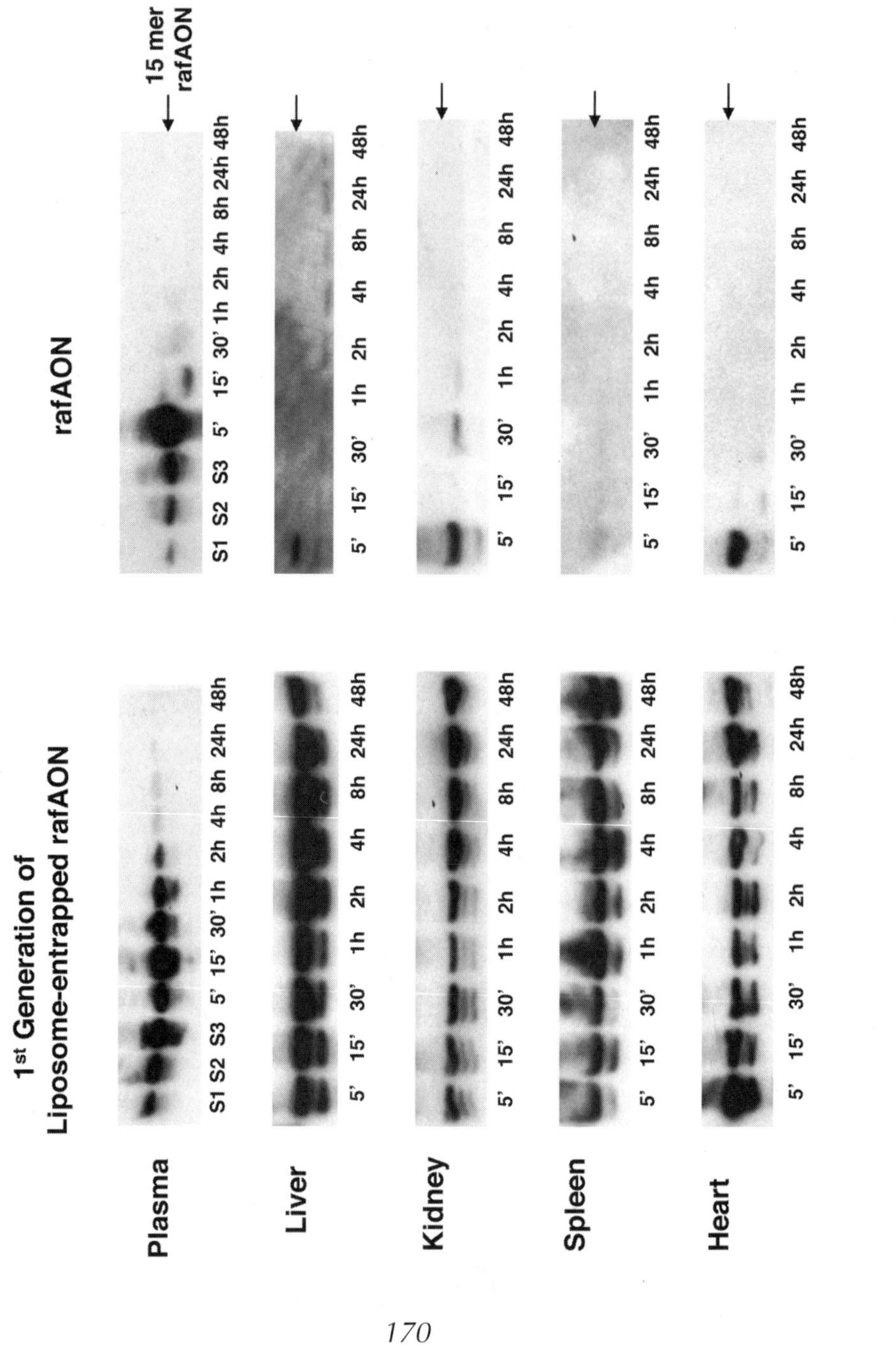

1st Generation of Liposome-entrapped rafAON

rafAON

15 mer rafAON

Plasma

S1 S2 S3 5' 15' 30' 1h 2h 4h 8h 24h 48h

Liver

5' 15' 30' 1h 2h 4h 8h 24h 48h

Kidney

5' 15' 30' 1h 2h 4h 8h 24h 48h

Spleen

5' 15' 30' 1h 2h 4h 8h 24h 48h

Heart

5' 15' 30' 1h 2h 4h 8h 24h 48h

170

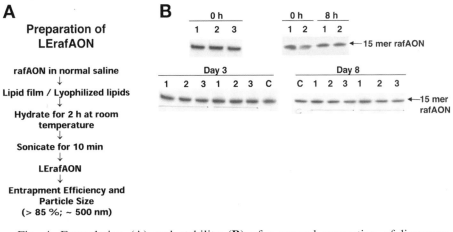

Fig. 4. Formulation (**A**) and stability (**B**) of a second generation of liposome-entrapped 15-mer *raf* antisense oligodeoxynucleotide (rafAON) with PS linkage of one base at 5'- and 3'-ends (LErafAON). The assays of LErafAON preparation, entrapment efficiency, particle size, and stability at room temperature have been reported in details earlier *(26)*. The rafAON to lipid ratio was 1:15 (w/w). C, control freshly prepared LErafAON.

in LErafAON and blank liposome groups. No morbidity/mortality and changes in clinical chemistry or histopathology were observed in NZW rabbits using two dose groups (3.75 mg/kg/dose, iv, ×8; 6.5 mg/kg/dose, iv, ×6) or in cynomolgous monkeys (3.75 or 6.25 mg/kg/dose, iv, ×9). Transient decrease in total hemolytic complement activity (CH50, ~62–74%) and increases in C3a (3-fold) and Bb levels (~5- to 12-fold) were observed in LErafAON and blank liposome groups of monkeys.

A 30-mg/kg iv dose of LErafAON in human prostate tumor (PC-3)-bearing Balb/c athymic mice gave a terminal plasma half-life of 27 h, and intact rafAON could be detected in plasma, and in normal and tumor tissues for up to at least 48 h (**Fig. 5**). In monkeys, the terminal plasma half-life of 30.36 ± 23.87 h was

Fig. 3. *(Opposite page)* A comparison of the plasma pharmacokinetics and tissue distribution profiles of first generation of liposome-entrapped (LE-ATG-AS *raf* ODN) and unentrapped 15-mer rafAON (ATG-AS *raf* ODN) with PS linkage of one base at 5'- and 3'-ends. The dried lipids (DDAB:PC:CHOL in a molar ratio of 1:3.2:1.6) and rafAON (1.0 mg/mL) were hydrated overnight at 4°C in phosphate buffered saline, followed by vigorous vortexing and sonication for 5 min. The rafAON to lipid ratio was 1:30 (w/w). Balb/c nu/nu mice received 30 mg/kg, iv of LE-ATG-AS *raf* ODN or ATG-AS *raf* ODN. Blood and tissue samples were collected at indicated times postinjection, and antisense oligonucleotides concentrations in plasma and tissue samples were quantified by electrophoresis and autoradiography. (Modified from **ref. *34***).

LErafAON: Balb/c nu/nu Mice

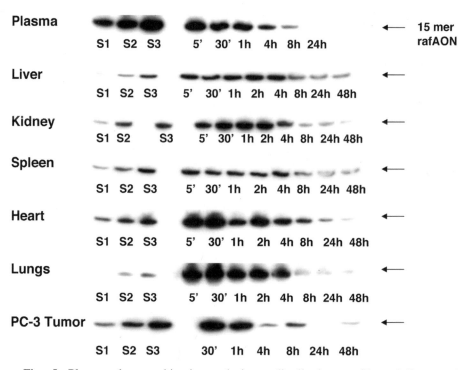

Fig. 5. Plasma pharmacokinetics and tissue distribution profiles of liposomal nanoparticle containing minimally modified *raf* antisense oligodeoxynucleotide (LErafAON). Balb/c nu/nu mice received 30 mg/kg, iv of LErafAON. Blood and tissue samples were collected at indicated times postinjection. Various samples may be differently diluted before electrophoresis to improve resolution of the bands following autoradiography. Different concentrations of the standard rafAON (S1, S2, S3) were used in different tissues. Antisense oligodeoxynucleotide concentrations in plasma and tissue samples were quantified as described earlier *(26)*.

observed at an iv dose of 6.25 mg/kg **(Fig. 6)** LErafAON treatment (25 mg/kg/dose, iv, ×10) caused inhibition of Raf-1 protein expression in normal and tumor tissues of PC-3 bearing athymic mice (>50%, vs controls) **(Fig. 7)**. A combination of LErafAON and ionizing radiation (IR) treatment of PC-3-tumor bearing athymic mice led to tumor growth arrest, whereas a combination of LErafAON and IR treatments resulted in tumor regression *(26)*. Enhanced tumor growth inhibition in response to LErafAON and IR was also observed in athymic mice bearing human pancreatic tumor (Aspc-1) or hormone-independent breast tumor (MDA-MB 435) **(Fig. 8)**. Previously, we have demonstrated enhanced antitumor effects of a combination of LErafAON and

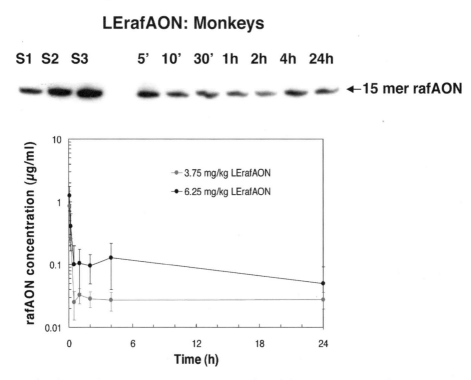

Fig. 6. The plasma concentration-time profile of liposomal nanoparticle containing minimally modified *raf* antisense oligodeoxynucleotide (LErafAON) in cynomolgus monkeys. Monkeys received a slow bolus injection of LErafAON via saphenous vein. Heparinized blood samples were collected at indicated time points postinjection and rafAON concentration was determined as described earlier *(26)*. Top, representative autoradiograph showing intact rafAON in plasma at various time points after administration of 6.25 mg/kg, iv, LErafAON in a male monkey. S1, S2, and S3, different concentrations of the standard rafAON. Bottom, plasma concentration–time curve of LErafAON. Each point represents mean ± SD (3.75 mg/kg LErafAON, *n* = 3; 6.25 mg/kg LErafAON, *n* = 6).

chemotherapeutic drugs against PC-3, pancreatic (Aspc-1 and Colo-357), lung (A549), and breast tumor xenografts grown in athymic mice (MDA-MB231) *(27,28)*. Similar observations were made in a different hormone-independent breast tumor model (MDA-MB 435) **(Fig. 9)**. These data have formed a basis of the clinical phase I studies of LErafAON for cancer treatment.

4.3. Clinical Studies

LErafAON is a recent addition to the slowly growing number of ASO in the clinical trials **(Table 3)**. It is also the first liposomal ASO drug tested in humans *(29,31)*.

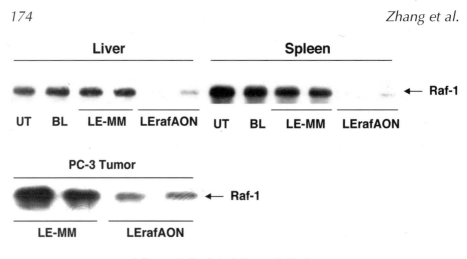

Fig. 7. LErafAON treatment inhibits Raf-1 expression in normal and tumor tissues of BALB/c nu/nu mice. Mice bearing human prostate tumor xenografts (PC-3) (>50 mm³) received liposomal nanoparticle containing minimally modified *raf* antisense oligodeoxynucleotide (LErafAON) (25.0 mg/kg/dose, iv, ×10), a liposome-entrapped mismatch oligonucleotide, (25.0 mg/kg/dose, iv, ×10) (LE-MM), blank liposomes (iv, at the same dosing and schedule) (BL), or were left untreated (UT). Normal and tumor tissues were excised within 6–12 h after the last dose and Raf-1 expression was determined in tissue homogenates by immunoprecipitation (I.P.) followed by immunoblotting (I.B.) using anti-Raf-1 antibody as described earlier *(26)*.

Prestudy validated methods were established to determine pharmacokinetics of LErafAON, and biomarker expression (c-*raf*-1 mRNA and Raf-1 protein) in clinical specimens. Bioanalytical method validation experiments were performed to quantify rafAON in human plasma using a gel electrophoresis method. Concentration standards were prepared by adding known amounts of rafAON to blank human plasma, followed by extraction of rafAON using the phenol chloroform extraction method. The validation experiments determined the precision and accuracy of the limits of quantification of rafAON in experiments, and the effects of dilution, freeze–thaw cycles, and storage at –80°C and 4°C. Other parameters included the integrity of rafAON during sample processing, specificity of rafAON sequence, and interference of lipids in the assays. The acceptance criteria were <25% coefficient of variation for precision and 100 ± 25% analytical recovery (AR). A maximum dilution of 500-fold from a 5-µg/mL rafAON specimen was acceptable in clinical studies. The rafAON samples could be stored at –80°C for up to 14 d. Three cycles of freeze–thaw did not impair the quality of the rafAON specimens at tested concentrations. The integrity of 15-mer rafAON was determined in two independent experiments

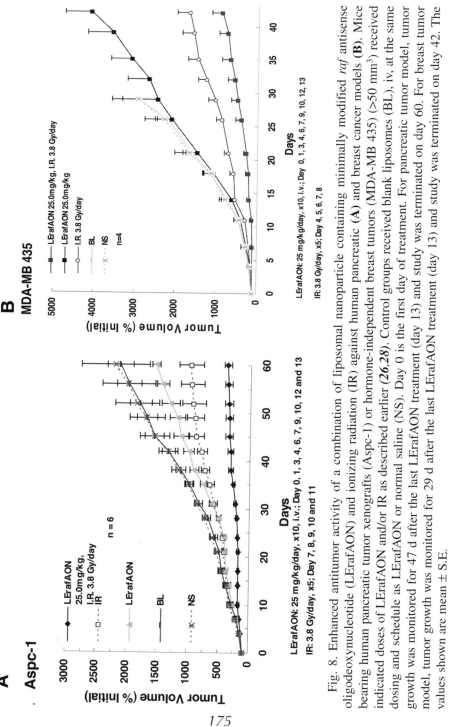

Fig. 8. Enhanced antitumor activity of a combination of liposomal nanoparticle containing minimally modified *raf* antisense oligodeoxynucleotide (LErafAON) and ionizing radiation (IR) against human pancreatic (**A**) and breast cancer models (**B**). Mice bearing human pancreatic tumor xenografts (Aspc-1) or hormone-independent breast tumors (MDA-MB 435) (>50 mm³) received indicated doses of LErafAON and/or IR as described earlier (*26,28*). Control groups received blank liposomes (BL), iv, at the same dosing and schedule as LErafAON or normal saline (NS). Day 0 is the first day of treatment. For pancreatic tumor model, tumor growth was monitored for 47 d after the last LErafAON treatment (day 13) and study was terminated on day 60. For breast tumor model, tumor growth was monitored for 29 d after the last LErafAON treatment (day 13) and study was terminated on day 42. The values shown are mean ± S.E.

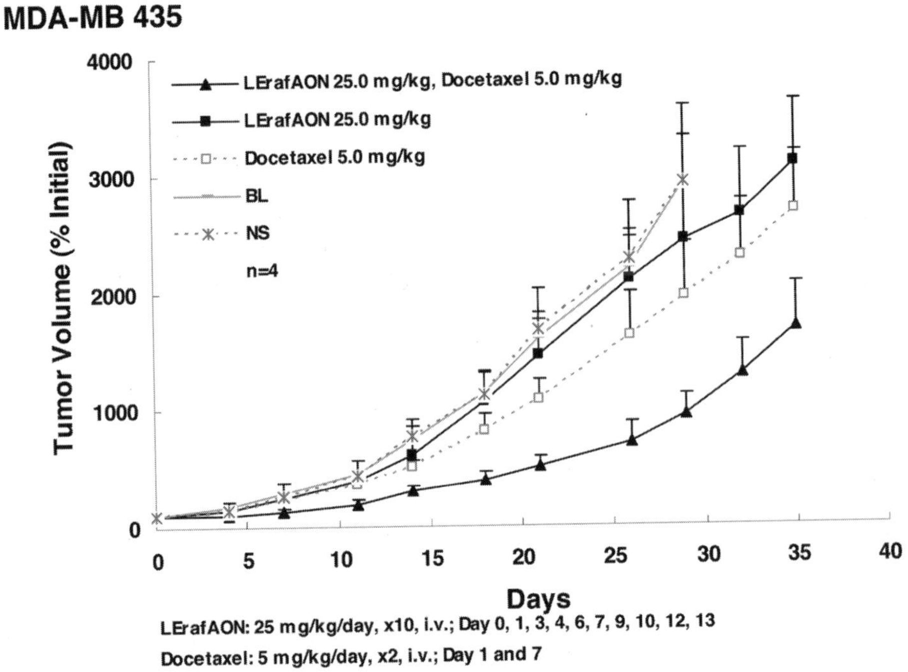

MDA-MB 435

LErafAON: 25 mg/kg/day, x10, i.v.; Day 0, 1, 3, 4, 6, 7, 9, 10, 12, 13
Docetaxel: 5 mg/kg/day, x2, i.v.; Day 1 and 7

Fig. 9. Enhanced antitumor activity of a combination of liposomal nanoparticle containing minimally modified *raf* antisense oligodeoxynucleotide (LErafAON) and docetaxel (Taxotere) against human breast cancer model (MDA-MB 435). Mice bearing human hormone-independent breast tumors (MDA-MB 435) (>50 mm³) received indicated doses of LErafAON and/or docetaxel as described earlier *(28)*. Control groups received blank liposomes (BL), iv, at the same dosing and schedule as LErafAON or normal saline (NS). Day 0 is the first day of treatment. Tumor growth was monitored for at least 22 d after the last LErafAON treatment (day 13). The values shown are mean ± S.E.

by comparing the size of the 15-mer rafAON with a size marker representing a mixture of 15-mer, 14-mer, and 13-mer rafAON. The sample processing procedure was acceptable with accuracy of the 15-mer rafAON controls in the 84.0– 90.0% AR range. Overall, lipids do not interfere in the quantification of rafAON in human plasma.

Experiments were also performed to establish certified methods for expression of biomarkers, c-*raf*-1 mRNA and Raf-1 protein in human peripheral blood lymphocytes. Relative levels of c-*raf*-1 mRNA and Raf-1 protein in human lymphocytes were quantified using a RT-PCR method for RNA and a Western blotting method for protein. The acceptance criteria were <25% coefficient of variation for precision and 100 ± 25% AR. For the mRNA validation experiments, leukocytes were isolated from heparinized human blood obtained from

Table 3
Summary of Antisense Oligonucleotides in Clinical Oncology Trials

Molecular target	Drug	Company	Size, ASO chemistry[a]	Cancer type	Clinical status (ref.)
Bcl-2	G3139	Genta	18-mer, PS	Solid tumors, MM, AML, HRPC, melanoma	Phase I–II *69–74*
PKA-R1α	GEM 231	Hybridon	18-mer, MBO	Refractory solid tumors	Phase I–II *75–77*
PKC-α	ISIS 3521	ISIS	20-mer, PS	Solid tumors, non-Hodgkin's lymphoma	Phase I–II *78–80*
Raf-1	ISIS 5132	ISIS	20-mer, PS	Solid tumors	Phase I–II *81,82*
LErafAON	NeoPharm		15-mer, liposome-entrapped, minimally modified	Solid tumors	Phase I *29,31*
LErafAON-ETU	NeoPharm		15-mer, liposome-entrapped, minimally modified	Advanced cancer	Phase I *33*
RNR (R2)	GTI-2040	Lorus	20-mer, PS	Solid tumors	Phase I *83*

[a]PS, phosphorothioate; MBO, mixed-backbone; minimally modified, one base at 5′- and 3′-ends has PS-linkage; MM, multiple myeloma; AML, acute myeloid leukemia; HRPC, hormone-refractory prostate cancer.

LErafAON: Humans

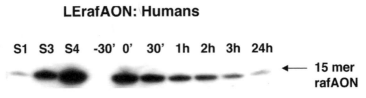

Fig. 10. Plasma pharmacokinetics of liposomal nanoparticle containing minimally modified *raf* antisense oligodeoxynucleotide (LErafAON) in clinical specimens. Representative autoradiograph showing intact circulating rafAON at various time points in a patient treated with LErafAON (Week1:2 mg/kg/wk dose level) as described earlier *(29)*. Sample aliquots were diluted as follows: 0', 4X; and 24 h, 0.5X; or left undiluted before electrophoresis. S1, S3, and S4 represent 0.01, 0.1, and 0.5 µg/mL of rafAON standard, respectively. –30', predose sample.

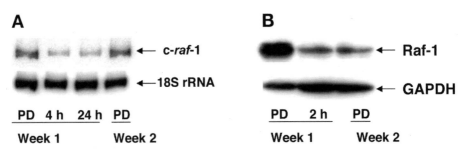

Fig. 11. Expression of c-*raf*-1 in clinical specimens. (**A**) Representative autoradiographs showing inhibition of c-*raf*-1 mRNA relative to the predose (PD) at 4 and 24 h in peripheral blood mononuclear cells of a patient treated with LErafAON (Week1:6 mg/kg/wk dose level) as described before *(29)*. The c-*raf*-1 mRNA expression was determined by quantitative RT-PCR using *raf*-1 and 18S specific primers. (**B**) Representative immunoblot showing inhibition of Raf-1 expression relative to the predose (PD) at 2 h in a different patient in the same cohort as (**A**). Raf-1 protein expression was analyzed in peripheral blood mononuclear cells by Western blotting using anti-Raf-1 antibody followed by reprobing of the same blot with anti-GAPDH antibody.

healthy donors. Based on the data obtained, lowest and highest amounts of total RNA to be used in clinical studies were 40 and 160 ng, respectively. Total RNA samples were unacceptable for expression analysis following three cycles of freeze–thaw and/or storage at –80°C for 3 wk prior to analysis.

The Raf-1 protein validation experiments were performed using whole cell lysates from donor human lymphocytes. Based on the data obtained, lowest and highest amounts of total protein to be used in clinical studies were 100 and 300 µg, respectively. Lymphocytes subjected to three cycles of freeze–thaw were unacceptable for Raf-1 expression determinations in clinical studies. However, lymphocytes stored frozen at −80°C for approx 2 mo prior to assay were found to be acceptable for Raf-1 expression in clinical studies.

In a phase I clinical study of LErafAON in patients with advanced solid tumors, dose-independent hypersensitivity reactions and dose-dependent thrombocytopenia were observed *(29)*. In this report, pharmacokinetic studies of LErafAON showed persistence of circulating rafAON for up to 24 h **(Fig. 10)**. Inhibition of *c-raf*-1 expression was seen in peripheral blood mononuclear cells in some of the evaluable clinical specimens **(Fig. 11)**. An improved formulation of LErafAON (LErafAON-ETU) is being tested in a clinical study *(32,33)*.

Acknowledgments

The authors thank colleagues and collaborators for their contributions to studies discussed in this review. The number of citations included does not reflect all of the literature in this field. The research work was supported by grants from the National Institutes of Health and NeoPharm, Inc.

References

1. Zamecnik, P. C. and Stephenson, M. L. (1978) Inhibition of Rous sarcoma virus replication and cell transformation by a specific oligodeoxynucleotide. *Proc. Natl. Acad. Sci. USA* **75**, 280–284.
2. Kasid, U., Pfeifer, A., Brennan, T., et al. (1989) Effect of antisense *c-raf*-1 on tumorigenicity and radiation sensitivity of a human squamous carcinoma. *Science* **243**, 1354–1356.
3. Pirrollo, K. F., Rait, A., Sleer, L. S., and Chang, E. H. (2003) Antisense therapeutics: from theory to clinical practice. *Pharmacol. Ther.* **99**, 55–77.
4. Kurreck, J. (2003) Antisense technologies. Improvement through novel chemical modifications. *Eur. J. Biochem.* **270**, 1628–1644.
5. Kasid, U. and Dritschilo, A. (2003) RAF antisense oligonucleotide as a tumor radiosensitizer. *Oncogene* **22**, 5876–5884.
6. Agrawal, S. and Kandimalla, E. R. (2004) Antisense and siRNA as agonists of Toll-like receptors. *Nat. Biotechnol.* **22**, 1533–1537.
7. Crooke, S. T. (2004) Progress in antisense technology. *Annu. Rev. Med.* **55**, 61–95.
8. Gleave, M. E. and Monia, B. P. (2005) Antisense therapy for cancer. *Nat. Rev. Cancer* **5**, 468–479.
9. Monia, B. P., Johnston, J. F., Geiger, T., Muller, M., and Fabbro, D. (1996) Antitumor activity of a phosphorothioate antisense oligodeoxynucleotide targeted against C-raf kinase. *Nat. Med.* **6**, 668–675.
10. Mullen, P., McPhillips, F., MacLeod, K., Monia, B., Smyth, J. F., and Langdon, S. P. (2004) Antisense oligonucleotide targeting of Raf-1: Importance of Raf-1 mRNA expression levels and Raf-1-dependent signaling in determining growth response in ovarian cancer. *Clin. Cancer Res.* **10**, 2100–2108.
11. Williams, N. G. and Roberts, T. M. (1994) Signal transduction pathways involving the Raf proto-oncogene. *Cancer Metastasis Rev.* **13**, 105–116.

12. Kasid, U., Suy, S., Dent, P., Ray, S., Whiteside, T. L., and Sturgill, T. W. (1996) Activation of Raf by ionizing radiation. *Nature* **382,** 813–816.

13. Suy, S., Anderson, W. B., Dent, P., Chang, E., and Kasid, U. (1997) Association of Grb2 with Sos and Ras with Raf-1 upon gamma irradiation of breast cancer cells. *Oncogene* **15,** 53–61.

14. Le Mellay, V., Houben, R., Troppmair, J., et al. (2002) Regulation of glycolysis by Raf protein serine/threonine kinases. *Adv. Enzyme. Regul.* **42,** 317–332.

15. Patel, S., Wang, F. -H., Whiteside, T. L., and Kasid, U. (1997) Constitutive modulation of Raf-1 protein kinase is associated with differential gene expression of several known and unknown genes. *Mol. Med.* **3,** 674–685.

16. Kasid, U. (2001) Raf-1 protein kinase, signal transduction, and targeted intervention of radiation response. *Exp. Biol. Med.* **226,** 624–625.

17. Kasid, U. and Suy, S. (1998) Stress-responsive signal transduction: emerging concepts and biological significance. In: *Apoptosis Genes,* (Potten, C. S., Booth, C., and Wilson, J., eds.), Kluwer Academic Publishers, Boston, MA, pp. 85–118.

18. Odabaei, G., Chatterjee, D., Jazirehi, A. R., Goodglick, L., Yeung, K., and Bonavida, B. (2004) Raf-1 kinase inhibitor protein: structure, function, regulation of cell signaling, and pivotal role in apoptosis. *Adv. Cancer Res.* **91,** 169–200.

19. Hindley, A. and Kolch, W. (2002) Extracellular signal regulated kinase (ERK)/mitogen activated protein kinase (MAPK)-independent functions of Raf kinases. *J. Cell Sci.* **115,** 1575–1581.

20. Rasouli-Nia, A., Liu, D., Perdue, S., and Britten, R. A. (1998) High Raf-1 kinase activity protects human tumor cells against paclitaxel-induced cytotoxicity. *Clin. Cancer Res.* **4,** 1111–1116.

21. Weinstein-Oppenheimer, C. R., Henriquez-Roldan, C. F., Davis, J. M., et al. (2001) Role of the Raf signal transduction cascade in the in vitro resistance to the anticancer drug doxorubicin. *Clin. Cancer Res.* **7,** 2898–2907.

22. Nimmanapalli, R., O'Bryan, E., Kuhn, D., Yamaguchi, H., Wang, H. G., and Bhalla, K. N. (2003) Regulation of 17-AAG-induced apoptosis: role of Bcl-2, Bcl-XL, and Bax downstream of 17-AAG-mediated down-regulation of Akt, Raf-1, and Src kinases. *Blood* **102,** 269–275.

23. Pfeifer, A., Mark, G., Leung, S., Dougherty, M., Spillare, E., and Kasid, U. (1998) Effects of c-*raf*-1 and c-*myc* expression on radiation response in an *in vitro* model of human small-cell-lung-carcinoma. *Biochem. Biophy. Res. Comm.* **252,** 481–486.

24. Tang, W. Y., Chau, S. P., Tsang, W. P., Kong, S. K., and Kwok, T. T. (2004) The role of Raf-1 in radiation resistance of human hepatocellular carcinoma Hep G2 cells. *Oncol. Rep.* **12,** 1349–1354.

25. Pal, A., Ahmad, A., Khan, S., et al. (2005) Systemic delivery of RafsiRNA using cationic cardiolipin liposome silences Raf-1 expression and inhibits tumor growth in xenograft model of human prostate cancer. *Int. J. Oncology.* **26,** 1087–1091.

26. Gokhale, P. C., Zhang, C., Newsome, J., et al. (2002) Pharmacokinetics, toxicity, and efficacy of ends-modified raf antisense oligodeoxyribonucleotide encapsulated in a novel cationic liposome (LErafAON). *Clin. Cancer Res.* **8,** 3611–3621.

27. Mewani, R. R., Tang, W., Rahman, A., et al. (2004) Enhanced therapeutic effects of doxorubicin and paclitaxel in combination with liposome-entrapped ends-modified raf antisense oligonucleotide against human prostate, lung and breast tumor models. *Int. J. Onc.* **24,** 1181–1188.

28. Pei, J., Zhang, C., Gokhale, P. C., et al. (2004) Combination with liposome-entrapped, ends-modified raf antisense oligonucleotide (LErafAON) improves the anti-tumor efficacies of cisplatin, epirubicin, mitoxantrone, docetaxel, and gemcitabine. *Anti-Cancer Drugs* **15,** 243–253.

29. Rudin, C. M., Marshall, J. L., Huang, C. H., et al. (2004) Delivery of a liposomal c-raf-1 antisense oligonucleotide by weekly bolus dosing in patients with advanced solid tumors: a phase I study. *Clin. Cancer Res.* **10,** 7244–7251.

30. Soldatenkov, V. A., Dritschilo, A., Wang, F. -H., Olah, Z., Anderson, W. B., and Kasid, U. (1997) Inhibition of Raf-1 protein kinase by antisense phosphorothioate oligodeoxyribonucleotide is associated with sensitization of human laryngeal squamous carcinoma cells to gamma radiation. *Can J. Sci. Am.* **3,** 13–20.

31. Dritschilo, A., Huang, C. H., Fleming, C., et al. (2003) Infusion of liposome-encapsulated c-*raf* antisense oligodeoxynucleotide (LErafAON) during radiation therapy in patients with advanced malignancies: a phase I study. *Proceedings of the American Society of Clinical Oncology.* **22,** p. 224.

32. Lei, Y., Ahmad, A., Sheikh, S., Zhang, A., and Ahmad, I. (2004) Enhanced therapeutic efficacy of a novel liposome-based formulation of c-raf AON in combination with Taxol against human ovarian tumor model in SCID mice. *Proc. Am. Assoc. Cancer Res.* **45,** 147.

33. Steinberg, J. L., Mendelson, D. S., Block, H., et al. (2005) Phase I study of LErafAON-ETU, an easy-to-use formulation of liposome entrapped c-raf antisense oligonucleotide, in advanced cancer patients. *J. Clin. Oncol.* **23 (Suppl.),** 244S.

34. Gokhale, P. C., Soldatenkov, V., Wang, F. -H., Rahman, A., Dritschilo, A., and Kasid, U. (1997) Antisense *raf* oligodeoxyribonucleotide is protected by liposomal encapsulation and inhibits Raf-1 protein expression *in vitro* and *in vivo*: implications for gene therapy of radioresistant cancer. *Gene Therapy* **4,** 1289–1299.

35. Gleave, M., Tolcher, A., Miyake, H., et al. (1999) Progression to androgen independence is delayed by adjuvant treatment with antisense Bcl-2 oligodeoxynucleotides after castration in the LNCaP prostate tumor model. *Clin. Cancer Res.* **5,** 2891–2898.

36. Taylor, J. K., Zhang, Q. Q., Monia, B. P., Marcusson, E. G., and Dean, N. M. (1999) Inhibition of Bcl-X$_L$ expression sensitizes normal human keratinocytes and epithelial cells to apoptotic stimuli. *Oncogene* **18,** 4495–4504.

37. Taylor, J. K., Zhang, Q. Q., Wyatt, J. R., and Dean, N. M. (1999) Induction of endogenous Bcl-xS through the control of Bcl-x pre-mRNA splicing by antisense oligonucleotides. *Nat. Biotechnol.* **17,** 1097–1100.

38. Zangemeister-Wittke, U., Leech, S. H., Olie, R. A., et al. (2000) A novel bispecific antisense oligonucleotide inhibiting both *bcl-2* and *bcl-xL* expression efficiently indues apoptosis in tumor cells. *Clin. Cancer Res.* **6,** 2547–2555.

39. Simões-Wüst, A. P., Hopkins-Donaldson, S., Sigrist, B., Belyanskaya, L., Stahel, R. A., and Zahgemeister-Wittke, U. (2004) A functionally improved locked nucleic acid antisense oligonucleotide inhibits Bcl-2 and Bcl-xL expression and facilitates tumor cell apoptosis. *Oligonucleotides* **14,** 199–209.
40. Rapozzi, V., Burm, B. E. A., Cogoi, S., et al. (2002) Antiproliferative effect in chronic myeloid leukaemia cells by antisense peptide nucleic acids. *Nucleic Acids Res.* **30,** 3712–3721.
41. Zellweger, T., Miyake, H., Cooper, S., et al. (2001) Antitumor activity of antisense clusterin oligonucleotides is improved in vitro and in vivo by incorporation of 2'-*O*-(2-methoxy)ethyl chemistry. *J. Pharmacol. Exp. Ther.* **298,** 934–940.
42. Park, Y. G., Nesterova, M., Agrawal, S., and Cho-Chung, Y. S. (1999) Dual blockade of cyclic AMP response element-(CRE) and AP-1-directed transcription by CRE-transcription factor decoy oligonucleotide. *J. Biol. Chem.* **274,** 1573–1580.
43. Aharinejad, S., Paulus, P., Sioud, M., et al. (2004) Colony-stimulating factor-1 blockade by antisense oligonucleotides and small interfering RNAs suppresses growth of human mammary tumor xenografts in mice. *Cancer Res.* **64,** 5378–5384.
44. Rait, A. S., Pirollo, K. F., Rait, V., Krygier, J. E., Xiang, L., and Chang, E. H. (2001) Inhibitory effects of the combination of HER-2 antisense oligonucleotide and chemotherapeutic agents used for the treatment of human breast cancer. *Cancer Gene Ther.* **8,** 728–739.
45. Shadidi, M. and Sioud, M. (2003) Identification of novel carrier peptides for the specific delivery of therapeutics into cancer cells. *FEBS J.* **17,** 256–258.
46. Thallinger, C., Wolschek, M. F., Maierhofer, H., et al. (2004) Mcl-1 is a novel therapeutic target for human sarcoma: Synergistic inhibition of human sarcoma xenotransplants by a combination of Mcl-1 antisense oligonucleotides with low-dose cyclophosphamide. *Clin. Cancer Res.* **10,** 4185–4191.
47. Zhang, Z., Wang, H., Prasad, G., et al. (2004) Radiosensitization by antisense anti-MDM2 mixed-backbone oligonucleotide in *in vitro* and *in vivo* human cancer models. *Clin. Cancer Res.* **10,** 1263–1273.
48. Shiraishi, T. and Nielsen, P. E. (2004) Down-regulation of MDM2 and activation of p53 in human cancer cells by antisense 9-aminoacridine-PNA (peptide nucleic acid) conjugates. *Nucleic Acids Res.* **32,** 4893–4902.
49. Zupi, G., Scarsella, M., Semple, S. C., Mottolese, M., Natali, P. G., and Leonetti, C. (2005) Antitumor efficacy of *bcl-2* and *c-myc* antisense oligonucleotides in combination with cisplatin in human melanoma xenografts: relevance of the administration sequence. *Clin. Cancer Res.* **11,** 1990–1998.
50. Cutrona, G., Carpaneto, E. M., Ponezanelli, A., et al. (2003) Inhibition of the translocated *c-myc* in Burkitt's lymphoma by a PNA complementary to the $E\mu$ enhancer. *Cancer Res.* **63,** 6144–6148.
51. Wang, H., Cai, Q., Zeng, X., Yu, D., Agrawall, S., and Zhang, R. (1999) Antitumor activity and pharmacokinetics of a mixed-backbone antisense oligonucleotide targeted to the RIα subunit of protein kinase A after oral administration. *Proc. Natl. Acad. Sci. USA* **96,** 13,989–13,994.

52. Dean, N., Mckay, R., Miraglia, L., et al. (1996) Inhibition of growth of human tumor cell lines in nude mice by an antisense of oligonucleotide inhibitor of protein kinase C-α expression. *Cancer Res.* **56,** 3499–3507.

53. Mologni, L., Marchesi, E., Nielsen, P. E., and Gambacorti-Passerini, C. (2001) Inhibition of promyelocytic leukemia (PML)/retinoic acid receptor-α and PML expression in acute promyelocytic leukemia cells by anti-PML peptide nucleic acid. *Cancer Res.* **61,** 5468–5473.

54. Tanami, H., Imoto, I., Hirasawa, A., et al. (2004) Involvement of overexpressed wild-type *BRAF* in the growth of malignant melanoma cell lines. *Oncogene* **23,** 8796–8804.

55. Kasid, U., Olah, Z., Anderson, W., and Dritschilo, A. (1991) Inhibition of c-*raf*-1 protein kinase activity by antisense phosphorothioate oligonucleotides in human radiation resistant squamous carcinoma cells. *Proceedings of the International Congress of Radiation Research,* no. P16-03, p. 242.

56. Lee, Y., Vassilakos, A., Feng, N., et al. (2003) GTI-2040, and antisense agent targeting the small subunit component (R2) of human ribonucleotide reductase, shows potent antitumor activity against a variety of tumors. *Cancer Res.* **63,** 2802–2811.

57. Elayadi, A. N., Demieville, A., Wancewicz, E. V., Monia, B. P., and Corey, D. R. (2001) Inhibition of telomerase by 2'-O-(2-methoxyethyl) RNA oligomers: effect of length, phosphorothioate substitution and time inside cells. *Nucleic Acids Res.* **29,** 1683–1689.

58. McManus, D. C., Lefebvre, C. A., Cherton-Horvat, G., et al. (2004) Loss of XIAP protein expression by RNAi and antisense approaches sesitizes cancer cells to functionally diverse chemotherapeutics. *Oncogene* **23,** 8105–8117.

59. Agrawal, S., Jiang, Z., Zhao, Q., et al. (1997) Mixed-backbone oligonucleotides as second generation antisense oligonucleotides: *in vitro* and *in vivo* studies. *Proc. Natl. Acad. Sci. USA* **94,** 2620–2625.

60. Gokhale, P. C., McRae, D., Monia, B. P., et al. (1999) Antisense *raf* oligodeoxyribonucleotide is a radiosensitizer *in vivo. Antisense Nucleic Acid Drug Dev.* **9,** 191–201.

61. Johnson, J. L., Guo, W., Zang, J., et al. (2004) Quantification of raf antisense oligonucleotide (rafAON) in biological matrices by LC-MS/MS to support pharmacokinetics of a liposome-entrapped rafAON formulation. *Biomed. Chromatogr.* **19,** 272–278.

62. Rait, A. S., Pirollo, K. F., Xiang, L., Ulick, D., and Chang, E. H. (2002) Tumor-targeting, systemically delivered antisense HER-2 chemosensitizes human breast cancer xenografts irrespective of HER-2 levels. *Mol. Med.* **8,** 475–486.

63. Xu, L., Huang, C. C., Huang, W., et al. (2002) Systemic tumor-targeted gene delivery by anti-transferrin receptor scFv-immunoliposomes. *Mol. Cancer Ther.* **1,** 337–346.

64. Pastorino, F., Brignole, C., Marimpietri, D., et al. (2003) Targeted liposomal c-*myc* antisense oligodeoxynucleotides induce apoptosis and inhibit tumor growth and metastases in human melanoma models. *Clin. Cancer Res.* **9,** 4595–4605.

65. Brignole, C., Pastorino, F., Marimpietri, D., et al. (2004) Immune cell-mediated antitumor activities of GD$_2$- targeted liposomal c-myb antisense oligonucleotides containing CpG motifs. *J. Natl. Cancer Inst.* **96,** 1171–1180.

66. Schwab, G., Chavany, C., Duroux, I., et al. (1994) Antisense oligonucleotides adsorbed to polyalkylcyanoacrylate nanoparticles specifically inhibit mutated Ha-*ras*-mediated cell proliferation and tumorigenicity in nude mice. *Proc. Natl. Acad. Sci. USA* **91,** 10,460–10,464.

67. Lamber, G., Bertrand, J. R., and Fattal, E. (2000) EWS Fli-1 antisense nanocapsules inhibits ewing sarcoma-related tumor in mice. *Biochem. Biophys. Res. Commun.* **279,** 401–406.

68. Leonetti, C., Biroccio, A., Benassi, B., et al. (2001) Encapsulation of c-myc antisense oligodeoxynucleotides in lipid particles improves antitumoral efficacy *in vivo* in a human melanoma line. *Cancer Gene Ther.* **8,** 459–468.

69. Rudin, C. M., Kozloff, M., Hoffman, P. C., et al. (2004) Phase I study of G3139, a *bcl*-2 antisense oligonucleotide, combined with carboplatin and etoposide in patients with small-cell lung cancer. *J. Clin. Oncol.* **22,** 1110–1117.

70. Marshall, J., Chen, H., Yang, D., et al. (2004) A phase I trial of a Bcl-2 antisense (G3139) and weekly docetaxel in patients with advanced breast cancer and other solid tumors. *Ann. Oncol.* **15,** 1274–1283.

71. Marcucci, G., Stock, W., Dai, G., et al. (2005) Phase I study of oblimersen sodium, an antisense to Bcl-2, in untreated older patients with acute myeloid leukemia: Pharmacokinetics, pharmacodynamics, and clinical activity. *J. Clin. Oncol.* **23,** 3404–3411.

72. Badros, A. Z., Goloubeva, O., Rapoport, A. P., et al. (2005) Phase II study of G3139, a Bcl-2 antisense oligonucleotide, in combination with dexamethasone and thalidomide in relapsed multiple myeloma patients. *J. Clin. Oncol.* **23,** 1–11.

73. Tolcher, A. W., Chi, K., Kuhn, J., et al. (2005) A phase II, pharmacokinetic, and biological correlative study of oblimersen sodium and docetaxel in patients with hormone-refractory prostate cancer. *Clin. Cancer Res.* **11,** 3854–3861.

74. Jansen, B., Wacheck, V., Heere-Ress, E., et al. (2000) chemosensitisation of malignant melanoma by BCL2 antisense therapy. *Lancet* **356,** 1728–1733.

75. Chen, H. X., Marshall, J. L., Ness, E., et al. (2000) A safety and pharmacokinetic study of a mixed-backbone oligonucleotide (GEM231) targeting the type I protein kinase A by two-hour infusions in patients with refractory solid tumors. *Clin. Cancer Res.* **6,** 1259–1266.

76. Goel, S., Desai, K., Bulgaru, A., et al. (2003) A safety study of a mixed-backbone oligonucleotide (GEM231) targeting the type I regulatory subunit α of protein kinase A using a continuous infusion shedule in patients with refractory solid tumors. *Clin. Cancer Res.* **9,** 4069–4076.

77. Mani, S., Goel, S., Nesterova, M., et al. (2003) Clinical studies in patients with solid tumors using a second-generation antisense oligonucleotide (GEM231) targeted against protein kinase A type I. *Ann. N.Y. Acad. Sci.* **1002,** 252–262.

78. Marshall, J. L., Eisenberg, S. G., Johnson, M. D., et al. (2004) A phase II trial of ISIS 3521 in patients with metastatic colorectal cancer. *Clin. Colorectal Cancer* **4,** 268–274.

79. Mani, S., Rudin, C. M., Kunkel, K., et al. (2002) Phase I clinical and pharmacokinetic study of protein kinase C-α antisense oligonucleotide ISIS 3521 administered in combination with 5-fluorouracil and leucovorin in patients with advanced cancer. *Clin. Cancer Res.* **8,** 1042–1048.

80. Rao, S., Watkins, D., Cunningham, D., et al. (2004) Phase II study of ISIS 3521, an antisense oligodeoxynucleotide to protein kinase C alpha, in patients with previously treated low-grade non-Hodgkin's lymphoma. *Ann. Oncol.* **15,** 1413–1418.

81. Stevenson, J. P., Yao, K. S., Gallagher, M., et al. (1999) Phase I clinical/pharmacokinetic and pharmacodynamic trial of the c-*raf*-1 antisense oligonucleotide ISIS 5132 (CGP 69846A). *J. Clin. Oncol.* **17,** 2227–2236.

82. Rudin, C. M., Holmlund, J., Fleming, G. F., et al. (2001) Phase I Trial of ISIS 5132, an antisense oligonucleotide inhibitor of c-*raf*-1, administered by 24-hour weekly infusion to patients with advanced cancer. *Clin. Cancer Res.* **7,** 1214–1220.

83. Desai, A. A., Schilsky, R. L., Young, A., et al. (2005) A phase I study of antisense oligonucleotide GTI-2040 given by continuous intravenous infusion in patients with advanced solid tumors. *Ann. Oncol.* **16,** 958–965.

8

Nucleic Acid-Based Aptamers as Promising Therapeutics in Neoplastic Diseases

Laura Cerchia and Vittorio de Franciscis

Summary

Isolated through combinatorial libraries by an iterative in vitro selection process, small single-stranded nucleic acid compounds, named aptamers, have been developed as high-affinity ligands for a variety of targets, ranging from small chemical compounds to large proteins. In the last years, an increasing number of aptamers has been generated that represent potential antagonists of the disease-associated target proteins. These molecules have been shown to discriminate between even closely related targets, thus representing a valid alternative to antibodies or other biomimetic receptors for the development of biosensors and other bioanalytical methods. Moreover, they can be easily stabilized by chemical modifications for in vivo applications and numerous examples have shown that stabilized aptamers against extracellular targets such as growth factors, receptors, hormones, or coagulation factors are very effective inhibitors of the corresponding protein function, thus resulting as useful reagents for target validation in a variety of diseases, including cancer. Indeed, many signaling proteins involved in diverse functions such as cell growth and differentiation can act as oncogenes and cause cellular transformation, thus making these high affinity ligands promising tools for cancer diagnosis or therapy.

Key Words: Aptamer; RNA ligand; SELEX; therapy; cancer.

1. Introduction

Cancers are generally considered to be a result of the accumulation of multiple genetic alterations that affect the activity and/or expression of proteins involved in the cellular signaling pathways, confering proliferative and invasive characteristics of growth on tumor cells (*1, see* Chapters 1 and 2).

The completion of the sequence of the human genome has provided us with a partial list of known and putative human genes, the total number of which is estimated between 30,000 and 45,000 *(2,3)*. Based on this knowledge, the

From: *Methods in Molecular Biology, vol. 361, Target Discovery and Validation Reviews and Protocols*
Volume 2, Emerging Molecular Targets and Treatment Options
Edited by: M. Sioud © Humana Press Inc., Totowa, NJ

availability of such novel genomic and proteomic techniques as the high-throughput screens and microarrays analysis has led in the last few years to the accumulation of huge amounts of information about genes that are potential targets in cancers. These include proteins already known to govern different functions in tumor progression, such as cell cycle, proliferation, survival, invasion, or angiogenesis. Indeed, in malignant tumors the expression and function of key cellular proteins, including the loss of tumor-suppressor genes or activation oncogenes, is altered through multiple mechanisms such as enhanced or ectopic expression, deletions, single-point mutations, and generation of chimeric proteins *(1)*. These proteins may thus provide primary targets in the rational approach to target cancer cells.

Despite the intrinsic genetic complexity of the neoplastic phenotype, in several cases highly selective molecular ligands have been developed as target-specific therapeutics to stop or delay the growth of cancers *(4)*, thus encouraging the ongoing search for oncogenes as selective targets for diagnosis or therapy. Indeed, the nature and the role played by the oncogene products largely vary across cancer types, and some tumors show a surprisingly tight dependence on the continued activity of a specific oncogene, even in the presence of additional tumorigenic lesions. This is best illustrated by targeting the Bcr/Abl oncoprotein, generated by the fusion of c-Bcr and the tyrosine kinase c-Abl, that is responsible for a wide range of human leukemias *(4,5)*. In chronic myeloid leukemia, the tyrosine kinase inhibitor, imatinib mesylate (known as Gleevec®), can cause complete regression of advanced tumors by specifically inhibiting the tyrosine kinase activity of the overexpressed Bcr-Abl oncoprotein *(6,7)*. Other paradigmatic examples of these target proteins are cell surface receptors with an intrinsic intracellular tyrosine kinase activity as for example the epidermal growth factor receptor that is frequently over-expressed in non-small cell lung carcinoma, bladder, cervical, ovarian, kidney, and pancreatic carcinoma *(4,5)*. Similarly, overexpression and/or gene amplification of the HER-2/neu receptor is found in various types of cancers, including breast (where it occurs in 30% of early stage cases), ovarian, gastric, lung, bladder, and kidney carcinomas *(4,5)*. Somatic rearrangements of the *Ret* gene are frequently associated to the papillary histiotype of the thyroid carcinoma, and germ-line mutations of the Ret receptor cause inheritance of multiple endocrine neoplasia type 2A and 2B and familial medullary thyroid carcinoma *(8)*. Single point mutations, which are frequently found in dominant oncogenes, often affect members of the Ras family. Activating mutations in Ras proteins (accounting for almost 30% of all human cancers) result in constitutive signaling, thereby stimulating cell proliferation and inhibiting apoptosis *(9)*. In Burkitt's lymphoma, a malignancy of immune B cells, the cancer is characterized by huge overexpression of Myc because the *Myc* gene is translocated next to the regulatory sequences for the immunoglobulin gene. As this latter gene is often switched on in B cells, the *Myc* gene itself is switched on *(10)*.

Hence, finding specific ligands capable to detect and inhibit the expression of all these proteins is a strategic objective for the diagnosis and therapy of cancer.

Different types of molecules have been shown to be of potential utility for cancer diagnosis and therapy, including small chemical compounds, peptides, antibodies, small-interfering RNAs, and the short nucleic acid-based ligands, named aptamers. Because of their high selectivity, monoclonal antibodies have been developed against tumor-specific antigens as highly promising molecules that have proven their worth as therapeutics. Aptamers are a new class of ligand molecules that, like antibodies, bind to their targets by complementary shape interactions. Single-stranded RNAs or DNAs-based aptamers function by folding into unique globular three-dimensional shapes that dictates high-affinity binding to a variety of targets, each structure being unique and determined by the sequence of the nucleic acid. Aptamers revealed useful for many of the applications for which antibodies are already employed because of their own definite characteristics: (1) capacity to discriminate between oncogenic and nononcogenic forms of the proteins involved in signaling pathways; (2) capacity to quantify the level of expression of the oncogenic forms; (3) are usable both for in vitro and in vivo purposes; and (4) may act as inhibitors to block the activity of the target oncogene product. Furthermore, aptamers are poor or not immunogenic when administered in animal models or in humans for therapeutic applications.

Protocols have been also developed that allow the targeting of intracellular proteins with inhibitory aptamers (named intramers) that are delivered into intracellular compartments either by direct transfection or through the use of expression systems for the aptamer sequences *(11–13)*. Once expressed inside the cell, aptamers retain their function and can alter the phenotype of a cell by modulating the biological function of the targeted protein.

In this review, we will summarize the current status on the possible applications of aptamers as tools to understand the biological function of proteins and as novel agents in therapy and diagnosis.

2. Systematic Evolution of Ligands by Exponential Enrichment Technology to Generate Nucleic Acid Aptamers

Aptamers are single-stranded nucleic acids routinely isolated from combinatorial oligonucleotide libraries using in vitro selection methods, referred as systematic evolution of ligands by exponential enrichment (SELEX) *(14,15)*.

By starting with a synthetic oligonucleotide library, containing up to 10^{15} different sequences (thus, virtually, 10^{15} different specific shapes), those oligonucleotides that bind with high affinity and specificity to the target molecule of interest are enriched in the library and, after several rounds, selected. The selection scheme is based on the property of single-stranded nucleic acids to fold up into unique three dimensional shapes, thus providing a limited number of specific contact points for the target molecule. The SELEX method includes the following steps (**Fig. 1**): (1) incubating the library with the target molecule under conditions favourable for binding; (2) partitioning from other sequences those molecules that, under the conditions employed, adopt conformations that permit better binding to a specific target; (3) dissociating the nucleic acid–protein complexes; and (4) amplifying of the nucleic acids pool to generate a library of reduced complexity enriched in sequences that bind to the target. This library will be then used as starting pool for the next round of selection. After reiterating these steps for a variable number of cycles, the resulting oligonucleotides are subjected to DNA sequencing. The sequences corresponding to the initially variable region of the library are screened for conserved sequences and structural elements indicative of potential binding sites and subsequently tested for their ability to bind specifically to the target molecule.

3. Target Validation

A crucial step to validate the most promising molecular targets for drug development is to determine their biological relevance for a given disease. The possible strategies that are usually used to understand the function of a specific gene in a cell are: (1) either based on techniques that impair the expression of the candidate target gene, or alternatively (2) rely on the use of products that act by specifically interfering or inhibiting the function, but not the expression, of the final product. In both cases, the resulting phenotype turns out as a powerful source of information on the function of the target protein.

The generation of null mutants by homologous recombination of a given gene in a single cell or in an entire organism has been extensively used to create models of several human diseases, including cancer. Using this technique (known as gene knockout), in which the gene of interest is irreversibly disrupted and the synthesis of the encoded products abolished, allowed to make an incredible and rapid progress in our understanding of the function of several oncogenes and tumor suppressor genes. As an alternative strategy for highly specific gene silencing the use of RNA interference has proven to be a precious approach that permits loss-of-function phenotypic screens in mammalian somatic cells or in whole animals (*see* Chapters 9, 10, and 11). Indeed, it is now feasible to design RNAi constructs against virtually any transcript in the genome. Furthermore, in contrast to the knockout approach, the RNA interference-based RNA strategies achieve loss-of-function phenotypes without the loss of genomic information of the targeted gene (recently reviewed in **ref. 16**).

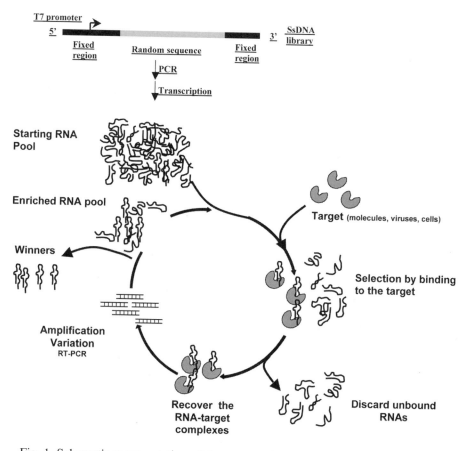

Fig. 1. Schematic representation of the systematic evolution of ligands by exponential enrichment (SELEX) process. The single-stranded (ss) DNA library is amplified by PCR to generate the double-stranded DNA pool that will be transcribed by T7 RNA polymerase. The pool of RNA molecules with different conformations will be used for the selection process.

This leaves the possibility to restore the exact expression of the endogenous gene once the RNAi vector is silenced or removed.

However, a major disadvantage of the gene silencing approaches to obtain functional data on a given protein is that, in most cases, proteins and enzymes involved in crucial functions, such as cell growth and differentiation, act in concert with various protein partners thus forming large stable complexes. Therefore, depleting a single key protein from the cell will change, or even disrupt, one or more of these multiprotein complexes recruited by the target protein. As a consequence, the resulting phenotype will be produced by the simultaneous impairment of several protein functions and the understanding frequently ambiguous. Furthermore, silencing a gene gives no information about which part or domain of the protein is important for its function. Therefore, to overcome these problems, additional approaches have been favored that enable to interfere with a given protein function without interfering with its expression. Indeed, addressing the process of target validation using inhibitors of protein function that directly target the protein in a drug-like manner has the advantage to interfere with a protein activity with low destabilization of the proteomic status of the cell. As excellent alternatives to monoclonal antibodies, peptides and small-molecule inhibitors, RNA-based aptamers have recently proven to be efficient inhibitors of a wide variety of protein implicated in cancer. Indeed, aptamers can recognize within the same protein different domains, or posttranslational modifications, which allows functional analysis of proteins at the molecular level. Furthermore, the SELEX procedure permits to generate aptamers that display high selectivity for the target thus allowing to easily discriminate between even very close molecules. For instance, RNA aptamers with high selectivity have been generated that bind with nanomolar affinities the protein kinase C, a potential target in cancer medicine, and are capable of discriminating between the β II from the highly related β I isoenzymes *(17)*. DNA aptamers have been obtained that recognize both the native and the denatured state of ERK-2, a member of the family of mitogen-activated protein kinases, which are central transducers of extracellular signals *(18)*. RNA ligands with high affinity for the Ras-binding domain of Raf-1 have been isolated and shown to inhibit either Ras binding to Raf-1 and Ras-induced Raf-1 activation, but they did not affect the interaction of Ras with B-Raf, a Raf-1 related protein *(19)*. Furthermore, highly specific aptamer has been generated against platelet-derived growth factor that suppress platelet-derived growth factor B-chain but not the epidermal- or fibroblast-growth-factor-2-induced proliferation *(20)*.

Among the proteins that have been reported as targets of biomedical interest for development of aptamers as therapeutics, particularly relevant is Tenascin-C (TN-C). It is a large, extracellular matrix glycoprotein that is overexpressed during tissue remodeling such as wound healing, atherosclerosis, psoriasis, and tumor growth *(21)*. To isolate oligonucleotide that can target anticancer drug delivery, selection yielded an aptamer that bound to TN-C with a Kd of 5 n*M* *(22)*. The TN-C aptamer is currently being developed for tumor-imaging applications *(23)*.

Furthermore, two aptamers have been selected against the prostate-specific membrane antigen (PSMA) overexpressed by the prostate cancer cells *(24)*. The aptamers inhibited the target with a Ki of 2.1 and 11.9 n*M*. One of the aptamers has been truncated and fluorescently end-labeled to evaluate its ability to bind PSMA-expressing cancer cells. The aptamer bound to LNCaP cells but not

PC-3, showing its specificity for PSMA and its potential in therapeutic development for this target.

Other proteins for aptamer targeting are: human epidermal growth factor receptor-3 (ErbB3/HER3; *[25]*) and the IFN-γ-inducible CXCL10 chemokine *(26)*. In the latter case, Marro et al. *(26)* identified a series of nuclease-resistant RNA aptamers with high binding affinity for human and/or mouse CXCL10. CXCL10 is a chemokine involved in a variety of inflammatory diseases. Because some of the aptamers are highly selective for CXCL10, they represent a powerful tool to further elucidate the complex cross-talk between the CXCL10/ CXCR3 receptor and other chemokine/receptor system.

As reported in **Table 1**, several aptamers are actually in clinical trials *(27)* and the Food and Drug Administration has recently approved one aptamer developed by Eyetech (Macugen™) that inhibits the human vascular endothelial growth factor 165 (VEGF165), for the treatment of age-related macular degeneration *(28)*. In addition to preventing ocular neovascularization, a logical potential therapy for aptamers to VEGF is in cancer. The aptamer isolated and optimized by Ruckman et al. *(28)* was tested in a mouse model of Wilm's tumor or nephroblastoma *(29)*. Renal histopathology revealed an 84% reduction in tumor weight in the aptamer-treated kidneys compared to the controls. Furthermore, lung metastases were seen in 20% of the aptamer-treated mice compared to 60% of control animals. The aptamer was also tested in a murine model of neuroblastoma, where it resulted in 53% reduction in tumor growth compared to control *(30)*.

Even though a large number of aptamers have been selected for preferential targeting of extracellular proteins or protein epitopes the use of living cells as complex target has been recently described to develop a differential whole-cell SELEX protocol to target cell-surface-bound proteins in their natural physiological environment *(31)*. The selection procedure was performed by using as target the RET^C634Y mutant expressed on PC12 cells. A library of 2'-F RNAs was incubated with parental PC12 cells to remove aptamers that bind nonspecifically to the cell surface. To select for aptamers that specifically bound the mutant receptor, the supernatant was incubated with PC12–RET^C634Y cells. Unbound sequences were washed off, the whole process reiterated 16 times and the bound winning sequences cloned. The resulting aptamers did not bind to a recombinant EC C634Y RET fragment highlighting the strength of the whole-cell approach. Among the selected aptamers, the best inhibitor (D4) binds specifically to the Ret receptor tyrosine kinase and blocks its downstream signaling effects on cell differentiation and transformation *(31)*. The results suggest that the differential whole-cell SELEX approach will be useful in the isolation of other lead therapeutic compounds and diagnostic cell-surface markers.

Table 1
Therapeutic Aptamers in Cancer Treatment

Aptamer	Aptamer activity		Therapeutic application
	in vitro	in vivo	
Macugen®	Inhibition of VEGF165	Inhibition of the VEGF-induced vascular permeability	Approved by FDA for treatment of age-related macular degeneration
PDGF-B aptamer	Inhibition of PDGF binding to PDGFR	Reduction of tumor interstitial fluid pressure	Administration in tumor-bearing rats
ProMune™	Agonist for Toll-like receptor 9 (TLR 9)	Activate the immune system through TLR 9 against cancer	Phase 2-melanoma; Phase 1-renal cell carcinoma; non-Hodgkin's lymphoma; cutaneous T-cell lymphoma, nonsmall-cell lung cancer
Agro 100	Binding to nucleolin	Antiproliferative activity in a broad array of tumor cell types; enhancement of chemotherapeutic agents effects	Phase 1; Phase 2 launched in 2005 for advanced solid malignancies
HYB2055	Agonist for TLR 9	Antitumor activity in nude mouse xenografts with colon, breast, lung cancer, and glioma cell lines	Phase 2 for advanced solid malignancies
VaxImmune™ adjuvant	Agonist for TLR 9	Elicits a powerful immune response against infectious disease and cancers	Phase 2 for several different cancer indications

Aptamers that have high affinity and specificity for tissues have also been produced *(32)*, demonstrating that complex targets, including tumor tissue, are compatible with the SELEX process. "Tissue SELEX" methodology could be favourable when the precise molecular target is unknown but the target is, for example, a specific type of cells. Using human red blood cell membranes as model system, DNA aptamers binding to multiple targets have been isolated simultaneously *(32)*. A fluorescence-based SELEX-procedure was applied against transformed endothelial cells as a complex target to detect microvessels of rat experimental glioma, a fatal brain tumor, which is highly vascularized. A secondary selection scheme, named deconvolution-SELEX, was carried out to facilitate the isolation of ligands for components of interest within the targeted mixture *(33)*.

4. In Vivo Applications of the Aptamers

To be of practical use, in vivo aptamers must possess defined molecular properties, for instance, adequate stability in the biological situation in which it will be employed, or sufficient systemic clearance in the case of aptamers used as imaging reagents.

One of the major limitations of the use of aptamers, especially RNA-based aptamers, in cell culture and animal models, is their rapid degradation by nucleases. To date, several chemical modifications have been employed to overcome this issue and a variety of approaches have been developed to improve aptamers stability. Initially, attention focused on "post-SELEX modifications", i.e., the substitution of nucleotides with the corresponding 2'-fluoro, 2'-amino or 2'-O-alkyl variants *(34,35)*. However, owing to the fact that folding rules for single stranded oligonucleotides regions change when these modifications are introduced, the binding properties of an aptamer selected in the presence of standard nucleotides might be completely different when the same sequence is synthesized with nucleotides containing a different 2'-substituent *(33,35,36)*. To circumvent this limitation selections can be performed directly in the presence of 2'-modified nucleotides, as long as the modified nucleotides are accepted by T7 RNA polymerase for the in vitro reaction steps of the selection *(28,36)*. In addition, restricted nucleotides, locked nucleic acid, have been characterized to improve further the stability against nucleases *(37)*.

An interesting application of the SELEX process is based on the selection of RNA aptamers binding to the mirror-image of an intended target molecule (e.g., an unnatural D-aminoacid peptide), followed by the chemical synthesis of the mirror-image of the selected sequence. As a consequence of molecular symmetry, the mirror-image aptamer (made from L-ribose) binds to the natural target molecule. Because of the substitution of the natural D-ribose with L-ribose, the mirror image aptamer (referred as a Spiegelmer) is totally stable. For example, Spiegelmers that bind to gonadotropin-releasing hormone I, a decapeptide associated with several malignant diseases, have been isolated and characterized *(38)*.

Despite the increasing number of aptamers isolated of potential medical importance their use in therapy is still lagging behind because of the lack of an efficient and safe delivery system to target specific cells with adequate amounts of aptamer. For therapy applications, aptamers have to cross the collagen microfibrillar network of the extracellular matrix, and reach the target tissue or cells and, most importantly, also penetrate the cell membrane. Coupling aptamers to inert large molecules, as cholesterol or polyethylene glycol, have been used to keep them in circulation anchored to liposome bilayers *(39)*.

The application for in vivo imaging is especially promising owing to the very wide range of possibilities available to introduce changes in their structure that will enhance the bioavailability and tune the pharmacokinetics properties. Indeed, apart those previously mentioned, there are very few drawbacks for the use of aptamers in vivo, also considering the absence of immunogenicity, a very useful property for reagents that need to be administered repeatedly to the same individual for therapy or diagnostic when studying disease progression.

5. Cancer Signature Measurement

Developing methods that allow clinicians and researchers to translate signature discoveries to routine clinical use by looking simultaneously at a large number of biomarkers has now become a major challenge in cancer diagnostics. Indeed, because they are readily accessible without any need of invasive intervention measuring molecules expressed in serum or plasma is highly preferable. However, many potential cancer biomarkers in biological fluids are present at low concentrations, presumably in the low nanomolar range. Therefore, the capability to measure multiple protein markers simultaneously depends on methods having low limits of detection with elevated signals, but also coupled to very low noise, thus capable to distinguish specific protein signaling in the presence of a huge excess of unrelated proteins.

To this aim Petach et al. at SomaLogic, Inc. *(40,41)* have developed an aptamer-based array technology for analysis of multiplexed proteins. PhotoSelex technology *(42)* permits to derive a new class of capture aptamer molecules, named photoaptamers. These modified aptamers (either DNA or RNA) at specific locations include, in place of Thymdine residues, the photoreactive 5-bromodeoxyuridine (BrdU) that can form a specific covalent cross-link with the target proteins. Indeed, short pulses of ultraviolet light at 308 nm induce a chemical cross-link between the BrdU residue and the electron-rich amino acid on the target protein that is in a specific location in proximity and in the correct juxtaposition of the BrdU. Because this cross-linking event is dependent on the correct juxtaposition of the BrdU and the target amino acid, it conveys specificity to the photoaptamer–protein complex. This gives rise to multiplicative specificity by a photochemical cross-link that follows the initial affinity binding event.

To measure simultaneously large numbers of proteins, even thousands, in biological fluids multiple capture photoaptamers can be deposited and covalently linked to the appropriate chip surface. Therefore, because photoaptamers covalently bind to their targets before staining, the photoaptamer arrays can be vigorously washed to remove background proteins, thus providing the needed potential for elevated signal-to-noise ratios. Proteins captured on the array are then measured by staining either with universal protein stain or with specific antibodies.

The aptamer array technology combined with bioinformatics could allow to discover disease-specific biomarkers and protein signatures and to verify drug compounds efficacy. Using an aptamer array, the measurement of the concentrations of a large number of proteins in a complex biological mixture, such as a clinical sample, could be obtained *(43)*. A protein profile is likely to change in the presence of disease, and different profiles may be associated with varying responses to therapeutics or other clinically relevant parameters. In this context, DNA and RNA aptamers have been used, in a study carried out at the company Archemix, as biorecognition element in optical sensors for multiplex analysis of proteins related to cancer *(44)*. Four fluorescently labeled aptamers (RNA-based aptamers against basic fibroblast growth factor, inosine monophosphate dehydrogenase, and VEGF, and an antithrombin DNA-based aptamer) were immobilized onto a glass surface within a flow cell and fluorescence polarization anisotropy was used for solid-phase measurements of target protein binding. It has been demonstrated specific detection and quantification of inosine monophosphate dehydrogenase II, VEGF, and basic fibroblast growth factor in the context of human serum as well as in cellular extracts.

To date, some photoaptamer-based chips are commercially available as highly sensitive and specific capture agents to discover disease-specific biomarkers and protein signatures (Somalogic Inc.). Furthermore, a continuous and crescent consideration is given to the challenges involved in producing multiplex aptamer chips composed of aptamers taken from disparate literature sources, and to the development of standardized methods for characterizing the performance of capture reagents used in biosensors.

6. Concluding Remarks

The encouraging results obtained with aptamers combined with their intrinsic properties make them promising candidates for diagnostic and even therapeutic applications. Several aptamers are actually in clinical trials and the Food and Drug Administration has recently approved one aptamer (Macugen) for the treatment of age-related macular degeneration *(45)*. Furthermore, the ability of aptamers to discriminate between two closely related targets even sharing common structural domains make these specific and stable ligands attractive as imaging reagents for noninvasive diagnostic procedures.

It is noteworthy that in addition to the use of aptamers in cancer medicine, in the past few years aptamers have been identified as powerful antagonists of proteins, which are associated with a number of other diseases thus emphasizing the versatility of these molecules *(45)*.

Acknowledgments

This work was supported by the European Molecular Imaging Laboratory (EMIL) Network, the MIUR-FIRB grant (no. RBIN04J4J7).

References

1. Hanahan, D., and Weinberg, R. A. (2000) The hallmarks of cancer. *Cell* **100**, 57–70.
2. Lander, E. S., Linton, L. M., Birren, B., et al. (2001) Initial sequencing and analysis of the human genome. *Nature* **409**, 860–921.
3. Venter, J. C., Adams, M. D., Myers, E. W., et al. (2001) The sequence of the human genome. *Science* **291**, 1304–1351.
4. Felsher, D. W. (2003) Cancer revoked: oncogenes as therapeutic targets. *Nat. Rev. Cancer.* **3**, 375–380.
5. Weinstein, I. B. (2002) Cancer. Addiction to oncogenes–the Achilles heal of cancer. *Science* **297**, 63–64.
6. Huettner, C. S., Zhang, P., Van Etten, R. A., and Tenen, D. G. (2000) Reversibility of acute B-cell leukaemia induced by BCR-ABL1. *Nat. Genet.* **24**, 57–60.
7. Martinelli, G., Soverini, S., Rosti, G., and Baccarani, M. (2005). Dual tyrosine kinase inhibitors in chronic myeloid leukaemia. *Leukemia* **19**, 1872–1879.
8. Mulligan, L. M. (2004) From genes to decisions: evolving views of genotype-based management in MEN 2. *Cancer Treat Res.* **122**, 417–428.
9. Chin, L., Tam, A., Pomerantz, J., et al. (1999) Essential role for oncogenic Ras in tumour maintenance. *Nature* **400**, 468–472.
10. Jain, M., Arvanitis, C., Chu, K., et al. (2002) Sustained loss of a neoplastic phenotype by brief inactivation of MYC. *Science* **297**, 102–104.
11. Klug, S. J., Huttenhofer, A., Kromayer, M., Famulok, M. (1997) In vitro and in vivo characterization of novel mRNA motifs that bind special elongation factor SelB. *Proc. Natl. Acad. Sci. USA* **94**, 6676–6681.
12. Blind, M., Kolanus, W., and Famulok, M. (1999) Cytoplasmic RNA modulators of an inside-out signal-transduction cascade. *Proc. Natl. Acad. Sci. USA* **30**, 3606–3610.
13. Famulok, M. and Mayer, G. (2005) Intramers and aptamers: applications in protein-function analyses and potential for drug screening. *Chem. Bio. Chem.* **6**, 19–26.
14. Ellington, A. D. and Szostak, J. W. (1990) In vitro selection of RNA molecules that bind specific ligands. *Nature* **346**, 818–822.
15. Tuerk, C. and Gold, L. (1990) Systematic evolution of ligands by exponential enrichment: RNA ligands to bacteriophage T4 DNA polymerase. *Science* **249**, 505–510.
16. Dykxhoorn, D. M. and Lieberman, J. (2005) The silent revolution: RNA Interference as Basic Biology, Research Tool, and Therapeutic. *Annu. Rev. Med.* **56**, 401–423.
17. Conrad, R., Keranen, L. M., Ellington, A. D., and Newton, A. C. (1994) Isozyme-specific inhibition of protein kinase C by RNA aptamers. *J. Biol. Chem.* **269**, 32,051–32,054.

18. Bianchini, M., Radrizzani, M., Brocardo, M. G., Reyes, G. B., Gonzalez Solveyra, C., Santa-Coloma, T. A. (2001) Specific oligobodies against ERK-2 that recognize both the native and the denatured state of the protein. *J. Immunol. Methods* **252**, 191–197.

19. Kimoto, M., Shirouzu, M., Mizutani, S., et al. (2002) Anti-(Raf-1) RNA aptamers that inhibit Ras-induced Raf-1 activation. *Eur. J. Biochem.* **269**, 697–704.

20. Floege, J., Ostendorf, T., Janssen, U., et al. (1999) Novel approach to specific growth factor inhibition in vivo: antagonism of platelet-derived growth factor in glomerulonephritis by aptamers. *Am. J. Pathol.* **154**, 169–179.

21. Erickson, H. P. and Bourdon, M. A. (1989) Tenascin: an extracellular matrix protein prominent in specialized embryonic tissues and tumors. *Annu. Rev. Cell Biol.* **5**, 71–92.

22. Hicke, B. J., Marion, C., Chang, Y. F., et al. (2001) Tenascin-C aptamers are generated using tumor cells and purified protein. *J. Biol. Chem.* **276**, 48,644–48,654.

23. Hicke, B. J. and Stephens, A. W. (2000) Escort aptamers: a delivery service for diagnosis and therapy. *J. Clin. Invest.* **106**, 923–928.

24. Lupold, S. E., Hicke, B. J., Lin, Y., and Coffey, D. S. (2002) Identification and characterization of nuclease stabilized RNA molecules that bind human prostate cancer cells via the prostate-specific membrane antigen. *Cancer Res.* **62**, 4029–4033.

25. Chen, C. H., Chernis, G. A., Hoang, V. Q., and Landgraf, R. (2003) Inhibition of heregulin signaling by an aptamer that preferentially binds to the oligomeric form of human epidermal growth factor receptor-3. *Proc. Natl. Acad. Sci. USA* **100**, 9226–9231.

26. Marro, M. L., Daniels, D. A., McNamee, A., et al. (2005) Identification of potent and selective RNA antagonists of the IFN-gamma-inducible CXCL10 chemokine. *Biochemistry* **44**, 8449–8460.

27. Thiel, K. (2004) Oligo oligarchy: the surprisingly small world of aptamers. *Nat. Biotechnol.* **22**, 649–665.

28. Ruckman, J., Green, L. S., Beeson, J., et al. (1998) 2'-Fluoropyrimidine RNA-based aptamers to the 165-amino acid form of vascular endothelial growth factor (VEGF165). Inhibition of receptor binding and VEGF-induced vascular permeability through interactions requiring the exon 7-encoded domain, *J. Biol. Chem.* **273**, 20,556–20,567.

29. Huang, J., Moore, J., Soffer, S., et al. (2001) Highly specific antiangiogenic therapy is effective in suppressing growth of experimental Wilms tumors. *J. Pediatr. Surg.* **36**, 357–361.

30. Kim, E. S., Serur, A., Huang, J., et al. (2002) Potent VEGF blockade causes regression of coopted vessels in a model of neuroblastoma. *Proc. Natl. Acad. Sci. USA* **99**, 11,399–11,404.

31. Cerchia, L., Ducongé, F., Pestourie, C., et al. (2005) Neutralizing aptamers from whole-cell SELEX inhibit the RET receptor tyrosine kinase. *PLoS Biology* **3(4)**, 697–704.

32. Morris, K. N., Jensen, K. B., Julin, C. M., Weil, M., and Gold, L. (1998) High affinity ligands from in vitro selection: complex targets. *Proc. Natl. Acad. Sci. USA* **95**, 2902–2907.

33. Blank, M., Weinschenk, T., Priemer, M., and Schluesener, H. (2001) Systematic evolution of a DNA aptamer binding to rat brain tumor microvessels. selective targeting of endothelial regulatory protein pigpen *J. Biol. Chem.* **276,** 16,464–16,468.
34. Hicke, B. J. and Stephens, A. W. (2000) Escort aptamers: a delivery service for diagnosis and therapy. *J. Clin. Invest.* **106,** 923–928.
35. Usman, N. and Blatt, L. M. (2000) Nuclease-resistant synthetic ribozymes: developing a new class of therapeutics *J. Clin. Invest.* **106,** 1197–1202.
36. Aurup, H., Williams, D. M., and Eckstein, F. (1992) 2'-Fluoro- and 2'-amino-2'-deoxynucleoside 5'-triphosphates as substrates for T7 RNA polymerase *Biochemistry* **31,** 9636–9641.
37. Petersen M, Wengel J. (2003) LNA: a versatile tool for therapeutics and genomics. *Trends Biotechnol.* **21,** 74–81.
38. Wlotzka, B., Leva, S., Eschgfaller, B., et al. (2002) In vivo properties of an anti-GnRH Spiegelmer: an example of an oligonucleotide-based therapeutic substance class *Proc. Natl. Acad. Sci. USA* **99,** 8898–8902.
39. Willis, M. C., Collins, B. D., Zhang, T., et al. (1998) Liposome-anchored vascular endothelial growth factor aptamers. *Bioconjug. Chem.* **9,** 573–582.
40. Petach, H., Ostroff, R., Greef, C., and Husar, G. M. (2004) Processing of photoaptamer microarrays. *Methods Mol. Biol.* **264,** 101–110.
41. Gander, T. R. and Brody, E. N. (2005) Photoaptamer chips for clinical diagnostics. *Expert Rev. Mol. Diagn.* **5,** 1–3.
42. Golden, M. C., Collins, B. D., Willis, M. C., and Koch, T. H. (2000) Diagnostic potential of PhotoSELEX-evolved ssDNA aptamers *J. Biotechnol.* **81,** 167–178.
43. Bock, C., Coleman, M., Collins, B., et al. (2004) Photoaptamer arrays applied to multiplexed proteomic analysis. *Proteomics* **4,** 609–618.
44. McCauley, T. G., Hamaguchi, N., and Stanton, M. (2003) Aptamer-based biosensor arrays for detection and quantification of biological macromolecules. *Anal. Biochem.* **319,** 244–250.
45. Nimjee, S. M., Rusconi, C. P., and Sullenger, B. A. (2005) Aptamers: an emerging class of therapeutics. *Annu. Rev. Med.* **56,** 555–583.

9

Guidelines for the Selection of Effective Short-Interfering RNA Sequences for Functional Genomics

Kumiko Ui-Tei, Yuki Naito, and Kaoru Saigo

Summary

To avoid long-double-stranded-RNA-dependent interferon response, short-interfering RNAs (siRNAs) are widely used for RNA interference (RNAi) in mammalian cells. siRNA-based RNAi, however, may not be readily available for the large-scale gene silencing essential for systematic functional genomics, because only a limited fraction of siRNAs is capable of inducing effective mammalian RNAi. siRNAs correctly designed for the knockdown of a particular gene may also destroy the functions of unrelated genes. Here, we describe algorithms by which these serious setbacks can be eliminated in mammalian functional genomics using RNAi and a Web-based online software system for computing highly functional siRNA sequences with maximal target-specificity in mammalian RNAi.

Key Words: Mammalian RNAi; functional siRNA; off-target effects; target assay; siDirect.

1. Introduction

RNA interference (RNAi) is the process of nucleotide-sequence-specific posttranscriptional gene silencing (1–4). In this process, long double-stranded RNA (dsRNA), either introduced into or produced within cells, is converted to many short interfering RNAs (siRNAs) 21- to 23-nt long through cytoplasmic-dicer-dependent RNase activity (5,6). siRNA is a 19- to 21-bp duplex associated with 2-nt 3'-overhangs at both ends. Twenty-one-base pair-long siRNA synthesized in vitro and incorporated into cells still possesses the capability to induce RNAi (7). The introduction of long dsRNA into mammalian cells frequently induces fatal interferon response, though siRNA may not do so (8), indicating that siRNA is more promising as a reagent for mammalian RNAi (9)

From: *Methods in Molecular Biology, vol. 361, Target Discovery and Validation Reviews and Protocols Volume 2, Emerging Molecular Targets and Treatment Options*
Edited by: M. Sioud © Humana Press Inc., Totowa, NJ

than long dsRNA *(10–14)*. siRNA generated in vivo or synthesized in vitro and introduced into cells via transfection is considered to form an RNA-induced silencing complex (RISC) with PIWI protein (Argonaute 2) and possibly other relevant proteins *(15–19)*. Active RISC as a silencing effector complex includes siRNA antisense strands (AS) but not sense strands (SS), and thus double-stranded siRNA is considered to undergo unwinding *(20)* during active RISC formation. Target mRNA is recognized by cognate siRNA AS serving as a guide strand via Watson–Crick hydrogen bonding. RISC cleaves target mRNA at a site corresponding to the center of the guide strand of siRNA in mammalian and *Drosophila* cells *(7,9,20,21)*.

siRNA-based RNAi, however, may not always be available for the large-scale gene silencing essential for mammalian systematic functional genomics, because only a limited fraction of siRNAs is capable of inducing effective RNAi in mammalian cells *(22–24)*. Thus, the first major problem when considering the use of siRNA as a mammalian RNAi reagent is the absence of a definitive way to identify functional siRNAs among hundreds or thousands of possible candidates, all homologous in sequence to a given target mRNA.

To approach this problem, examination was made of arbitrarily chosen siRNAs targeting for the firefly luciferase gene (*luc*) for their ability to induce RNAi in mammalian cells *(23)*, using human (HeLa, HEK293 and colo205), Chinese hamster ovary (CHO-K1), and mouse ES (E14TG2a) cells. As shown in **Fig. 1**, hardly any or no difference in RNAi-inducing activity was found in these cell types, suggesting that siRNA-based RNAi in mammalian cells is subject to the same rules for siRNA sequence preference. As schematically shown in **Fig. 2A** (algorithm I), all data obtained indicated four immediately apparent features of the siRNA sequence to possibly serve to discriminate highly functional siRNAs from those nonfunctional. First, the 5'-AS end of highly functional siRNAs may always be A or U, with the counterpart of nonfunctional siRNA being C or G. Second, the 5'-SS ends of highly functional siRNAs are preferably G or C, with the counterpart of nonfunctional siRNAs being A or U. Third, in the case of highly functional siRNAs, the 5'-terminal AS are A/U-rich whereas the corresponding region of nonfunctional siRNAs are G/C-rich. Fourth, highly functional siRNAs lack a long G/C stretch in the 5'-terminal two-thirds of SS. Most siRNAs associated with mixed features appeared to belong to a siRNA class with intermediate RNAi activity. From these findings, we classified siRNAs as follows: class I consisting of siRNAs possessing (1) A/U at the 5'-AS end, (2) G/C at the 5'-SS end, (3) more than four A/U nucleotides in a 7-nt 5'-terminal AS end, and (4) lacking a long G/C stretch in the 5'-terminal two-thirds of SS (*see* **Note 1**). Class III siRNAs were defined as siRNAs with opposite features except for condition 4. All other siRNAs belong to class II. Class I was subdivided into classes Ia and Ib. Class I siRNAs with

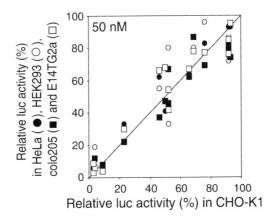

Fig. 1. Comparison of short-interfering RNAs (siRNAs)-dependent RNA interference (RNAi) activity induced in five mammalian cells. Cells were transfected with 1 of 16 arbitrarily chosen siRNAs at 50 nM and RNAi activity was measured using the luciferase assay 1 d after transfection. The horizontal axis shows relative *luc* activity in Chinese hamster cells, CHO-K1, whereas the vertical axis indicates *luc* activity in three human cells, HeLa, HEK293, colo205, and mouse ES cells, E14TG2a.

five to seven A/U residues in 5'-terminal one-third of AS were assumed to belong to class Ia and the remainder to class Ib. Initial experiments indicated class Ia siRNAs are highly functional, whereas class III siRNAs are inactive. Subsequent experiments showed that class Ib siRNAs possess RNAi-inducing activity almost identical to that of class Ia (Naito, Ui-Tei, and Saigo unpublished data; *see also* **Fig. 3**).

To demonstrate the validity of the previously described algorithm (algorithm I in **Fig. 2A**), 34 class Ia, 5 class Ib, and 13 class III siRNAs targeting for 2 exogeneous and 2 endogenous genes were arbitrarily chosen and assessed for their ability to give rise to RNAi in mammalian cells (*[23]*; K.U.-T., et al., unpublished data). As anticipated, all class Ia and class Ib siRNAs brought about highly effective RNAi, whereas little or no effective RNAi could be detected by transfection of class III siRNAs. The importance of base preference at the 5'-ends of both AS and SS and A/U-richness in 5'-AS-terminal one-third has been demonstrated by site-directed mutagenesis of both target and siRNA sequences (Ui-Tei et al. unpublished data). **Figure 3** shows the relationship of RNAi activity to A/U content in the 5'-terminal one-third of AS. It should be noted that, in siRNAs with A/U and G/C at the 5'-ends of AS and SS, respectively, RNAi-inducing activity dramatically decreases when the A/U content is equal to or less than 43% (3/7). It would follow then that both functional and nonfunctional siRNAs for mammalian RNAi can be quite effectively designed provided that the present algorithm, algorithm I, is used. **Figure 3** also shows that a small fraction of class II

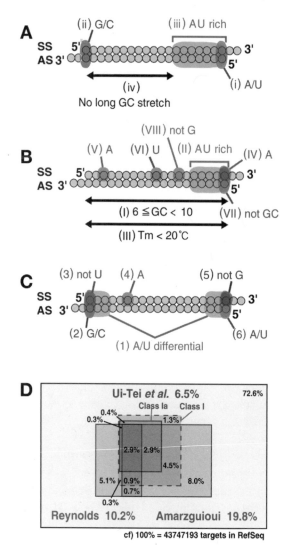

Fig. 2. Three algorithms for short-interfering RNAs (siRNA) design for functional RNA interference (RNAi) in mammalian cells. (**A**) Algorithm I. This algorithm was published by Ui-Tei et al. *(23)*. According to this algorithm, highly functional siRNAs simultaneously satisfy the following four conditions: (i) A/U at the 5' antisense strand (AS) end, (ii) G/C at the 5' sense strand (SS) end and (iii) more than four A/U nucleotides in the 5'-terminal one-third of AS, and (iv) lacking a long G/C stretch in the 5-terminal two-thirds of SS. (**B**) Algorithm II, siRNA design algorithm proposed by Reynolds et al. *(24)*. This includes eight requirements: (I) low G/C contents (30–52%), (II) three or more A/U at the SS 3'-terminus 5 bp, (III) low internal stability lacking stable inverted repeats, (IV–VIII) base preferences at SS positions 3, 10, 13, and 19. (**C**) Algorithm III, an algorithm proposed by Amarzguioui and Prydz *(25)*. This requires that A/U content in the

siRNAs is still associated with high RNAi activity, indicating that a small fraction of functional siRNAs may not be predicted by algolithm I.

Figure 2B,C shows other algorithms that have been proposed for selection of functional siRNA sequences for mammalian RNAi. Reynolds et al. *(24)* performed systematic analysis on 180 siRNAs targeting the mRNA of two genes and suggest the following characteristics to be associated with siRNA functionality: low G/C content, bias toward low internal stability at the SS 3'-terminus and lack of inverted repeats. Their algorithm (algorithm II) also maintains that the SS preferably uses A, U, and A residues at SS positions 3, 10, and 19, respectively, and that G may not be present at position 13 **(Fig. 2B)**. But it is significant that only 1 of 23 highly functional class I siRNAs shown in **Fig. 3** satisfies all SS base preferences. Sixteen functional class I siRNAs exhibited none of the base preferences at both position 3 and 10.

Amarzguioui and Prydz *(25)* carried out statistical analysis on 46 siRNAs and identified some features of functional siRNAs (algorithm III). As in our study, A/U at the 5'-AS terminus and its SS partner and G/C at the 5'-SS terminus and its AS partner in functional siRNAs were noted to be important, opposite combination of terminal bases was maintained to cause lack of functionality. Their algorithm includes asymmetry in siRNA duplex end stability. That is, the A/U content differential for the three terminal nucleotides at both ends of the duplex is assumed essential for determining siRNA functionality. Amarzguioui and Prydz also found A to be preferably used at position 6 of functional siRNAs **(Fig. 2C)**. Only 5 of 23 highly functional class I siRNAs shown in **Fig. 3** exhibited A residue at SS position 6.

Algorithms I–III may specify different siRNA sequences that are functional. Thus, using about 4.4×10^7 potential targets derived from RefSeq human sequences, determination was made of percent of siRNAs predicted to be functional by algorithm I (class Ia) that can be repredicted as functional by algorithms II or III or vice versa (Naito et al., unpublished). In **Fig. 2D**, 73% of the total possible siRNA sequences (3.2×10^7 sequences) are scored as nonfunctional ones. Class Ia was found to represent 6.5% of the total, whereas algorithms II and III, respectively, predicted 10.2 and 19.8% as functional siRNAs. About 90% of siRNAs predicted to be functional by algorithm I could be repredicted to be functional by either algorithm II or III or both. More than 60% of

Fig. 2. *(Continued)* 5'-AS end should be higher than that in the 5'-SS end. Base preferences are also required at position labeled with (2–6). **(D)** Difference in functional siRNA prediction. 97,475,268 siRNA sequences were collected from human sequences deposited in RefSeq and classified using three algorithms. About 6.5 and 13.5% of siRNAs, respectively, were assigned to class Ia and class I siRNAs by algorithm I, whereas about 10 and 20% were predicted to be functional by algorithms II and III.

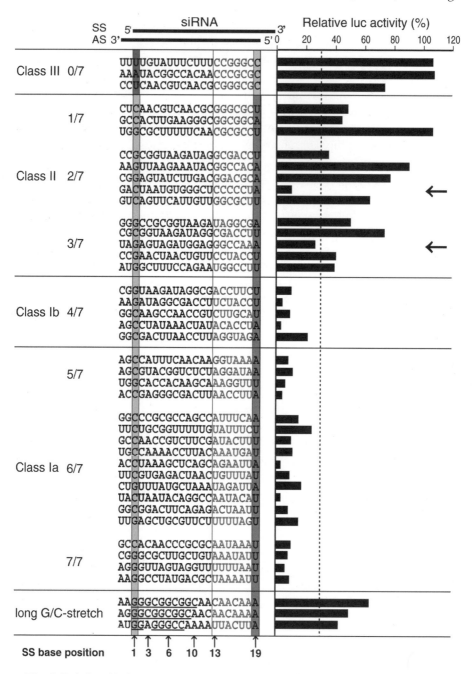

Fig. 3. Relationship between RNA interference (RNAi) activity and A/U content in the 5'-terminal one-third of AS. Thirty-nine short-interfering RNAs (siRNA) sequences, which target *luc* and possess A/U and G/C, respectively, at 5'- antisense strand (AS) and

siRNAs simultaneously predicted to be functional by algorithms II and III could be repredicted to be functional by algorithm I. This value increases to 85% in the case of class I. More than 50 and 40% of siRNAs predicted to be functional by algorithms II and III, respectively, could not be supported by other algorithms. Algorithm I is thus shown capable of predicting more reliably the functionality of siRNAs than algorithm II or III.

Our computational analysis also showed that class Ia can provide at least one functional siRNA to 99.6% of human mRNA sequences registered in RefSeq **(Fig. 4)**. Algorithm I is thus sufficient to search functional siRNAs for genome-wide gene silencing. As described previously *(23)*, class Ia siRNAs are comprised of heterogeneous members with more than 10 times the capacity to induce RNAi. Thus, it may reasonably be considered that only siRNAs predicted simultaneously to be functional by three algorithms should be used for functional genomics. This class of siRNAs represents more than 44% of class Ia **(Fig. 2D)** and most of genes are capable of generating more than 10 class Ia siRNAs as shown in **Fig. 4**. This approach should accordingly be applicable in most cases. Note that human *src* and *vimentin* sequences, respectively, generate 27 and 64 class Ia siRNAs **(Fig. 4)**.

Mammalian Argonaute proteins (eIF2Cs) are each composed of an N-terminal proline-arginine-proline (PRP) motif and Piwi Argonaute Zwelle (PAZ) and PIWI domains *(26)*. Crystal structural analysis of the Argonaute protein from *Pyrococcus farious* indicated the PIWI domain to have essentially the same three-dimensional structure as ribonuclease H, with a conserved active site Asp-Asp-Glu motif and that Argonaute may serve as "Slicer," the enzyme that cleaves mRNA *(27)*. Both ends of siRNA appear to be separately recognized by two domains of the Argonaute protein. Ma et al. *(28)* reported the crystal structure of the complex of the PAZ domain from human Argonaute eIF2C1 and a 9-mer siRNA-like duplex and indicated that, in a sequence-independent manner, the PAZ domain is anchored to the 2-nucleotide 3' overhang of the siRNA-like duplex. The PIWI domain from *Archaeoglobus fulgidus* in complex with a siRNA-like duplex has been shown to contain a highly conserved metal-binding site that anchors the 5'-nt of the guide RNA in a sequence-independent manner *(29)*. The first base pair of the duplex is unwound and the base at the 5'-unpaired AS end stacks on the aromatic ring of invariant Tyr 123 so that interactions between the 5'-AS end and the PIWI domain may possibly be nonsequence specific. The remaining base-paired nucleotides assume an A-form helix.

Fig. 3. *(Continued)* 5'-sense strand (SS) ends, were chosen and their RNAi inducing activity were compared at 5 n*M*. All class Ia and class Ib siRNA were found to be highly functional. siRNA functionality significantly dropped upon A/U content reduction from four to three. Arrows indicate two exceptional type II siRNAs associated with high RNAi activity.

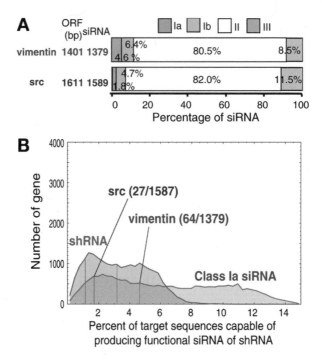

Fig. 4. Fraction of targets capable of producing functional short-interfering RNAs (siRNA) or short-hairpin RNAs (shRNA). (**A**) From vimentin and src ORF sequences, respectively, 1379 and 1589 siRNA sequences can be generated. Algorithm I predicted that 64 (4.6%) and 152 (11%) of 1379 vimentin sequences belong to class Ia and class I, respectively. Only 27 (1.8%) class Ia siRNAs can be designed from the *src* ORF sequence. (**B**) Genome-wide distribution of fraction of targets capable of producing functional siRNA or shRNA. All human sequences registered in RefSeq were examined and it was found that 99.6% of "human genes" possess at least one target sequence capable of producing class Ia sequence.

As previously described, algorithms I and III predict that functional siRNAs possess A/U and G/C at the 5′-AS and SS ends, respectively. Algorithm II maintains that the 5′-end of AS should be A. Because the GC pair is thermodynamically much more stable than the AU pair, difference in stability in terminal base pair of the siRNA duplex may determine terminal sequence preference in highly effective and ineffective siRNAs most probably by stimulating the asymmetric binding of the PIWI and PAZ domains to siRNA ends. We assume that the presence of an A/U pair at the siRNA end including the 5′-AS end is much more preferable for PIWI binding than that of the G/C pair.

The guide stand of siRNA is always designed so as to be complementary in sequence to that of its target. However, siRNA designed for a particular mRNA may also inactivate certain targets of other mRNA most probably through incomplete

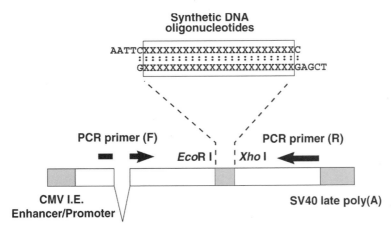

Fig. 5. Structure near the oligonucleotide insertion site of pTREC, a vector for target cleavage assay. For typical target assay, 29-bp-long single-stranded complementary oligonucleotides are annealed and the resultant double-stranded DNA oligonucleotide is inserted into *Eco*RI and *Xho*I sites of the vector. Cells are cotransfected with pTREC construct and suitable siRNA and possible change in mRNA content is examined using real time PCR.

Watson–Crick base paring. These silencing effects are collectively called off-target silencing effects. The second major problem in siRNA designing thus becomes how to eliminate possible off-target silencing effects. Molecular mechanisms of off-target effects have yet to be clarified. In some cases, even a single mismatch in the center of an siRNA appears to eliminate target mRNA silencing (*[30,31]*; our unpublished observation), whereas siRNAs with 11 contiguous matches can give rise to off-target effects *(32)*. To experimentally determine how incomplete base pairing between AS and nontargeted mRNA sequences affects silencing as a result of mRNA breakdown, a new plasmid vector, pTREC, was made, as shown in **Fig. 5**. Our unpublished observations (Naito et al.) indicate that, if the target sequence possesses three or more internal mismatches to the AS sequence, off-target effects on RNA stability should be virtually negligible.

Based on these observations on off-target silencing effects and algorithm I for selection of highly functional siRNAs for mammalian cells, a web-based online software system, siDirect *(33)* was constructed and by which it is possible to easily and very rapidly identify functional siRNAs exhibiting the least off-target effect for any human and mouse genes.

2. Materials

2.1. Small-Interfering RNAs

Sense and antisense RNA oligonucleotides, whose sequences have been selected by siDirect, are chemically synthesized, mixed in a 1:1 fashion in 10 m*M* NaCl and 20 m*M* Tris-HCl, pH 7.5, and annealed by incubating at 95°C for 15 min,

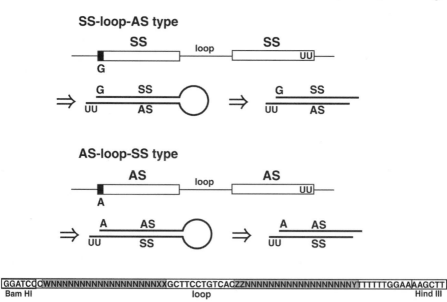

Fig. 6. Two types of DNA oligonucleotides encoding short-hairpin RNAs (shRNA). Functional short-interfering RNAs (siRNA) may be generated from two different types of shRNA. In the sense strand (SS)-loop-antisense strand (AS) type (**A**), DNA near the *Hind*III site codes for AS, whereas in the AS-loop-SS type (**B**), DNA near the *Bam*HI site encodes AS. The loop sequence is presumed to be eliminated by cytoplasmic dicer activity.

at 37°C for 30 min and at 25°C for 30 min. Annealed products may be examined using 3% agarose gel electrophoresis in TBE buffer, which can separate 21-bp-long double-stranded siRNA from 21-bp-long single stranded RNA (*see* **Note 2**).

2.2. DNA Plasmid

pSilencer 3.0-H1 (Ambion) is a plasmid vector for DNA-based RNAi *(34)*. Double-stranded oligonucleotides to be inserted vary depending on shRNA types (*see* **Fig. 6**). pTREC is a derivative of pCI-neo with cytomegalovirus immediate-early enhancer/promoter and SV40 late polyadenylation signal and can be used to express various target sequences within cells (Naito, Ui-Tei, and Saigo manuscript in preparation).

3. Methods

3.1. Identification of Functional Small-Interfering RNA and Short-Hairpin RNA Sequences for Mammalian RNA Interference

3.1.1. Design for Small-Interfering RNA

Highly functional class Ia siRNAs with maximal target-specificity for mammalian RNAi can be designed by using the web-based online software system, siDirect (http://design.RNAi.jp/) *(33)*, which is driven by algorithm I *(23)* and an accelerated off-target search algorithm developed by Yamada and Morishita *(35)*. In siDirect, functional siRNAs for human and mouse RNAi (*see* **Note 3**) are easily designed under default conditions.

1. First, enter the accession number (GenBank or RefSeq accession number) of any human or mouse gene to be knocked down in the open box on the first page of siDirect (*see* the arrow in **Fig. 7A**).

2. Click "retrieve sequence." The nucleotide sequence of the gene corresponding to the accession number entered is automatically downloaded from the GenBank database, and full sequence appears in the box, which is labeled with double arrows in **Fig. 7A**.

3. For a off-target search for all human mRNA sequences, "Homo sapiens" should be selected in the "Off-target search" (*see* **Note 4**). For a off-target search for mouse genes, select "Mus musculus."

4. Click "design siRNA." Then, as shown in **Fig. 7B**, selected functional siRNA sequences appear on the next page with the sense DNA sequence of the target gene. The size and location of target sequences which exhibit the least off-target effect to both sense and AS are colored in blue (*see* **Fig. 7B**), whereas those with the least off-target effect only to the SS are colored in light blue (*see* **Note 5**). The sequence of siRNA selected (class Ia; *see* **Note 6**) and its off-target candidates are shown on the next page of siDirect (**Fig. 7C**) upon clicking the number in the box of the siRNA.

3.1.2. Design for Short-Hairpin RNA for DNA-Based RNA Interference

As described previously *(23)*, our algorithm (algorithm I) is successfully applicable to functional shRNA design for DNA-based mammalian RNAi. However, additional sequence conditions are required for shRNA design, because RNA polymerase III is usually used for RNA synthesis in DNA-based mammalian RNAi. For shRNA design, following steps (**steps 1** and **2**) should be inserted between aforementioned steps for siRNA design, **Subheading 3.1.1.**, **steps 1–3** and **4**.

1. Check the small box of "Custom rule," and then enter "NNGNNNNNNNNNNNN NNNNNNNNN" in the right long rectangle, which accommodate a 23-nt-long target sequence corresponding to both 21-bp-long AS and SS, if shRNA to be designed belongs to the 5'-SS-loop-AS type (**Fig. 6A**). For design of shRNAs belonging to the 5'-AS-loop-SS type (**Fig. 6B**) insert "NNNNNNNNNNNNN NNNNNNNTNN" (*see* **Note 7**). Note that the 5'-end of SS corresponds to the third nucleotide of the 23-bp-long sequence.

2. Check the small box labeled with As or Ts and then select numeral 4 in the right box (*see* **Note 8**).

3.2. RNA Interference in Mammalian Cells

RNAi experiments using mammalian cultured cells should be carried out essentially as described previously (*[23]*; *see* **Note 9**)

A

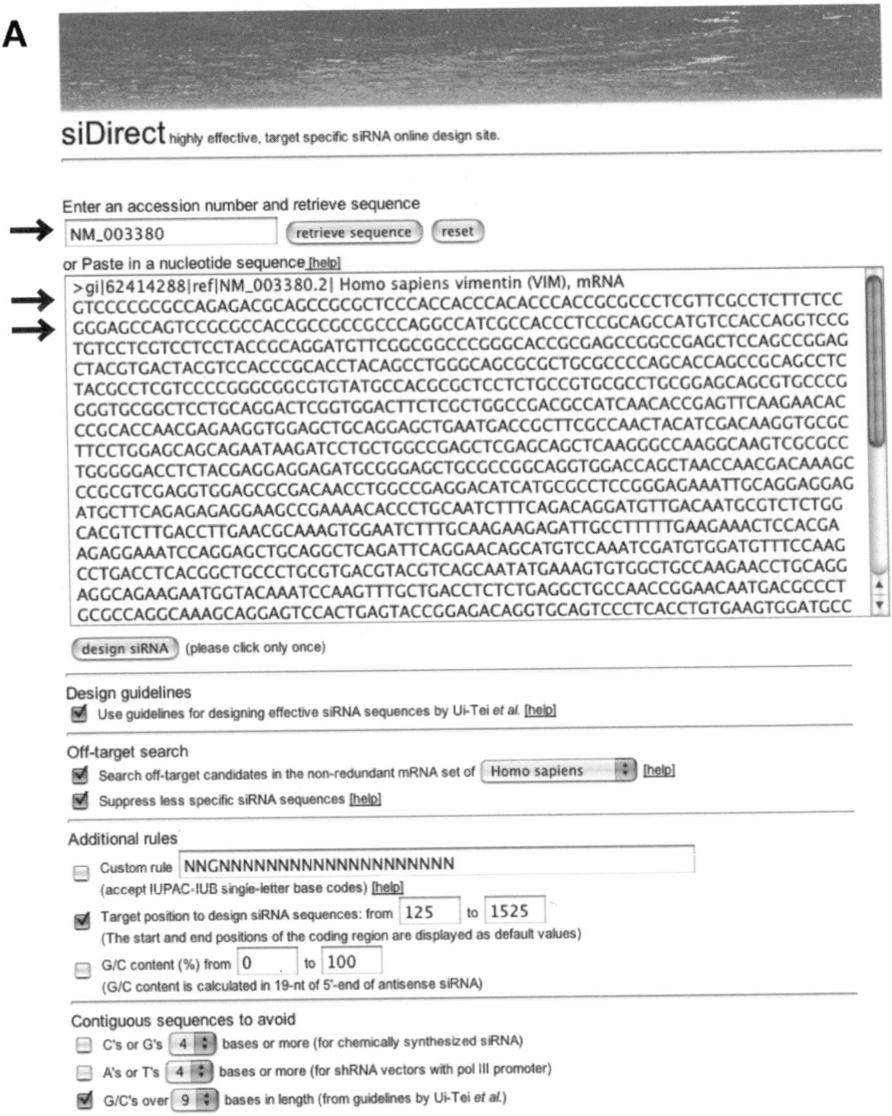

siDirect *highly effective, target specific siRNA online design site.*

Enter an accession number and retrieve sequence

→ | NM_003380 | (retrieve sequence) (reset)

or Paste in a nucleotide sequence [help]

```
>gi|62414288|ref|NM_003380.2| Homo sapiens vimentin (VIM), mRNA
GTCCCCGCGCCAGAGACGCAGCCGCGCTCCCACCACCCACACCCACCGCGCCCTCGTTCGCCTCTTCTCC
GGGAGCCAGTCCGCGCCACCGCCGCCGCCCAGGCCATCGCCACCCTCGCAGCCATGTCCACCAGGTCCG
TGTCCTCGTCCTCCTACCGCAGGATGTTCGGCGGCCCGGGCACCGCGAGCCGGCCGAGCTCCAGCCGGAG
CTACGTGACTACGTCCACCCGCACCTACAGCCTGGGCAGCGCGCTGCGCCCCAGCACCAGCCGCAGCCTC
TACGCCTCGTCCCCGGGCGGCGTGTATGCCACGCGCTCCTCTGCCGTGCGCCTGCGGAGCAGCGTGCCCG
GGGTGCGGCTCCTGCAGGACTCGGTGGACTTCTCGCTGGCCGACGCCATCAACACCGAGTTCAAGAACAC
CCGCACCAACGAGAAGGTGGAGCTGCAGGAGCTGAATGACCGCTTCGCCAACTACATCGACAAGGTGCGC
TTCCTGGACGCAGCAGAATAAGATCCTGCTGGCCGAGCTCGAGCAGCTCAAGGGCCAAGGCAAGTCGCGCC
TGGGGGACCTCTACGAGGAGGAGATGCGGGAGCTGCGCCGGCAGGTGGACCAGCTAACCAACGACAAAGC
CCGCGTCGAGGTGGAGCGCGACAACCTGGCCGAGGACATCATGCGCCTCCGGGAGAAATTGCAGGAGGAG
ATGCTTCAGAGAGAGGAAGCCGAAAACACCCTGCAATCTTTCAGACAGGATGTTGACAATGCGTCTCTGG
CACGTCTTGACCTTGAACGCAAAGTGGAATCTTTGCAAGAAGAGATTGCCTTTTTGAAGAAACTCCACGA
AGAGGAAATCCAGGAGCTGCAGGCTCAGATTCAGGAACAGCATGTCCAAATCGATGTGGATGTTTCCAAG
CCTGACCTCACGGCTGCCCTGCGTGACGTACGTCAGCAATATGAAAGTGTGGCTGCCAAGAACCTGCAGG
AGGCAGAAGAATGGTACAAATCCAAGTTTGCTGACCTCTCTGAGGCTGCCAACCGGAACAATGACGCCCT
GCGCCAGGCAAAGCAGGAGTCCACTGAGTACCGGAGACAGGTGCAGTCCCTCACCTGTGAAGTGGATGCC
```

(design siRNA) (please click only once)

Design guidelines
☑ Use guidelines for designing effective siRNA sequences by Ui-Tei *et al.* [help]

Off-target search
☑ Search off-target candidates in the non-redundant mRNA set of (Homo sapiens ▼) [help]
☑ Suppress less specific siRNA sequences [help]

Additional rules
☐ Custom rule | NNGNNNNNNNNNNNNNNNNNNNNN |
   (accept IUPAC-IUB single-letter base codes) [help]
☑ Target position to design siRNA sequences: from | 125 | to | 1525 |
   (The start and end positions of the coding region are displayed as default values)
☐ G/C content (%) from | 0 | to | 100 |
   (G/C content is calculated in 19-nt of 5'-end of antisense siRNA)

Contiguous sequences to avoid
☐ C's or G's [4 ▼] bases or more (for chemically synthesized siRNA)
☐ A's or T's [4 ▼] bases or more (for shRNA vectors with pol III promoter)
☑ G/C's over [9 ▼] bases in length (from guidelines by Ui-Tei *et al.*)

Fig. 7. The first (**A**), second (**B**) and third (**C**) pages of siDirect. *See* **Subheading 3.1.1.** for details.

3.3. Experimental Evaluation of Off-Target Effects

Although siDirect is capable of predicting highly functional siRNA sequences along with the most dangerous off-target candidate sequences against any given functional siRNA, it is important to observe how much mRNA derived from the target gene or putative off-target genes is really destroyed within cells upon siRNA transfection (*see* **Note 10**). pTREC is a newly developed target-activity assay vector capable of accommodating any siRNA target sequence between *Eco*RI and *Xho*I sites (Naito, Ui-Tei, and Saigo in preparation). In mammalian cells transfected with pTREC, the inserted target sequence is transcribed most probably without translation.

1. Insert a desired target sequence into the *Eco*RI/*Xho*I site of pTREC (**Fig. 5**).
2. Introduce the resultant pTREC construct (0.5 μg) into cells through transfection with or without cognate siRNA and examine RNAi effects 24 h after transfection using real time PCR.
3. Total RNA is purified from transfected cells using RNeasy 96 (Qiagen) and DNase treatment (*see* **Note 11**). cDNA corresponding to extracted mRNA is synthesized using SuperScript First-Strand Synthesis System for RT-PCR (Invitrogen).
4. Real time PCR is carried out using ABI PRISM 7000 (Applied Biosystems) with SYBR Green PCR master mix (Applied Biosystems). The quantity of unbroken target or off-target mRNA is normalized with neomycin resistant mRNA simultaneously transcribed from the same construct. Universal PCR primers for any target RNA derived from the transfected construct are 5'AGGCACTGGG CAGGTGTC and 5'TGCTCGAAGCATTAACCCTCACTA, and those for neomycin gene expression are 5'ATCAGGATGATCTGGACGAAG and 5'CTCT CAGCAATATCACGGGT.

4. Notes

1. Previously, class I and class Ia siRNAs were defined as siRNAs simultaneously satisfying three conditions (*see* **Subheading 1.**). Here, for simplicity, this definition is somewhat modified by considering the fourth condition concerning to the absence of a long G/C stretch in the 5'-terminal two-thirds of SS. The permissible length of G/C stretch may vary depending on the concentration of siRNA used for transfection. In the case of RNAi with 50 n*M* siRNA, this value is 10 *(23)*, whereas it may reduce to 7–8 when 5 n*M* siRNA is used (*see* **Fig. 3**).
2. Under the condition used here, almost all single-stranded siRNA appears transformed to double-stranded siRNA, possibly suggesting that the gel electrophoresis step may be eliminated.
3. siDirect predicts class Ia sequences corresponding to both open reading frame (ORF) and untranslated regions of the target gene, whereas requirements for functional siRNA sequences were established only based on experiments with siRNAs homologous in sequence to the ORF of the target genes. Thus, class Ia siRNAs homologous in sequence to the target-gene ORF might serve as more effective RNAi reagents.
4. At present, only "Homo sapiens" and "Mus musculus" are selections. In the planned new version, "Rattus norvegicus" and "Gallus gallus" and "Canis familiaris" will be added.
5. Theoretically, siRNA transfection may produce two types of RISCs, SS-RISC containing SS as a guide strand, and AS-RISC with AS guide within cells. In mammalian cells transfected with highly functional siRNAs, AS-RISC is considered to be

predominant. In addition, highly functional siRNAs are asymmetric in sequence preference. Thus, off-target effects owing to putative SS RISCs may not be prominent.

6. Algorithm for selection for class I siRNAs will be included in a planned new version of siDirect.

7. RNA polymerase III requires purine nucleotides for RNA start and accordingly, the first base of shRNA should be A or G. 5'-end of shRNA should be A if shRNA begins with AS, whereas it should be G if shRNA begins with SS (**Fig. 6**). Both configurations can be functional, but the latter may induce somewhat more effective RNAi (Ui-Tei unpublished data).

8. RNA polymerase III-dependent RNA polymerization is terminated in a region with continuous U residues, indicating shRNA possessing four or more nucleotide-long A stretches or U stretches is prematually terminated.

9. For RNAi assay of endogenous gene or RNAi activity observation in cells with a low-transfection efficiency, transfected cells are recommended to be preselected through cotransfection with a selective-marker-containing plasmid DNA such as pCAGIpuroEGFP possessing puromycin resistant and enhanced green fluorescent protein (EGFP) genes. pCAGIpuroEGFP plasmid DNA (0.2–0.4 µg) is simultaneously introduced into mammalian cells with siRNA via transfection. Twenty-four hours after transfection, puromycin (2 µg/mL) is added to the medium and puromycin-susceptible cells (untransfected cells) are removed 24 h after puromycin treatment. Cells are harvested 3 d after transfection for RNAi assay.

10. RNAi reaction might be prevented by secondary structures of and/or protein binding to the target mRNA.

11. DNase treatment is essential for eliminating a small amount of DNA, which cannot be eliminated by RNeasy 96.

Acknowledgments

We thank Dr. S. Nishihara for supplying colo205 cells, A. Juni and A. Tanaka for technical assistance. This work was partially supported by Special Coordination Fund for promoting Science and Technology to K.S., and grants from the Ministry of Education, Culture, Sports, Science and Technology of Japan to K.S. and K.U.-T.

References

1. Fire, A., Xu, S., Montgomery, M. K., Kostas, S. A., Driver, S. E., and Mello, C. C. (1998) Potent and specific genetic interference by double-stranded RNA in *Caenorhabditis elegans*. *Nature* **391,** 806–811.

2. Dykxhoorn, D. M., Novina, C. D., and Sharp, P. A. (2003) Killing the messenger: short RNAs that silence gene expression. *Nat. Rev. Mol. Cell Biol.* **4,** 457–467.

3. Mello, C. C. and Conte Jr, D. (2004) Revealing the world of RNA interference. *Nature* **431,** 338–342.

4. Meister, G. and Tuschl, T. (2004) Mechanisms of gene silencing by double-stranded RNA. *Nature* **431,** 343–349.

5. Bernstein, E., Caudy, A. A., Hammond, S. M., and Hannon, G. J. (2001) Role for a bidentate ribonuclease in the initiation step of RNA interference. *Nature* **409,** 363–366.

6. Ketting, R. F., Fischer, S. E. J., Bernstein, E., Sijen, T., Hannon, G. J., and Plasterk, R. H. A. (2001) Dicer functions in RNA interference and in synthesis of small developmental timing in *C. elegans. Genes Dev.* **15,** 2654–2659.

7. Elbashir, S. M., Lendeckel, W., and Tuschl, T. (2001) RNA interference is mediated by 21 and 22 nt RNAs. *Genes Dev.* **15,** 188–200.

8. Stark, G. R., Kerr, I. M., Williams, B. R., Silverman, R. H., and Schreiber, R. D. (1998) How cells respond to interferons. *Annu. Rev. Biochem.* **67,** 227–264.

9. Elbashir, S. M., Harborth, J., Lendeckel, W., Yalcin, A., Weber, K., and Tuschl, T. (2001) Duplexes of 21-nucleotide RNAs mediate RNA interference in cultured mammalian cells. *Nature* **411,** 494–498.

10. Ui-Tei, K., Zenno, S., Miyata, Y., and Saigo, K. (2000) Sensitive assay of RNA interference in *Drosophila* and chinese hamster cultured cells using firefly luciferase gene as target. *FEBS Lett.* **479,** 79–82.

11. Billy, E., Brondani, V., Zhang, H., Müller, U., and Filipowicz, W. (2001) Specific interference with gene expression induced by long, double-stranded RNA in mouse embryonal teratocarcinoma cell lines. *Proc. Natl. Acad. Sci. USA* **98,** 14,428–14,433.

12. Paddison, P. J., Caudy, A. A., and Hannon, G. J. (2002) Stable suppression of gene expression by RNAi in mammalian cells. *Proc. Natl. Acad. Sci. USA* **99,** 1443–1448.

13. Yang, S., Tutton, S., Pierce, E., and Yoon, K. (2001) Specific double-stranded RNA interference in undifferentiated mouse embryonic stem cells. *Mol. Cell. Biol.* **21,** 7807–7816.

14. Wianny, F. and Zernicka-Goetz, M. (1999) Specific interference with gene function by double-stranded RNA in early mouse development. *Nat. Cell Biol.* **2,** 70–75.

15. Hammond, S. M., Bernstein, E., Beach, D., and Hannon, G. J. (2000) An RNA-directed nuclease mediates post-transcriptional gene silencing in *Drosophila* cells. *Nature* **404,** 293–296.

16. Nykänen, A., Haley, B., and Zamore, P. D. (2001) ATP requirements and small interfering RNA structure in the RNA interference pathway. *Cell* **107,** 309–321.

17. Zamore, P. D., Tuschl, T., Sharp, P. A., and Bartel, D. P. (2000) RNAi: double-stranded RNA directs the ATP-dependent cleavage of mRNA at 21 to 23 nucleotide intervals. *Cell* **101,** 25–33.

18. Hammond, S. M., Boettcher, S., Caudy, A. A., Kobayashi, R., and Hannon, G. J. (2001) Argonaute2, a link between genetic and biochemical analyses of RNAi. *Science* **293,** 1146–1150.

19. Caudy, A. A., Myers, M., Hannon, G. J., and Hammond, S. M. (2002) Fragile X-related protein and VIG associated with the RNA interference machinery. *Genes Dev.* **16,** 2491–2496.

20. Martinez, J., Patkaniowska, A., Urlaub, H., Lührmann, R., and Tuschl, T. (2002) Single-stranded antisense siRNAs guide target RNA cleavage in RNAi. *Cell* **110,** 563–574.

21. Elbashir, S. M., Martinez, J., Patkaniowska, A., Lendeckel, W., and Tuschl, T. (2001) Functional anatomy of siRNAs for mediating efficient RNAi in *Drosophila melanogaster* embryo lysate. *EMBO J.* **20,** 6877–6888.

22. Holen, T., Amrzguioui, M., Wiiger, M. T., Babaie, E., and Prydz, H. (2002) Positional effects of short interfering RNAs targeting the human coagulation trigger tissue factor. *Nucleic Acids Res.* **30,** 1757–1766.

23. Ui-Tei, K., Naito, Y., Takahashi, F., et al. (2004) Guidelines for the selection of highly effective siRNA sequences for mammalian and chick RNA interference. *Nucleic Acids Res.* **32,** 936–948.

24. Reynolds, A., Leake, D., Boese, Q., Scaringe, S., Marshall, W. S., and Khvorova, A. (2004) Rational siRNA design for RNA interference. *Nat. Biotech.* **22,** 326–330.

25. Amarzguioui, M. and Prydz, H. (2004) An algorithm for selection of functional siRNA sequences. *Biochem. Briophys. Res. Commun.* **316,** 1050–1058.

26. Doi, N., Zenno, S., Ueda, R., Ohki-Hamazaki, H., Ui-Tei, K., and Saigo, K. (2003) Short-interfering-RNA mediated gene silencing in mammalian cells requires Direr and eIF2C translation initiation factors. *Curr. Biol.* **13,** 41–46.

27. Song, J. -J., Smith, S. K., Hannon, G. J., and Joshua-Tor, L. (2004) Crystal structure of Argonaute and its implications for RISC slicer activity. *Science* **305,** 1434–1437.

28. Ma, J. -B., Ye, K., and Patel, D. J. (2004) Structural basis for overhang-specific small interfereing RNA recognition by the PAZ domain. *Nature* **429,** 318–322.

29. Ma, J. -B., Yuan, Y. -R., Meister, G., Pei, Y., Tuschl, T., and Patel, D. J. (2005) Structural basis for 5'-end-specific recognition of guide RNA by the *A. fulgidus* Piwi protein. *Nature* **434,** 666–670.

30. Ding, H., Schwarz, D. S., Keene, A., et al. (2003) Selective silencing by RNAi of a dominant allele that causes amyotrophic lateral sclerosis. *Aging Cell* **2,** 209–217.

31. Du, Q., Thonberg, H., Wang, J., Wahlestedt, C., and Liang, Z. (2005) A systematic analysis of the silencing effects of an active siRNA at all single-nucleotide mismatched target sites. *Nucleic Acids Res.* **33,** 1671–1677.

32. Jackson, A. L., Bartz, S. R., Schelter, J., et al. (2003) Expression profiling reveals off-target gene regulation by RNAi. *Nat. Biotech.* **21,** 635–637.

33. Naito, Y., Yamada, T., Ui-Tei, K., Morishita, S., and Saigo, K. (2004) siDirect: highly effective, target-specific siRNA design software for mammalian RNA interference. *Nucleic Acids Res.* **32,** W124–W129.

34. Brummelkamp, T. R., Bernards, R., and Agami, R. (2002) A system for stable expression of short interfering RNAs in mammalian cells. *Science* **296,** 550–553.

35. Yamada, T. and Morishita, S. (2005) Accelerated off-target search algorithm for siRNA. *Bioinformatics* **21,** 1316–1324.

10

Suppression of Apoptosis in the Liver by Systemic and Local Delivery of Small-Interfering RNAs

Lars Zender and Stefan Kubicka

Summary

RNA interference (RNAi) is a sequence-specific gene-silencing mechanism triggered by double-stranded RNA. RNAi was shown to allow transient or stable knockdown of gene expression in a broad range of species and has been used successfully for functional genomic screens in mammalian cells and *Caenorhabditis elegans*. Standard therapeutic use of RNAi in clinical settings in humans has been hampered by the lack of effective methods to deliver the small-interfering RNAs (siRNAs) or short-hairpin RNA expression vectors into the diseased organs. In mice, systemic delivery of siRNAs by hydrodynamic intravascular injection leads to highly efficient uptake of siRNAs into the liver. Several groups demonstrated therapeutic use of RNAi in mouse models of acute liver failure or hepatitis B virus replication. This chapter will focus on the technical background of hydrodynamic and portal vein delivery techniques in mice and will give practical guidance for using these techniques for siRNA delivery into the liver.

Key Words: siRNA; RNA interference; hydrodynamic intravascular injection; apoptosis; acute liver failure.

1. Introduction

RNA interference (RNAi) has been shown to be a powerful tool to study gene function in a broad range of different organisms. It overcomes the limitations of classical genetic methods to knockdown gene expression in mammalian cells. Most recently, RNAi has been exploited as a high-throughput genomics tool in mammals *(1–3)*. Furthermore, RNAi holds great promise as a therapeutic tool. Applications of RNAi directed against targets in diseases, for example cancer, infectious diseases, or dominant genetic diseases, are conceivable. Although the therapeutic use in humans is

From: *Methods in Molecular Biology, vol. 361, Target Discovery and Validation Reviews and Protocols*
Volume 2, Emerging Molecular Targets and Treatment Options
Edited by: M. Sioud © Humana Press Inc., Totowa, NJ

still some time from becoming routine in the clinic, use of experimental delivery methods in mice currently allows the study of RNAi in preclinical therapeutic settings *(4–7)*.

Because numerous comprehensive reviews about RNAi are available in the literature, this chapter will not give a detailed background on the discovery of RNAi but will focus on practical aspects of using RNAi in mice.

1.1. Efficient Delivery: the Holy Grail of Gene Therapeutic Approaches

The holy grail of all in vivo gene therapeutic approaches is to deliver effective amounts of the therapeutic gene into the desired target cells. Currently, viral vectors are most widely used for delivery of therapeutic genes in vivo. However, vector-associated side effects limit their value as a tool for clinical use.

Systemic application of plasmid DNA or antisense oligonucleotides (ASO), however, leads to very low uptake in most tissues. In part, this is owing to the fact that nucleic acids are rapidly degraded after systemic intravascular application in vivo. With regard to future therapeutic applications in humans, it is promising that under certain conditions short-interfering RNA (siRNA) duplexes seem to be more stable than chemically modified ASO *(8)*. Several approaches have been described to achieve more efficient uptake of naked DNA or ASO into tissues in vivo. Among these are direct injection into the target organ, as shown for muscle and liver *(9,10)* and electroporation *(11,12)*.

1.2. Hydrodynamic Intravascular Injection

The large volume hydrodynamic delivery technique was a major advance in the in vivo delivery of nucleic acids into mice and rats. In principle, it means the injection of a high volume into the vascular system within a short period of time. The first report that this delivery method can be even more effective than direct injection into the target organ is from Budker et al. *(13)*, who injected high volumes of either lacZ or luciferase reporter plasmids into the portal vein of mice. Using this approach approx 1% of all hepatocytes throughout the whole liver showed uptake of the plasmid. Remarkably, reporter activity was undetectable in endothelial and bile duct cells.

Because surgery on mice and intraportal injection is not feasible in every laboratory, it was an important discovery that injection of a high volume of plasmid DNA into the tail vein also leads to a very efficient uptake of DNA into the liver *(14)*. In 2002, McCaffrey et al. showed that the hydrodynamic tail-vein delivery technique could be used to effectively deliver siRNA into hepatocytes *(15)*. Subsequent studies showed that the siRNA uptake into the liver after hydrodynamic tail-vein delivery is much more effective than the uptake of plasmid DNA using this technique; uptake of siRNA in up to 70–90% of all hepatocytes was achieved *(16,17)*.

The physiological mechanisms of the hydrodynamic intravascular injection technique are still not fully elucidated. Intravascular delivery of a large bolus of fluid is thought to result in an accumulation of the liquid in the caval vein. As the heart is swamped with the high amount of liquid, a temporary right heart failure with subsequent backflow into the liver is the consequence. In the liver, the fluid is thought to be extravasated through the pores (fenestrate) in the liver endothelium (sinusoids). It is well known that liver endothelium has a much bigger average pore size than endothelium of other organs. The observation that siRNA uptake into the liver after hydrodynamic tail-vein injection is much higher than the uptake of plasmid DNA is in line with the idea that extravasation through the endothelial pores is a prerequisite for uptake into hepatocytes. After passing the endothelium, the siRNA molecules or plasmid DNA are in direct contact with the hepatocytes. Whether the molecules are finally internalized by receptor mediated *(18)* or receptor independent processes like membrane rupture *(19)* remains unclear.

1.3. Therapeutical Use of siRNA to Prevent and Treat Acute Liver Failure in Mice

As the first demonstrations of a therapeutic application of siRNA in vivo were done in mouse models of acute liver failure (ALF), the next paragraphs will give a brief introduction into this disease, followed by a discussion of the therapeutic use of siRNA to suppress apoptosis in this model.

ALF is defined as a dramatic clinical syndrome in which a previously normal liver fails within days or weeks. Three subgroups of ALF can be distinguished, hyperacute, acute, and subacute liver failure. Despite the frequent occurrence of cerebral edema and renal failure in patients with hyperacute liver failure, prognosis without transplantation is relatively good. Survival rates in patients with acute and subacute liver failure, however, are at best 15% *(20,21)*. The etiology of ALF shows marked worldwide variation: in underdeveloped countries viral causes predominate, whereas drug-induced hepatotoxicity and seronegative hepatitis predominate in most countries of the Western world *(22)*. To this day, the management of these varying clinical scenarios is essentially supportive. It aims to identify and remove the insult that led to destruction of the liver, whereas preventing associated complications, such as acute renal and respiratory failure, bleeding diatheses, severe sepsis, cerebral edema, and encephalopathy. Overall mortality in patients with severe ALF remains high, ranging from 40 to 80%. Although liver support devices or hepatocyte transplantation may in time have a place in treatment, currently liver transplantation remains the only therapeutic option that has been shown to significantly improve the outcome of patients with ALF. Because of limitations of donor organs and the requirement of lifelong and life-limiting immunosuppression, liver transplantation should be only performed in patients who are unlikely to recover from ALF. In patients who recover from ALF with medical support, the liver almost always returns to normal, both structurally and functionally. Consequently, prevention of destruction of liver cells in the time-course of ALF and support of liver regeneration are the most important goals in management of ALF by molecular therapies in the future.

Several molecular mechanisms can initiate liver cell injury and can further aggravate ongoing damage processes *(23)*. Mitochondria are the prominent targets for hepatotoxicity of many drugs, leading to impairment of energy metabolism and intracellular oxidative stress. Once hepatocellular function is impaired, accumulation of hydrophobic bile acids causes additional cytotoxicity. Although drug-induced hepatotoxicity appears to be mediated by both apoptosis and necrosis, viral infection predominantly induces cell death of hepatocytes by apoptosis. In contrast to necrosis, apoptosis is a highly conserved physiological process important in normal development and tissue homeostasis of multicellular organisms. Apoptosis occurs by two pathways: a death receptor pathway and a mitochondrial pathway. Signals released from the cytoplasm and/or from the cell membrane activate a well-characterized cascade of caspases (cysteine aspartase), which execute apoptotic cell death *(24–27)*. Receptor-mediated apoptosis, as triggered by the tumor necrosis factor-R, Fas-, or TNF-related apoptosis-inducing ligand (TRAIL)-receptor 1, has been reported to be involved in the pathogenesis of different liver diseases like viral hepatitis, ALF, autoimmune hepatitis, ischemia-reperfusion injury, nonalcoholic steatohepatitis, and toxic liver damage like Wilson's disease or bile acid-induced hepatotoxicity *(28–33)*. Therefore, the apoptotic pathway provides attractive targets for molecular therapy to prevent further liver damage and provides a condition for successful liver regeneration in ALF.

Recently, Song et al. *(16)* and our group *(34)* reported the therapeutic use of siRNA in mouse models of ALF. Song et al. used siRNA duplexes targeting the Fas (CD95) receptor. Three consecutive applications of Fas-siRNA led to an uptake of siRNA in more than 80% of all hepatocytes resulting in an 8- to 10-fold downregulation of Fas mRNA expression in the liver. To note, comparable downregulation of Fas had been shown before using ASO *(35)*, however, this required treating the mice with an approx 14-fold higher amount of anti-Fas ASO (6 mg/kg body weight for 12 consecutive days). In accordance with the results from Zhang et al. *(35)*, inhibition of Fas expression by siRNA protected the hepatocytes against treatment with the Fas-activating antibody Jo-2 and resulted in significantly increased survival. Remarkably, Fas-siRNA also conferred protection against ConA-mediated acute liver damage, whereas Fas-antisense did not.

As it is well established that in addition to FasL, tumor necrosis factor α and TRAIL are also involved in the pathogenesis of viral hepatitis *(36,37)*, we reasoned that an essential early downstream mediator of all death receptors would be the most suitable target to achieve the best therapeutic effects in preclinical animal models of viral hepatitis and ALF. To test this, we directed siRNA against caspase-8, which is a key downstream effector in receptor-mediated apoptosis. A single dose of 0.45–0.6 nmol/g body weight of caspase-8-siRNA resulted in very effective inhibition of caspase-8 expression in the liver, thus leading to protection against Jo-2-mediated liver damage or liver damage induced by an adenovirus overexpressing Fas ligand (Ad-FasL). With regard to potential clinical applications, it is noteworthy that caspase-8-siRNA not only prevented acute liver damage but was also highly effective when delivered into an ongoing ALF. Furthermore, it is of particular interest that in our study the therapeutic efficiency of caspase-8-siRNA was shown in acute viral hepatitis that was triggered by wild-type adenovirus, which better resembles the multiple molecular events in human acute hepatitis.

2. Materials

2.1. Preparation for Hydrodynamic Tail-Vein Injection in Mice

1. Restraining device for mice.
2. Paper towels, warm water, or alternatively heating lamp.
3. 3-mL Syringe with screw thread, 21- to 27-gauge needle.
4. 0.9% Saline or Ringer's solution.
5. siRNA duplexes (0.5–1.0 nmol/g body weight).

2.2. Preparation for Portal Vein Injection in Mice

1. Surgery pad for mice.
2. Antiseptic solution.
3. 24-Gauge iv catheter.
4. Gauze.
5. Surgical instruments (scissors, tweezers, and retractors).
6. Ketamine/xylazine, alternatively gas-anesthsia (e.g., isoflurane may be used).
7. Suture material, 4–0.
8. Optional Fibrine/Thrombine adhesive solution (*see* **Subheading 3.**).
9. 0.9% Saline or Ringer's solution.
10. Lipiodol.
11. Microvascular clamps (optional).

12. Adapter tube and infusion pump (optional).
13. siRNA duplex (0.5–1.0 nmol/g body weight).

3. Methods
3.1. Hydrodynamic/High Volume Tail-Vein Injection in Mice (see Note 1)

In principle, any mouse strain can be used for this technique. BALB/c or other strains with white fur are preferred as visualization and puncture of the tail vein, especially with bigger needles, is more difficult in black mice.

We prefer to perform standard hydrodynamic tail-vein injection without anesthesia, as the combination of the high-volume injection together with anesthesia can lead to complications in some mice. If anesthesia is used, a gentle gas-anesthesia (e.g., isoflurane) should be preferred.

First, the injection solution is prepared. In our hands, best results are obtained with desalted, lyophilized siRNA duplexes, as siRNA duplexes lyophilized in annealing buffer can result in higher morbidity of the mice. Most of the "siRNA-companies" provide siRNA duplexes in a desalted "ready-to-go" option. The desired amount of siRNA duplex is dissolved in 0.9% saline or Ringer's solution. Effective siRNAs should work in a dose of 0.5–1.0 nmol per gram body weight. The total injection volume can be calculated by dividing the mouse body weight by 10 (*see* **Note 2**).

The mouse is restrained using a suitable restraining device (numerous Plexiglas versions are available from different manufacturers) and a tail vein is dilated by application of warm water. Alternatively, some researchers dilate the tail vessels by placing the whole mouse under a heating lamp for 10 min. A 3-mL syringe with a screw thread is connected to a needle. Needles from 21- to 27-gauges are suitable. Using syringes without a screw thread can lead to disconnection during hydrodynamic injection. A tail vein is punctured approximately midway between the tail tip and middle of the tail. If the first puncture is not successful, a more proximal puncture site can be tried. After injecting a small test volume to ensure that the needle is safely placed in the vein, the whole volume is applied within 4–10 s. Longer injection times will lead to less effective uptake of siRNA into the liver. Some mice will show heavy breathing and reduced activity after injection. These symptoms should not last longer than 30 min.

3.2. Intraportal Delivery of siRNA in Mice

The hydrodynamic tail-vein injection technique leads to high and reproducible siRNA uptake into the liver. It offers the possibility to investigate the effects of siRNA-mediated gene knockdown in the "target organ" liver in different physiological and pathophysiological settings (*see* **Note 3**). However, a criticism against hydrodynamic tail-vein injection is that it is an experimental procedure that is not feasible in the clinical situation in humans. Therefore, it is desirable to have an experimental setting in the mouse model that can resemble the clinical situation in humans.

In humans the portal vein can be reached without open surgery by puncturing the jugular vein and placing a catheter from the inferior caval vein through the liver. Thus, the direct portal vein injection in mice can serve as a model for this procedure.

Animals are anesthetized with ketamine/Xxlazine or, if preferred, with gas-anesthesia (e.g., isoflurane). The abdominal wall is cleaned with antiseptic solution. A midline ventral incision is made and the abdominal cavity is kept open with retractors. The bowels are wrapped in saline soaked gauze and placed sideward of the operation field to obtain a good view on the portal vein. The desired amount of siRNA (0.5–1.0 nmol) is dissolved in saline or Ringer's solution containing 10% lipiodol as an embolizing agent. The use of an embolizing agent leads to a temporary stasis of the siRNA solution in the liver and, therefore, enhances the siRNA uptake into the liver. Alternatively, some researchers place microvascular clamps on the suprahepatic inferior caval vein during the injection procedure. This likewise prevents a fast flow-through of the siRNA solution through the liver. The portal vein is punctured with a 24-gauge iv catheter. After the plastic catheter is placed in a safe position the needle is removed. To avoid accidental movement of the catheter during injection, the portal vein is looped with a 4–0 ligature to tighten the catheter. A total volume of up to 5% of mouse body weight can be injected within 10 s. Inexperienced researchers may find it easier to use an adapter tube to connect the catheter to an infusion-pump instead of injecting free hand. Before removing the needle, an adhesive solution of Fibrine/Thrombine is spread on the puncture site to prevent bleeding. The abdominal cavity is closed with two separate layers of 4–0 suture material (*see* **Note 4**). **Fig. 1** shows the inhibition of endogenous expression of *LacZ* gene by hydrodynamic-derived siRNAs.

4. Notes

1. Researchers who are inexperienced with hydrodynamic tail-vein injection in mice may want to test their technical proficiency by using transgenic mice carrying a reporter gene like *lacZ* or green fluorescent protein (GFP). Using this approach with established siRNA duplexes against lacZ or GFP, the efficiency of siRNA delivery into the liver can be quantified (*see also* **Fig. 1**). Alternatively, Cy-5-labeled siRNAs can be injected. An easy and precise way to quantify the percentage of liver cells with siRNA uptake is to prepare a single-cell suspension of liver cells using standard collagenase perfusion (*38*) and subsequently determine the Cy-5-positive fraction of hepatocytes by flow cytometry. In this context it is

siRNA-scrambled   **siRNA-lacZ**

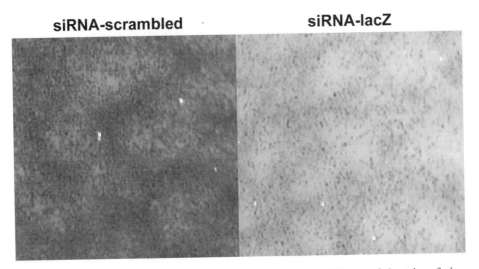

Fig. 1. Hydrodynamic tail-vein injection leads to efficient delivery of short-interfering RNAs (siRNA)-lacZ into the liver of *lacZ*-transgenic mice. Shown are photographs of the liver surface of *lacZ*-transgenic mice (C57BL/6J-TgN [MtnlacZ]) after hydrodynamic tail-vein injection of either siRNA-scrambled or siRNA-*lacZ*. *LacZ* staining was performed on whole liver (*see* **Note 5**).

   important to mention that some siRNA duplexes lose their functionality when they are Cy-5-labeled.
2. To rule out off-target effects of siRNA, two independent siRNAs against every target should be used.
3. Although siRNA duplexes are effectively delivered to a target organ, the efficiency of knockdown of a specific gene must be quantified by assaying mRNA and protein expression.
4. Researchers who want to use the hydrodynamic tail-vein injection technique to deliver plasmid DNA to the liver are advised to work with supercoiled plasmid DNA that can be obtained easily by cesium chloride DNA preparations.
5. For experiments that need sustained knockdown of the target gene in the mouse liver, stability of the respective siRNA in the liver must be tested individually. Depending on the siRNA duplex, the duration of in vivo knockdown can be variable ranging from 2 d to more than 1 wk.

Acknowledgments

   The authors would like to thank Drs. Mona S. Spector and Jesus Gil for critical reading of the manuscript.

References

1. Paddison, P. J., Silva, J. M., Conklin, D. S., et al. (2004) A resource for large-scale RNA-interference-based screens in mammals. *Nature* **428,** 427–431.

2. Berns, K., Hijmans, E. M., Mullenders, J., et al. (2004) A large-scale RNAi screen in human cells identifies new components of the p53 pathway. *Nature* **428,** 431–437.

3. Brummelkamp, T. R., Nijman, S. M., Dirac, A. M., and Bernards, R. (2003) Loss of the cylindromatosis tumour suppressor inhibits apoptosis by activating NF-kappaB. *Nature* **424,** 797–801.

4. Zender, L., Hutker, S., Liedtke, C., et al. (2003) Caspase 8 small interfering RNA prevents acute liver failure in mice. *Proc. Natl. Acad. Sci. USA* **100,** 7797–7802.

5. Song, E., Lee, S. K., Wang, J., et al. (2003) RNA interference targeting Fas protects mice from fulminant hepatitis. *Nat. Med.* **9,** 347–351.

6. Klein, C., Bock, C. T., Wedemeyer, H., et al. (2003) Inhibition of hepatitis B virus replication in vivo by nucleoside analogues and siRNA. *Gastroenterology* **125,** 9–18.

7. McCaffrey, A. P., Nakai, H., Pandey, K., et al. (2003) Inhibition of hepatitis B virus in mice by RNA interference. *Nat. Biotechnol.* **21,** 639–644.

8. Bertrand, J. R., Pottier, M., Vekris, A., Opolon, P., Maksimenko, A., and Malvy, C. (2002) Comparison of antisense oligonucleotides and siRNAs in cell culture and in vivo. *Biochem. Biophys. Res. Commun.* **296,** 1000–1004.

9. Danko, I., Williams, P., Herweijer, H., et al. (1997) High expression of naked plasmid DNA in muscles of young rodents. *Hum. Mol. Genet.* **6,** 1435–1443.

10. Hickman, M. A., Malone, R. W., Lehmann-Bruinsma, K., et al. (1994) Gene expression following direct injection of DNA into liver. *Hum. Gene Ther.* **5,** 1477–1483.

11. Hartikka, J., Sukhu, L., Buchner, C., et al. (2001) Electroporation-facilitated delivery of plasmid DNA in skeletal muscle: plasmid dependence of muscle damage and effect of poloxamer 188. *Mol. Ther.* **4,** 407–415.

12. Somiari, S., Glasspool-Malone, J., Drabick, J. J., et al. (2000) Theory and in vivo application of electroporative gene delivery. *Mol. Ther.* **2,** 178–187.

13. Budker, V., Zhang, G., Knechtle, S., and Wolff, J. A. (1996) Naked DNA delivered intraportally expresses efficiently in hepatocytes. *Gene Ther.* **3,** 593–598.

14. Zhang, G., Budker, V., and Wolff, J. A. (1999) High levels of foreign gene expression in hepatocytes after tail vein injections of naked plasmid DNA. *Hum. Gene Ther.* **10,** 1735–1737.

15. McCaffrey, A. P., Meuse, L., Pham, T. T., Conklin, D. S., Hannon, G. J., and Kay, M. A. (2002) RNA interference in adult mice. *Nature* **418,** 38–39.

16. Song, E., Lee, S. K., Wang, J., et al. (2003) RNA interference targeting Fas protects mice from fulminant hepatitis. *Nat. Med.* **9,** 347–351.

17. Zender, L., Hutker, S., Liedtke, C., et al. (2003) Caspase 8 small interfering RNA prevents acute liver failure in mice. *Proc. Natl. Acad. Sci. USA* **100,** 7797–7802.

18. Budker, V., Budker, T., Zhang, G., Subbotin, V., Loomis, A., and Wolff, J. A. (2000) Hypothesis: naked plasmid DNA is taken up by cells in vivo by a receptor-mediated process. *J. Gene Med.* **2,** 76–88.

19. Kobayashi, N., Kuramoto, T., Yamaoka, K., Hashida, M., and Takakura, Y. (2001) Hepatic uptake and gene expression mechanisms following intravenous administration of plasmid DNA by conventional and hydrodynamics-based procedures, *J. Pharmacol. Exp. Ther.* **297,** 853–860.

20. O'Grady, J. G., Schalm, S. W., and Williams, R. (1993) Acute liver failure: redefining the syndromes. *Lancet* **342,** 273–275.

21. Plevris, J. N., Schina, M., and Hayes, P. C. (1998) Review article: the management of acute liver failure. *Aliment. Pharmacol. Ther.* **12,** 405–418.

22. Bernal, W. (2003) Changing patterns of causation and the use of transplantation in the United Kingdom. *Semin. Liver Dis.* **23,** 227–237.

23. Jaeschke, H., Gores, G. J., Cederbaum, A. I., Hinson, J. A., Pessayre, D., and Lemasters, J. J. (2002) Mechanisms of hepatotoxicity. *Toxicol. Sci.* **65,** 166–176.

24. Adams, J. M. and Cory, S. (1998) The Bcl-2 protein family: arbiters of cell survival. *Science* **281,** 1322–1326.

25. Ashkenazi, A. and Dixit, V. M. (1998) Death receptors: signaling and modulation, *Science* **281,** 1305–1308.

26. Evan, G. and Littlewood, T. (1998) A matter of life and cell death. *Science* **281,** 1317–1322.

27. Green, D. R. and Reed, J. C. (1998) Mitochondria and apoptosis. *Science* **281,** 1309–1312.

28. Galle, P. R., Hofmann, W. J., Walczak, H., et al. (1995) Involvement of the CD95 (APO-1/Fas) receptor and ligand in liver damage. *J. Exp. Med.* **182,** 1223–1230.

29. Strand, S., Hofmann, W. J., Grambihler, A., et al. (1998) Hepatic failure and liver cell damage in acute Wilson's disease involve CD95 (APO-1/Fas) mediated apoptosis. *Nat. Med.* **4,** 588–593.

30. Kuhnel, F., Zender, L., Paul, Y., et al. (2000) NFkappaB mediates apoptosis through transcriptional activation of Fas (CD95) in adenoviral hepatitis. *J. Biol. Chem.* **275,** 6421–6427.

31. Faubion, W. A., Guicciardi, M. E., Miyoshi, H., et al. (1999) Toxic bile salts induce rodent hepatocyte apoptosis via direct activation of Fas. *J. Clin. Invest.* **103,** 137–145.

32. Feldstein, A. E., Canbay, A., Angulo, P., et al. (2003) Hepatocyte apoptosis and fas expression are prominent features of human nonalcoholic steatohepatitis. *Gastroenterology* **125,** 437–443.

33. Yin, X. M. and Ding, W. X. (2003) Death receptor activation-induced hepatocyte apoptosis and liver injury. *Curr. Mol. Med.* **3,** 491–508.

34. Zender, L., Hutker, S., Liedtke, C., et al. (2003) Caspase 8 small interfering RNA prevents acute liver failure in mice. *Proc. Natl. Acad. Sci. USA* **100,** 7797–7802.

35. Zhang, H., Cook, J., Nickel, J., et al. (2000) Reduction of liver Fas expression by an antisense oligonucleotide protects mice from fulminant hepatitis. *Nat. Biotechnol.* **18,** 862–867.

36. Mundt, B., Kuhnel, F., Zender, L., et al. (2003) Involvement of TRAIL and its receptors in viral hepatitis. *FASEB J.* **17,** 94–96.

37. Streetz, K. L., Luedde, T., Manns, M. P., and Trautwein, C. (2000) Interleukin 6 and liver regeneration. *Gut* **47,** 309–312.

38. Seglen, P. O., Schwarze, P. E., and Saeter, G. (1986) Changes in cellular ploidy and autophagic responsiveness during rat liver carcinogenesis. *Toxicol. Pathol.* **14,** 342–348.

11

Target Validation Using RNA Interference in Solid Tumors

Seyedhossein Aharinejad, Mouldy Sioud, Trevor Lucas, and Dietmar Abraham

Summary

Reverse genetics is one strategy that is currently used to establish a link between a target gene and a disease phenotype. In this process, the function of a gene is inhibited and the consequence of its loss on a desired biological function, such as tumor growth and metastasis, is monitored. RNA interference (RNAi) has been found to be the most effective method to specifically inhibit gene expression. Notably, interactions between cancer cells, stromal cells, and the extracellular matrix (ECM) are crucial to angiogenesis and tumorigenesis. Tumor cells and the surrounding stroma are the principle source of growth factors and cytokines, which induce remodeling of the ECM mediated by metalloproteases (MMPs) secreted by macrophages. The production of macrophages is regulated by colony-stimulating factor (CSF)-1, which is overexpressed in several tumors. When short-interfering RNAs (siRNAs) targeting either the CSF-1 or its receptors were delivered into colon and breast cancer xenografts in mice, tumor growth was inhibited. Associated with this suppression, we observed decreased tumor vascularity, reduced expression of angiogenic factors and MMPs, and decreased macrophage recruitment to the tumors. The suppression of CSF-1 by RNA interference is therefore a powerful tool to block gene function and influence tumor–stroma interactions in solid tumor development.

Key Words: Reverse genetics; breast cancer; RNAi; siRNA; CSF-1.

1. Introduction
1.1. The Microenvironment of Cancer Cells

The development of cancer is a complex, multistage process during which a normal cell undergoes genetic changes that result in phenotypic alterations and acquisition of the ability to invade and colonize distant sites *(1,2)*. Solid tumors are composed of both malignant and normal cells. Targeting the complex

From: *Methods in Molecular Biology, vol. 361, Target Discovery and Validation Reviews and Protocols*
Volume 2, Emerging Molecular Targets and Treatment Options
Edited by: M. Sioud © Humana Press Inc., Totowa, NJ

interaction between genetically unstable neoplastic cells, the surrounding extracellular matrix (ECM), and stromal cells such as fibroblasts and inflammatory cells is a key obstacle to the cure of human cancers *(1,2)*. Changes in the tumor microenvironment can lead to ECM modification, infiltration of inflammatory cells, and alteration in the activity of matrix metalloproteases (MMPs), which are essential regulatory factors in tumor growth and invasion *(3)*. In addition, mediators released from both the stroma and tumor cells can lead to the induction of angiogenesis by shifting the balance between factors that promote and inhibit angiogenesis *(4–7)*, allowing the growth of tumors to macroscopic levels *(8–11)*.

1.2. Macrophages, Angiogenesis, and the Extracellular Matrix

Macrophages are common components of the tumor stroma *(11)* that modify the ECM and influence new capillary growth by several different mechanisms *(12,13)*. Macrophages can produce growth factors, cytokines, proteolytic enzymes, and matrix molecules that act directly to stimulate vascularization by stimulating endothelial cell proliferation, migration, and differentiation in vitro and angiogenesis in vivo *(11,12)*. Macrophages can also modify the ECM either through the direct production of ECM components or the production of proteases that alter ECM structure and composition *(14,15)*. The composition of the ECM dramatically influences endothelial cell shape and morphology and profoundly influences capillary growth *(16)*. Importantly, recruitment of macrophages to tumors can significantly increase metastatic progression *(17)*. Macrophages can also secrete cytokines that stimulate other cells to synthesize or degrade ECM molecules. Remodeling of the ECM is crucial to both angiogenesis and tumorigenesis and primarily involves the MMP family of proteolytic enzymes. MMPs degrade the ECM including the basement membrane and in conjunction with soluble growth factors, foster the migration and proliferation of endothelial cells. This process promotes angiogenesis and also allows tumors to spread locally and distantly *(3)*. Strict regulation of MMP expression is critical for maintenance of proper ECM homeostasis, however, in malignancies high levels of MMPs are often synthesized not only by cancer cells but also by adjacent and intervening stromal cells *(18)*.

2. CSF-1 Biology

2.1. CSF-1 and Macrophages

The production of macrophages is regulated by colony-stimulating factor (CSF)-1 also called macrophage-CSF (M-CSF) *(19)*. CSF-1 is produced by a variety of cell types such as fibroblasts or macrophages and prevents the death of monocytes and promotes their differentiation into macrophages *(20,21)*. CSF-1 also induces or augments the production of a variety of cytokines by macrophages such as tumor necrosis factor-α *(22)*. Macrophages most likely enhance tumor progression through paracrine circuits involving the production of CSF-1 by tumor cells *(11)* or other host-derived stromal cells and by ECM-modulating functions mediated by MMPs *(12)* to accelerate angiogenesis in vivo *(23)*. Consistent with a proangiogenic effect, recent work suggests that CSF-1 also stimulates monocytes to secrete biologically active vascular endothelial growth factor (VEGF) *(24)*. VEGF is a key factor in tumor angiogenesis and is upregulated in numerous malignant tumors. The biological effects of VEGF are mediated by VEGF-receptor 1 (VEGF-R1, Flt-1) and VEGF-R2 (KDR/Flk-1).

2.2. CSF-1 Signaling Pathways

CSF-1 is a disulfide-linked homodimeric growth factor, which binds the integral membrane receptor tyrosine kinase (CSF-1R) product of the c-*fms* proto-oncogene *(25)*. Similar to other tyrosine kinase receptors, ligand binding stabilizes CSF-1R dimerization to activate the receptor through autophosphorylation *in trans*, thereby initiating a series of membrane-proximal tyrosine phosphorylation cascades leading to rapid stimulation of cytoskeletal remodeling, gene transcription, and protein translation *(26)*. Many of the downstream tyrosine-phosphorylated proteins, such as the p85 regulatory subunit of phosphatidyl-inositol 3-kinase, Cbl, and Gab3, have been shown to be important in regulating macrophage survival, differentiation, and motility *(27)*.

2.3. CSF-1 and Solid Tumors

CSF-1 is widely overexpressed in tumors of the reproductive system. In breast cancer, CSF-1 expression has been shown to correlate with high grade and poor prognosis associated with dense leukocytic infiltration *(28,29)*. High levels of CSF-1R mRNA have been observed in ovarian and endometrial cancers and elevated levels correlated with high histological grade and advanced clinical presentation *(30)*. Over half of invasive ovarian adenocarcinomas and endometrial cancers coexpress CSF-1 and CSF-1R *(31)*. Constitutive production of CSF-1 has been reported in normal ovarian epithelial cultures at levels comparable with ovarian cancer cell lines *(32)*. However, the coexpression of CSF-1 and CSF-1R may establish an autocrine loop that plays a role in metastatic progression. Serum levels of CSF-1 are markedly elevated in patients with endometrial cancer associated with active or recurrent disease *(33)*. Increased serum CSF-1 levels also characterize most clinical cases of epithelial ovarian cancers *(34)* and CSF-1 is considered a tumor marker for ovarian germ cell tumors *(35)*.

2.4. CSF-1 and Tumor Cell Invasion

Osteopetrotic CSF-1(op) *(op/op)* mice that have a CSF-1 gene defect and a profound macrophage deficiency *(36)* have been used as a model to examine tumor growth. These mice show an impaired tumor development (Lewis lung carcinoma) when compared to normal littermates, which is reversed by CSF-1 treatment *(37)*. Crossing CSF-1(op) mice with a transgenic mouse susceptible to mammary cancer prevented macrophage accumulation in mammary tumors. In the macrophage-deficient mice, the incidence and initial rates of growth of primary tumors were not different from those seen in normal mice, but the rate of tumor progression was slowed and metastatic ability was almost completely abrogated when compared with mice that contained normal numbers of macrophages. Overexpression of CSF-1 in wild-type mice also accelerated tumor progression and increased rates of metastasis *(17)*. Another study has shown that CSF-1 promotes tissue invasion by enhancing ECM-degrading proteinase MMP-2 production by lung cancer cells *(38)*. In some instances, malignant cells coexpress CSF-1 and CSF-1R, raising the possibility of autocrine growth control by CSF-1 in the development of these malignancies *(39)*.

3. Target Validation of CSF-1 in Cancer

3.1. CSF-1 Antisense Treatment Suppresses Growth of Human Embryonic and Colon Carcinoma Xenografts in Mice

3.1.1. Human Embryonic Cancer Cells Upregulate Host CSF-1 Production

Human embryonic cancer cells (CRL-2073) show no detectable mRNA or protein for human CSF-1 or CSF-1R in vitro. When these cells are xenografted into the testis of SCID mice, however, mouse tissue CSF-1 gene and protein expression increases significantly compared to untreated mice. Associated with increasing CSF-1 tissue expression is an enhanced infiltration of macrophages within and surrounding the tumor. These findings indicate that human embryonic cancer cells stimulate increased host tissue expression of CSF-1. Correlated with these results, increased mouse CSF-1R expression is seen in tumor lysates *(40)*.

3.1.2. CSF-1 Oligodeoxyribonucleotide Treatment Suppresses CSF-1 Expression and the Growth of Embryonic Tumor Xenografts

Severe combined immunodeficient (SCID) mice bearing established human embryonic tumors were treated systemically with CSF-1 antisense oligodeoxyribonucleotides (ODNs), scrambled ODN or Ringer's solution. Antisense ODN treatment was well tolerated. Local inflammatory reactions were not observed and no significant changes in the complete blood count (CBC) of treated mice were seen. Treatment with CSF-1 antisense ODN significantly downregulated tissue CSF-1 mRNA and protein levels and suppressed the growth of embryonic tumors to dormant levels. Marked differences were found in the testicular weight between SCID mice with embryonic tumors treated with CSF-1 ODN for 2 wk

(89 ± 32 mg tumor weight) and those treated with Ringer's solution (285 ± 31 mg) or scrambled ODN (278 ± 27 mg) *(40)*.

3.1.3. CSF-1 Antisense ODN Decreases Angiogenic Activity and MMP-2 Expression in Embryonic Tumor Xenografts

In human embryonic cancer cell xenografts, both intravital video microscopy and histomorphometry of embryonic tumors showed a significantly increased density of vascular sprouts in controls compared to untreated mice that returned to baseline levels after CSF-1 antisense ODN treatment in mouse testis. Similarly, VEGF-A, KDR/flk-1 and Ang-1 mRNA levels were significantly reduced in CSF-1 antisense ODN-treated mice. Protein expression of MMP-2, a key molecule in mediating tumor metastasis and angiogenesis, increased significantly in controls compared to untreated animals. Treatment with CSF-1 antisense ODN but not scrambled ODN, significantly downregulated MMP-2 protein expression in testicular tissue. Positive MMP-2 antigen staining was primarily observed in the intertubular interstitium, the capsule of testicular tubules and less frequently in the walls of vessels in untreated and ODN-treated mice, whereas in control mice, MMP-2 expression was primarily intratubular *(40)*.

3.1.4. CSF-1 Antisense Treatment Suppresses the Growth of a Human Colon Carcinoma Xenografts and Increases Survival in Mice

The promising results with CSF-1 antisense treatment in the mouse model of human embryonic tumorogenicity encouraged us to test CSF-1 antisense treatment in other human tumor models. We chose colon carcinoma because of its poor prognosis, short median survival, and high incidence, and utilized SW-620 human colon carcinoma cells that lack expression of CSF-1 or CSF-1R. Using an established flank model in nude mice, we showed that host CSF-1 tissue mRNA and protein levels increase with tumor progression. After 2 wk of CSF-1 antisense ODN treatment at 5 mg/kg/d, CSF-1 mRNA and protein expression was significantly downregulated compared to controls. Tumor growth was markedly retarded in mice following CSF-1 blockade and tumor weights were significantly decreased compared to controls. Similar to mice bearing embryonic tumors, CSF-1 treatment was well tolerated in nude mice bearing colon carcinoma and the CBC was not significantly influenced by the treatment. MMP-2 protein expression in tumor lysates markedly increased with tumor progression and declined significantly following CSF-1 inhibition. CSF-1 ODN, but not scrambled ODN treatment, resulted in downregulation of mRNA levels of Ang-1 and the VEGF-A receptors Flt-1 and KDR/flk-1 associated with decreased angiogenesis. Long-term (6 mo) survival was observed in 8 of 14 mice following CSF-1 blockade, whereas all mice were dead after 65 d in the control groups. At sacrifice 6 mo after therapy, no metastases were detected. At

65 d (at which time the last animal in the control groups died), 85.7% of CSF-1 antisense-treated mice were still alive.

3.2. CSF-1 in Breast Cancer

The mechanism by which mammary epithelial cells undergo genetic changes that result in acquisition of the ability to invade and colonize distant sites is complex *(2,41,42)*. Normal and malignant mammary epithelium and the surrounding stromal cells produce and respond to various growth factors. Among the stromal cells, macrophages play a unique role because they are recruited into mammary gland carcinomas *(43,44)*. The fact that in the absence of such tumor-associated macrophages, metastatic progression of mammary gland tumors is profoundly reduced *(17)* as well as the fact that CSF-1 blockade suppresses tumor growth, MMP production, and macrophage recruitment in embryonic tumors and colon cancer *(40)* support the paradigm that CSF-1 enhances progression of malignancies through effects on the recruitment and control of macrophages that regulate tumor cell growth, angiogenesis, and the ECM. The recent discovery of highly specific, small-interfering (siRNA) molecules as promising candidate therapeutics to specifically and potently modify gene expression led us to hypothesize that blocking CSF-1 using this approach would efficiently suppress breast cancer development.

3.2.1. MCF-7 Cells Upregulate Mouse CSF-1 Production But Lose Their Ability to Express Human CSF-1 After Xenografting to Mice

Expression analysis showed that human MCF-7 mammary carcinoma cells express both mRNA and protein for human CSF-1 and CSF-1R in vitro. When MCF-7 cells were xenografted to immunodeficient nude mice, cancer cell expression of CSF-1 was lost but host (mouse) cells were stimulated to overexpress CSF-1.

3.2.2. CSF-1 siRNA Against CSF-1 and c-fms Downregulate Target Proteins and Suppress Mammary Tumor Growth

CSF-1 and CSF-1R siRNAs suppress target gene expression in a sequence and dose dependent manner in vitro. Mice bearing human MCF-7 mammary carcinoma xenografts were treated with five intratumoral injections of CSF-1 siRNA, CSF1-R siRNA, scrambled control siRNA, or Ringer's solution (control). siRNA treatment was well tolerated and no significant changes in the CBC of treated mice were observed. siRNA treatment against CSF-1 and CSF-1R suppressed mammary tumor growth by 45 and 40%, respectively, and selectively downregulated target protein expression in tumor lysates.

3.2.3. CSF-1 and CSF-1R Blockade Downregulate Mouse MMP-2 and MMP-12 Expression and Decrease Angiogenic Activity in MCF-7 Mammary Tumor Xenografts

After human MCF-7 cell xenografting in mice, macrophage invasion in the tumor xenografts was observed. In association with this, host (mouse) MMP-2 and MMP-12 (a macrophage-specific protease involved in ECM remodeling) were strongly expressed during tumor progression in control animals. Treatment with CSF-1 siRNA or CSF-1R siRNA reduced macrophage recruitment to the tumor and intratumoral levels of both MMP-2 and MMP-12.

Histomorphometrical analysis of mammary tumors showed an increased density of proliferating endothelial cells with tumor progression that was decreased after CSF-1 and CSF-1R siRNA blockade. In addition, VEGF-A mRNA levels increased with tumor progression and were reduced in CSF-1 and CSF-1R siRNA-treated mice. CSF-1 and CSF-1R blockade, however, did not significantly affect tissue mRNA expression of the VEGF-A receptors Flt-1 and KDR. These data indicated that blocking CSF-1 or CSF-1R is associated with decreased VEGF-A expression and reduced angiogenic activity in mammary tumor xenografts.

3.2.4. CSF-1 Blockade Increases Survival in Mice With Mammary Tumor Xenografts

The median survival of animals in the control group was 62 d, which was significantly increased in mice after treatment with CSF-1 siRNA (103 d) and slightly (but not significantly) increased after treatment with CSF-1R siRNA (76 d).

4. Conclusions

Using antisense oligonulcleotides and siRNAs, we have demonstrated that CSF-1 plays a crucial role in tumor growth and angiogenesis. Indeed, inhibition of upregulated host CSF-1 in human embryonic, colon, and breast cancer xenografts in mice suppressed tumor growth, leading to inhibition of tumor vascularity, angiogenic factors, and MMPs expression. Additionally, recruitment of host macrophages to tumors was significantly reduced (40,42). These results combined with the recently recognized role of macrophages as VEGF-secreting cells (24), suggest that certain cancer cells upregulate host CSF-1 by mechanisms that have yet to be identified leading to macrophage modification of the ECM and facilitating angiogenesis and tumor development. Moreover, some cancer cells produce CSF-1 and directly influence macrophages (45). Thus, interaction between cancer cells and the surrounding tumor microenvironment leads to upregulation of CSF-1, which in turn leads to macrophage recruitment. The tumor microenvironment educates these tumor-associated macrophages to

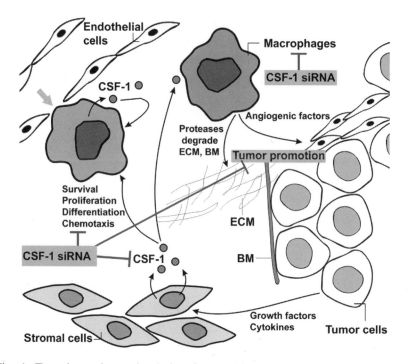

Fig. 1. Targeting colony-stimulating factor (CSF)-1 in tumor progression. Tumor cells may produce CSF-1 or secrete growth factors that upregulate CSF-1 production by stromal cells, thereby recruiting macrophages to the tumor. Tumor-associated macrophages also produce CSF-1 and stimulate angiogenesis by secreting factors such as vascular endothelial growth factor (VEGF). Macrophages also promote tumor invasion by producing proteases such as metalloproteases (MMP)-2 and MMP-9 that break down the basement membrane (BM), remodel the extracellular matrix (ECM) and promote angiogenesis. This creates a microenvironment that promotes tumor progression and invasion. CSF-1 blockade inhibits tumor progression by influencing the macrophages that regulate angiogenesis and the ECM illustrated by decreased macrophage recruitment to the tumors associated with diminished VEGF-A and MMP expression and reduced angiogenic activity. siRNA, small-interfering RNA.

perform supportive roles that promote tumor progression and metastasis *(46)*. Together, these studies demonstrate that CSF-1 and CSF-1R can be used as therapeutic targets in the treatment of solid tumors **(Fig. 1)**.

The fact that five injections of siRNA at much lower doses than antisense ODNs required for a comparable effect can block the function of the target genes effectively favors the use of these nucleic acid-based constructs for large-scale human studies *(47)* whereby a more sustained therapeutic modality may be required to increase therapeutic efficacy. Moreover, although reduction of CSF-1 by phosphorothioate antisense ODN in human tumor xenografts has the potential to suppress tumor growth *(40,42)*, absolute sequence specificity is not attainable using oligonucleotide with phosphorothioate linkages *(48)*, which again favors the use of siRNAs that induce sequence-specific gene silencing *(49)*. RNA interference is therefore a powerful tool to block gene function and influence solid tumor development. The continuing development of stable siRNA constructs optimized to target solid tumors by systemic application therefore hold great promise for the future in cancer therapy (*see* Chapters 9 and 10).

References

1. Aharinejad, S., Marks, S. C., Jr., Bock, P., et al. (1995) CSF-1 treatment promotes angiogenesis in the metaphysis of osteopetrotic (toothless, tl) rats. *Bone* **16,** 315–324.
2. Aharinejad, S., Abraham, D., Paulus, P., et al. (2002) Colony-stimulating factor-1 antisense treatment suppresses growth of human tumor xenografts in mice. *Cancer Res.* **62,** 5317–5324.
3. Aharinejad, S., Paulus, P., Sioud, M., et al. (2004) Colony-stimulating factor-1 blockade by antisense oligonucleotides and small interfering RNAs suppresses growth of human mammary tumor xenografts in mice. *Cancer Res.* **64,** 5378–5384.
4. Baiocchi, G., Kavanagh, J. J., Talpaz, M., Wharton, J. T., Gutterman, J. U., and Kurzrock, R. (1991) Expression of the macrophage colony-stimulating factor and its receptor in gynecologic malignancies. *Cancer* **67,** 990–996.
5. Bast, R. C., Jr., Boyer, C. M., Jacobs, I., et al. (1993) Cell growth regulation in epithelial ovarian cancer. *Cancer* **71,** 1597–1601.
6. Caplen, N. J., Parrish, S., Imani, F., Fire, A., and Morgan, R. A. (2001) Specific inhibition of gene expression by small double-stranded RNAs in invertebrate and vertebrate systems. *Proc. Natl. Acad. Sci. USA* **98,** 9742–9747.
7. Coussens, L. M. and Werb, Z. (1996) Matrix metalloproteinases and the development of cancer. *Chem. Biol.* **3,** 895–904.
8. Eubank, T. D., Galloway, M., Montague, C. M., Waldman, W. J., and Marsh, C. B. (2003) M-CSF induces vascular endothelial growth factor production and angiogenic activity from human monocytes. *J. Immunol.* **171,** 2637–2643.
9. Farber, E. (1984) The multistep nature of cancer development. *Cancer Res.* **44,** 4217–4223.
10. Fidler, I. J. and Ellis, L. M. (1994) The implications of angiogenesis for the biology and therapy of cancer metastasis. *Cell* **79,** 185–188.
11. Folkman, J., Watson, K., Ingber, D., and Hanahan, D. (1989) Induction of angiogenesis during the transition from hyperplasia to neoplasia. *Nature* **339,** 58–61.
12. Folkman, J. (1995) Angiogenesis in cancer, vascular, rheumatoid and other disease. *Nat. Med.* **1,** 27–31.
13. Folkman, J. (1995) Angiogenesis inhibitors generated by tumors. *Mol. Med.* **1,** 120–122.
14. Goswami, S., Sahai, E., Wyckoff, J. B., et al. (2005) Macrophages promote the invasion of breast carcinoma cells via a colony-stimulating factor-1/epidermal growth factor paracrine loop. *Cancer Res.* **65,** 5278–5283.

15. Ingber, D. E. and Folkman, J. (1989) How does extracellular matrix control capillary morphogenesis? *Cell* **58**, 803–805.
16. James, S. L., Cook, K. W., and Lazdins, J. K. (1990) Activation of human monocyte-derived macrophages to kill schistosomula of Schistosoma mansoni in vitro. *J. Immunol.* **145**, 2686–2690.
17. Kacinski, B. M., Chambers, S. K., Stanley, E. R., et al. (1990) The cytokine CSF-1 (M-CSF) expressed by endometrial carcinomas in vivo and in vitro, may also be a circulating tumor marker of neoplastic disease activity in endometrial carcinoma patients. *Int. J. Radiat. Oncol. Biol. Phys.* **19**, 619–626.
18. Kascinski, B. (2002) Expression of CSF-1 and its receptor CSF-1R in nonhematopoietic neoplasms. *Cancer Treat. Res.* **107**, 285–292.
19. Lidor, Y. J., Xu, F. J., Martinez-Maza, O., et al. (1993) Constitutive production of macrophage colony-stimulating factor and interleukin-6 by human ovarian surface epithelial cells. *Exp. Cell. Res.* **207**, 332–339.
20. Lin, E. Y., Nguyen, A. V., Russell, R. G., and Pollard, J. W. (2001) Colony-stimulating factor 1 promotes progression of mammary tumors to malignancy. *J. Exp. Med.* **193**, 727–740.
21. Lin, E. Y., Gouon-Evans, V., Nguyen, A. V., and Pollard, J. W. (2002) The macrophage growth factor CSF-1 in mammary gland development and tumor progression. *J. Mammary Gland. Biol. Neoplasia.* **7**, 147–162.
22. Liotta, L. A., Steeg, P. S., and Stetler-Stevenson, W. G. (1991) Cancer metastasis and angiogenesis: an imbalance of positive and negative regulation. *Cell* **64**, 327–336.
23. Liotta, L. A. and Kohn, E. C. (2001) The microenvironment of the tumour-host interface. *Nature* **411**, 375–379.
24. Lopez, M., Martinache, C., Canepa, S., Chokri, M., Scotto, F., and Bartholeyns, J. (1993) Autologous lymphocytes prevent the death of monocytes in culture and promote, as do GM-CSF, IL-3 and M-CSF, their differentiation into macrophages. *J. Immunol. Methods* **159**, 29–38.
25. Mantovani, A., Bottazzi, B., Colotta, F., Sozzani, S., and Ruco, L. (1992) The origin and function of tumor-associated macrophages. *Immunol. Today* **13**, 265–270.
26. Nowicki, A., Szenajch, J., Ostrowska, G., et al. (1996) Impaired tumor growth in colony-stimulating factor 1 (CSF-1)-deficient, macrophage-deficient op/op mouse: evidence for a role of CSF-1-dependent macrophages in formation of tumor stroma. *Int. J. Cancer* **65**, 112–119.
27. Pei, X. H., Nakanishi, Y., Takayama, K., Bai, F., and Hara, N. (1999) Granulocyte, granulocyte-macrophage, and macrophage colony-stimulating factors can stimulate the invasive capacity of human lung cancer cells. *Br. J. Cancer* **79**, 40–46.
28. Pixley, F. J. and Stanley, E. R. (2004) CSF-1 regulation of the wandering macrophage: complexity in action. *Trends Cell Biol.* **14**, 628–638.
29. Pollard, J. W. (2004) Tumour-educated macrophages promote tumour progression and metastasis. *Nat. Rev. Cancer* **4**, 71–78.

30. Polverini, P. J., Cotran, P. S., Gimbrone, M. A., Jr., and Unanue, E. R. (1977) Activated macrophages induce vascular proliferation. *Nature* **269,** 804–806.
31. Roth, P. and Stanley, E. R. (1992) The biology of CSF-1 and its receptor. *Curr. Top. Microbiol. Immunol.* **181,** 141–167.
32. Russo, J. and Russo, I. H. (2001) The pathway of neoplastic transformation of human breast epithelial cells. *Radiat. Res.* **155,** 151–154.
33. Scholl, S. M., Pallud, C., Beuvon, F., et al. (1994) Anti-colony-stimulating factor-1 antibody staining in primary breast adenocarcinomas correlates with marked inflammatory cell infiltrates and prognosis. *J. Natl. Cancer Inst.* **86,** 120–126.
34. Sherr, C. J., Rettenmier, C. W., Sacca, R., Roussel, M. F., Look, A. T., and Stanley, E. R. (1985) The c-fms proto-oncogene product is related to the receptor for the mononuclear phagocyte growth factor, CSF-1. *Cell* **41,** 665–676.
35. Sioud, M. (2004) Therapeutic siRNAs. *Trends Pharmacol. Sci.* **25,** 22–28.
36. Stanley, E. (1992) Interleukins, in *Human Cytokines,* (Aggarwal, B. and Gutterman, J., eds.), Blackwell, Boston, MA, pp. 196–220.
37. Nowicki A, Szenajch J, Ostrowska G, et al. (1996). Impaired tumor growth in colony-stimulating factor 1 (CSF-1)-deficient, macrophage-deficient op/op mouse: evidence for a role of CSF-1-dependent macrophages in formation of tumor stroma. *Int J. Cancer.* **65,** 112–119.
38. Stein, C. A. (2001) The experimental use of antisense oligonucleotides: a guide for the perplexed. *J. Clin. Invest.* **108,** 641–644.
39. Stetler-Stevenson, W. G. and Yu, A. E. (2001) Proteases in invasion: matrix metalloproteinases. *Semin. Cancer Biol.* **11,** 143–152.
40. Sunderkotter, C., Goebeler, M., Schulze-Osthoff, K., Bhardwaj, R., and Sorg, C. (1991) Macrophage-derived angiogenesis factors. *Pharmacol. Ther.* **51,** 195–216.
41. Sunderkotter, C., Steinbrink, K., Goebeler, M., Bhardwaj, R., and Sorg, C. (1994) Macrophages and angiogenesis. *J. Leukoc. Biol.* **55,** 410–422.
42. Suzuki, M., Ohwada, M., Aida, I., Tamada, T., Hanamura, T., and Nagatomo, M. (1993) Macrophage colony-stimulating factor as a tumor marker for epithelial ovarian cancer. *Obstet. Gynecol.* **82,** 946–950.
43. Suzuki, M., Kobayashi, H., Ohwada, M., Terao, T., and Sato, I. (1998) Macrophage colony-stimulating factor as a marker for malignant germ cell tumors of the ovary. *Gynecol. Oncol.* **68,** 35–37.
44. Weidner, N., Semple, J. P., Welch, W. R., and Folkman, J. (1991) Tumor angiogenesis and metastasis—correlation in invasive breast carcinoma. *N. Engl. J. Med.* **324,** 1–8.
45. Weidner, N., Carroll, P. R., Flax, J., Blumenfeld, W., and Folkman, J. (1993) Tumor angiogenesis correlates with metastasis in invasive prostate carcinoma. *Am. J. Pathol.* **143,** 401–409.
46. Weinberg, R. A. (1989) Oncogenes, antioncogenes, and the molecular bases of multistep carcinogenesis. *Cancer Res.* **49,** 3713–3721.
47. Werb, Z., Banda, M. J., and Jones, P. A. (1980) Degradation of connective tissue matrices by macrophages. I. Proteolysis of elastin, glycoproteins, and collagen by proteinases isolated from macrophages. *J. Exp. Med.* **152,** 1340–1357.

48. Yeung, Y. G. and Stanley, E. R. (2003) Proteomic approaches to the analysis of early events in colony-stimulating factor-1 signal transduction. *Mol. Cell. Proteomics* **2,** 1143–1155.

49. Yoshida, H., Hayashi, S., Kunisada, T., et al. (1990) The murine mutation osteopetrosis is in the coding region of the macrophage colony stimulating factor gene. *Nature* **345,** 442–444.

12

Validation of Telomerase and Survivin as Anticancer Therapeutic Targets Using Ribozymes and Small-Interfering RNAs

Nadia Zaffaroni, Marzia Pennati, and Marco Folini

Summary

In recent years expanding knowledge about basic biology and a detailed understanding of the molecular pathways involved in tumor cell growth and progression have allowed the identification of numerous genes as potential therapeutic targets. Studies in which the expression of these genes was manipulated by antisense strategies have provided clues as to how we can intervene to specifically kill tumor cells or sensitize them to conventional chemical and physical antitumor therapies. Such tumor specificity can only be obtained by exploiting a basic difference between normal and malignant cells. In this context, targeting cytoprotective factors such as telomerase and survivin is particularly attractive because of their almost selective expression in tumor cells and their proven association with disease progression. This chapter summarizes the results obtained with ribozymes and small-interfering RNAs in the functional validation of these two targets in cell cultures and animal tumor models.

Key Words: Human cancer; ribozyme; survivin; siRNA; telomerase.

1. Introduction

1.1. Telomerase

During the past decade we have seen fundamental changes in the approaches used by researchers to identify and validate therapeutic targets (1–3). Human telomeres are specialized DNA-protein structures that cap the ends of linear chromosomes and are essential for the maintenance of genome integrity. Specifically, telomeres prevent the ends of linear chromosomes from being recognized as double-strand breaks, protect chromosomes from end-to-end fusion and degradation, and contribute to the organization of chromosomes during cell

From: *Methods in Molecular Biology, vol. 361, Target Discovery and Validation Reviews and Protocols*
Volume 2, Emerging Molecular Targets and Treatment Options
Edited by: M. Sioud © Humana Press Inc., Totowa, NJ

division *(4)*. Telomeres consist of double-stranded DNA tandem repeats $(T_2AG_3)_n$ that terminate with a 3'-single-strand overhang, which folds back onto duplex telomeric DNA, generating a T-loop structure *(4)*. In addition to the repeated sequences, several DNA-binding proteins regulate telomere structure *(5)*. Specifically, the telomeric repeat-binding factor 1 (TRF1), which interacts with double-stranded DNA, plays an important role in the negative regulation of telomere length; the related protein TRF2 is essential for the protection of telomere integrity by maintaining the T-loop *(6)* and preventing the T-loop insertion site from being recognized as an intermediate for the homologous recombination *(7)*. In addition, TRF2 plays a pivotal role in preventing nonhomologous end joining as demonstrated by the occurrence of telomeric fusion in cells expressing a TRF2 dominant-negative mutant *(8)*. Several other proteins bind to telomeric DNA via TRF1 and TRF2: the polyadenosine diphosphate ribosylase tankyrase and the TRF1-interacting nuclear protein 2 (Tin2) contribute to regulate TRF1 functions, whereas Rap1 and the Mre11 complex, which are involved in the control of telomere length and in the cellular response to DNA-damaging agents, interact with TRF2 *(6,7)*. The human telomere-binding protein 1 (hPOT1), which binds single-stranded DNA, has been recently identified *(9)*. The exact role of this protein in telomere dynamics is far from being completely understood *(10)*. A possible role as a negative regulator of telomerase for hPOT1 via its interaction with the TRF1 complex has been proposed. Conversely, other authors suggest that the protein acts as a telomerase-dependent positive regulator of telomere length because its forced expression in telomerase-positive human cell line lengthened telomeres, whereas hPOT1 was unable to lengthen telomeres in a telomerase-negative cell line *(11)*.

Telomeres act as a mitotic clock by which cells count divisions *(12)*. During each round of cellular replication, telomeres undergo sequence loss as a consequence of the incomplete DNA lagging-strand replication (the "end replication problem") *(13)*, which results in critically short telomeres that lead to replicative senescence and ultimately cell death. To compensate for telomere attrition, different mechanisms have evolved to maintain telomere homeostasis, and they seem to play a pivotal role for the development of human malignancies.

Telomere maintenance is mainly performed in human cells by telomerase *(14)*. The main core of telomerase consists of two subunits: a catalytic subunit, the human telomerase reverse transcriptase (hTERT) *(15)*, and the human telomerase RNA component (hTR) *(16)*. The *hTR* gene is located on chromosome 3 and encodes for the telomerase RNA component, which consists of a 451-nt-long RNA. hTR bears a sequence located at its 5'-end, which is exploited as a template for the addition of telomeric repeats at the 3'-terminus of the linear chromosomes during the enzyme's catalytic cycle. The human telomerase RNA component is consistently expressed in almost all human tissues and, for this reason, does not represent a limiting factor for telomerase activity but is essential for the enzyme's catalytic activity through its association with the catalytic subunit *(14)*.

The catalytic subunit of human telomerase hTERT is a 127-kDa protein comprising a specific telomerase domain (T-motif) and shares structural and functional properties with reverse transcriptases. It is encoded by a 37-kb-long gene located on chromosome 5 and composed of 16 exons and 15 introns. The catalytic component of telomerase is typically expressed in telomerase-positive tumor tissues and in those normal cells that transiently acquire telomerase activity. Such evidence has suggested that hTERT is the limiting factor for the restoration of telomerase activity and its expression is strictly regulated at multiple levels *(14)*. In fact, the *hTERT* gene undergoes transcriptional regulation that is mediated by different transcription factors. The hTERT pre-mRNA is posttranscriptionally modified by alternative splicing, a process which generates different hTERT transcripts with opposite functions. Specifically, the α-variant (which lacks conserved residues from the catalytic core of the protein) acts as a dominant negative *(17)*. In addition, the activity of the hTERT protein is regulated by different posttranslational mechanisms such as the assembly of telomerase in a large complex holoenzyme mediated by Hsp90 and p23 *(14)*. The hTERT protein undergoes cellular relocalization from the cytoplasm to the nucleus (a process presumably mediated by the 14-3-3 protein) and can be sequestered in a form of enzymatically inactive complex into the nucleolus through its interaction with PinX1 *(18)*. The activity of hTERT is also regulated through phosphorylation/dephosphorylation of specific amino acid residues, catalyzed by protein kinases (e.g., PKC, Akt, and c-Abl tyrosine kinase) and protein phosphatase 2A *(14)*.

The reactivation of telomerase is involved in the attainment of immortality in cancer cells and therefore may contribute to tumorigenesis and neoplastic progression *(19)*. Several lines of evidence indicate that telomerase is present in 85–90% of human cancers *(20)* but is generally absent in somatic cells, with a few exceptions (i.e., germ line cells, embryonic stem cells, activated lymphocytes, endometrial tissue during the menstrual cycle, and cells from the basal layer of the epidermis). Because telomerase reactivation has been identified as one of the six hallmarks of cancer *(21)* due to its ability to provide cancer cells with an unlimited proliferative potential and owing to its specific expression in cancer tissues, approaches aimed to inhibit the enzyme's catalytic activity in tumor cells could represent promising and innovative anticancer therapies *(22)*. Furthermore, recent evidence has suggested that telomerase reactivation contributes to tumorigenesis by means of mechanisms other than the enzyme's catalytic activity. Specifically, it has been proposed that the hTERT serves as a physical "cap" for the telomere that can shift from a capped to an uncapped state *(23)*. The appropriate response to uncapped telomeres is action by telomerase, which protects the telomere from signaling into cell-cycle arrest or apoptosis pathways *(23)*. Additional novel functions of telomerase, which are distinct from its telomere-maintenance activity and might have potentially important consequences in tumor cells, are related to the ability of hTERT to cross-link telomere and enhance genomic stability and DNA repair *(24)*. Moreover, it has been suggested that hTERT is involved in the maintenance of cell survival and proliferation via enzymatic activity-independent intermolecular interactions involving p53 and poly(ADP-ribose) polymerase *(25)*. The evolving understanding of telomerase composition and functions and of its interaction with telomeres is expected to contribute to improve the knowledge of the tumorigenisis process and has prompted the formulation of distinct rationales for the development of enzyme inhibitors *(22)*. Telomerase inhibitors include antisense oligonucleotides that target hTR or hTERT mRNA *(22)*, traditional reverse transcriptase inhibitors, and agents able to promote and/or stabilize high-order DNA tetraplex (G-quartet) formation in telomeres *(26)*.

1.2. Survivin

Survivin is a member of the inhibitor of apoptosis (IAP) gene family, which is positioned at the interface between mitotic progression and apoptosis inibition *(27)*.

The human *survivin* gene spans 14.7 kb on the telomeric position of chromosome 17 and is localized to band q25 *(28)*. It comprises three introns and four exons, a TATA-less proximal promoter, and approx 200-nt GC-rich regions upstream of exon 1 *(29)*. The gene encodes a 16.5-kD protein of 142 amino acids. Structurally, it is composed of a single baculovirus IAP repeat domain and an extended COOH-terminal α-helical coiled-coil domain *(30)*. Moreover, it does not contain a RING-finger domain, found in other IAPs. Splicing variants of survivin have been identified. Survivin-2B is generated by insertion of an alternative exon, survivin-ΔEx3 arises from the removal of the exon 3, and survivin-3B results from the introduction of a novel exon 3B *(31,32)*. Very recently, an additional splice variant, survivin 2α, has been identified. Structurally, the transcript consists of two exons: exon 1 and exon 2, as well as a 3' 197-bp region of intron 2. Acquisition of a new in-frame stop codon within intron 2 results in an open reading frame of 225 nt, predicting a truncated 74-amino acid protein *(33)*. Little is known about the differential functions of survivin alternative splice forms. However, preliminary data would suggest that heterodimerization of survivin with survivin-ΔEx3 is essential for the inhibition of mitochondrial-dependent apoptosis *(34)*. Moreover, it has been demonstrated in exogenous expression assays that survivin 2α attenuates the antiapoptotic activity of survivin *(33)*.

Survivin is regulated in a highly cell cycle-dependent manner, with a marked increase in the G_2/M phase *(35)*. During this phase, survivin associates with and is phosphorylated by p34^{cdc2}/cyclin B1 kinase *(36)*. It has been demonstrated that survivin exists in two immunohistochemically distinct pools, with a nuclear pool localized to kinetochores of metaphase chromosomes and to the central spindle midzone at anaphase, and a cytosolic pool associated with interphase microtubules, centrosomes, spindle poles, and mitotic spindle microtubules at metaphase and anaphase *(37)*. However, the microtubule-associated pool appears to be quantitatively predominant and functionally relevant. These findings, together with the phenotype of knockout mice (which is characterized by a catastrophic defect of microtubule assembly, with absence of mitotic spindle, formation of multinucleated cells and 100% embryonic lethality *[38]*), are consistent with a critical role of survivin in mitosis to preserve the mitotic apparatus and to allow normal mitotic progression. In fact, it has been demonstrated that survivin downregulation causes pleiotropic cell-division defects *(39,40)*. Moreover, Giodini et al. *(41)* showed that forced expression of survivin in HeLa epithelial carcinoma cells profoundly influenced microtubule dynamics and also caused stabilization of microtubules against nocodazole-induced depolymerization, thus indicating that survivin may facilitate evasion from checkpoint mechanisms of growth arrest and, consequently, promote resistance to drugs targeting the mitotic spindle. Additional evidence indicates that survivin also participates in the regulation of chromosome segregation *(42)*, and that the protein cooperates together with the chromosomal passenger proteins INCENP and Aurora-B to perform its mitotic duties *(43)*. The existence of a mitochondrial pool of survivin, which is able to orchestrate a novel pathway of apoptosis inhibition in tumor cells, has been recently reported *(44)*. Specifically, it was found that, in response to cell death stimulation, mitochondrial survivin is rapidly discharged in the cytosol, where it prevents caspase activation and inhibits apoptosis.

It has been demonstrated that Hsp90, a molecular chaperone that is the central regulator of cellular stress response, associates with survivin. Such a physical interaction, which involves the Hsp90 ATPase domain and the survivin baculovirus IAP repeat domain, is required for survivin stability and function. In fact, targeted antibody-mediated disruption of the survivin-Hsp90 complex in cancer cells resulted in proteasomal degradation of survivin *(45)*.

In regard to the precise role of survivin in cell death, at present it is still controversial whether this protein inhibits caspases through direct binding, as other IAPs do, or indirectly, requiring intermediate proteins. In this context, a possible direct interaction of survivin with caspase-9 has been reported by O'Connor et al. *(46)* whereas more recently Song et al. *(47)* suggested an alternative model for indirect inhibition of caspases by survivin, which requires Smac/Diablo as intermediate protein. This mitochondrial factor, that is released into the cytosol in response to different apoptotic stimuli, was found to bind to some IAPs (including XIAP, cIAP$_1$, cIAP$_2$, and livin), thus preventing them from inhibiting caspases (48). The ability of survivin to physically interact with Smac/Diablo and, as a consequence, sequester it would allow other IAPs to block caspases without being antagonized.

Survivin is strongly expressed in embryonic and fetal organs but not in differentiated normal tissues with the exception of thymus, basal colonic epithelium (49) endothelial cells, and neural stem cells during angiogenesis (50). Several reports have demonstrated survivin expression in the majority of human tumor types including lung, breast, colon, gastric, oesophageal, pancreatic, liver, bladder, uterine, and ovarian cancers, large-cell non-Hodgkin's lymphomas, leukemias, neuroblastoma, brain tumors, pheochromocytoma, soft-tissue sarcomas, melanomas, and other skin cancers (49). Moreover, the expression of survivin has been also detected in a variety of preneoplastic and/or benign lesions including polyps of the colon, breast adenomas, Bowen's disease, and hypertrophic actinic keratosis (49), suggesting that reexpression of survivin may occur early during malignant transformation or following disturbance in the balance between cell proliferation and death. The upregulation of survivin at the transcriptional level in human tumors has been confirmed in genome-wide searches, which indicated survivin as the fourth top "transcriptome" in cancers of various histology (51). At least for some tumor types, molecular abnormalities have been described that may account for the increased expression of survivin in cancer compared to normal tissue. Specifically, in neuroblastoma a gain of 17q25 containing the survivin locus represents a frequent genetic abnormality (52). Moreover, in most ovarian cancers survivin exon 1, which is silenced by methylation in normal ovarian epithelium, becomes unmethylated and, consequently, transcriptionally active (53). Survivin overexpression in tumors has been recently linked to the loss of wild-type p53 (54). Specifically, it was seen that accumulation of wild-type p53 in human ovarian cancer cells induced survivin transcriptional repression, which did not require direct sequence-specific DNA binding of p53 to the survivin promoter. Modifications of chromatin structure within the promoter could be the molecular explanation for silencing of the survivin gene by wild-type p53.

In the majority of tumors investigated for survivin expression (including breast, lung, colorectal, gastric, liver, bladder, and kidney cancers, neuroblastoma, gliomas, soft tissue sarcomas, leukemias, and lymphomas), high levels of the protein were predictive of tumor progression, either in terms of disease-free survival or overall survival, thus providing prognostically relevant informations (49). In several neoplasms, the association with tumor progression has been also corroborated in the context of comprehensive analysis of gene-expression profiling by DNA microarray or PCR-based assays.

Considering that apoptosis is the primary mode of cell death induced by several classes of anticancer agents and ionizing radiation, a possible general role of survivin in determining the chemo- and radio-sensitivity profiles of tumor cells has been hypothesised. Moreover, because survivin is associated with microtubules and with the mitotic spindle it is likely that this protein can specifically contribute to the response of cells to microtubule-interacting agents. Li et al. *(55)* first demonstrated that transfection of wild-type survivin efficiently protected murine NIH3T3 fibroblasts from apoptosis induced by the microtubule-stabilizing agent taxol. In agreement with this observation, Giodini et al. *(41)* reported that infection of HeLa cells with an adenoviral vector expressing survivin suppressed apoptosis induced by taxol. Based on this finding, our laboratory performed a parallel investigation on cell lines and clinical specimens from ovarian carcinomas to determine whether survivin is involved in regulating cell sensitivity to taxanes. The OAW42 and IGROV-1 human ovarian cancer cell lines were transfected with the human survivin cDNA. Stable transfection with survivin cDNA was able to protect these cells from the cytotoxic effects induced by taxol and taxotere *(56)*. In the clinical setting, when we analyzed the response of advanced ovarian cancer patients to a taxol/platinum-based regimen as a function of survivin expression, we found a significantly higher clinical or pathologic response rate in cases with absent/low protein expression than in those expressing high levels of survivin *(56)*.

Regarding the possible role of survivin in determining the radiation response of human tumor cells, Asanuma et al. *(57)* reported that survivin acts as a constitutive radio-resistance factor in pancreatic cancer cells. Specifically, in a panel of established cell lines they found an inverse relationship between survivin mRNA expression and in vitro sensitivity to X-irradiation. Moreover, these authors also demonstrated that survivin mRNA expression was increased by sublethal doses of X-irradiation, which would suggest that the protein also acts as an inducible radio-resistance factor.

Very recently, Zhang et al. *(58)* showed that survivin mediates resistance to antiandrogen therapy with flutamide in prostate cancer cells. Specifically, these authors suggested that upregulation of survivin via insulin-like growth factor-1/AKT signaling during androgen blockade may be one of the mechanisms by which prostate cancer cells develop resistance to antiandrogens.

Overall, the results obtained in the different studies indicate survivin to be a cellular factor potentially involved in the chemo- and radio-resistant phenotypes of human tumors cells and suggest that approaches designed to inhibit survivin expression may lead to human tumor sensitization to chemical and physical agents. In recent years, considerable efforts have been made by researchers to develop strategies for modulating apoptosis in cancer and other human diseases *(59,60)*. In this context, approaches to counteract survivin in tumor cells have been proposed with the dual aim to inhibit tumor growth through an increase of spontaneous apoptosis, and to enhance tumor cell response to apoptosis-inducing agents *(61)*. Different kinds of survivin molecular inhibitors, including antisense oligonucleotides, dominant negative mutants, and cyclin-dependent kinase inhibitors have been used.

2. Hammerhead Ribozymes

Ribozymes are small RNA molecules that possess specific endonucleolytic activity and catalyze the hydrolysis of phosphodiester bonds, thereby leading to cleavage of RNA targets *(62)*. Naturally occurring ribozymes mediate sequence-specific RNA processing through Watson-Crick base pairing. Several catalytic domains derived from natural ribozymes have been identified, the most common of which are the hammerhead and hairpin structures *(63)*. Owing to their inherent simplicity and relatively small size, hammerhead ribozymes have received much attention in view of their potential therapeutic usefulness and ability to be incorporated into a variety of flanking sequence motifs without changing site-specific cleavage capacities. In fact, the hammerhead ribozyme consists of a 40-nt-long, highly conserved catalytic core, which cleaves substrate RNA at 5'-NHH-3' consensus sequence, where N is any nucleotide and H is any nucleotide but guanidine *(64)*. The catalytic potential of such a ribozyme can be exploited to cleave any NHH consensus sequence in a given RNA substrate by the addition of flanking arms bearing nucleotide sequences, which are complementary to the specific RNA target. Moreover, after the cleavage reaction, the substrate becomes more accessible to ribonucleases, which leads to its degradation. In addition to the catalytic activity, ribozymes possess binding capacity to the target RNA ("antisense effect") and can induce the RNase-mediated degradation of the target as a consequence of double stranded RNA formation. Because one of the major limitations to the therapeutic use of hammerhead ribozymes is the problem of their intracellular delivery different strategies have been developed. There are two main ways to deliver a ribozyme within cells. The exogenous delivery, which exploited presynthesized ribozymes that are introduced directly into the cells with the aid of conventional transfection agents, and the endogenous delivery by which the intracellular transcription of a ribozyme coding sequence is accomplished through transfection/infection of ribozyme-expressing vectors (e.g., plasmid or viruses). Using both approaches, several studies focused on experimental human tumor models have shown the possibility to obtain efficient ribozyme-mediated downregulation of cancer-associated genes *(64)*.

2.1. Ribozymes Targeting Telomerase

Telomerase is an exploitable target for strategies based on the use of antisense oligonucleotides. In fact, the template region of hTR, which naturally binds to the 3' single-strand overhang of the telomere end to add new telomeric repeats, is inherently accessible to incoming nucleic acids and represents a suitable target site for these approaches. A number of studies on experimental human tumor models have shown the possibility to obtain efficient inhibition of telomerase through the use of hammerhead ribozymes targeting hTR. The first developed hammerhead ribozyme was engineered to target a consensus sequence located at the end of the telomerase template *(65)*. When added to cell extracts from two hepatocellular carcinoma cell lines (HepG2 and Huh-7), the ribozyme induced dose-dependent inhibition of telomerase activity. The potential use of chemically stabilized hammerhead ribozymes to inhibit telomerase activity by cleaving the hTR component was also pursued. Specifically, hammerhead ribozymes containing 2'-*O*-methyl ribonucleotides for enhanced biologic stability and designed to be complementary to the RNA component of human telomerase exhibited dose-dependent inhibition of telomerase activity in human glioma cell lysates and induced the cleavage of the full-length hTR in intact U87-MG cells *(66)*.

The catalytic sequence described by Kanazawa et al. *(64)* was exploited in our laboratory to downregulate telomerase activity in intact human tumor cells. Specifically, the JR8 human melanoma cells were transfected with the ribozyme sequence inserted into a mammalian expression vector *(67)*. Ribozyme transfectants successfully expressing the ribozyme and characterized by reduced telomerase activity and a decreased level of telomerase RNA expression compared with mock transfectants were selected. Ribozyme-expressing clones grew more slowly than parental cells and also expressed an altered morphology with a dendritic appearance in monolayer cultures. A small but significant fraction of the cell population also expressed an apoptotic phenotype. However, no telomere shortening was observed in these clones even after a prolonged period (50 d) of growth in culture *(67)*.

In a further study, three hammerhead ribozymes targeting GUC sequences from the 5'-end of telomerase RNA were described *(68)*. In a cell-free system, all the ribozymes efficiently cleaved the RNA substrate. However, when the ribozymes were introduced into intact endometrial carcinoma Ishikawa cells, only the ribozyme targeting the template region was able to attenuate telomerase activity. The ribozyme sequence was then inserted into an expression vector subsequently used to transfect the endometrial carcinoma cell line AN3CA. Ribozyme-expressing clones obtained after in vitro selection showed reduced telomerase activity and telomerase RNA expression. A marked reduction of telomere length was observed in some of these clones. However, even after 30 passages in vitro, these cells still maintained their ability to proliferate. To search for more potent ribozymes targeting telomerase, the same group recently reported the use of a divalent ribozyme (referred to as 36- to 59-divalent ribozyme) designed to cleave simultaneously the GUC triplet (which represents the most exploited target site in the template region of hTR) and the closest target sequence GUA, located 23 nt downstream from the GUC in the template region of hTR *(69)*. Data obtained by in vitro cleavage assay showed that the 36- to 59-divalent ribozyme cleaved telomerase RNA more efficiently than the related monovalent ribozymes (36- and 59-ribozyme). However, when the divalent ribozyme was introduced into Ishikawa endometrial carcinoma cells, its inhibitory effect on telomerase activity was less than that of the 36-ribozyme, whereas the 59-ribozyme did not show a significant activity on telomerase.

Recently, hammerhead ribozymes were designed against seven NHH sequences located in open loops of the hTR secondary structure and introduced through an expression vector into human breast tumor MCF-7 cells. Results showed that stable transfectants of ribozyme R1 targeting the template region of hTR induced the degradation of target and attenuated telomerase activity in breast cancer cells. Moreover, the ribozyme R1 transfectant displayed a significant telomere shortening and a lower proliferation rate than parental cells. Clones with reduced proliferation capacity showed enlarged senescence-like shapes and the occurrence of apoptotic cells was observed *(70)*.

Because the expression of hTERT is almost completely confined to tumor cells and its presence represents the rate-limiting step for telomerase activity, the antisense-mediated attenuation of hTERT mRNA expression would represent an excellent means to regulate the enzyme's activity in cancer cells *(14)*. However, hTERT is a more challenging target than hTR for antisense-based strategies. In fact, its mRNA possesses a complex secondary structure that makes it difficult to accurately predict which target site will be most accessible for hybridization. As a consequence, there are still few studies based on the use of antisense-mediated approaches to achieve telomerase inhibition through hTERT downregulation.

However, the possibility to downregulate telomerase activity by the use of hammerhead ribozymes that target the mRNA of hTERT has been exploited. Specifically, seven presynthesized ribozymes, directed against 5'-NHH-3' consensus sequences within the hTERT mRNA, were delivered into endometrial carcinoma cells by cationic lipids and demonstrated to significantly inhibit telomerase activity in intact cells *(71)*. However, a stable transfection of endometrial carcinoma cells carried out by cloning the ribozyme sequences into expression vectors confirmed the ability of only one ribozyme to suppress telomerase activity. In another study, Ludwig et al. *(72)* developed a hammerhead ribozyme directed against the consensus sequence within the T-motif of the hTERT mRNA that was able to attenuate telomerase activity in stable transfected clones of the immortal, telomerase-positive human breast epithelial cell line HBL-100 and the breast cancer cell line MCF-7. After a significant lag phase, in ribozyme-expressing clones the decline of the enzyme's catalytic activity resulted in telomere shortening, inhibition of cell proliferation, and induction of apoptosis. In addition, such clones demonstrated an increased susceptibility to topoisomerase II inhibitors such as doxorubicin, etoposide, and mitoxantrone. Successively, the same ribozyme sequence was transduced through an adenoviral vector into four ovarian cancer cell lines with widely different telomere lengths *(73)*. The authors observed massive cell loss in mass cultures from all cell lines tested 3 d after transduction.

2.2. Ribozymes Targeting Survivin

We first demonstrated the possibility to efficiently inhibit survivin expression through the use of ribozymes. Specifically, we designed two hammerhead ribozymes targeting the 3'-end of the CUA_{110} (RZ7) and the GUC_{294} (RZ1) triplets in the survivin mRNA and transfected them into the JR8 human melanoma cell line over expressing survivin. Stably transfected clones proven to endogenously express the active ribozyme RZ1 or RZ7 were characterized by a markedly lower survivin protein level than JR8 parental cells, whereas a negligible reduction of survivin expression was observed in cells expressing a mutant ribozyme (which was produced by introducing a mutation in the catalytic core of the active ribozyme RZ1). These cells demonstrated an increased caspase-9-dependent apoptotic response to cisplatin treatment *(74)*. JR8 cells expressing RZ1 also showed a significantly increased sensitivity to the topoisomerase-I inhibitor topotecan (as detected by clonogenic cell survival) as a consequence of an enhanced rate of drug-induced caspase-9-dependent apoptosis. Moreover, an increased antitumor activity of oral topotecan was observed in ribozyme-expressing JR8 cells grown as xenograft tumors in athymic nude mice *(75)*. JR8 cells endogenously expressing the active RZ7 ribozyme also showed significantly increased sensitivity to γ-irradiation *(76)*. More recently, we constructed a Moloney-based retroviral vector expressing the RZ7 ribozyme, encoded as a chimeric RNA within adenoviral VA1 RNA. Polyclonal cell populations, obtained by infection with the retroviral vector, of two androgen-independent human prostate cancer cell lines (DU145 and PC-3) were characterized by a significant reduction of survivin expression; the cells became polyploid, underwent caspase-9-dependent apoptosis, and showed an altered pattern of gene expression, as detected by oligonucleotide array analysis. Survivin inhibition also increased the susceptibility of these cells to cisplatin-induced apoptosis and prevented tumor formation when cells were xenografted into athymic nude mice *(77)*.

Choi et al. *(78)* recently showed that two hammerhead ribozymes, able to cleave the human survivin mRNA at nucleotide position +279 and +28 and cloned into a replication-deficient adenoviral vector, were able to increase the apoptotic response to etoposide in transduced MCF-7 breast cancer cells.

3. RNA Interference

RNA interference (RNAi) is a natural mechanism of sequence-specific, post-transcriptional gene silencing. RNAi may play an important role in protecting the genome against instability caused by transposons and repetitive sequences, and it represents an evolutionary conserved antiviral defense pathway in animals and plants *(79)*. Moreover, RNAi has emerged as a powerful mechanism for sequence-specific modulation of gene expression and seems to provide a higher potency than conventional antisense strategies, presumably because it relies on natural site-directed cleavage machinery *(79)*.

In mammalian cells RNAi can be triggered by several double-stranded RNAs (dsRNA) or dsRNA domain-containing molecules. Endogenously expressed dsRNA domains are converted into the nucleus by specific ribonucleases in the form of precursors that are successively processed in the cytoplasm to give rise to microRNAs (miRNAs). The miRNAs are believed to bind to sites that have partial sequence complementarity in the 3' untranslated region of their target mRNA, causing repression of translation and inhibition of protein synthesis *(80,81)*. By contrast, exogenously introduced dsRNA (e.g., viral genome) are processed in the cytoplasm by the endoribonuclease dicer into small duplex RNAs, the 21- to 23-nt-long terminal effectors molecule, known as small-interfering RNAs (siRNA), characterized by a 2- to 3-nt overhang at the 3'-terminus *(80,81)*. The resulting siRNAs are then assembled to form an RNA/protein complex, referred to as the RNA-induced silencing complex (RISC). The double-stranded siRNA is then unwound, leaving the antisense strand to guide RISC to its homologous target mRNA for endonucleolytic cleavage. The target mRNA is cleaved in the center of the duplex region arising from the annealing of the antisense strand of siRNA and the target mRNA, a process that ultimately results in the target degradation. To date, different effectors molecules have been identified as inductors of gene expression silencing in mammalian cells through the activation of the RNAi pathway. Specifically, short-hairpin RNAs (shRNAs) are transcribed from plasmid- or viral-based vectors as a pre-siRNA in which the sense and antisense strands are linked by a short spacer. The pre-siRNA is then predicted to form a 19-nt-long stem-loop structure, the terminal effectors shRNA. shRNAs are usually coded downstream of an RNA polymerase III promoter (e.g., U6 small nucleolar RNA or human RNase H1 promoters) although the use of inducible or tissue-specific RNA polymerase II promoters has been described *(80,81)*. By contrast, presynthesized siRNA are RNA duplexes formed by two complementary single strands. In this case, a siRNA may be obtained by the annealing of two in vitro transcribed 21-nt-long single strands leaving two nucleotides unpaired at the 3' terminus *(80,81)* or as preformed duplexes, usually provided by specialized companies. Presynthesized siRNAs are delivered to cells by conventional transfection approaches *(80,81)*. To date, the siRNA technology has been validated in several mammalian experimental models but its therapeutic usefulness for human diseases is still under intensive investigation. In fact, although the effect of siRNAs on gene expression has been demonstrated to be rapid and persistent (days/weeks), the main limitation to be overcome before such technology will be exploited in the clinical practice is represented by the selectivity for the target RNA, delivery and stability inside cells, similarly to ribozyme- and antisense-based approaches.

3.1. Telomerase Silencing Through RNAi

Kosciolek et al. *(82)* first described the exploitation of siRNAs as telomerase inhibitors. Two types of RNA molecules targeted to the hTR and hTERT components of human telomerase were developed: chemically synthesized siRNAs and a long dsRNA expressed in the target cells as a hairpin construct. The ability of chemically synthesized siRNAs to inhibit telomerase activity was assessed in a panel of human cancer cell lines. Results showed that the siRNA targeting the hTR component was more effective in inducing inhibition of the enzyme's catalytic activity than that designed to target the catalytic component hTERT. The antitelomerase effect was concentration-dependent and relied on the transfection schedule. Furthermore, transfectant clones expressing the siRNA construct directed against the hTR subunit were characterized by a marked inhibition of the enzyme's catalytic activity, the downregulation of the hTR RNA expression levels and a reduction of telomeric DNA content. Unfortunately, the authors did not attempt to analyze the effects of specific telomerase inhibition on tumor cell proliferative potential.

It has been recently reported that a shRNA, expressed from a lentiviral vector and targeting the sequence encompassing the 11-nt template region of hTR, quickly inhibited the growth of p53-wild type, p53-null HCT116 colon cancer cells and LOX melanoma cells, independently of p53 status or telomere length, and without bulk telomere shortening. By contrast, no effect was detected in the immortalized, telomerase-negative VA13 cell line. Moreover, hTR downregulation did not cause telomere uncapping in these experimental models, but induced a modulation of the global gene expression profile, including suppression of specific genes implicated in angiogenesis and metastasis. This finding could be indicative of a novel response pathway distinct from the expression profile changes previously reported by the same authors and induced by telomere-uncapping mutant-template telomerase RNAs *(83)*.

3.2. Survivin Silencing Through RNAi

Carvalho et al. *(43)* first used RNAi to specifically repress survivin in HeLa cells. These authors showed that survivin was no longer detectable in cultures a few days after transfection with specific siRNA and that survivin-depleted cells were delayed in mitosis and accumulated in prometaphase with mis-aligned chromosomes. In this model, loss of survivin activated the mitotic checkpoint, which was mediated by induction of p53 and was associated with the increase of its downstream target, p21^{Waf1}. Survivin ablation also caused loss of mitochondrial membrane potential, enhanced caspase-9 proteolytic activation and spontaneous apoptosis *(43)*. More recently, survivin downregulation, accomplished through the use of siRNAs, was seen to reduce clonogenic potential and increase the percentage of multinucleated cells in a panel of human sarcoma cell lines independently of p53 gene status *(84)*. Moreover, survivin knockdown caused radio-sensitization, which was paralleled by an increased activity of caspase-3 and caspase-7, in wild-type-p53 but not in mutant-p53 sarcoma cells *(85)*. An enhanced apoptotic response to APO2L/TRAIL treatment was also observed in melanoma and renal carcinoma cell lines transfected with survivin-specific siRNAs *(86)*. Finally, Coma et al. *(87)* recently demonstrated that transfection of endothelial cells with survivin specific siRNAs induced a marked increase in the apoptotic rate, a dose-dependent inhibition of their migration on vitronectin and a decrease in capillary formation.

To prevent nonphysiological responses associated with persistent suppression of a gene that is essential for cell survival and cell cycle progression such as survivin, systems allowing an inducible regulation of RNAi have been developed. Coumoul et al. *(88)* recently demonstrated that inducible suppression of survivin was efficiently achieved in ES cells by regulating RNAi using a *Cre-Lox*P approach, as indicated by the decrease level of gene expression and reduced proliferative potential.

4. Comparison of Technologies

The new wave of interest in the antisense field arises from the discovery that dsRNAs can induce a potent targeted degradation of complementary RNA sequences, a process referred to RNAi, and that the effectors components of the RNAi pathway (siRNAs or shRNAs) can be chemically synthesized or expressed from plasmid/viral vectors, similarly to ribozymes *(79)*. There is a widely diffused opinion that RNAi provides a powerful tool for targeted inhibition of gene expression, with respect to conventional antisense strategies (i.e., ribozymes), presumably because it relies on a natural process. Despite the unique assumed potential of RNAi, limitations in the use of such an approach, such as the possibility that some mammalian cells may not be susceptible to RNAi, have been described. However, it is possible to identify many factors that most likely influence the biological efficacy of ribozymes and siRNAs *(89)*. The use of synthetic or expressed ribozymes/siRNAs to induce gene knockdown in mammalian cells requires the consideration of several common issues. To provide effectors molecules with both selectivity and specificity for the target sequence, nontarget sequence homologies of ribozyme or both strands of a siRNA must be avoided. Moreover, thermodynamic parameters that can influence the catalytic cycle of a ribozyme and the efficiency with which siRNA is unwound and assembled into RISC complex need to be carefully determined. In addition, sequence constraints allowing the expression of ribozymes and shRNAs, from plasmid or viral vectors, that could influence the efficiency with which they are folded into an effective molecule should be taken into account *(90)*. Finally, the presence of a suitable target site in a given RNA represents a major determinant for the biological activity of both molecules. A significant obstruction of gene knockdown mediated by ribozymes and siRNA arises from structural features of the substrate RNA. In fact, a direct correlation between the extent of gene downregulation and the local free energy in the RNA target regions has been described *(91)*. To this purpose, the selection of accessible target sites can be made by a systematic testing of a large number of oligomers (i.e., RNase H mapping) or, alternatively, by means of specific bioinformatics tools based on thermodynamic algorithms *(79)*. As a consequence, a systemic structural analysis of local RNA target regions can significantly improve the design of biologically active molecules *(92)*.

Cellular uptake and colocalization to the specific target site within cells represent another main hurdle that has to be overcome for an efficient therapeutic inhibition of gene expression and the exploitation of ribozymes and siRNAs in clinical trials. To date, there are still no means to improve colocalization to the target site and to increase the efficacy of siRNAs in the presence of hardly accessible target RNA. As a consequence, the siRNA delivery is usually achieved by employing conventional methods such as cationic-lipid formulations, electroporation, or conjugation to peptides *(80,81,90)*. In contrast, a number of specific strategies have been demonstrated to be effective in inducing a sequence-directed colocalization of ribozymes and to improve their efficacy at the target site *(93)*.

Data reported in the literature have demonstrated that RNAi is a process that occurs in the cytoplasm. In contrast, ribozymes can act not only against cytoplasmic mRNAs but can also be exploited to target sequences localized in the nucleus (i.e., introns). This characteristic has been applied for the RNA repair, a process based on a transsplicing version of group I ribozymes, which demonstrated to be effective in inducing the repair of mutant transcripts such as sickle β-globin, p53, and mutant RNAs associated to myotonic muscular dystrophy *(89,94)*.

The introduction of chemical modifications aimed to improve the half-life of chemically synthesized ribozymes and siRNAs makes these molecules useful for short-term experiments. In particular, modifications made at the 2' position of specific ribose residues or the introduction of inverted thymidine at the 3'-terminus can stabilize ribozymes without affecting their biological activities.

Recently, the use of phosphorothioate backbone for siRNA has shown to increase their toxicity and to reduce the silencing activity. As a consequence, alternative backbone and nucleotide modifications have been pursued, such as the introduction of boranophosphate or the incorporation of few locked nucleic acid modifications. Alternatively, the stability and delivery of siRNAs have also been improved by complexing them with polyethyleneimmine or cholesterol. Other chemical modifications, aimed to improve the stability of siRNA and to reduce the ability to induce non specific effects without affecting their biological functions, have been developed by different companies, such as the Stealth siRNAs (Invitrogen, San Giuliano Milanese, Italy) or siSATBLE siRNAs, recently developed by researchers from Dharmacon Inc. (Lafayette, CO) *(22)*.

Ribozymes as well as siRNAs can lead to nonsequence-specific effects (off-target effects) that are strongly dependent on the concentration of oligomers. However, it should be stressed that the double-stranded siRNAs may result in two single-stranded oligomers, which yield more pronounced off-target effects than those obtained with an equal molar amount of ribozymes *(89)*. Furthermore, it has been reported that ribozymes are much more sensitive to polymorphisms at the cleavage site level *(89)*. This phenomenon can contribute to reduce the possibility of ribozyme-mediated off-target effects with respect to siRNAs. Although in a large number of studies reported thus far siRNAs have been shown to be effective in a broad range of experimental models, they can be potent inducers of stress-response pathways. Such a phenomenon that could depend on the different cellular environments would compromise the efficacy of the siRNA-mediated gene silencing. In fact, it has been demonstrated that antiluciferase siRNAs were highly effective at inhibiting luciferase activity when transfected into HeLa cells, but the presence of siRNA in PC-3 prostate cancer cells led to strong nonspecific effects, as shown by the significant downregulation of luciferase expression in the presence of a scramble siRNA *(95)*. Moreover, transfection of siRNAs can result in a global upregulation of interferon-stimulated genes as well as the activation of genes independent of an interferon response, such as the interferon-regulatory factor 3 *(96,97)*. In this regard, mammalian cells display a number of nonsequence-specific responses triggered by dsRNAs, such as those involved in viral host defense *(98)*. The effectors of such a pathway are mainly represented by the dsRNA-dependent protein-kinase PKR and 2'-5' oligoadenilate synthetase, whose activation is dependent on the size and concentration of dsRNA. Although siRNAs were initially thought to be too short to induce dsRNA-initiated response, it is becoming evident that nonspecific effects are consistent for a wide range of chemically synthesized siRNA *(96)*. Moreover, it is possible that dsRNA-response pathways are not only activated by siRNA, but may also mediate the specific gene-silencing effects of RNAi, that ultimately result in nonspecific degradation of cellular

RNAs and general repression of protein synthesis *(96,98)*. Overall, siRNAs seem to induce complex signaling responses in target cells beyond the selective silencing of specific genes *(96)*. The relative efficacy and specificity of a given siRNA as well as the use of stringent controls need to be carefully established for each individual experimental model.

In conclusion, the lack of studies aimed to comparatively evaluate the efficacy of ribozymes and siRNAs in inhibiting the expression of the same genes on the same experimental systems makes it difficult to predict which is the better approach to be exploited for therapeutic purposes. It should also be stressed that hybrid RNAs, carrying ribozyme and siRNA sequences, could provide a much more powerful tool to achieve gene expression knockout with respect to ribozyme and siRNAs alone, as recently proposed *(22)*.

5. Concluding Remarks

As reported in this review, ribozyme- and siRNA-based approaches have been demonstrated to efficiently inhibit telomerase activity by targeting the RNA component hTR or the reverse transcriptase catalytic subunit hTERT. It is now well established that hTR represents a suitable target to achieve the inhibition of telomerase activity because of its natural accessibility to binding by different antisense oligonucleotides. Despite recent evidences reported by Li et al. *(83)*, a remarkable number of studies have emphasized that targeting hTR results in cancer cell growth arrest and reduced viability only after several population doublings as a consequence of interference with the telomere lengthening activity of the enzyme. Such evidence is in keeping with the classical mechanism by which telomerase inhibition would induce a delayed cell growth arrest and apoptosis as a result of critically shortened telomeres *(22)*. Such a cellular response has been proved to be largely dependent on the initial telomere length in a given tumor cell population. As a consequence, single-agent therapies based on inhibitors targeted to hTR would need long-term treatment to induce effective impairment of cancer cell growth with relatively long telomeres, thereby allowing a significant progression of the neoplastic disease *(99)*.

Conversely, recent studies have shown that treatment with telomerase inhibitors targeting hTERT was able to induce programmed cell death within a few days in different telomerase-positive tumor cell models *(22)*. Such results cannot be explained by the classical model, which predicts that long-term exposure of tumor cells to telomerase inhibitors should induce telomere shortening after a certain number of rounds of cells division and growth arrest. In fact, it is unlikely that cell death was related to telomere attrition because the cells would not have undergone enough divisions to significantly shorten their telomeres. Interference with telomerase activity might therefore affect aspects of the control of cell proliferation and apoptosis other than telomere length. Such results would suggest that abrogation of telomerase activity may affect cell proliferation also through pathways that are not dependent on telomere erosion. In fact, it has been reported that antitelomerase approaches based on the modulation of hTERT expression could lead to an early and pronounced biological response. Such evidence gains support from recent data demonstrating that the downregulation of hTERT expression levels quickly induced programmed cell death in human breast cancer cells and that such an apoptotic response could be counteracted by the expression of an hTERT mutant lacking telomerase activity *(25)*. This finding has conferred to hTERT a putative prosurvival and antiapoptotic function, which could be independent of the specific enzymatic activity of telomerase. Such a cytoprotective function of hTERT has been confirmed by us in a recent study demonstrating that oligonucleotide-mediated inhibition of hTERT, but not of hTR, induced rapid cell growth decline and programmed cell death in the absence of telomere shortening in human prostate cancer cells *(100)*.

It should be also taken into account that prolonged treatments with telomerase inhibitors could lead to the occurrence of specific mechanisms of resistance, such as the emergence of the alternative lengthening of telomeres (ALT) phenotype *(101)*. In fact, it has been reported that some eukaryotic organisms make use of telomerase-independent pathways to maintain their telomeres and that the ALT mechanisms may often occur when telomerase is repressed. The ALT phenotype is present in a small fraction (about 10%) of tumor tissues mainly of mesenchymal origin that are telomerase negative *(101,102)*. Moreover, it has been recently demonstrated that ALT- and telomerase-based pathways may coexist in the same tumor cells *(102)*. Such evidence would suggest that even in cells that stabilize their telomeres through telomerase, a marked and prolonged inhibition of the enzyme's catalytic activity could be responsible for the selection of mutant clones that are resistant to antitelomerase agents via reactivation of the ALT pathway and emphasize the notion that all tumor cells require a solution to the "end replication problem."

Even though the efficacy of telomerase inhibitors needs to be further validated in vivo tumor models before entering clinical practice, the availability of effective antisense-based telomerase inhibitors will give further insight about the role(s) of telomerase (beyond the classical mechanism of telomere lengthening) in the tumorigenesis process. It will also provide a better rationale for developing new anticancer therapies based on the use of antitelomerase inhibitors, also in the context of combined treatments.

Through the contribution of several groups the survivin pathway has emerged as a complex and essential cellular infrastructure controlling spindle microtubule function, chromosome segregation and also the initiation of mitochondrial-dependent apoptosis. Results obtained by different experimental studies aimed at targeting survivin by means of different molecular approaches clearly demonstrated that downregulation of this protein results in anticancer activity potentially suitable for clinical testing.

As far as the actual cellular targets of survivin antagonists are concerned, it appears that inhibition of survivin results in apoptosis of the proliferating tumor cell compartment. However, there is evidence that survivin may provide a broader cytoprotective role for the tumor microenvironment as a whole. This hypothesis is supported by the observation that survivin becomes strongly expressed in endothelial cells during the proliferating as well as the remodelling phases of angiogenesis and mediates the apoptosis resistance of these cells *(103)*.

The evidence that survivin plays a crucial role also in tumor angiogenesis would suggest that molecular targeting of survivin may provide a dual advantage for anticancer strategies in vivo as a consequence of the ability to increase the overall tumor response to treatment not only through direct interference with the apoptotic pathways in cancer cells but also by favoring the apoptotic involution of newly formed tumor vasculature *(104)*. Clinical testing of survivin antisense oligonucleotides is currently underway.

References

1. Jansen, B. and Zangemeister-Wittke, U. (2002) Antisense therapy for cancer—the time of truth. *Lancet Oncol.* **3**, 672–683.
2. Kyo, S. and Inoue, M. (2002) Complex regulatory mechanisms of telomerase activity in normal and cancer cells: how can we apply them for cancer therapy? *Oncogene* **21**, 688–697.
3. Altieri, D. C. (2003) Survivin and apoptosis control. *Adv. Cancer Res.* **88**, 31–52.
4. Hahn, W. C. (2003) Role of telomeres and telomerase in the pathogenesis of human cancer. *J. Clin. Oncol.* **21**, 2034–2043.
5. Smogorzewska, A. and de Lange, T. (2004) Regulation of telomerase by telomeric proteins. *Annu. Rev. Biochem.* **73**, 177–208.
6. Karlseder, J. (2003) Telomere repeat binding factor: keeping the ends in check. *Cancer Lett.* **194**, 189–197.
7. Wright, W. E. and Shay, J. W. (2005) Telomere-binding factors and general DNA repair. *Nat. Genet.* **37**, 116–118.
8. Smogorzewska, A., Karlseder, J., Holtgreve-Grez, H., Jauch, A., and de Lange, T. (2002) DNA ligase IV-dependent NHEJ of deprotected mammalian telomeres in G1 and G2. *Curr. Biol.* **12**, 1635–1644.
9. Baumann, P. and Cech, T. R. (2001) Pot1, the putative telomere end-binding protein in fission yeast and humans. *Science* **292**, 1171–1175.
10. Lundblad, V. (2003) Telomeres: taking the measure. *Nature* **423**, 926–927.
11. Colgin, L. M., Baran, K., Baumann, P., Cech, T. R., and Reddel, R. R. (2003) Human POT1 facilitates telomere elongation by telomerase. *Curr. Biol.* **13**, 942–946.
12. Keith, W. N., Evans, T. R. J., and Glasspool, R. M. (2001) Telomerase and cancer: time to move from a promising target to a clinical reality. *J. Pathol.* **195**, 404–414.

13. Olovnikov, A. M. (1973) A theory of marginotomy. The incomplete copy of template margin in enzymatic synthesis of polynucleotides and biological significance of the phenomenon. *J. Theor. Biol.* **41,** 181–190.

14. Cong, Y. S., Wright, W. E., and Shay, J. W. (2002) Human telomerase and its regulation. *Microbiol. Mol. Biol. Rev.* **66,** 407–425.

15. Harrington, L., Zhou, W., McPhail, T., et al. (1997) Human telomerase contains evolutionarily conserved catalytic and structural subunits. *Genes Dev.* **11,** 3109–3115.

16. Feng, J., Funk, W. D., Wang, S. S., et al. (1995) The RNA component of human telomerase. *Science* **269,** 1236–1241.

17. Yi, X., White, D. M., Aisner, D. L., Baur, J. A., Wright, W. E., and Shay, J. W. (2000) An alternate splicing variant of the human telomerase catalytic subunit inhibits telomerase activity. *Neoplasia* **2,** 433–440.

18. Blackburn, E. H. (2005) Telomeres and telomerase: their mechanisms of action and the effects of altering their functions. *FEBS Lett.* **579,** 859–862.

19. Hahn, W. C. and Meyerson, M. (2001) Telomerase activation, cellular immortalization and cancer. *Ann. Med.* **2,** 123–129.

20. Shay, J. W. and Bacchetti, S. (1997) A survey of telomerase activity in human cancer. *Eur. J. Cancer* **33,** 787–791.

21. Hanahan, D. and Weinberg, R. A. (2000) The hallmarks of cancer. *Cell* **100,** 57–70.

22. Folini, M. and Zaffaroni, N. (2005) Targeting telomerase by antisense-based approaches: perspectives for new anti-cancer therapies. *Curr. Pharm. Des.* **11,** 1105–1117.

23. Blackburn, E. H. (2000) Telomere states and cell fates. *Nature* **408,** 53–56.

24. Sharma, G. G., Gupta, A., Wang, H., et al. (2003) hTERT associates with human telomeres and enhances genomic stability and DNA repair. *Oncogene* **22,** 131–146.

25. Cao, Y., Li, H., Deb, S., and Liu, J. P. (2004) TERT regulates cell survival independent of telomerase enzymatic activity. *Oncogene* **21,** 3130–3138.

26. Kelland, L. R. (2005) Overcoming the immortality of tumor cells by telomere and telomerase based cancer therapeutics—current status and future prospects. *Eur. J. Cancer* **41,** 971–979.

27. Altieri, D. (2004) Molecular circuits of apoptosis regulation and cell division control: the survivin paradigm. *J. Cell. Biochem.* **92,** 656–663.

28. Ambrosini, G., Adida, C., Sirugo, A., and Altieri, D. C. (1998) Induction of apoptosis and inhibition of cell proliferation by survivin gene targeting. *J. Biol. Chem.* **273,** 11,177–11,182.

29. Ambrosini, G., Adida, C., and Altieri, D. C. (1997) A novel anti-apoptosis gene, survivin, expressed in cancer and lymphoma. *Nat. Med.* **3,** 917–921.

30. LaCasse, E. C., Baird, S., Korneluk, R. G., and MacKenzie, A. E. (1998) The inhibitors of apoptosis (IAPs) and their emerging role in cancer. *Oncogene* **17,** 3247–3259.

31. Mahotka, C., Wenzel, M., Springer, E., Gabbert, H. E., and Gerharz, C. D. (1999) Survivin-ΔEx3 and survivin-2B: two novel splice variants of the apoptosis inhibitor survivin with different antiapoptotic properties. *Cancer Res.* **59,** 6097–6102.

32. Badran, A., Yoshida, A., Ishikawa, K., et al. (2004) Identification of a novel splice variant of the human anti-apoptopsis gene survivin *Biochem. Biophys. Res. Commun.* **314**, 902–907.
33. Caldas, H., Honsey, L. E., and Altura, R. A. (2005) Survivin 2alpha: a novel Survivin splice variant expressed in human malignancies. *Mol. Cancer* **4**, 11.
34. Caldas, H., Jiang, Y., Holloway, M. P., et al. (2005) Survivin splice variants regulate the balance between proliferation and cell death. *Oncogene* **24**, 1994–2007.
35. Li, F. and Altieri, D. C. (1999) The cancer anti-apoptosis mouse survivin gene: characterization of locus and transcriptional requirements of basal and cell cycle-dependent expression. *Cancer Res.* **59**, 3143–3151.
36. O'Connor, D. S., Grossman, D., Plescia, J., et al. (2000) Regulation of apoptosis at cell division by p34cdc2 phosphorylation of survivin. *Proc. Natl. Acad. Sci.* **97**, 13,103–13,107.
37. Fortugno, P., Wall, N. R., Giodini, A., et al. (2002) Survivin exists in immuno-chemically distinct subcellular pools and is involved in spindle microtubule function. *J. Cell Sci.* **115**, 575–585.
38. Uren, A. G., Wong, L., Pakusch, M., et al. (2000) Survivin and the inner centromere protein INCENP show similar cell-cycle localization and gene knockout phenotype. *Curr. Biol.* **10**, 1319–1328.
39. Li, F., Ackermann, E. J., Bennett, C. F., et al. (1999) Pleiotropic cell-division defects and apoptosis induced by interference with survivin function. *Nat. Cell Biol.* **1**, 461–466.
40. Chen, J., Wu, W., Tahir, S. K., et al. (2000) Down-regulation of survivin by antisense oligonucleotides increases apoptosis, inhibits cytokinesis and anchorage-dependent growth. *Neoplasia* **2**, 235–241.
41. Giodini, A., Kallio, M. J., Wall, N. R., et al. (2002) Regulation of microtubule stability and mitotic progression by survivin. *Cancer Res.* **62**, 2462–2467.
42. Kallio, M. J., Nieminen, M., and Eriksson, J. E. (2001) Human inhibitor of apoptosis protein (IAP) survivin participates in regulation of chromosome segregation and mitotic exit. *FASEB* **15**, 2721–2723.
43. Carvalho, A., Carmena, M., Sambade, C., Earnshaw, W. C., and Wheatley, S. P. (2003) Survivin is required for stable checkpoint activation in taxol-treated HeLa cells. *J. Cell. Sci.* **116**, 2987–2998.
44. Dohi, T., Beltrami, E., Wall, N. R., Plescia, J., and Altieri, D. C. (2004) Mitochondrial survivin inhibits apoptosis and promotes tumorigenesis. *J. Clin. Invest.* **114**, 1117–1127.
45. Fortugno, P., Beltrami, E., Plescia, J., et al. (2003) Regulation of survivin function by Hsp90. *Proc. Natl. Acad. Sci. USA* **100**, 13,791–13,796.
46. O'Connor, D. S., Grossman, D., Plescia, J., et al. (2000) Regulation of apoptosis at cell division by p34cdc2 phosphorylation of survivin. *Proc. Natl. Acad. Sci.* **97**, 13,103–13,107.
47. Song, Z., Yao, X., and Wu, M. (2003) Direct interaction between survivin and Smac/DIABLO is essential for the anti-apoptotic activity of survivin during taxol-induced apoptosis. *J. Biol. Chem.* **278**, 23,130–23,140.

48. Shiozaki, E. N. and Shi, Y. (2004) Caspases, IAPs and Smac/DIABLO: mechanisms from structural biology. *Trends Biochem. Sci.* **29**, 486–494.
49. Altieri, D. C. (2003) Survivin, versatile modulation of cell division and apoptosis in cancer. *Oncogene* **22**, 8581–8589.
50. O'Connor, D. S., Schechner, J. S., Adida, C., et al. (2000) Control of apoptosis during angiogenesis by survivin expression in endothelial cells. *Am. J. Pathol.* **156**, 393–398.
51. Velculescu, V. E., Madden, S. L., Zhang, L., et al. (1999) Analysis of human transcriptomes. *Nat. Gen.* **23**, 387–388.
52. Plantaz, D., Mohapatra, G., Matthay, K. K., Pellarin, M., Seeger, R. C., and Feuerstein, B. G. (1997) Gain of chromosome 17 is the most frequent abnormality detected in neuroblastoma by comparative genomic hybridization. *Am. J. Pathol.* **150**, 81–89.
53. Hattori, M., Sakamoto, H., Satoh, K., and Yamamoto, T. (2001) DNA demethylase is expressed in ovarian cancers and the expression correlates with demethylation of CpG sites in the promoter region of c-erbB-2 and survivin genes. *Cancer Lett.* **169**, 155–164.
54. Mirza, A., McGuirk, M., Hockenberry, T. N., et al. (2002) Human survivin is negatively regulated by wild-type p53 and participates in p53-dependent apoptotic pathway. *Oncogene* **21**, 2613–2622.
55. Li, F., Ambrosini, G., Chu, E. Y., et al. (1998) Control of apoptosis and mitotic spindle checkpoint by survivin. *Nature* **396**, 580–584.
56. Zaffaroni, N., Pennati, M., Colella, G., et al. (2002) Expression of the anti-apoptotic gene survivin correlates with taxol resistance in human ovarian cancer. *Cell. Mol. Life Sci.* **59**, 1406–1412.
57. Asanuma, K., Moriai, R., Yajima, T., et al. (2000) Survivin as a radio-resistance factor in pancreatic cancer. *Jap. J. Cancer Res.* **91**, 1204–1209.
58. Zhang, M., Latham, D. E., Delaney, M. A., and Chakravarti, A. (2005) Survivin mediates resistance to antiandrogen therapy in prostate cancer. *Oncogene* **24**, 2474–2482.
59. Nicholson, D. W. (2000) From bench to clinic with apoptosis-based therapeutic agents. *Nature* **407**, 810–816.
60. Fischer, U. and Schulze-Osthoff, K. (2005) New approaches and therapeutics targeting apoptosis in disease. *Pharmacol. Rev.* **57**, 187–215.
61. Altieri, D. C. (2003) Validating survivin as a cancer therapeutic target. *Nat. Rev. Cancer* **3**, 46–54.
62. Puerta-Fernandez, E., Romer-Lopez, C., Barroso-delJesus, A., and Berzal-Herranz, A. (2003) Ribozymes: recent advances in the development of RNA tools. *FEMS Microbiol. Rev.* **27**, 75–97.
63. Kore, A. R., Vaish, N. K., Kutzke, U., and Eckstein, F. (1998) Sequence specificity of the hammerhead ribozyme revisited: the NHH rule. *Nucleic Acids Res.* **26**, 4116–4120.
64. Kurreck, J. (2003) Antisense technologies. Improvement through novel chemical modifications. *Eur. J. Biochem.* **270**, 1628–1644.

65. Kanazawa, Y., Ohkawa, K., Ueda, K., et al. (1996) Hammerhead ribozyme-mediated inhibition of telomerase activity in extracts of human hepatocellular carcinoma cells. *Biochem. Biophys. Res Commun.* **225,** 570–576.
66. Wan, M. S., Fell, P. L., and Akhtar, S. (1998) Synthetic 2'-O-methyl-modified hammerhead ribozymes targeted to the RNA component of telomerase as sequence-specific inhibitors of telomerase activity. *Antisense Nucleic Acid Drug Dev.* **8,** 309–317.
67. Folini, M., Colella, G., Villa, R., Lualdi, S., Daidone, M. G., and Zaffaroni, N. (2000) Inhibition of telomerase activity by a hammerhead ribozyme targeting the RNA component of telomerase in human melanoma cells. *J. Invest. Dermatol.* **114,** 259–267.
68. Yokoyama, Y., Takahashi, Y., Shinohara, A., et al. (1998) Attenuation of telomerase activity by a hammerhead ribozyme targeting the template region of telomerase RNA in endometrial carcinoma cells. *Cancer Res.* **58,** 5406–5410.
69. Yokoyama, Y., Wan, X., Takahashi, Y., Shinohara, A., Liulin, T., and Tamaya, T. (2002) Divalent hammerhead ribozyme targeting template region of human telomerase RNA has potent cleavage activity, but less inhibitory activity on telomerase. *Arch. Biochem. Biophys.* **405,** 32–37.
70. Yeo, M., Rha, S. Y., Jeung, H. C., et al. (2005) Attenuation of telomerase activity by hammerhead ribozyme targeting human telomerase RNA induces growth retardation and apoptosis in human breast tumor cells. *Int. J. Cancer* **114,** 484–489.
71. Yokoyama, Y., Takahashi, Y., Shinohara, A., et al. (2000) The 5'-end of hTERT mRNA is a good target for hammerhead ribozyme to suppress telomerase activity. *Biochem. Biophys. Res Commun.* **273,** 316–321.
72. Ludwig, A., Saretzki, G., Holm, P. S., et al. (2001) Ribozyme cleavage of telomerase mRNA sensitizes breast epithelial cells to inhibitors of topoisomerase. *Cancer Res.* **61,** 3053–3061.
73. Saretzki, G., Ludwig, A., von Zglinicki, T., and Runnebaum, I. B. (2001) Ribozyme-mediated telomerase inhibition induces immediate cell loss but not telomere shortening in ovarian cancer cells. *Cancer Gene Ther.* **8,** 827–834.
74. Pennati, M., Colella, G., Folini, M., Citti, L., Daidone, M. G., and Zaffaroni, N. (2002) Ribozyme-mediated attenuation of survivin expression sensitizes human melanoma cells to cisplatin-induced apoptosis. *J. Clin. Invest.* **109,** 285–286.
75. Pennati, M., Binda, M., De Cesare, M., et al. (2004) Ribozyme-mediated down-regulation of survivin expression sensitizes human melanoma cells to topotecan in vitro and in vivo. *Carcinogenesis* **25,** 1129–1136.
76. Pennati, M., Binda, M., Coltella, G., et al. (2003) Radiosensitization of human melanoma cells by ribozyme-mediated inhibition of survivin expression. *J. Invest. Dermatol.* **120,** 648–654.
77. Pennati, M., Binda, M., Coltella, G., et al. (2004) Ribozyme-mediated inhibition of survivin expression increases spontaneous and drug-induced apoptosis and decreases the tumorigenic potential of human prostate cancer cells. *Oncogene* **23,** 386–394.

78. Choi, K. S., Lee, T. H., and Jung, M. H. (2003) Ribozyme-mediated cleavage of the human survivin mRNA and inhibition of antiapoptotic function of survivin in MCF-7 cells. *Cancer Gene Ther.* **10,** 87–95.

79. Elbashir, S. M., Harborth, J., Weber, K., and Tuschl, T. (2002) Analysis of gene function in somatic mammalian cells using small interfering RNAs. *Methods* **26,** 199–213.

80. Dykxhoorn, D. M., Novina, C. D., and Sharp, P. A. (2003) Killing the messenger: short RNAs that silence gene expression. *Nat. Rev. Mol. Cell. Biol.* **4,** 457–467.

81. Izquierdo, M. (2005) Short interfering RNAs as a tool for cancer gene therapy. *Cancer Gene Ther.* **12,** 217–227.

82. Kosciolek, B. A., Kalantidis, K., Tabler, M., and Rowley, P. T. (2003) Inhibition of telomerase activity in human cancer cells by RNA interference. *Mol. Cancer Ther.* **2,** 209–216.

83. Li, S., Crothers, J., Haqq, C. M., and Blackburn, E. H. (2005) Cellular and gene expression responses involved in the rapid growth inhibition of human cancer cells by RNA interference-mediated depletion of telomerase RNA. *J. Biol. Chem.* **280,** 23,709–23,717.

84. Kappler, M., Bache, M., Bartel, F., et al. (2004) Knockdown of survivin expression by small interfering RNA reduces the clonogenic survival of human sarcoma cell lines independently of p53. *Cancer Gene Ther.* **11,** 186–193.

85. Kappler, M., Taubert, H., Bartel, F., et al. (2005) Radiosensitization, after a combined treatment of survivin siRNA and irradiation, is correlated with the activation of caspases 3 and 7 in a wt-p53 sarcoma cell line, but not in a mt-p53 sarcoma cell line. *Oncol. Rep.* **13,** 167–172.

86. Chawla-Sarkar, M., Bae, S. I., Reu, F. J., Jacobs, B. S., Lindner, D. J., and Borden, E. C. (2004) Downregulation of Bcl-2, FLIP or IAPs (XIAP and survivin) by siRNAs sensitizes resistant melanoma cells to Apo2L/TRAIL-induced apoptosis. *Cell Death Differ.* **11,** 915–923.

87. Coma, S., Noe, V., Lavarino, C., et al. (2004) Use of siRNAs and antisense oligonucleotides against survivin RNA to inhibit steps leading to tumor angiogenesis. *Oligonucleotides* **14,** 100–113.

88. Coumoul, X., Li, W., Wang, R. H., and Deng, C. (2004) Inducible suppression of Fgfr2 and Survivin in ES cells using a combination of the RNA interference (RNAi) and the Cre-LoxP system. *Nucleic Acids Res.* **32,** e85.

89. Scherer, L. J. and Rossi, J. J. (2003) Approaches for the sequence-specific knockdown of mRNA. *Nature Biotechnol.* **21,** 1457–1465.

90. Caplen, N. J. (2004) Gene therapy progress and prospects. Downregulating gene expression: the impact of RNA interference. *Gene Ther.* **11,** 1241–1248.

91. Schubert, S., Grünweller, A., Erdmann, V. A., and Kurreck, J. (2005) Local RNA target structure influences siRNA efficacy: systematic analysis of intentionally designed binding regions. *J. Mol. Biol.* **348,** 883–893.

92. Overhoff, M., Alken, M., Far, R. K., et al. (2005) Local RNA target structure influences siRNA efficacy: a systematic global analysis. *J. Mol. Biol.* **348,** 871–881.

93. Lee, N. S., Lee, N. S., Bertrand, E., and Rossi, J. (1999) mRNA localizasion signals can enhance the intracellular effectiveness of hammerhead ribozymes. *RNA* **5,** 1200–1209.
94. Sullenger, B. A. and Gilboa, E. (2002) Emerging clinical application of RNA. *Nature* **418,** 252–258.
95. Bantounas, I., Phylactou, L. A., and Uney, J. B. (2004) RNA interference and the use of small interfering RNA to study gene function in mammalian systems. *J. Mol. Endocrinol.* **33,** 545–557.
96. Sledz, C. A. and Williams, B. R. G. (2004) RNA interference and double-stranded-RNA-activated pathways. *Biochem. Soc. Trans.* **32,** 952–956.
97. Sledz, C. A., Holko, M., de Veer, M. J., Silverman, R. H., and Williams, R. G. (2003) Activation of interferon system by short-interfering RNAs. *Nat. Cell. Biol.* **5,** 834–839.
98. Huppi, K., Martin, S. E., and Caplen, N. J. (2005) Defining and assaying RNAi in mammalian cells. *Mol. Cell.* **17,** 1–10.
99. Shay, J. W. and Wright, W. E. (2002) Telomerase: a target for cancer therapeutics. *Cancer Cell* **2,** 257–265.
100. Folini, M., Brambilla, C., Villa, R., et al. (2005) Antisense oligonucleotide-mediated inhibition of hTERT, but not hTERC, induces rapid cell growth decline and apoptosis in the absence of telomere shortening in human prostate cancer cells. *Eur. J. Cancer* **41,** 624–634.
101. Henson, J. D., Neumann, A. A., Yeager, T. R., and Reddel, R. R. (2002) Alternative lengthening of telomeres in mammalian cells. *Oncogene* **21,** 598–610.
102. Reddel, R. R. and Bryan, T. M. (2003) Alternative lengthening of telomeres: dangerous road less travelled. *Lancet* **361,** 1840.
103. Tran, J., Master, Z., Yu, J. L., Rak, J., Dumont, D. J., and Kerbel, R. S. (2002). A role for survivin in chemoresistance of endothelial cells mediated by VEGF. *Proc. Natl. Acad. Sci. USA* **99,** 4349–4354.
104. Mesri, M., Morales-Ruiz, M., Ackermann, E. J., et al. (2001) Suppression of vascular endothelial growth factor-mediated endothelial cell protection by survivin targeting. *Am. J. Pathol.* **158,** 1757–1765.

13

Collagen-Induced Arthritis in Mice

A Major Role for Tumor Necrosis Factor-α

Richard O. Williams

Summary

Collagen-induced arthritis is the most widely used animal model for the evaluation of novel therapeutic strategies for rheumatoid arthritis. The disease is induced by immunization of genetically susceptible strains of mice or rats with type II collagen in adjuvant. Susceptibility to collagen-induced arthritis is associated with major histocompatibility complex (MHC) class II genes, although non-MHC genes also play a role. Both B- and T-lymphocytes are important in the pathogenesis of collagen-induced arthritis, with the peak of the T-cell response occurring around the time of disease onset. Histopathological assessment of the joints of animals with collagen-induced arthritis reveal a proliferative synovitis with infiltration of polymorphonuclear and mononuclear cells, the formation of an erosive pannus, cartilage degradation, and fibrosis. As in human rheumatoid arthritis, a number of both pro- and anti-inflammatory cytokines are expressed in the joints of mice with collagen-induced arthritis, including tumor necrosis factor-α (TNFα) and interleukin (IL)-1β, IL-6, IL-1Ra, IL-10, and transforming growth factor β. The use transgenic and knockout strains of mice, as well as biological inhibitors, have revealed important pathological roles for multiple cytokines. Of these, TNFα emerged as a valid therapeutic target for rheumatoid arthritis and this led to the setting up of clinical trials of anti-TNFα antibody therapy. Three anti-TNFα biologics (infliximab, etanercept, and adalimumab) are now approved for use and TNFα blockade therefore represents an important advance in our ability to treat rheumatoid arthritis.

Key Words: Rheumatoid arthritis; TNFα; autoimmunity; experimental animal models; collagen-induced arthritis; type II collagen.

1. Introduction

1.1. Rheumatoid Arthritis

Rheumatoid arthritis (RA) is an inflammatory disease of unknown etiology with a world-wide prevalence of approx 1%. The disease is often progressive

From: *Methods in Molecular Biology, vol. 361, Target Discovery and Validation Reviews and Protocols*
Volume 2, Emerging Molecular Targets and Treatment Options
Edited by: M. Sioud © Humana Press Inc., Totowa, NJ

and results in pain, stiffness, and swelling of joints. In late stages, deformity and ankylosis develop. RA is one of the most common causes of disability in the Western world and has a female to male ratio of around 3 to 1. The age of onset of RA is typically between 25 and 50, although it can strike at any age. The chief pathological features of the disease include the formation of an inflammatory erosive synovitis that ultimately leads to destruction of cartilage, bone, and soft tissues resulting in loss of joint function. Although joints are the main target of the disease process in RA, the disease is usually classified as a nonorgan specific autoimmune disease, because of the occurence of extraarticular features, such as subcutaneous nodules, vasculitis, and pulmonary fibrosis, especially in the more severe cases.

There has been considerable progress recently in characterizing the mediators that contribute to the pathogenesis of RA and a number of studies have pointed to a pivotal role for tumor necrosis factor (TNF)α. Indeed, the successful introduction of infliximab, a chimeric anti-TNFα monoclonal antibody (mAb) *(1–3)*, etanercept, a soluble p75 TNF receptor-Fc fusion protein *(4,5)*, and adalimumab, a monoclonal human antibody produced by phage display *(6–8)* into the clinic confirms the importance of TNFα in RA. However, the underlying cause of RA is still unknown and there remains an urgent need for more effective and durable remedies with low toxicity profiles. It is for this reason that animal models of arthritis are being studied.

1.2. Collagen-Induced Arthritis

Animal models of arthritis have been used in many different kinds of experiments, including the evaluation of novel therapies, the identification of proinflammatory cytokines, the identification of genes associated with disease susceptibility, and in the identification of markers of disease progression *(9)*. Collagen-induced arthritis (CIA) is probably the most widely used model for studies of therapeutic intervention although data arising from such studies should be interpreted with caution because much depends on the timing of treatment (i.e., before or after onset of arthritis). For example, a number of T-cell-targeted therapies (e.g., anti-CD4, anti-interleukin [IL]-12, CTLA4-Ig) have been shown to be effective when given at the time of immunization but ineffective when given in established disease *(10–13)*.

CIA exhibits many pathological similarities to RA *(14)*, including similar patterns of synovitis, pannus formation, erosion of cartilage and bone, fibrosis, and loss of joint function *(15)*. In addition, susceptibility to both human RA and murine CIA is associated with genes encoding major histocompatibility complex (MHC) class II molecules, implying the involvement of CD4$^+$ T cells in the pathogenesis of both forms of arthritis. Thus, susceptibility to CIA is restricted to mouse strains bearing MHC types I-A^q and I-A^r, the mouse homologs of human leukocyte antigen (HLA)-DQ, whereas in human RA certain subtypes of HLA-DR4 and -DR1 are associated with disease susceptibility. Another similarity is that humoral responses are thought to play a significant role in the pathogenesis of both CIA and RA *(14)* although there is a lack of convincing data pointing to a role for type II collagen-specific autoantibodies in the majority of RA patients as elevated levels of anticollagen antibody are detected only in 10–15% of patients *(16)*. Another extremely important feature of CIA that makes it a valid model for RA is the expression of proinflammatory cytokines, including TNFα, and IL-1β, in the joints of mice with arthritis *(17)*.

CIA induced by immunization of DBA/1 mice with chicken, rat, or bovine type II collagen usually leads to a relatively acute and self-remitting form of arthritis in which arachidonic acid metabolites, such as prostaglandin E$_2$, play an important pathological role in the development of arthritis. This was shown in a study in which cytosolic phospholipase A2α (cPLA2α) knockout mice were backcrossed onto the arthritis susceptible DBA/1 background. cPLA2α is responsible for releasing arachidonic acid from cell membranes, which is the first step in the production of prostaglandins and leukotrienes. The development of arthritis was profoundly inhibited in cPLA2α knockout mice compared with wild-type littermates, despite the fact that levels of type II collagen-specific antibodies were comparable in the two groups *(18)*. However, immunization of DBA/1 mice with mouse collagen results in a more chronic form of arthritis *(19–21)*, which is resistant to nonsteroidal anti-inflammatory drugs, such as indomethacin *(21)*. However, the drawback to the use of autologous type II collagen is that it is less arthritogenic than heterologous collagen and therefore produces a less reproducible form of arthritis. The relative lack of arthritogenicity of mouse collagen has been attributed to the low affinity of specific epitope of murine collagen (CII256-270) for I-A^q, which results in a low level of CII-specific T-cell activation *(22)*.

1.3. The Role of Proinflammatory Cytokines in Arthritis

1.3.1. Evidence From Transgenic Strains of Mice

Mice expressing a human TNFα transgene in which the 3' AU-rich region has been replaced by the 3' untranslated region of the human β-globin gene, resulting in increased mRNA stability and increased TNFα expression **(Fig. 1)**, were shown to develop arthritis spontaneously *(23)*. The arthritis could be prevented by continuous administration of neutralizing antihuman TNFα mAb.

Histopathological studies of the joints of hTNFα transgenic mice revealed that the arthritis was highly erosive in nature, with subchondral bone being

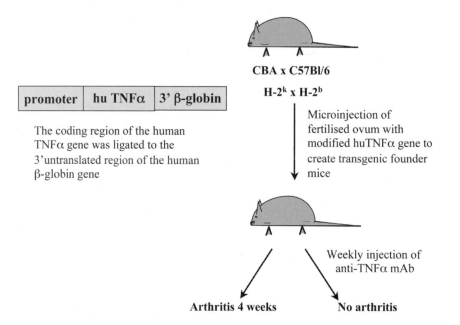

Fig. 1. Generation of trangenic mice expressing a modified human tumor necrosis factor (TNF)α gene. The replacement of the 3'-AU-rich region of the TNFα gene by the 3'-region of the β-globin gene stabilizes mRNA, resulting in over-expression of TNFα protein *(23)*.

particularly affected **(Fig. 2)**. hTNFα was found to be overexpressed in various tissues, including lung, spleen, and the joint and it is not obvious why the joint should be affected pathologically whereas other tissues were apparently normal. Indeed, a second strain of TNFα over-expressing mice was generated in which the AU-rich region of the TNFα transgene was deleted by targeted disruption and these mice developed not only arthritis but also inflammatory bowel disease *(24)*. It is noteworthy that TNFα over-producing mice can be back-crossed to RAG$^{-/-}$ mice without altering the arthritis phenotype, indicating that TNFα is mostly "downstream" of the T- or B-cell response. Furthermore, we have been unable to detect autoantibodies to cartilage-derived proteins (type II collagen, type IX collagen, type XI collagen, or aggrecan) in hTNFα transgenic mice on a DBA/1 background (unpublished data).

It is of interest that treatment of hTNFα transgenic mice with an antagonistic anti-IL-1R antibody prevented the development of spontaneous arthritis *(25)*. This is compatible with studies in human RA synovial cell cultures where blockade of TNFα was found to reduce IL-1 production *(26)*, indicating that IL-1 production is downstream of TNFα.

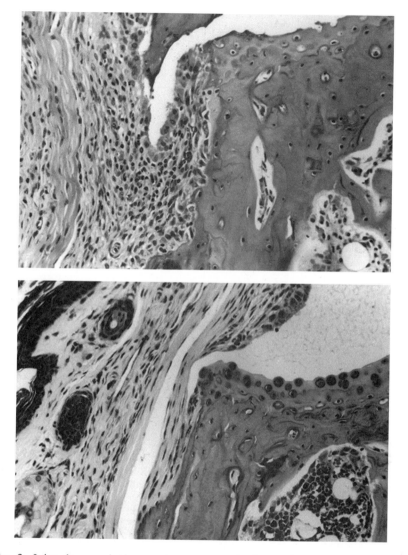

Fig. 2. Joint damage in human tumor necrosis factor (hTNF)α-transgenic mice. **(Top)** Erosive changes in the cartilage-bone-pannus region of a proximal interphalangeal joint from a hTNFα-transgenic mouse with arthritis. Note the focal erosion of subchondral bone. **(Bottom)** Normal joint from a nontransgenic littermate. Hematoxylin and eosin.

In addition to TNFα, it is also recognized that IL-1 is a major pathological mediator in arthritis and this is confirmed by the observation that IL-1α-transgenic mice develop severe polyarthritis spontaneously at around 4 wk of age *(27)*. Synovitis was observed at 2 wk of age and after 6 wk synovial lining layer hyperplasia and the formation of pannus were seen. The cartilage was also shown to exhibit degradative changes and this confirms previous findings regarding the importance of IL-1 in cartilage breakdown *(28–30)*.

1.3.2. Evidence From Knockout Mice

The generation of gene-targeted strains of mice has provided important insights into the roles played by different cytokines in arthritis. For example, the role of IL-12 was investigated by studying the progression of CIA in IL-12$^{-/-}$ mice on a DBA/1 genetic background and the incidence and severity of disease were both found to be significantly reduced, although disease was not completely abolished *(31)*. Collagen-specific IgG2a antibodies were reduced and IFNγ production by collagen-stimulated splenocytes was inhibited, consistent with a diminished Th1 response. These results demonstrate an important role for IL-12 in the development of Th1 responses and in the pathogenesis of CIA *(31)*. This was subsequently confirmed in wild-type mice given neutralizing anti-IL-12 antibodies twice weekly from the time of collagen immunization. It was found that anti-IL-12 blockade dramatically reduced the severity of arthritis, both clinically and histopathologically *(13)*.

In a similar study, the development of CIA was followed in IL-18$^{-/-}$ mice on a DBA/1 background. IL-18$^{-/-}$ mice developed markedly reduced incidence and severity of arthritis compared with wild-type mice and this was accompanied by reduced serum anticollagen IgG2a levels and reduced proinflammatory cytokine production by spleen and lymph node cells in vitro *(32)*. Treatment of IL-18$^{-/-}$ mice with rIL-18 restored the development of arthritis to that of wild-type mice. These findings demonstrate a role for IL18 in CIA and this was subsequently confirmed in further studies in which anti-IL-18 IgG or rIL-18-binding protein were found to reduce the severity of established CIA *(33)*.

Targeted deletion of the *IL-6* gene has given conflicting results. IL-6$^{-/-}$ mice, backcrossed onto the DBA/1 genetic background for five generations were completely protected from CIA and there was a reduction in the anticollagen IgG response and an absence of inflammatory cells and tissue destruction in the joints *(34)*. In contrast, in another study in which IL-6$^{-/-}$ mice were backcrossed onto the DBA/1 genetic background for eight generations, overt arthritis developed in all of the IL-6 knockout mice, although there was a delay in disease onset and a reduction in severity *(35)*. This latter study would suggest that IL-6 is important, though not essential for the development of CIA and this is supported by therapeutic studies showing that blockade of the IL-6 receptor reduces the severity of collagen-induced arthritis in mice and cynomolgus monkeys *(36,37)*.

IL-17 is a T-cell-derived cytokine that is expressed at elevated levels in synovial tissues of RA patients and postulated to play a pathogenic role in arthritis. This was subsequently confirmed by the finding that CIA was markedly suppressed in IL-17$^{-/-}$ mice *(38)* and that blockade of IL-17 using neutralizing antibodies was effective in reducing the severity of disease *(39,40)*.

An important pathological feature of CIA (and to a lesser extent, RA) is the preponderance of granulocytes in the joints of arthritic mice therefore it is not surprising that G-CSF-deficient mice were protected from arthritis *(41)*. The reduced arthritis severity was associated with inhibited mobilization of granulocytic cells from the bone marrow and reduced cellular infiltration in the joints. More surprising, however, was the observation that G-CSF blockade in established CIA in wild-type DBA/1 mice reduced disease severity *(41)*. These findings clearly point to a role for G-CSF in driving arthritis in the CIA model and should therefore be regarded as a potential therapeutic target for human disease.

Although the majority of gene knockout studies in CIA have focused on genes encoding proinflammatory cytokines, at least two groups have analyzed the progression of CIA in mice lacking the inflammatory cytokine, IL-10. Cuzzocrea et al. reported enhanced clinical and histological development of CIA in IL-10$^{-/-}$ mice *(42)*. In another study, IL-10$^{-/-}$ mice displayed increased incidence and severity of CIA compared to IL-10$^{+/-}$ littermates. Surprisingly, however, IL-10$^{-/-}$ were less susceptible to arthritis induced by passive transfer of anticollagen antibodies. It was concluded that endogenous IL-10 has a protective role in CIA, but exacerbates antibody-mediated joint inflammation *(43)*. However, the net effects of administration of exogenous IL-10 appears to be anti-inflammatory because daily injections of recombinant IL-10 were found to inhibit the progression of established CIA in wild-type DBA/1 mice *(44)*.

CIA is regarded as a strongly Th1-biased disease with high levels of IFNγ production in draining lymph node cells that peak at around the time of onset of disease *(45)*. Hence, one of the least anticipated findings to come out of studies of gene knockout mice was the increased severity, accelerated onset, and increased cumulative incidence of CIA in IFNγ receptor knockout mice, compared to wild-type littermates *(46,47)*. These findings are also supported by our own studies, which demonstrated enhanced progression of CIA in DBA/1 mice treated with IFNγ neutralizing mAb *(48)* and those of Boissier et al. which showed increased disease severity following blockade of IFNγ in late CIA *(49)*. Clearly, the pro- and anti-inflammatory properties of IFNγ are complex and a more comprehensive analysis will be required to elucidate the role of this cytokine in arthritis.

1.3.3. TNFα is a Valid Therapeutic Target for Rheumatoid Arthritis

There has been considerable progress in recent years in our elucidation of the pathological processes in RA and the roles played by the many cytokines, chemokines, and growth factors have come to be appreciated. Two cytokines in particular, TNFα and IL-1, have been shown to be major inducers of both inflammation and tissue destruction. Subsequently, it was shown that blockade of TNFα in cultured synovial cells from RA patients prevented the expression of IL-1 and other proinflammatory cytokines (26,50–52), suggesting a cytokine cascade in which TNFα was responsible for driving the production of multiple mediators of inflammation.

In the light of these findings a number of studies have analyzed the effect of TNFα blockade in CIA. For example, a number of studies showed that treatment of mice with monoclonal or polyclonal anti-TNFα antibodies, or soluble TNF receptors, reduced the severity of arthritis when administered before the onset of clinical arthritis (53–55). Subsequently, we assessed the effect of anti-TNFα treatment in mice with established CIA (54). DBA/1 mice were immunized with type II collagen in CFA. The mice were inspected daily and each mouse that exhibited clinical signs of arthritis was randomly assigned to one of three treatment groups. The mice were then given twice-weekly injections of TN3-19.12 (anti-TNFα mAb), L2 (isotype control) or PBS over a period of 14 d. The half-life of TN3-19.12 in mice had been previously estimated to be around 7 d (56). There was found to be a dose-dependent reduction in the severity of arthritis following treatment with anti-TNFα mAb (**Fig. 3**). At the end of the treatment period, arthritic paws were processed for histology and it was confirmed that anti-TNFα treatment had reduced the histological severity of arthritis and protected joints from erosive changes (**Fig. 4**).

Soluble TNF receptors play an important physiological role in regulating the activity of TNFα, and two studies showed that the administration of recombinant soluble TNFRs is effective in established CIA. In the first study, a p75 TNFR–Fc fusion protein was found to reduce the severity of arthritis whether given before or after the onset of the disease (57). We then showed that a p55 TNFR–Ig fusion protein was effective in reducing both the clinical and histological severity of established CIA (58).

It was concluded from these studies was that TNFα is involved in the pathogenesis of CIA and this provided part of the rationale for the testing of anti-TNFα mAb therapy in human RA.

1.3.4. Effect of TNFα Blockade in Other Models of Arthritis

Although CIA is probably the most widely utilized animal model of arthritis, many other models exist, all of which mimic human RA to a greater or lesser extent (9). Issekutz et al. (59) used neutralizing antibodies to assess the respective roles of TNFα, IL-1α, and IL-1β in adjuvant arthritis in rats. Treatment with anti-IL-1α and anti-IL-1β on day 5 of arthritis did not significantly affect infiltration of polymorphonuclear leukocytes (PML) or T-cell infiltration into the joint. In contrast, anti-TNFα treatment reduced clinical scores,

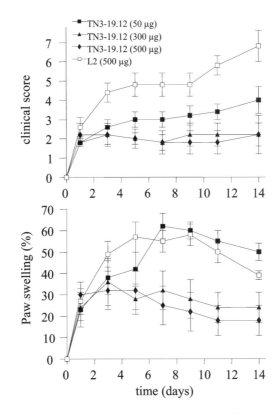

Fig. 3. Effect of antitumor necrosis factor monoclonal antibody (mAb) (TN3-19.12) on clinical progression of established collagen-induced arthritis. Arrows indicate time of injection. L2 is an isotype control mAb. There were 10 mice per group. **(Top)** Clinical score (0 = normal, 1 = slight swelling and/or erythema, 2 = pronounced edematous swelling, 3 = ankylosis). Each limb is graded, giving a maximum score of 12 per mouse. **(Bottom)** paw swelling (expressed as the percentage increment in paw-width relative to the paw-width before the onset of arthritis). (Adapted from **ref. 54**.)

inhibited infiltration of PML by 40–50% and T lymphocytes by 30–50%. It was concluded from this study that leucocyte infiltration in adjuvant arthritis is a strongly TNFα-dependent disease with IL-1 playing a relatively minor role. This clearly differs from CIA, in which IL-1 plays a major role in both inflammatory and destructive processes *(60,61)*.

Neutralization of TNFα in antigen-induced arthritis in rabbits was found to inhibit inflammatory changes in the joint during the acute phase of the disease but had only a minor effect on proteoglycan loss from cartlilage in the long-term *(62)*. Similarly, anti-TNFα treatment failed to prevent changes in cartilage proteoglycan synthesis or proteoglycan loss in antigen-induced arthritis, zymosan-induced arthritis, immune complex-mediated arthritis, or streptococcal cell wall-induced

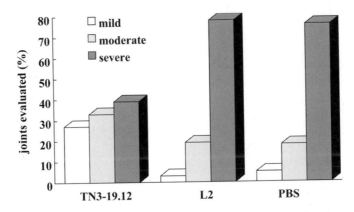

Fig. 4. Histopathological assessment of joints of arthritic DBA/1 mice treated with antitumor necrosis factor (TN3-19.12). L2 is an isotype control monoclonal antibody . The scoring system was as follows. Mild, minimal synovitis, erosions limited to discrete foci, cartilage surface intact. Moderate, synovitis, and erosions present but normal joint architecture intact. Severe, extensive erosions, joint architecture disrupted. Approximately 60 joints were examined per treatment group. (Adapted from **ref. 54**.)

arthritis in mice *(63,64)*. It can concluded from these findings that arthritis models differ in terms of their response to TNFα blockade. Given that human RA is a relatively heterogenous disease, it seems likely that individual patients will also show different levels of response to anti-TNFα therapy.

1.3.5. What is the Effect of IL-1 Blockade?

Although this review has focused primarily on the therapeutic effect of TNFα blockade in CIA, it is clear that neutralization of anti-IL-1 also has a pronounced therapeutic effect *(60,61,65–67)*. In contrast, continuous infusion with IL-1 receptor antagonist (IL-1Ra) was found to be relatively ineffective in adjuvant arthritis *(66)* and neutralization of IL-1 in streptococcal cell wall-induced arthritis failed to affect the clinical severity of disease, although a reduction in cartilage proteoglycan depletion was observed microscopically *(64)*. In human RA, clinical trials with IL-1Ra have shown only modest reductions in disease activity *(68)* although in view of the poor pharmacokinetics of IL-1Ra, this may be owing to incomplete neutralization of IL-1 *(66)*. In the light of these conflicting findings, we evaluated the effects of anti-TNFα, anti-IL-1β, and anti-IL-1α/β therapy in CIA. Anti-TNFα, anti-IL-1β and anti-IL-1R (which blocks the activity of both IL-1α and IL-β) were all found to be effective in reducing the clinical and histological severity of arthritis, with anti-IL-1R and anti-IL-1β showing somewhat greater efficacy than anti-TNFα *(69)*. Anti-IL-1β was equally as effective as anti-IL-1R, suggesting that IL-1β plays a more important pathological role than IL-1α in CIA. An additive effect was observed between anti-TNFα and anti-IL-1R in the prevention of joint erosion and in reduction of the levels of the acute phase protein, serum amyloid P (69). On the basis of these findings it is concluded that, in addition to TNFα, IL-1 is a valid therapeutic for RA.

2. Materials

2.1. Purification of Type II Collagen

1. Powdered cartilage (see **Note 1**).
2. 4 M Guanidine-HCl, 0.05 M Tris-HCl, pH 7.5.
3. 0.5 and 0.1 M Acetic acid.
4. Sodium chloride (powder).
5. 70% (v/v) Formic acid.
6. Pepsin from porcine gastric mucosa (3X crystalized; Sigma-Aldrich).
7. 0.02 M Na$_2$HPO$_4$, pH 9.4.

2.2. Immunization of Mice

1. Male DBA/1 mice, 8–12 wk old (Harlan-Olac).
2. Type II collagen.
3. 0.1 M Acetic acid.
4. *Mycobacterium tuberculosis* H37 RA (Difco).
5. Incomplete Freund's adjuvant (IFA; Difco).
6. 0.2 mg/mL Fentanyl and 10 mg/mL fluanisol (Hypnorm®).

2.3. Measurement of Anticollagen IgG

1. Type II collagen.
2. 0.05 M Tris-HCl, 0.2 M NaCl, pH 7.4.
3. Nunc-immuno microtiter plates (Nalge-Nunc).
4. 0.05% (v/v) Tween-20 in phosphate buffered saline (PBS).
5. 2% (w/v) Bovine serum albumin (BSA) in PBS.
6. Test sera.
7. Standard serum sample.
8. HRP-conjugated anti-IgG, IgG1, and IgG2a (BD Biosciences).
9. TMB microwell peroxidase substrate system (Kirkegaard and Perry).
10. 4.5 N H$_2$SO$_4$.

2.4. Analysis of T-Cell Responses

1. Type II collagen immunized DBA/1 mice.
2. 70-μm Cell strainers (Falcon).
3. Hanks' balanced salt solution (HBSS).
4. Complete medium: RPM1 1640 containing 10% (v/v) heat-inactivated fetal calf serum or 1% (v/v) mouse serum, 100 U/mL penicillin, 100 μg/mL streptomycin, 2×10^{-5} M 2-mercaptoethanol, and 20 mM L-glutamine.
5. 0.05% (v/v) Tween-20 in PBS.

6. 2% (w/v) BSA in PBS.
7. Recombinant IL-5, IL-10, and IFNγ (Peprotech).
8. The following capture/biotinylated detect antibody pairs. IL-5, TRFK5/TRFK4; IL-10, JES5-16E3/JES5-2A5; IFNγ, R4-6A2/XMG1.2 (Immunokontact).
9. Streptavidin-HRP (BD Biosciences).
10. TMB microwell peroxidase substrate system (Kirkegaard and Perry).
11. 4.5 N H$_2$SO$_4$.
12. [^{3}H]thymidine (Amersham).

3. Methods
3.1. Purification of Type II Collagen

The method of purification of type II collagen from cartilage is based on the studies of Miller *(70)* and Herbage et al. *(71)*.

1. Powder cartilage in a liquid nitrogen freezer mill (Spex, Metuchen, NJ). If unavailable, the cartilage may be ground to a fine powder using a pestle and mortar placed in a bath of dry ice and liquid nitrogen.
2. To remove proteoglycans, suspend powdered cartilage in 5 vol of 4 M guanidine-HCl, 0.05 M Tris-HCl, pH 7.5, for 24 h at 4°C. Centrifuge at 14,000g for 1 h at 4°C.
3. Discard supernatant and wash cartilage pellet with 0.5 M acetic acid to remove guanidine-HCl. Centrifuge at 14,000g for 1 h at 4°C.
4. To solubilize collagens, resuspend cartilage pellet in 20 vol of 0.5 M acetic acid. Adjust pH of the suspension to 2.8 using 70% formic acid. Add 1 g of pepsin for every 20 g of cartilage (wet weight). Leave stirring for 48 h at 4°C.
5. Centrifuge at 14,000g for 1 h at 4°C and discard pellet. To precipitate type II collagen from the supernatant, add NaCl (powder) gradually with stirring to give a final concentration of 0.89 M. Leave to equilibriate overnight at 4°C then centrifuge at 14,000g for 1 h at 4°C.
6. Dissolve pellet in 0.1 M acetic acid. Then inactivate residual pepsin by dialyzing against 0.02 M Na$_2$HPO4, pH 9.4. The collagen will form a precipitate.
7. Centrifuge at 14,000g for 1 h at 4°C, then redissolve pellet in 0.1 M acetic acid.
8. Dialyze against 0.1 M acetic acid and freeze-dry. Store at 4°C in a dessicator.
9. Purity of the collagen can be assessed on a-5% SDS-polyacrilamide gel. In addition, the presence of contaminating proteoglycans (which may not be detected by gel electrophoresis) can be assessed according to the method of Ratcliffe *(72)*. In brief, 40 µL of sample is added to 250 µL of 1,9-dimethylmethylene blue in formate buffer, pH 3.5, in a 96-well microtiter plate. The absorbance is then read immediately at 600 nm using an ELISA plate reader. A standard curve is constructed by titrating a known concentration of chondroitin sulfate.

3.2. Induction and Assessment of Arthritis

1. Dissolve type II collagen at 4 mg/mL in 0.1 M acetic acid overnight at 4°C, with vigorous stirring. Collagen dissolved in this way may be stored at –20°C (*see* **Note 2**).

2. To produce CFA, grind *M. tuberculosis* with a pestle and mortar to produce a fine powder, then suspend in IFA (approx 3 mg *M. tuberculosis*/mL of IFA). This should be carried out in a fume hood and with a face mask to prevent inhalation of *M. tuberculosis* powder.

3. Emulsify dissolved type II collagen with an equal volume of CFA on ice, using a syringe (preferably glass) or an Ultra-Turrax (IKA) in short bursts to prevent heating. The emulsion should be thick enough not to drip out of the vessel when inverted.

4. Sedate mice by intraperitoneal injection of 100 µL of 10% (v/v) Hypnorm, diluted in distilled water.

5. Shave rumps of mice using electric clippers to facilitate the injection.

6. Inject emulsion intradermally (as far as possible) at two or more sites at the base of the tail using a glass syringe or a latex-free syringe and a 27-gauge needle. The needle becomes blunt easily and should be changed frequently. Each mouse should receive 0.1 mL of emulsion in total. The emulsion should be shallow enough to be visible under the skin (*see* **Note 3**).

7. Some workers boost the mice with a second intraperitoneal injection of 100 µg type II collagen in 100 µL of 0.1 *M* acetic acid, 21 d after primary immunization. However, we have not found this to be necessary.

8. Monitor mice for arthritis every day from day 14 after immunization. The peak time of arthritis onset is around day 30.

9. To compare the clinical severity of arthritis a scoring system may be used where 0 = normal, 1 = slight swelling and/or erythema, 2 = pronounced swelling, 3 = ankylosis. Each limb is graded in this way, giving a maximum score of 12 per mouse. In addition, paw swelling can be monitored using calipers (Poco 2T, Kroeplin).

10. To compare histological severity, paws are removed at post mortem, fixed in buffered formalin (10% v/v), then decalcified in EDTA in buffered formalin (5.5% w/v). The tissues are then embedded in paraffin, sectioned, and stained with hematoxylin and eosin. The severity of arthritis may be graded as mild, moderate, or severe based on the following criteria: mild = minimal synovitis, cartilage loss, and bone erosions limited to discrete foci; moderate = synovitis and erosions present but normal joint architecture intact; severe = synovitis, extensive erosions, joint architecture disrupted. Alternatively, the proportion of joints with erosions (defined as demarcated defects in cartilage or bone filled with inflammatory tissue) can be determined.

3.3. Measurement of Anticollagen IgG

Serum levels of anticollagen IgG provide a marker of the magnitude of the humoral anticollagen response whereas levels of IgG1 and IgG2a serve as extremely valuable in vivo markers of Th2 and Th1 responses, respectively.

1. Make up stock solution of type II collagen in 0.05 *M* Tris-HCl, 0.2 *M* NaCl, pH 7.4, at 1 mg/mL. Aliquot and store at –20°C (*see* **Note 2**).

2. Coat ELISA plate with type II collagen at 2–5 µg/mL in 0.05 *M* Tris-HCl, 0.2 *M* NaCl, pH 7.4, overnight at 4°C.

3. Block for 1 h at room temperature with 2% BSA.

4. Incubate test sera (diluted in PBS/Tween-20) for 2 h at room temperature. Levels of anticollagen IgG may vary enormously between mice and it is important to serially dilute samples to ensure that comparisons are made based on the linear portion of the titration curve. A suggested starting dilution is 1/100, with seven three- to fivefold dilution steps. Include a standard serum sample on each plate. Pooled serum from collagen-immunized mice or affinity purified anticollagen IgG can be used as a standard.
5. Wash 6X with PBS/Tween-20, then detect bound IgG with HRP-conjugated anti-mouse IgG, IgG1 or IgG2a.
6. Develop with TMB substrate. Stop reaction with 4.5 N H_2SO_4 and read at 450 nm.

3.4. Analysis of Cell Responses

1. Proliferative responses may be measured by incorporation of [^{3}H]thymidine in response to stimulation of lymph node cells with type II collagen. Alternatively, cytokines in culture supernatants can be measured by ELISA.
2. Make up stock solution of type II collagen in 0.05 M Tris-HCl, 0.2 M NaCl, pH 7.4, at 1 mg/mL. Collagen in solution can be kept at 4°C for up to 3 mo (for stimulation of T cells only; *see* **Note 2**).
3. Remove draining (inguinal) lymph nodes from collagen-immunized mice.
4. Push through cell strainer using syringe plunger, then wash three times in HBSS.
5. Resuspend at 5×10^6 cells/mL in complete medium and culture for 72 h (37°C; 5% CO_2) in the presence or absence of type II collagen (50 µg/mL).
6. Remove supernatant for measurement of IL-5, IL-10, and IFNγ (*see* **Note 5**). Coat ELISA plates with relevant capture mAb (overnight at 4°C), block with 2% BSA (1 h at room temperature), then add supernatants (overnight at 4°C). Generate standard curve using appropriate recombinant cytokine at a range of 10,000 to 14 pg/mL for IL-5 and IL-10 and 100,000–137 pg/mL for IFNγ. Wash six times with PBS/Tween-20, then incubate with biotinylated detection mAb. Wash six times with PBS/Tween-20, then add HRP-conjugated streptavidin (1 h at room temperature), and develop with TMB substrate. Stop the reaction with 4.5 N H_2SO_4 and read at 450 nm.
7. To determine the rate of T-cell proliferation, pulse cells with [^{3}H]thymidine and culture for a further 16 h. Harvest cells and assess for incorporation of radioactivity.

4. Notes

1. For immunization of mice, type II collagen from bovine, porcine, or chick cartilage is normally used. Alternatively, mouse collagen (derived from mouse sternums) may be used, which results in a more chronic relapsing form of arthritis, which is reported to be more similar to human RA than conventional CIA induced with heterologous collagen (*21*). The yield and solubility of the type II collagen is greater when derived from young animals owing to the reduced level of cross-linking. The sternum, nasal septum, or articular cartilage may be used. A good source is femoral head cartilage from a young calf. Peel off the cartilage from the surface of the bone using a scalpel wearing chain mail gloves and eye protection for safety. The cartilage is white. Avoid the underlying bone, which is pink. In the case

of sternum or nasal septum the cartilage should be chopped into small pieces. Type II collagen for immunization is also commercially available.

2. Once in solution, it is important for type II collagen to be maintained at low temperature to prevent denaturation. This is important for successful immunization and for measurement of anticollagen antibody levels whereas T-cell activity is less sensitive to the conformational state of the collagen molecule.

3. Two factors of importance in determining incidence of arthritis are the concentrations of *M. tuberculosis* in the adjuvant and collagen in the acetic acid. To establish the system, high concentrations can be used, e.g., 3 mg mycobacterium per milliliter of IFA and collagen at 4 mg/mL of acetic acid. This invariably induces high incidence but the arthritis is severe and acute in nature, therefore the amounts can subsequently be reduced once the system is known to be working.

    The most likely reasons for a failure to induce a high incidence of arthritis include the following: (1) the collagen preparation is of low purity or in a denatured form. (2) There is concurrent infection in the mouse colony, the mice are immature (less than 8 wk of age), or females rather than males are used. (3) The concentration of type II collagen or *M. tuberculosis* in the emulsion used for immunization is insufficient and the emulsion is not thick enough or is injected too deeply.

4. Following immunization, mice will develop arthritis of varying degrees of severity and novel treatment regimens may produce unexpected adverse effects. Hence, mice should be monitored on a daily basis for signs of ill-health or distress. Clearly defined humane endpoints should be strictly enforced. For example, any mouse showing severe and sustained paw swelling should be humanely killed. Any mouse which has lost 20% or more of its body weight should be humanely killed. Any mouse with severe lameness should be humanely killed. Any mouse with dyspnoea, ruffled fur, weakness, dehydration, or a hunched appearance should be humanely killed. Any mouse showing blistering at the injection site should be humanely killed. In addition, the duration of experiments involving arthritic animals should be minimized, compatible with the aims of the study.

5. In general, IL-5, IL-10, and IFNγ can be measured in culture supernatants of collagen-stimulated T cells taken from mice with active disease, whereas IL-2 and IL-4 are difficult to detect, probably because of consumption of these cytokines by proliferating T cells. An alternative is therefore to study cytokine expression by intracellular staining and fluorescence-activated cell sorting (FACS) analysis. Another important factor is that Th2 cells are usually found in low abundance in DBA/1 mice immunized with CFA, although immunomodulatory treatments may influence the Th1:Th2 ratio.

References

1. Elliott, M. J., Maini, R. N., Feldmann, M., et al. (1993) Treatment of rheumatoid arthritis with chimeric monoclonal antibodies to tumor necrosis factor α. *Arthritis Rheum.* **36,** 1681–1690.
2. Elliott, M. J., Maini, R. N., Feldmann, M., et al. (1994) Treatment with a chimeric monoclonal antibody to tumour necrosis factor α suppresses disease activity in

rheumatoid arthritis: results of a multi-centre, randomised, double blind trial. *Lancet* **344,** 1105–1110.

3. Elliott, M. J., Maini, R. N., Feldmann, M., et al. (1994) Repeated therapy with a monoclonal antibody to tumour necrosis factor α in patients with rheumatoid arthritis. *Lancet* **344,** 1125–1127.

4. Moreland, L. W., Baumgartner, S. W., Schiff, M. H., et al. (1997) Treatment of rheumatoid arthritis with a recombinant human tumor necrosis factor receptor (p75)-Fc fusion protein. *N. Engl. J. Med.* **337,** 141–147.

5. Weinblatt, M. E., Kremer, J. M., Bankhurst, A. D., et al. (1999) A trial of etanercept, a recombinant tumor necrosis factor receptor: Fc fusion protein, in patients with rheumatoid arthritis receiving methotrexate. *N. Engl. J. Med.* **340,** 253–259.

6. Kempeni, J. (1999) Preliminary results of early clinical trials with the fully human anti-TNF monoclonal antibody D2E7. *Ann. Rheum. Dis.* **58,** I70–I72.

7. den Broeder, A., van de Putte, L., Rau, R., et al. (2002) A single dose, placebo controlled study of the fully human anti-tumor necrosis factor-alpha antibody adalimumab (D2E7) in patients with rheumatoid arthritis. *J. Rheumatol.* **29,** 2288–2298.

8. Weinblatt, M. E., Keystone, E. C., Furst, D. E., et al. (2003) Adalimumab, a fully human anti-tumor necrosis factor alpha monoclonal antibody, for the treatment of rheumatoid arthritis in patients taking concomitant methotrexate: the ARMADA trial. *Arthritis Rheum.* **48,** 35–45.

9. Williams, R. O. (1998) Rodent models of arthritis: relevance for human disease. *Clin. Exp. Immunol.* **114,** 330–332.

10. Ranges, G. E., Sriram, S., and Cooper, S. M. (1985) Prevention of type II collageninduced arthritis by in vivo treatment with anti-L3T4. *J. Exp. Med.* **162,** 1105–1110.

11. Hom, J. T., Butler, L. D., Riedl, P. E., and Bendele, A. M. (1988) The progression of the inflammation in established collagen-induced arthritis can be altered by treatments with immunological or pharmacological agents which inhibit T cell activities. *Eur. J. Immunol.* **18,** 881–888.

12. Webb, L. M., Walmsley, M. J., and Feldmann, M. (1996) Prevention and amelioratrion of collagen-induced arthritis by blockade of the CD28 co-stimulatory pathway: requirement for both B7-1 and B7-2. *Eur. J. Immunol.* **26,** 2320–2328.

13. Malfait, A. -M., Butler, D. M., Presky, D. H., Maini, R. N., Brennan, F. M., and Feldmann, M. (1998) Blockade of IL-12 during the induction of collagen-induced arthritis (CIA) markedly attenuates the severity of the arthritis. *Clin. Exp. Immunol.* **111,** 377–383.

14. Holmdahl, R., Andersson, M. E., Goldschmidt, T. J., et al. (1989) Collagen induced arthritis as an experimental model for rheumatoid arthritis. Immunogenetics, pathogenesis and autoimmunity. *APMIS* **97,** 575–584.

15. Trentham, D. E. (1982) Collagen arthritis as a relevant model for rheumatoid arthritis: evidence pro and con. *Arthritis Rheum.* **25,** 911–916.

16. Williams, R. O., Williams, D. G., and Maini, R. N. (1992) Anti-type II collagen ELISA. Increased disease specificity following removal of anionic contaminants from salt-fractionated type II collagen. *J. Immunol. Methods* **147,** 93–100.

17. Marinova-Mutafchieva, L., Williams, R. O., Mason, L. J., Mauri, C., Feldmann, M., and Maini, R. N. (1997) Dynamics of proinflammatory cytokine expression in the joints of mice with collagen-induced arthritis (CIA). *Clin. Exp. Immunol.* **107,** 507–512.
18. Hegen, M., Sun, L., Uozumi, N., et al. (2003) Cytosolic phospholipase A2alpha-deficient mice are resistant to collagen-induced arthritis. *J. Exp. Med.* **197,** 1297–1302.
19. Holmdahl, R., Jansson, L., Larsson, E., Rubin, K., and Klareskog, L. (1986) Homologous type II collagen induces chronic and progressive arthritis in mice. *Arthritis Rheum.* **29,** 106–113.
20. Boissier, M. C., Feng, X. Z., Carlioz, A., Roudier, R., and Fournier, C. (1987) Experimental autoimmune arthritis in mice. I. Homologous type II collagen is responsible for self-perpetuating chronic polyarthritis. *Ann. Rheum. Dis.* **46,** 691–700.
21. Malfait, A. M., Williams, R. O., Malik, A. S., Maini, R. N., and Feldmann, M. (2001) Chronic relapsing homologous collagen-induced arthritis in DBA/1 mice as a model for testing disease-modifying and remission-inducing therapies. *Arthritis Rheum.* **44,** 1215–1224.
22. Huang, J. C., Vestberg, M., Minguela, A., Holmdahl, R., and Ward, E. S. (2004) Analysis of autoreactive T cells associated with murine collagen-induced arthritis using peptide-MHC multimers. *Int. Immunol.* **16,** 283–293.
23. Keffer, J., Probert, L., Cazlaris, H., et al. (1991) Transgenic mice expressing human tumour necrosis factor: a predictive genetic model of arthritis. *EMBO J.* **10,** 4025–4031.
24. Kontoyiannis, D., Pasparakis, M., Pizarro, T. T., Cominelli, F., and Kollias, G. (1999) Impaired on/off regulation of TNF biosynthesis in mice lacking TNF AU-rich elements: implications for joint and gut-associated immunopathologies. *Immunity* **10,** 387–398.
25. Probert, L., Plows, D., Kontogeorgos, G., and Kollias, G. (1995) The type I interleukin-1 receptor acts in series with tumor necrosis factor (TNF) to induce arthritis in TNF-transgenic mice. *Eur. J. Immunol.* **25,** 1794–1797.
26. Brennan, F. M., Chantry, D., Jackson, A., Maini, R., and Feldmann, M. (1989) Inhibitory effect of TNFα antibodies on synovial cell interleukin-1 production in rheumatoid arthritis. *Lancet* **2,** 244–247.
27. Niki, Y., Yamada, H., Seki, S., et al. (2001) Macrophage- and neutrophil-dominant arthritis in human IL-1 alpha transgenic mice. *J. Clin. Invest.* **107,** 1127–1135.
28. Fell, H. B. and Jubb, R. W. (1977) The effect of synovial tissue on the breakdown of articular cartilage in organ culture. *Arthritis Rheum.* **20,** 1359–1371.
29. Saklatvala, J., Pilsworth, L. M., Sarsfield, S. J., Gavrilovic, J., and Heath, J. K. (1984) Pig catabolin is a form of interleukin 1. Cartilage and bone resorb, fibroblasts make prostaglandin and collagenase, and thymocyte proliferation is augmented in response to one protein. *Biochem. J.* **224,** 461–466.
30. Saklatvala, J., Sarsfield, S. J., and Townsend, Y. (1985) Pig interleukin 1. Purification of two immunologically different leukocyte proteins that cause cartilage resorption, lymphocyte activation, and fever. *J. Exp. Med.* **162,** 1208–1222.

31. McIntyre, K. W., Shuster, D. J., Gillooly, K. M., et al. (1996) Reduced incidence and severity of collagen-induced arthritis in interleukin-12-deficient mice. *Eur. J. Immunol.* **26,** 2933–2938.

32. Wei, X. Q., Leung, B. P., Arthur, H. M., McInnes, I. B., and Liew, F. Y. (2001) Reduced incidence and severity of collagen-induced arthritis in mice lacking IL-18. *J. Immunol.* **166,** 517–521.

33. Plater-Zyberk, C., Joosten, L. A., Helsen, M. M., et al. (2001) Therapeutic effect of neutralizing endogenous IL-18 activity in the collagen-induced model of arthritis. *J. Clin. Invest.* **108,** 1825–1832.

34. Alonzi, T., Fattori, E., Lazzaro, D., et al. (1998) Interleukin 6 is required for the development of collagen-induced arthritis. *J. Exp. Med.* **187,** 461–468.

35. Sasai, M., Saeki, Y., Ohshima, S., et al. (1999) Delayed onset and reduced severity of collagen-induced arthritis in interleukin-6-deficient mice. *Arthritis Rheum.* **42,** 1635–1643.

36. Takagi, N., Mihara, M., Moriya, Y., et al. (1998) Blockage of interleukin-6 receptor ameliorates joint disease in murine collagen-induced arthritis. *Arthritis Rheum.* **41,** 2117–2121.

37. Mihara, M., Kotoh, M., Nishimoto, N., et al. (2001) Humanized antibody to human interleukin-6 receptor inhibits the development of collagen arthritis in cynomolgus monkeys. *Clin. Immunol.* **98,** 319–326.

38. Nakae, S., Nambu, A., Sudo, K., and Iwakura, Y. (2003) Suppression of immune induction of collagen-induced arthritis in IL-17-deficient mice. *J. Immunol.* **171,** 6173–6177.

39. Lubberts, E., Joosten, L. A., Oppers, B., et al. (2001) IL-1-independent role of IL-17 in synovial inflammation and joint destruction during collagen-induced arthritis. *J. Immunol.* **167,** 1004–1013.

40. Lubberts, E., Koenders, M. I., Oppers-Walgreen, B., et al. (2004) Treatment with a neutralizing anti-murine interleukin-17 antibody after the onset of collagen-induced arthritis reduces joint inflammation, cartilage destruction, and bone erosion. *Arthritis Rheum.* **50,** 650–659.

41. Lawlor, K. E., Campbell, I. K., Metcalf, D., et al. (2004) Critical role for granulocyte colony-stimulating factor in inflammatory arthritis. *Proc. Natl. Acad. Sci. USA* **101,** 11,398–11,403.

42. Cuzzocrea, S., Mazzon, E., Dugo, L., et al. (2001) Absence of endogeneous interleukin-10 enhances the evolution of murine type-II collagen-induced arthritis. *Eur. Cytokine Netw.* **12,** 568–580.

43. Johansson, A. C., Hansson, A. S., Nandakumar, K. S., Backlund, J., and Holmdahl, R. (2001) IL-10-deficient B10.Q mice develop more severe collagen-induced arthritis, but are protected from arthritis induced with anti-type II collagen antibodies. *J. Immunol.* **167,** 3505–3512.

44. Walmsley, M., Katsikis, P. D., Abney, E., et al. (1996) IL-10 inhibits progression of established collagen-induced arthritis. *Arthritis Rheum.* **39,** 495–503.

45. Mauri, C., Williams, R. O., Walmsley, M., and Feldmann, M. (1996) Relationship between Th1/Th2 cytokine patterns and the arthritogenic response in collagen-induced arthritis. *Eur. J. Immunol.* **26,** 1511–1518.

46. Vermeire, K., Heremans, H., Vandeputte, M., Huang, S., Billiau, A., and Matthys, P. (1997) Accelerated collagen-induced arthritis in IFN-gamma receptor-deficient mice. *J. Immunol.* **158,** 5507–5513.

47. Manoury-Schwartz, B., Chiocchia, G., Bessis, N., et al. (1997) High susceptibility to collagen-induced arthritis in mice lacking IFN-gamma receptors. *J. Immunol.* **158,** 5501–5506.

48. Williams, R. O., Williams, D. G., Feldmann, M., and Maini, R. N. (1993) Increased limb involvement in murine collagen-induced arthritis following treatment with anti-interferon-gamma. *Clin. Exp. Immunol.* **92,** 323–327.

49. Boissier, M. C., Chiocchia, G., Bessis, N., et al. (1995) Biphasic effect of interferon-gamma in murine collagen-induced arthritis. *Eur. J. Immunol.* **25,** 1184–1190.

50. Brennan, F. M., Zachariae, C. O., Chantry, D., et al. (1990) Detection of interleukin 8 biological activity in synovial fluids from patients with rheumatoid arthritis and production of interleukin 8 mRNA by isolated synovial cells. *Eur. J. Immunol.* **20,** 2141–2144.

51. Alvaro-Garcia, J. M., Zvaifler, N. J., Brown, C. B., Kaushansky, L., and Firestein, G. S. (1991) Cytokines in chronic inflammatory arthritis. VI. Analysis of the synovial cells involved in granulocyte-macrophage colony stimulating factor production and gene expression in rheumatoid arthritis and its regulation by IL-1 and TNFα. *J. Immunol.* **146,** 3365–3371.

52. Butler, D. M., Maini, R. N., Feldmann, M., and Brennan, F. M. (1995) Modulation of proinflammatory cytokine release in rheumatoid synovial membrane cell cultures. Comparison of monoclonal anti TNF-alpha antibody with the interleukin-1 receptor antagonist. *Eur. Cytokine Netw.* **6,** 225–230.

53. Thorbecke, G. J., Shah, R., Leu, C. H., Kuruvilla, A. P., Hardison, A. M., and Palladino, M. A. (1992) Involvement of endogenous tumor necrosis factor α and transforming growth factor β during induction of collagen type II arthritis in mice. *Proc. Natl. Acad. Sci. USA* **89,** 7375–7379.

54. Williams, R. O., Feldmann, M., and Maini, R. N. (1992) Anti-tumor necrosis factor ameliorates joint disease in murine collagen-induced arthritis. *Proc. Natl. Acad. Sci. USA* **89,** 9784–9788.

55. Piguet, P. F., Grau, G. E., Vesin, C., Loetscher, H., Gentz, R., and Lesslauer, W. (1992) Evolution of collagen arthritis in mice is arrested by treatment with anti-tumour necrosis factor (TNF) antibody or a recombinant soluble TNF receptor. *Immunology* **77,** 510–514.

56. Sheehan, K. C., Ruddle, N. H., and Schreiber, R. D. (1989) Generation and characterization of hamster monoclonal antibodies that neutralize murine tumor necrosis factors. *J. Immunol.* **142,** 3884–3893.

57. Wooley, P. H., Dutcher, J., Widmer, M. B., and Gillis, S. (1993) Influence of a recombinant human soluble tumour necrosis factor receptor Fc fusion protein on type II collagen-induced arthritis in mice. *J. Immunol.* **151,** 6602–6607.

58. Williams, R. O., Ghrayeb, J., Feldmann, M., and Maini, R. N. (1995) Successful therapy of collagen-induced arthritis with TNF receptor-IgG fusion protein and combination with anti-CD4. *Immunology* **84,** 433–439.

59. Issekutz, A. C., Meager, A., Otterness, I., and Issekutz, T. B. (1994) The role of tumour necrosis factor-alpha and IL-1 in polymorphonuclear leucocyte and T lymphocyte recruitment to joint inflammation in adjuvant arthritis. *Clin. Exp. Immunol.* **97,** 26–32.

60. Van den Berg, W. B., Joosten, L. A., Helsen, M., and van de Loo, F. A. (1994) Amelioration of established murine collagen-induced arthritis with anti-IL-1 treatment. *Clin. Exp. Immunol.* **95,** 237–243.

61. Joosten, L. A. B., Helen, M. M. A., van de Loo, F. A. J., and Van den Berg, W. B. (1996) Anticytokine treatment of established type II collagen-induced arthritis in DBA/1 mice: a comparative study using anti-TNFα, anti-IL-1α/β, and IL-1Ra. *Arthritis Rheum.* **39,** 797–809.

62. Lewthwaite, J., Blake, S., Hardingham, T., et al. (1995) Role of TNFα in the induction of antigen induced arthritis in the rabbit and the anti-arthritic effect of species specific TNFα neutralising monoclonal antibodies. *Ann. Rheum. Dis.* **54,** 366–374.

63. van de Loo, F. A., Joosten, L. A., van Lent, P. L., Arntz, O. J., and Van den Berg, W. B. (1995) Role of interleukin-1, tumor necrosis factor alpha, and interleukin-6 in cartilage proteoglycan metabolism and destruction. Effect of in situ blocking in murine antigen- and zymosan-induced arthritis. *Arthritis Rheum.* **38,** 164–172.

64. Kuiper, S., Joosten, L. A., Bendele, A. M., et al. (1998) Different roles of tumour necrosis factor alpha and interleukin 1 in murine streptococcal cell wall arthritis. *Cytokine* **10,** 690–702.

65. Geiger, T., Towbin, H., Cosenti-Vargas, A., et al. (1993) Neutralization of interleukin-1β activity in vivo with a monoclonal antibody alleviates collagen-induced arthritis in DBA/1 mice and prevents the associated acute-phase response. *Clin. Exp. Rheumatol.* **11,** 515–522.

66. Bendele, A., McAbee, T., Sennello, G., Frazier, J., Chlipala, E., and McCabe, D. (1999) Efficacy of sustained blood levels of interleukin-1 receptor antagonist in animal models of arthritis: comparison of efficacy in animal models with human clinical data. *Arthritis Rheum.* **42,** 498–506.

67. Bessis, N., Guery, L., Mantovani, A., et al. (2000) The type II decoy receptor of IL-1 inhibits murine collagen-induced arthritis. *Eur. J. Immunol.* **30,** 867–875.

68. Bresnihan, B., Alvaro-Gracia, J. M., Cobby, M., Doherty, M., Domljan, Z., Emery, P., et al. (1998) Treatment of rheumatoid arthritis with recombinant human interleukin-1 receptor antagonist. *Arthritis Rheum.* **41,** 2196–2204.

69. Williams, R. O., Marinova-Mutafchieva, L., Feldmann, M., and Maini, R. N. (2000) Evaluation of TNFα and IL-1 blockade in collagen-induced arthritis and comparison with combined anti-TNFα/anti-CD4 therapy. *J. Immunol.* **165,** 7240–7245.

70. Miller, E. J. (1972) Structural studies on cartilage collagen employing limited cleavage and solubilization with pepsin. *Biochemistry* **11,** 4903–4909.

71. Herbage, D., Bouillet, J., and Bernengo, J. C. (1977) Biochemical and physiochemical characterization of pepsin-solubilized type-II collagen from bovine articular cartilage. *Biochem. J.* **161,** 303–312.

72. Ratcliffe, A., Doherty, M., Maini, R. N., and Hardingham, T. E. (1988) Increased concentrations of proteoglycan components in the synovial fluids of patients with acute but not chronic joint disease. *Ann. Rheum. Dis.* **47,** 826–832.

14

Novel Opportunities for Therapeutic Targeting in Systemic Autoimmune Diseases

Meryem Ouarzane and Moncef Zouali

Summary

Systemic autoimmune diseases, such as systemic lupus erythematosus and rheumatoid arthritis, continue to cause significant morbidity in affected persons. In the past few years, significant progress was made in understanding their pathogenesis and the underlying molecular mechanisms. As a result, a number of new exciting therapeutic options have become available, and novel therapeutic targets have emerged, including B-cell depletion therapies, B cell-activating factor of tumor necrosis factor family (BAFF) antagonists, and FcγRIIB receptor antagonists. Also promising is the current interest centered on the development of inhibition of signal transduction pathways, such as pharmacological inhibitors that act at various levels of signal transduction pathways.

Key Words: Autoimmune diseases; B lymphocytes; TNFα; complement components; signaling; systemic lupus erythematosus; rheumatoid arthritis.

1. Introduction

The ability of the immune system to distinguish self from nonself is central to its capacity to protect against pathogens and, at the same time, maintains nonresponsiveness to its own components. This property is established at discrete checkpoints, both during early development and adulthood. To date, several early developmental checkpoint mechanisms have been identified. These include clonal deletion *(1–3)* of autoreactive lymphocytes during early development of the immune system, clonal anergy *(4)*, which converts autoreactive cells to a state that precludes them from becoming activated, and editing *(5–7)*, a mechanism for modifying self-reactive B cells that renders them nonautoreactive. Although these developmental checkpoints purge the immune repertoire from autoreactive cells, the processes of central

From: *Methods in Molecular Biology, vol. 361, Target Discovery and Validation Reviews and Protocols*
Volume 2, Emerging Molecular Targets and Treatment Options
Edited by: M. Sioud © Humana Press Inc., Totowa, NJ

tolerance remain incomplete, allowing self-reactive cells to escape into the periphery *(8,9)*.

Failure of one of these self-tolerance mechanisms results in pathogenic autoimmunity, such as systemic lupus erythematosus (SLE) and rheumatoid arthritis (RA). SLE is a chronic systemic autoimmune disease that results in inflammation of, and damage to a range of organ systems. Approximately one-third of lupus cases have a mild form of the disease characterized by elevated titers of antinuclear antibodies, arthritis, and skin and/or mucosal membrane involvement *(10)*. However, the majority of patients will suffer additional and more severe clinical manifestations, such as renal inflammation (nephritis), and central nervous system vasculitis (cerebritis). The disease aggregates in families, suggesting an important role for genetic predisposition, and woman are about 10 times more likely to develop SLE than men. Autoantibodies directed against nuclear antigens (e.g., histones, single-stranded DNA, double-stranded DNA, Ro, La) are found in virtually all cases. RA is a chronic, systemic autoimmune disease that targets synovial joints, and is often accompanied by an array of extra-articular manifestations. The immunopathogenesis of RA is multifactorial (*see* Chapter 13). Evidence suggests that the interaction between an unknown exogenous or endogenous antigen via antigen-presenting cells and CD4$^+$ T-helper cells is involved in the induction of the immune response in RA. Subsequent recruitment and activation of monocytes and macrophages occurs with secretion of proinflammatory cytokines, in particular tumor necrosis factor-α (TNFα) and interleukin (IL)-1 into the synovial cavity. Release of these cytokines mediates tissue destruction by activation of chondrocytes and fibroblasts, which release collagenases and metalloproteinases, resulting in cartilage loss and bone erosion. B-lymphocyte dysregulation with production of rheumatoid factor and other antibodies, formation of immune complexes and release of destructive mediators also contributes to this process *(11)*.

Drugs do exist for the majority of autoimmune illnesses, but the challenge is to design new drugs that prevent autoimmune attacks without seriously affecting the body's ability to defend itself against infection. Understanding the development of autoimmunity is therefore crucial toward improving the management of autoimmune diseases. As will be discussed below, the rapid expansion of knowledge on autoimmunity is fuelling the development of a novel approach known as targeted immunotherapy. Focusing on SLE and RA, we summarize therapeutic targets that offer promising avenues for future development in systemic autoimmune diseases.

2. The Key Role for B Lymphocytes in Autoimmune Diseases

For some time, autoimmune diseases have been considered to be mediated essentially by T cells. Of late, emerging data suggest that B cells play an important role in these diseases than previously thought. While it has long been known that levels of autoantibodies such those directed to the thyroid stimulating hormone receptor that correlate with disease severity and progression in Graves disease, and those directed to double-stranded DNA that are often elevated in lupus disease, it is becoming appreciated that B cells play more than one role in these diseases *(12)*. Not only are they the precursors of antibody-secreting plasma cells, but they also act as remarkably effective antigen-presenting cells, suggesting that they may play a potential role in autoimmunity via abnormal autoantigen presentation. B cells can also secrete cytokines, such as TNFα, that exacerbate the autoimmune and inflammatory responses. In addition, autoreactive B cells express ligands that bind costimulatory receptors on T cells. Along with presentation of self-derived peptides on cell surface major histocompatibility complex class II molecules, this can drive activation of autoreactive T cells. Therefore, targeting B cells may prove to be an effective avenue for the development of novel therapies for systemic autoimmune diseases.

2.1. B-Cell Depletion Therapy

The important role of B cells in SLE and RA etiologies is supported by the encouraging results of clinical trials aiming to eliminate B cells in affected patients. B-cell development is characterized by a series of changes of surface phenotypic markers. One of them CD20 is expressed at intermediate stages and is lost during terminal differentiation to immunoglobulin-producing plasma cells. A chimeric monoclonal antibody (MAb) against human CD20, called Rituximab, is now used in clinical trials of several autoimmune diseases. Its mode of action remains under investigation, but the available evidence suggests that this antibody acts via complement-mediated and antibody-dependent, cell mediated-toxicity, and induction of apoptosis *(13)*.

In RA, Rituximab is effective, and clinical benefits are observed 6 mo after only two infusions *(14)*. The treatment is accompanied with a major B-cell depletion and a large drop of rheumatoid factor titers, whereas total immunoglobulin levels show little changes *(15,16)*. In SLE too, the beneficial effect of Rituximab therapy has been demonstrated by a study that provides sufficient evidence of excellent tolerability and high efficacy *(17)*. Rituximab not only reduced B-cell numbers and IgG levels, but also downregulated CD40 and CD80 expression on B cells, suggesting a possible disturbance of T-cell activation through these costimulatory molecules *(18)*. Reduction of both the quantity and the functions of B cells suggest that Rituximab could improve the disease course in patients with SLE.

2.2. BAFF Antagonists

BAFF, also known as BLys, is a member of the TNF family that acts as an essential survival factor for B cells *(19,20)* and appears to play a central role in the development of some autoimmune diseases and B-cell malignancies. It has a potent effect on B cells, but also has direct effects on other cell types. This specificity is achieved at the molecular level by binding to three different receptors (TACI, BCMA, and the BAFF receptor *[19–22]*).

Two major avenues of evidence link BAFF to autoimmunity, namely studies in animal models and measurement of BAFF levels in patients with systemic autoimmune diseases. BAFF levels are elevated in autoimmune mice, notably the (NZB × NZW) F_1 and MLR-*lpr* strains *(21)*. In patients with RA, SLE and other systemic autoimmune diseases, BAFF levels are also elevated *(23)*. During the course of SLE, BAFF levels fluctuate *(24)*, and BAFF has been proposed to be a biomarker for SLE disease activity. This information is suggestive of a link between BAFF and development of autoimmunity, and implicates BAFF in the etiology and progression of autoimmune diseases. As such, antagonism to BAFF may provide a novel therapeutic approach to the treatment of autoimmune diseases. Two types of antagonists are currently in development. First, a fully human MAb against BAFF (LymphoStat-B) has entered clinical trials. Second soluble forms of the BAFF receptor, in which the extracellular domain of a BAFF receptor is fused with the Fc domain of an immunoglobulin molecule, are in various stages of development.

2.3. The Inhibitory Coreceptor FcγRIIB: A Potential Target

The balance between stimulatory and inhibitory signals regulates the activation and expansion of lymphoid cells. Inhibitory signaling, in particular, is a critical feature of peripheral tolerance, providing a means for establishing thresholds for stimulation and for active deletion of autoreactive cells from the peripheral repertoire.

Previous work has demonstrated that the expression of the inhibitory Fc receptor FcγRIIB is required for the maintenance of self-tolerance *(25)*. C57BL/6 mice deficient in this receptor develop spontaneous lupus-like autoimmunity. Several other stains of mice that develop spontaneous autoimmune disease, such as NZB, NOD, BXSB, and MLR, have also been shown to express reduced levels of FcγRIIB on activated or germinal center B cells. This reduced expression results from a polymorphism in the promoter of the corresponding gene. These results suggest that the levels of FcγRIIB expressed on some B cells may regulate their ability to maintain tolerance, and that relatively small changes in the expression of this inhibitory receptor may permit the survival and expansion of autoreactive cells *(26)*. Thus, changes in the surface expression of this receptor appear to be critical for determining disease progression, and these changes provide a rational basis for a therapeutic approach based on manipulating the expression of this receptor to restore self-tolerance in autoimmune diseases *(27)*.

3. The Role of the Complement in Autoimmune Diseases

In addition to its important roles in the innate immune system to foreign antigens, the complement system is increasingly recognized to be causally involved in tissue injury during ischemic, inflammatory and autoimmune diseases *(28,29)*. Studies of human diseases have provided clinical evidence for activation of the alternative pathway. Indeed, the presence of activated C3 or C4 fragments and other activated components of the alternative pathway in target organs has been described in several clinical settings *(29)*. The involvement of the complement in RA has been suggested by the observation that the complement activity of the joint fluid from patients is significantly lower than that of control subjects. In addition, significant increases in soluble complement activation fragments in the joint fluid, as well as enhanced local production of complement proteins in synovial tissue, are found *(30)*.

In SLE, the first solid evidence that complement inhibitors could ameliorate target organ damage came from the finding that an inhibitory anti-C5 MAb could block the development of glomerulonephritis in the (NZB × NZW) F_1 mouse model of lupus. With regard to the alternative pathway, MRL-*lpr* mice are also protected from renal disease, as are mice in which activation of the classical and alternative pathways of C3 is partially blocked *(28)*. Thus, it is anticipated that complement inhibitors will belong to the array of therapies available for disease management.

4. Interfering With Dendritic Cell Functions

Dendritic cells contribute to central tolerance in the thymus by presenting antigens to T cells and deleting the T cells that exhibit strong autoreactivity. However, dendritic cells also play a pivotal role in peripheral tolerance. In the absence of infection or inflammation, dendritic cells remain immature and capture antigens via a number of mechanisms, such as phagocytosis and macropinocytosis *(31)*. These immature dendritic cells contribute to deleting autoreactive lymphocytes and to expanding the population of regulatory T cells, thereby ensuring peripheral tolerance. Dendritic cells mature when they come into contact with antigen via surface receptors called Toll-like receptors (TLR) and via receptors belonging to the TNF family (TNFα and CD40 ligand). Dendritic cell activation leads to T-cell activation, in particular via expression of costimulatory molecules (B7, CD40), chemokines receptors (CCR-7), and cytokines (IL-12) *(31)*.

A major role for dendritic cells has been established in lupus. Dendritic cell dysfunction may account for the loss of peripheral tolerance that characterizes lupus. Peripheral blood CD14$^+$ monocytes from lupus patients, but not from normal controls, may act as mature dendritic cells that activate potentially autoreactive T cells. Maturation of these CD14$^+$ cells is induced by elevated circulating levels of interferon-α (INFα) produced by a population of dendritic cells that infiltrate lupus lesions. These crucial pieces of evidence suggest that INFα and dendritic cells may represent therapeutic targets in patients with lupus *(32,33)*.

5. Disruption of the Interferon-Activating Pathway

An important clue that interferon (INF) might contribute to lupus comes from a series of studies in patients who received INFα as a therapeutic agent for viral hepatitis or carcinoid tumors. Nearly a quarter of INFα-treated subjects (22%) developed a positive antinuclear antibodies blood test *(34)*, and one in five (19%) developed overt autoimmunity, including a small number who developed SLE *(35)*.

In one possible scenario, INF production promotes differentiation of SLE monocytes into activated, antigen-presenting dendritic cells, which migrate to lymph nodes and tissues, and activate autoreactive CD4+ T cells *(36)*. T cells in turn stimulate self-reactive B cells to produce autoantibodies, particularly those with specificities for nucleic acids and associated proteins. These autoantibodies bind endogenous nucleic acids and chromatin derived from apoptotic material to form chromatin-containing immune complexes that stimulate further INF production by plasmacytoid dendritic cells (pDCs), and B-cell proliferation and differentiation by cross-linking of both the B-cell receptor and TLR-9. Aside from TLRs, several proteins expressed on the pDC surface might also contribute to IFN production. Monoclonal antibodies against blood dendritic cell antigen 2 (BDCA-2), a c-type lectin expressed on pDCs, prevent the production of INF by both normal and SLE pDCs in response to SLE serum and viral inducers. However, ligation of CD40 on pDCs synergizes with TLR-9 signaling to induce INF. Interestingly, activated SLE T cells express increased levels of CD40 ligand (CD40L), and levels of soluble CD40L in lupus blood correlate with disease activity. Taken together, this proposed series of events suggests new targets for therapeutic intervention aimed at disrupting the IFN activation pathway in SLE *(37)*.

6. Antitumor-Necrosis-α Therapies in RA

TNFα is an inflammatory cytokine that plays a pivotal role in the pathogenic mechanisms of RA *(11,38)*. It binds to two widely expressed receptors, type 1 (p55) and type 2 (p75), and soluble receptors also influence the activity of the cytokine. The importance of this cytokine in RA is supported by its overexpression in RA synovium, by data from in vitro synovial cell cultures with the use of anti-TNFα antibody, and by animal studies, which demonstrated development of disease in mice transgenic for TNFα and amelioration of the symptoms after treatment with anti-TNFα agents. Currently, there are three agents available which inhibit the action of TNFα. First; Infliximab is a chimeric anti-TNFα antibody that binds soluble and membrane-bound TNFα, thereby impairing binding to its receptors. In addition, it also mediates killing of cells expressing TNFα *(39)*. Second, Adalimumab is a recombinant human MAb that binds TNFα, thereby precluding binding to its receptor. This antibody also lyses cells expressing the cytokine on their surface *(40)*. Third, Etanercept is a soluble TNFα receptor fusion protein composed of two dimers, each with a ligand-binding portion of the type 2 receptor linked to the Fc portion of human IgG1. The protein binds to both TNFα and TNFβ, preventing each from interacting with its respective receptor *(41)*.

7. RANK, RANKL, and Osteoprotegerin: New Target for RA Treatment

It has been known for some time that RA is characterized by destruction of joint cartilage and bone erosion. However, it is only recently that a major role in bone erosion has been attributed to the receptor activator of nuclear factor κB ligand (RANKL), released by activated lymphocytes and osteoblasts *(42)*. In vitro, binding of RANKL to the cognate RANK, expressed on the surface of osteoclasts, results in osteoclastrogenesis by differentiation of monocyte/macrophage progenitors to osteoclasts and activation of mature osteoclasts *(43)*.

Osteoprotegerin (OPG) produced by activated osteoblasts, is a soluble decoy receptor for RANKL and competes with RANK for RANKL binding *(44)*. Consequently, OPG is an effective inhibitor of osteoclast maturation and activation in vitro and in vivo *(45)*. These observations suggest that inhibition of the downstream RANKL effectors via OPG or other drugs should prevent bone destruction and cartilage damage in patients with RA. Therefore, modulation of these systems provides an opportunity to inhibit bone loss and deformity in chronic arthritis.

8. Anti-CD40 Ligand Therapy

Production of pathogenic antibodies in SLE requires T-cell help; along with ligation of the B-cell surface immunoglobulin receptor by antigen. It is likely that macrophages, dendritic cells, and endothelial cells are also activated by interaction with T-cells and contribute to lupus pathology. CD40 ligand (CD40L, CD154), a member of TNF family of cell surface molecules, mediates these contact-dependent signals delivered by CD4[+] T helper cells to CD40[+] target cells *(46)*.

Several tissue injuries and immune-mediated pathologies were found to involve CD40-CD40L signaling. Disruption of this pathway in animal models led to the improvement of graft survival. CD40–CD154 interactions were also shown to play a significant role in the progression of autoimmunity, and the production of auto-antibodies in SLE *(47)*. High-level expression of CD154 *(48)* has been detected in T cells from patient with SLE, RA, and other autoimmune disease, indicating that such cells could account for the high-level expression of immune accessory molecules on B cells of patients with active disease. An increased serum level of soluble CD154 was also reported in SLE and RA in correlation with the relevant autoantibodies and with disease activity. Anti-CD154 antibody therapy prevents autoantibody production and renal immune complex deposition in lupus nephritis, indicating that disruption of this pathway could be a beneficial treatment in SLE *(49)*. Clinical trials are under way *(50)*.

9. Signal Transduction Pathways: New Targets for Treating RA and SLE

The last few years have witnessed a radical change in the treatment of immune system-mediated joint diseases, with the advent of biotherapeutic agents directed at targets identified by basic research into the mechanism of inflammation *(51)*. These agents block the proinflammatory effects of cytokines such as TNFα and IL-1β. They fall into two categories: antibodies that bind specifically to a cytokine or cytokine receptor, and soluble receptors that capture a cytokine before it binds to the cell membrane receptor. Another strategy for preventing cell activation seeks to inhibit the intracellular transduction of signals produced when ligands bind to their membrane receptors.

When the receptors that are coupled to the signal transduction pathways are stimulated, they cause activation of transcription factors that control the production of cytokines, proteases, growth factors, and many other compounds involved in the inflammatory process. Signal transduction pathways closely involved in inflammation include the mitogen-activated protein kinase pathway, the phosphatidylinositol-3 protein kinase pathway, and Janus kinase-signal transducer and activator of transcription, and nuclear factor κB. Other signal transduction pathways are key to inflammation, such as those involving immunoreceptors (integrins, selectins), receptors coupled to G proteins (chemokine receptors), and steroid nucleocytoplasmic receptors.

10. Other Promising Potential Therapeutic Targets

Several inhibitory mechanisms can act at various levels of signal transduction pathways. At least three additional main strategies hold potential for inhibiting signal transduction pathways. One strategy consists in inhibiting an enzyme that activates a signal transduction pathway by administering a pharmacological inhibitor. First, Imatinib Mesylate (Gleevec®) is a tyrosine kinase inhibitor that is highly effective in several haematological malignancies. Second, the role of p38 mitogen-activated protein kinase in the various stages of inflammation has prompted the production of several imidazole compounds capable of inhibiting p38 (SB200765A, RWJ 67657, L-167307, VX-745, and RPR200765A). These pharmacological inhibitors are cytokine-suppressive anti-inflammatory drugs responsible for in vitro and in vivo inhibition of

Table 1
Some Biological Therapies in Clinical Rials for SLE and RA

Compound	Disease	Activity
B-cell directed therapies		
Rituximab	SLE and RA	Chimeric anti-CD20 MAb
Epratuzumab	SLE	Humanized anti-CD22 MAb
Lymphostat-B®	SLE and RA	Monoclonal anti-BAFF
Abetimus sodium (LJP 394)	SLE	Synthetic toleragen molecule specific for anti-DNA antibodies
TNF inhibitors		
Infliximab	RA	Chimeric anti-TNFα antibody
Adalimumab	RA	Recombinat human monoclonal anti-TNFα antibody
Etanercept	RA	Soluble TNFα receptor fusion protein
Pegsunercept	RA	PEGlated soluble TNF receptor type I
ISIS-104838	RA	TNFα antisense inhibitor
Signaling inhibitors		
Scio-469	RA	p38 MAP kinase inhibitor
Temsirolimus (CCI-779)	RA	Cell cycle inhibitor
Interleukin-based therapies		
Anakinra	SLE	Recombinant IL-1 receptor antagonist
Atlizumab	RA	Humanized anti-IL-6 receptor MAb
Cell-adhesion molecule inhibitors		
Natalizumab	RA	Humanized anti-α4 integrin MAb
Costimulation inhibitors		
CTLA4-Ig (BMS-188667)	RA/SLE	CD28/B7 pathway inhibitor
RG2077	SLE/RA	CD28/B7 interaction inhibitor

RA, rheumatoid arthritis; SLE, systemic lupus erythematosis; IL, interleukin.

lipopolysaccharide induced TNFα expression. Third, pharmacological inhibitors of C-Jun N-terminal kinase, extracellular signal-regulated protein kinase, and phosphatidylinositol-3 protein kinase have shown in vitro and in vivo efficacy in inhibiting the production of proinflammatory compounds. The specific C-Jun N-terminal kinase inhibitor SP600125 not only diminishes the production of TNFα, INFγ, and IL-6, but also decreases joint destruction in the adjuvant model of RA.

A second strategy involves increasing the expression of a naturally occurring signal transduction pathway inhibitor. This can be achieved either via direct administration of the recombinant protein or via gene therapy with a viral vector. A third strategy makes use of molecular biology techniques, such as antisense oligonucleotides or interfering RNAs, to directly block the synthesis of transcription factors or signaling molecules.

11. Conclusion

The last few years have been very exciting in understanding the pathogenesis of SLE and RA, with potential subsequent translation into effective treatment options. Some of the therapies reviewed here are relatively safe, more effective than placebo and slow disease progression. Research into newer pharmacological treatments and immunotherapies includes several compounds in development (**Table 1**) for patients with SLE or RA.

References

1. Kappler, J. W., Roehm, N., and Marrack, P. (1987) T cell tolerance by clonal elimination in the thymus. *Cell* **49,** 273–280.
2. Kappler, J. W., Staerz, U., White, J., and Marrack, P. C. (1988) Self-tolerance eliminates T cells specific for Mls-modified products of the major histocompatibility complex. *Nature* **332,** 35–40.
3. Nemazee, D. and Buerki, K. (1989) Clonal deletion of autoreactive B lymphocytes in bone marrow chimeras. *Proc. Natl. Acad. Sci. USA* **86,** 8039–8043.
4. Nossal, G. J. and Pike, B. L. (1980) Clonal anergy: persistence in tolerant mice of antigen-binding B lymphocytes incapable of responding to antigen or mitogen. *Proc. Natl. Acad. Sci. USA* **77,** 1602–1606.
5. Tiegs, S. L., Russell, D. M., and Nemazee, D. (1993) Receptor editing in self-reactive bone marrow B cells. *J. Exp. Med.* **177,** 1009–1020.
6. Radic, M. Z., Erikson, J., Litwin, S., and Weigert, M. (1993) B lymphocytes may escape tolerance by revising their antigen receptors. *J. Exp. Med.* **177,** 1165–1173.
7. Radic, M. Z. and Zouali, M. (1996) Receptor editing, immune diversification, and self-tolerance. *Immunity* **5,** 505–511.
8. Bouneaud, C., Kourilsky, P., and Bousso, P. (2000) Impact of negative selection on the T cell repertoire reactive to a self-peptide: a large fraction of T cell clones escapes clonal deletion. *Immunity* **13,** 829–840.
9. Yan, J. and Mamula, M. J. (2002) Autoreactive T cells revealed in the normal repertoire: escape from negative selection and peripheral tolerance. *J. Immunol.* **168,** 3188–3194.
10. Zouali, M. (2005) Taming lupus. *Sci. Am.* **292,** 70–77.
11. Choy, E. H. and Panayi, G. S. (2001) Cytokine pathways and joint inflammation in rheumatoid arthritis. *N. Engl. J. Med.* **344,** 907–916.

12. Viau, M. and Zouali, M. (2005) B-lymphocytes, innate immunity, and autoimmunity. *Clin. Immunol.* **114,** 17–26.
13. Uchida, J., Hamaguchi, Y., Oliver, J. A., et al. (2004) The innate mononuclear phagocyte network depletes B lymphocytes through Fc receptor-dependent mechanisms during anti-CD20 antibody immunotherapy. *J. Exp. Med.* **199,** 1659–1669.
14. Goldblatt, F. and Isenberg, D. A. (2005). New therapies for rheumatoid arthritis. *Clin. Exp. Immunol.* **140,** 195–204.
15. Leandro, M. J., Edwards, J. C., and Cambridge, G. (2002) Clinical outcome in 22 patients with rheumatoid arthritis treated with B lymphocyte depletion. *Ann. Rheum. Dis.* **61,** 883–888.
16. Edwards, J. C., Szczepanski, L., Szechinski, J., et al. (2004) Efficacy of B-cell-targeted therapy with rituximab in patients with rheumatoid arthritis. *N. Engl. J. Med.* **350,** 2572–2581.
17. Leandro, M. J., Edwards, J. C., Cambridge, G., Ehrenstein, M. R., and Isenberg, D. A. (2002) An open study of B lymphocyte depletion in systemic lupus erythematosus. *Arthritis Rheum.* **46,** 2673–2677.
18. Tokunaga, M., Fujii, K., Saito, K., et al. (2005) Down-regulation of CD40 and CD80 on B cells in patients with life-threatening systemic lupus erythematosus after successful treatment with rituximab. *Rheumatology (Oxford)* **44,** 176–182.
19. Zouali, M. (2002) B cell diversity and longevity in systemic autoimmunity. *Mol. Immunol.* **38,** 895–901.
20. Ng, L. G., Mackay, C. R., and Mackay, F. (2005) The BAFF/APRIL system: life beyond B lymphocytes. *Mol. Immunol.* **42,** 763–772.
21. Gross, J. A., Johnston, J., Mudri, S., et al. (2000) TACI and BCMA are receptors for a TNF homologue implicated in B-cell autoimmune disease. *Nature* **404,** 995–999.
22. Yan, M., Brady, J. R., Chan, B., et al. (2001) Identification of a novel receptor for B lymphocyte stimulator that is mutated in a mouse strain with severe B cell deficiency. *Curr. Biol.* **11,** 1547–1552.
23. Cheema, G. S., Roschke, V., Hilbert, D. M., and Stohl, W. (2001) Elevated serum B lymphocyte stimulator levels in patients with systemic immune-based rheumatic diseases. *Arthritis Rheum.* **44,** 1313–1319.
24. Stohl, W., Metyas, S., Tan, S. M., et al. (2003) B lymphocyte stimulator overexpression in patients with systemic lupus erythematosus: longitudinal observations. *Arthritis Rheum.* **48,** 3475–3486.
25. Bolland, S. and Ravetch, J. V. (2000) Spontaneous autoimmune disease in Fc(gamma)RIIB-deficient mice results from strain-specific epistasis. *Immunity* **13,** 277–285.
26. McGaha, T. L., Sorrentino, B., and Ravetch, J. V. (2005) Restoration of tolerance in lupus by targeted inhibitory receptor expression. *Science* **307,** 590–593.
27. Zouali, M. and Sarmay, G. (2004) B lymphocyte signaling pathways in systemic autoimmunity: implications for pathogenesis and treatment. *Arthritis Rheum.* **50,** 2730–2741.

28. Watanabe, H., Garnier, G., Circolo, A., et al. (2000) Modulation of renal disease in MRL/lpr mice genetically deficient in the alternative complement pathway factor B. *J. Immunol.* **164,** 786–794.

29. Holers, V. M. (2003) The complement system as a therapeutic target in autoimmunity. *Clin. Immunol.* **107,** 140–151.

30. Neumann, E., Barnum, S. R., Tarner, I. H., et al. (2002) Local production of complement proteins in rheumatoid arthritis synovium. *Arthritis Rheum.* **46,** 934–945.

31. Steinman, R. M. and Nussenzweig, M. C. (2002) Avoiding horror autotoxicus: the importance of dendritic cells in peripheral T cell tolerance. *Proc. Natl. Acad. Sci. USA* **99,** 351–358.

32. Blanco, P., Palucka, A. K., Gill, M., Pascual, V., and Banchereau, J. (2001) Induction of dendritic cell differentiation by IFN-alpha in systemic lupus erythematosus. *Science* **294,** 1540–1543.

33. Pascual, V., Banchereau, J., and Palucka, A. K. (2003) The central role of dendritic cells and interferon-alpha in SLE. *Curr. Opin. Rheumatol.* **15,** 548–556.

34. Kalkner, K. M., Ronnblom, L., Karlsson Parra, A. K., Bengtsson, M., Olsson, Y., and Oberg, K. (1998) Antibodies against double-stranded DNA and development of polymyositis during treatment with interferon. *Qjm* **91,** 393–399.

35. Ronnblom, L. E., Alm, G. V., and Oberg, K. (1991) Autoimmune phenomena in patients with malignant carcinoid tumors during interferon-alpha treatment. *Acta Oncol.* **30,** 537–540.

36. Ronnblom, L. and Alm, G. V. (2001) A pivotal role for the natural interferon alpha-producing cells (plasmacytoid dendritic cells) in the pathogenesis of lupus. *J. Exp. Med.* **194,** F59–F63.

37. Baechler, E. C., Gregersen, P. K., and Behrens, T. W. (2004) The emerging role of interferon in human systemic lupus erythematosus. *Curr. Opin. Immunol.* **16,** 801–807.

38. Taylor, P. C., Peters, A. M., Paleolog, E., et al. (2000) Reduction of chemokine levels and leukocyte traffic to joints by tumor necrosis factor alpha blockade in patients with rheumatoid arthritis. *Arthritis Rheum.* **43,** 38–47.

39. Voulgari, P. V., Alamanos, Y., Nikas, S. N., Bougias, D. V., Temekonidis, T. I., and Drosos, A. A. (2005) Infliximab therapy in established rheumatoid arthritis: an observational study. *Am. J. Med.* **118,** 515–520.

40. Emery, P. (2005) Adalimumab therapy: clinical findings and implications for integration into clinical guidelines for rheumatoid arthritis. *Drugs Today (Barc)* **41,** 155–163.

41. Sokol, M. C. (2005) Effective coverage and reim bursement strate etanercept and infliximab in the treatment of rheumatoid arthritis. *Manag. Care Interface* **18,** 32–37.

42. Bezerra, M. C., Carvalho, J. F., Prokopowitsch, A. S., and Pereira, R. M. (2005) RANK, RANKL and osteoprotegerin in arthritic bone loss. *Braz. J. Med. Biol. Res.* **38,** 161–170.

43. Boyle, W. J., Simonet, W. S., and Lacey, D. L. (2003) Osteoclast differentiation and activation. *Nature* **423,** 337–342.

44. Yun, T. J., Tallquist, M. D., Aicher, A., et al. (2001) Osteoprotegerin, a crucial regulator of bone metabolism, also regulates B cell development and function. *J. Immunol.* **166,** 1482–1491.
45. Kong, Y. Y., Yoshida, H., Sarosi, I., et al. (1999) OPGL is a key regulator of osteoclastogenesis, lymphocyte development and lymph-node organogenesis. *Nature* **397,** 315–323.
46. Cheng, G. and Schoenberger, S. P. (2002) CD40 signaling and autoimmunity. *Curr. Dir. Autoimmun.* **5,** 51–61.
47. Datta, S. K. and Kalled, S. L. (1997) CD40-CD40 ligand interaction in autoimmune disease. *Arthritis Rheum.* **40,** 1735–1745.
48. Crow, M. K. and Kirou, K. A. (2001) Regulation of CD40 ligand expression in systemic lupus erythematosus. *Curr. Opin. Rheumatol.* **13,** 361–369.
49. Toubi, E. and Shoenfeld, Y. (2004) The role of CD40-CD154 interactions in autoimmunity and the benefit of disrupting this pathway. *Autoimmunity* **37,** 457–464.
50. Grammer, A. C., Slota, R., Fischer, R., et al. (2003) Abnormal germinal center reactions in systemic lupus erythematosus demonstrated by blockade of CD154-CD40 interactions. *J. Clin. Invest.* **112,** 1506–1520.
51. Morel, J. and Berenbaum, F. (2004) Signal transduction pathways: new targets for treating rheumatoid arthritis. *Joint Bone Spine* **71,** 503–510.

15

Considerations for Target Validation and Industrial Approaches

Carlos R. Plata-Salamán and Sergey E. Ilyin

Summary

Target validation in health and disease integrates the modulation of a certain molecular target with an expected biological/biochemical/physiological or pathophysiological response or effect. The current state-of-the-art in target validation requires the interface of multiple complementary approaches and technologies to define the mechanistic connectivity between a molecular target and underlying micro- and macrobiotic processes. Target validation also represents the basis for "drug target validation" with focus on therapeutic applications. The concepts of "target validation" and "drug-based therapeutic intervention" continue to coevolve as new classes of therapeutic agents and delivery systems emerge and enable us to target or modulate previously inaccessible molecular entities.

Key Words: Allegro™; bioinformatics; biomarkers; functional informatics; gene expression; high-throughput screening; HTS; reverse transcription-PCR; RT-PCR; small-interfering RNA; siRNA; TaqMan; target validation.

1. Introduction

Target validation is a pivotal but sometimes exceedingly confusing subject in the biopharmaceutical definition compendium. In its simplest form, target validation relates to answering a question on whether modulation of a certain molecular target—such as an enzyme or receptor—would lead to an expected biological response or effect. This validation may involve confirmation in normal homeostatic regulation, involvement in a pathophysiological process or disease condition, or therapeutic applications of a molecule inducing a selective and specific modulation (e.g., inhibition or stimulation) (drug target validation). Part of the complexity and confusion of target validation arises from the multidimensional

From: *Methods in Molecular Biology, vol. 361, Target Discovery and Validation Reviews and Protocols*
Volume 2, Emerging Molecular Targets and Treatment Options
Edited by: M. Sioud © Humana Press Inc., Totowa, NJ

nature of the research directions and required data interpretation within various contexts. For example, studies performed in vitro by using functional genomic tools may not fully recapitulate the real situation in vivo, whereas the target can be modified with knockout or transgenic strategies to produce phenotypes of interest. Also, species-specific molecular, biochemical, and physiological mechanistic differences may be a potential source for the lack of translation to human clinical conditions. A concept in target validation that needs attention is the assumption that modulation of a certain molecular pathway may be fairly specific, whereas actually, in the in vivo situation, there are pleiotropic, divergent, and redundant processes and interactions that operate because of the cross-talk and connectivity of the signaling pathways. This cross-talk may result in additional biological effects (e.g., additivity, synergism, or antagonism) or in undesired side effects. Often, side effects and undesired toxicities may not be apparent in early and short-duration exploratory medicine or clinical studies.

Overall, target validation is a continuous process and the result of integrative approaches rather than a single step or a series of isolated events. One key consideration for target validation is the mechanistic connectivity between a molecular target and a biological process, which can be modulated and can be related to a pathophysiological pathway, where an association of a target with human genetics and functional genomics often exists. Technology platforms to identify and validate targets include multiple classes of tools with complementary principles, e.g., small molecules, peptides and antibodies, antisense, small-interfering RNA (siRNA), aptamers *(1)*, ribozymes, gene knockouts *(2,3)*, dominant negative mutants, and delivery systems, including vectors and carriers. However, there is no template for the application of various technologies to validate a particular target. The approach needs to be integrative with focus on incorporating scientific intuition with experience, e.g., into a flow scheme of testing while maintaining a flexible and continuous strategy of data-driven adjustments.

2. Automated High-Throughput Target Validation by Using siRNAs

Among multiple approaches, target validation often involves modulation of gene expression. Analysis of changes in gene expression could be achieved using various functional genomics tools, such as antisense, siRNA, and various viral vectors *(4*; Hahn; *see* Chapters 7, 9, 10, and 12). siRNA offers a compelling choice for in vitro target validation because of high potency, reliability, specificity, and a well defined mechanism of action at the mRNA level *(5,6)*. Changes in mRNA levels are relatively easy to follow with reverse transcription (RT)-PCR and microarray assays. From a technological standpoint, automation offers a compelling solution to increase throughput and improve testing consistency of siRNA applications. Automated transfections of siRNA

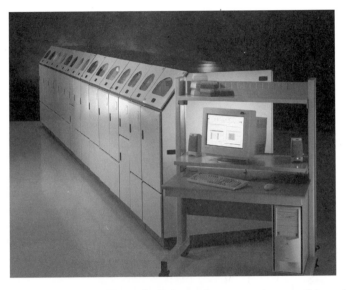

Fig. 1. The Allegro™ High Throughput Screening system is amenable and adaptable to high-throughput siRNA strategies to assay for target validation. The Allegro system consists of a host PC coupled to robotic stations for the purpose of sequentially processing a large number of samples residing in 96- or 384-well microplates. The system accepts these samples as its input, processes them through precise combinations with the user-supplied reagents, and provides information and processed samples as its output. (image is a courtesy of Zymark Corporation). (From **ref. 7** with permission.)

molecules have been reported previously *(7)*. In these experiments, fairly complex procedures were split into a series of relatively straightforward steps, each performed by an automated workstation. This approach is briefly illustrated by the following series of descriptions. **Figure 1** shows the automated high-throughput screening (HTS) platform that was used. For reliable application, the assays had been validated and reformulated in an automation-friendly format. **Figure 2** illustrates how a fairly complex experiment can be split in a series of relatively straightforward steps, each carried by an individual robotic workstation. Incorporation of reference controls allows for a quality control of each step in the process. A first step of high-throughput target validation may start with the delivery of a gene-modulating agent into the cells. This step can be monitored and verified by incorporating fluorescent tags into siRNA molecules. **Figure 3** illustrates this point. The successful transfection of siRNA molecules is not by itself a guarantee of gene-specific inhibition. The specific activity of siRNA needs to be validated using gene-specific RT-PCR assays to confirm downregulation of mRNA for the gene of interest. **Figure 4** demonstrates an example of RT-PCR analysis of siRNA-transfected

Carousel 1	Empty reagent plates input
Rapid plate 1	Enhancer R reagent addition
Transfer station 1	siRNA plates input and siRNA samples addition
Carousel 2	Incubation
Transfer station 2	TransMessenger transfection reagent addition
Carousel 3	Incubation
Rapid plate 2	Media w/o FBS addition
Barrier	Environment control unit
Transfer station 3	Cell plates input and final transfection reagent addition
Carousel 4	Transfection incubation
Washer	Wash the cell plates and stop transfection
Rapid plate 3	Fresh media addition
Barrier	Environment control unit

Fig. 2. The Allegro system (Zymark Corporation) modules and their operational specifics. The four modules enclosed by barrier units are environmentally controlled to maintain a temperature of 37°C. (From **ref. 7** with permission.)

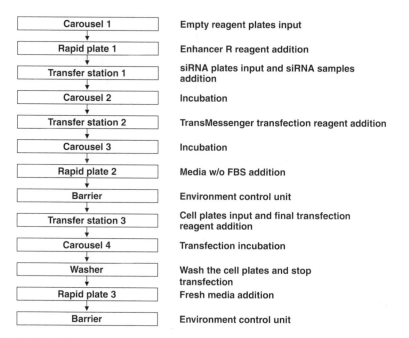

Fig. 3. Confocal laser scanning image of human embryonic kidney (HEK)293 cells transfected with siRNA. Incorporation of fluorescence at the 3' end on the sense strand allows for the monitoring of siRNA delivery. (From **ref. 7** with permission.)

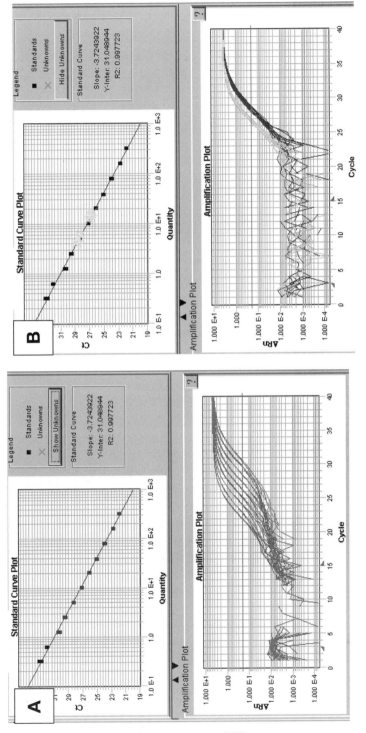

Fig. 4. TaqMan amplification plots showing amplification of reference samples and two groups of experimental samples. (**A**) Reference samples ranging from 625 ng of reverse transcriptase (RT) material to 61 pg of RT material were analyzed in triplicates. Threshold cycle (C_t) values were determined, and a standard curve plot was constructed using the SDS 2.0 Software package (Applied Biosystems, Foster City, CA). A linear relationship between amount of input material and C_t values was observed. (**B**) Standard curve plot was analyzed using SDS 2.0 to determine the amount of target transcripts in samples treated with control or target-specific siRNA. (From **ref. 7** with permission.)

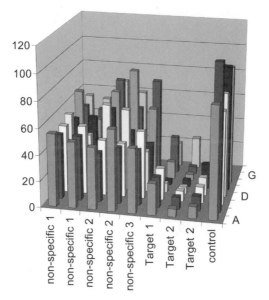

Fig. 5. Automated siRNA transfections were conducted in the 96-well format on the Allegro System. Target expression analysis was conducted on ABI Prism® 7900 HT (Applied Biosystems; http://home.appliedbiosystems.com). In this example, siRNA specifically and significantly downregulated appropriate transcripts, as detected by TaqMan quantitative RT-PCR. By designing functional assays to specific biological questions, siRNA can be used to validate targets in drug discovery. (From **ref. 7** with permission.)

cells. RT-PCR analysis is also important to distinguish between target-specific and off-target effects of siRNA. If a gene of interest regulates a biological process, a positive relationship between the ability to downregulate the expression of a target gene and impact a biological process is expected. Thus, it is advisable to have several different siRNAs for each gene of interest (**Figs. 5** and **6**). RT-PCR assays used to be fairly time-consuming and involved hard-to-automate procedures (*8*), but novel modifications such as those described by Maley et al. (*9*) take advantage of RNA capture plates, which simplify the assays. Modulation of gene expression is often linked to studies in in vitro and in vivo models that can be diverse and involve acute and chronic strategies where biological and behavioral observations can be associated with cellular and molecular outcomes.

It is important to note, however, that alternative splicing of a large number of genes and resulting protein isoforms with distinct posttranslational modifications increases significantly the number of potential molecular targets (individual proteins). Thus, focused inactivation of a single gene may have impact on multiple

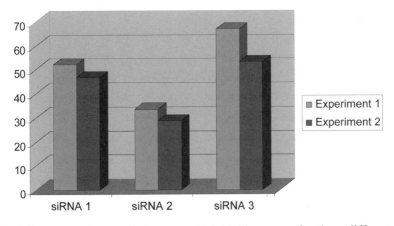

Fig. 6. Representative results in a growth inhibition assay for three different gene-specific siRNAs run in triplicate in two different experiments. Each bar represents the growth of siRNA-transfected cells as percentage of control (control or scramble siRNA-transfected cells, 100%). Growth inhibition was measured in vitro by using a sulforhodamine B assay. Cells were transfected with siRNA and allowed to grow for 72 h. (From **ref. 7** with permission.)

proteins and functions, and caution is required when interpreting the results of a single gene modulation as evidence to assess the potential relevance of a protein as a drug target. Reduction or loss-of-function approaches to assess a protein's target validation include inhibitory peptides, aptamers, and monoclonal antibodies. Overall, the integration of data—including genetic profiling, relationship of mRNA with target protein levels as well as protein–protein interactions and derived analyses, e.g., genomics, proteomics/pharmacoproteomics, and bioinformatics—is pivotal within the context of critical "path" studies for target validation.

Automated high-throughput target validation by using existing HTS equipment offers significant advantages in terms of speed and consistency *(10)*, but costs can be significant. For example, PCR confirmation, performed in triplicate, may cost US$0.8–$3.00, depending on the format of the assay for each of the transfected wells. Transfection and siRNA reagents further contribute to the cost, making large-scale, whole-genome experiments an expensive undertaking. An approach to cost reduction and improved efficiency is the transitioning of functional genomic studies to a microarray format. In this format, thousands or even tens of thousands of siRNAs or other gene expression-modulating reagents are printed on the slides in essentially the same way as DNA chip microarrays are fabricated. Several such systems have been successfully tested and described in the contemporary literature *(11–15)*. For example, Carpenter

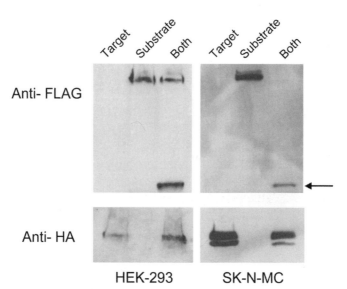

Fig. 7. Western blot analysis reveals a target-specific cleavage product. The target was detected by Western blot by using a hemagglutinin antibody conjugated to horseradish peroxidase (HRP); the substrate was detected using either a FLAG antibody–HRP conjugate (Sigma) or an HRP-conjugated antibody to the substrate. Cells (HEK293 or SK-N-MC) were infected with recombinant adenoviruses expressing either the target-green fluorescent protein (GFP)-HAHIS protein alone, or substrate-GFP-FLAGHIS protein alone, or coinfected with both of these adenoviruses. Western blots of crude cell lysates by using the anti-FLAG M2 monoclonal antibody (mAb) were used to visualize the pattern of substrate processed into C-terminal fragments (arrow). Representative Western blots are shown with the particular adenovirus, used to infect the two cell types, as indicated. The anti-HA mAb was used to detect the specific expression of the target-GFP-HAHIS recombinant protein. (From **ref. 4** with permission.)

and Sabatini *(13)*, described an imaging-based readout performed on an siRNA array. However, even though these advances represent a promising trend, the approaches are continuously evolving and improving to solve current limitations (e.g., current physical boundaries between spots that do not allow extraction of spot-specific material for downstream applications). Translation from in vitro to in vivo testing and validation is undoubtedly a serious challenge. Although there is no single technology to answer all of the questions that may arise during this translation, certain strategies may at least help to prioritize the most promising targets. One opportunity is direct delivery of a pharmacological tool to a suspected site of action in vitro and in vivo. For example, in vivo studies using implanted minipumps helped to elucidate regulatory systems involved in the control of feeding and energy balance regulation under normal and

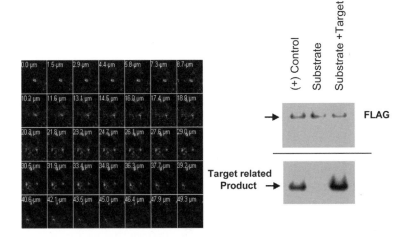

Fig. 8. GFP fluorescence in the mouse brain 48 h after intracerebral adenovirus infusion is visualized using laser scanning confocal microscopy. Western blot analysis reveals a target-specific cleavage product in samples prepared from brains cotransduced with both substrate and target protease-expressing adenoviruses. FLAG detection is used as a positive control. The positive control corresponds to the eluted fraction of the substrate and cleavage product purified using Anti-FLAG M2 agarose affinity gel target protease and substrate-expressing adenoviruses after transduction of HEK293 cells. (From **ref. *4*** with permission.)

pathophysiological conditions. These minipumps delivered precise doses of cytokines and peptides to target sites of action *(16–19)*. Similarly, viral-based expression systems could be used for target validation by modulating expression of targeted genes and for monitoring biological consequences of this perturbation (**Figs. 7** and **8**; *[4]*). In this example, expression of a target protease resulted in the accumulation of disease-specific biomarkers in several cell lines tested, and these findings were recapitulated in vivo by using intracranial injections of appropriate adenoviral constructs. Thus, this adenovirus-mediated gene transfer strategy resulted in an efficient and rapid target functionality validation, both in vitro and in vivo, and facilitated the transition between target validation and assay development for HTS.

Various examples of strategies and approaches for target validation have been briefly presented here. There are many others as well as permutations. Importantly, for human applicability, the definitive target validation occurs in normal biochemical and physiological homeostasis and in clinical medicine and clinical therapeutics.

References

1. Burgstaller, P., Girod, A., and Blind, M. (2002) Aptamers as tools for target prioritization and lead identification. *Drug Discov. Today* **7**, 1221–1228.
2. Zambrowicz, B. P., Turner, C. A., and Sands, A. T. (2003) Predicting drug efficacy: knockouts model pipeline drugs of the pharmaceutical industry. *Curr. Opin. Pharmacol.* **3**, 563–570.
3. Zambrowicz, B. P. and Sands, A. T. (2003) Knockouts model the 100 best-selling drugs—will they model the next 100? *Nat. Rev. Drug Discov.* **2**, 38–51.
4. Darrow, A. L., Conway, K. A., Vaidya, A. H., et al. (2003) Virus-based expression systems facilitate rapid target in vivo functionality validation and high-throughput screening. *J. Biomol. Screen.* **8**, 65–71.
5. Elbashir, S. M., Harborth, J., Lendeckel, W., Yalcin, A., Weber, K., and Tuschl, T. (2001) Duplexes of 21-nucleotide RNAs mediate RNA interference in cultured mammalian cells. *Nature* **411**, 494–498.
6. Hammond, S. M., Bernstein, E., Beach, D., and Hannon, G. J. (2000) An RNA-directed nuclease mediates post-transcriptional gene silencing in *Drosophila* cells. *Nature* **404**, 293–296.
7. Xin, H., Bernal, A., Amato, F. A., et al. (2004) High throughput siRNA-based functional target validation. *J. Biomol. Screen.* **9**, 286–293.
8. Pinhasov, A., Mei, J., Amaratunga, D., et al. (2004) Gene expression analysis for high throughput screening applications. *Comb. Chem. High Throughput Screen.* **7**, 133–140.
9. Maley, D., Mei, J., Lu, H., Johnson, D. L., and Ilyin, S.E. (2004) Multiplexed RT- PCR for high throughput screening applications. *Comb. Chem. High Throughput Screen.* **7**, 727–732.
10. Ilyin, S. E., Bernal, A., Horowitz, D., Derian, C. K., and Xin, H. (2004) Functional informatics: convergence and integration of automation and bioinformatics. *Pharmacogenomics* **5**, 721–730.
11. Wheeler, D. B., Carpenter, A. E., and Sabatini, D. M. (2005) Cell microarrays and RNA interference chip away at gene function. *Nat. Genet.* **37 (6 Suppl.)**, S25–S30.
12. Wheeler, D. B., Bailey, S. N., Guertin, D. A., Carpenter, A. E., Higgins, C. O., and Sabatini, D. M. (2004) RNAi living-cell microarrays for loss-of-function screens in *Drosophila melanogaster* cells. *Nat. Methods* **1**, 127–132.
13. Carpenter, A. E. and Sabatini, D. M. (2004) Systematic genome-wide screens of gene function. *Nat. Rev. Genet.* **5**, 11–22.
14. Mousses, S., Caplen, N. J., Cornelison, R., et al. (2003) RNAi microarray analysis in cultured mammalian cells. *Genome Res.* **13**, 2341–2347.
15. Wu, R. Z., Bailey, S. N., and Sabatini, D. M. (2002) Cell-biological applications of transfected-cell microarrays. *Trends Cell Biol.* **12**, 485–488.
16. Sonti, G., Ilyin, S. E., and Plata-Salaman, C. R. (1996) Neuropeptide Y blocks and reverses interleukin-1 beta-induced anorexia in rats. *Peptides* **17**, 517–520.

17. Sonti, G., Ilyin, S. E., and Plata-Salaman, C. R. (1996) Anorexia induced by cytokine interactions at pathophysiological concentrations. *Am. J. Physiol.* **270,** R1394–R1402.

18. Ilyin, S. E., Sonti, G., Gayle, D., and Plata-Salaman, C. R. (1996) Regulation of brain interleukin-1 beta (IL-1 beta) system mRNAs in response to pathophysiological concentrations of IL-1 beta in the cerebrospinal fluid. *J. Mol. Neurosci.* **7,** 169–181.

19. Plata-Salaman, C. R. and Ilyin, S. E. (1997) Interleukin-1beta (IL-1beta)-induced modulation of the hypothalamic IL-1beta system, tumor necrosis factor-alpha, and transforming growth factor-beta1 mRNAs in obese (fa/fa) and lean (Fa/Fa) Zucker rats: implications to IL-1beta feedback systems and cytokine-cytokine interactions. *J. Neurosci. Res.* **49,** 541–550.

16

Regulatory RNAs

*Future Perspectives in Diagnosis, Prognosis,
and Individualized Therapy*

**Marjorie P. Perron, Vincent Boissonneault, Lise-Andrée Gobeil,
Dominique L. Ouellet, and Patrick Provost**

Summary

With potentially up to 1000 microRNAs (miRNAs) present in the human genome, altogether regulating the expression of thousands of genes, one can anticipate that miRNAs will play a significant role in health and disease. Deregulated protein expression induced by a dysfunctional miRNA-based regulatory system is thus expected to lead to the development of serious, if not lethal, genetic diseases. A relationship among miRNAs, Dicer, and cancer has recently been suggested. Further investigations will help establish specific causal links between dysfunctional miRNAs and diseases. miRNAs of foreign origin, e.g., viruses, may also be used as specific markers of viral infections. In these cases, miRNA expression profiles could represent a powerful diagnostic tool. Regulatory RNAs may also have therapeutic applications, by which disease-causing genes or viral miRNAs could be neutralized, or functional miRNAs be restored. Will bedside miRNA expression profiling eventually assist physicians in providing patients with accurate diagnosis, personalized therapy, and treatment outcome?

Key Words: microRNAs; miRNAs; small-interfering RNAs; siRNAs; RNA interference; RNAi; Dicer; individualized therapy; gene expression.

1. microRNAs as Novel Regulators of Gene Expression

microRNAs (miRNA)-guided RNA silencing is a recently discovered gene regulatory process by which endogenous miRNAs mediate translational repression of specific mRNAs through imperfect complementarity; whereas, RNA interference (RNAi) is referred to as the process initiated by exogenous small-interfering RNAs (siRNAs) that are designed to induce cleavage and degradation

From: *Methods in Molecular Biology, vol. 361, Target Discovery and Validation Reviews and Protocols*
Volume 2, Emerging Molecular Targets and Treatment Options
Edited by: M. Sioud © Humana Press Inc., Totowa, NJ

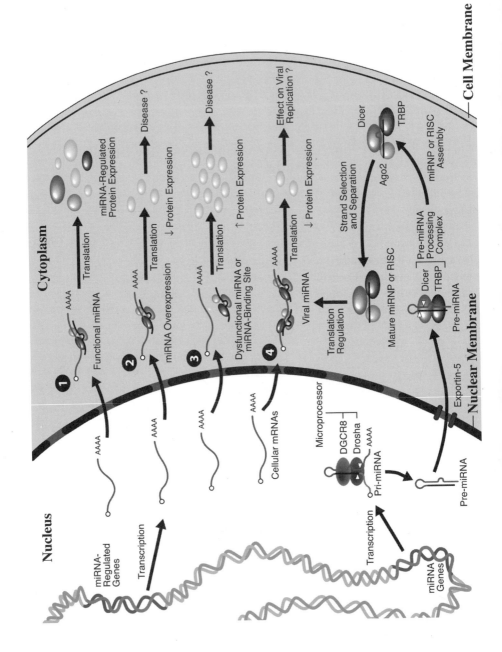

of specific mRNAs (*see* Chapter 9). siRNAs are thus a powerful tool to knock-down genes potently and specifically (*1*). Usually synthetized chemically, siRNAs are designed to be perfectly complementary to a targeted mRNA and are formed by two complementary strands of approx 21–23 nt with 2-nt 3' overhangs (*1*). siRNAs are phosphorylated at the 5' termini and hydroxylated at their 3'-ends (*2*), mimicking the endogenous miRNA:miRNA* duplexes resulting from Dicer processing of endogenous miRNA precursors (pre-miRNAs).

Several chemical modifications can be made to siRNAs to enhance some of their characteristics, such as their stability, cellular uptake, or intracellular distribution. Modifications affecting the second carbon of the pentose sugar have been widely characterized, such as 2'-*O*-methylation (2'OMe) and deoxynucleotides (*3*). siRNAs can also be obtained by the cleavage by Dicer of short-hairpin RNAs (shRNAs), which are transcribed from a vector or a PCR product containing this particular sequence. shRNAs are structurally homologous to the endogenous miRNAs precursors, with the difference that their stem is usually perfectly complementary. It is important to note that, when introduced into mammalian cells, siRNAs do not seem to induce an interferon response (*1*), opening up the possibilities for therapeutic applications.

miRNA genes can be found as clusters forming their own transcriptional units (*4,5*). For miRNAs that coincide with protein-encoding genes, the majority are found within introns (*6*). These observations strongly suggest that some miRNAs are coordinately expressed in parallel with their host proteins. Primary transcripts (pri-miRNAs) possess the signature of RNA polymerase (pol) II transcribed RNAs, characterized by a 5' methylguanosine cap and a 3' polyA tail (*7,8*). As shown in **Fig. 1**, the first processing step is initiated by the nuclear ribonuclease (RNase) III Drosha and produces an approx 60–70-nt stem loop named pre-miRNAs (*4,9*). The Drosha cleavage products harbor a classical 2-nt

---

Fig. 1. (*Opposite page*) Importance of microRNA (miRNA)-regulated gene expression in humans. (**1**) For more than 30% of the genes, miRNAs control the expression of their encoded proteins through recognition of their corresponding mRNAs. (**2**) miRNA overexpression may accentuate the degree of translation inhibition mediated by miRNAs. (**3**) Whereas loss of miRNA control, induced by a dysfunctional miRNA or miRNA-binding site, may lead to the overexpression of a specific protein and provoke the development of a disease. (**4**) miRNAs or small-interfering RNA can also originate from viruses and modulate host gene expression, which may result in facilitation of viral replication. Dysfunction of a protein involved in miRNA biosynthesis or function may affect miRNA expression globally and have more serious, if not lethal, consequences. TRBP, transactivating response RNA-binding protein; DGCR8, DiGeorge syndrome critical region 8.

3' overhang and a 5' phosphate that characterize cleavage of dsRNA substrates by members of the RNase III family *(10–12)*. This step is carried out in collaboration with the DiGeorge syndrome critical region 8 protein; this heterodimeric complex is known as the microprocessor *(13–16)*. The pre-miRNA is then exported from the nucleus to the cytoplasm by the Ran-GTP dependent transporter Exportin (Exp)-5 *(17–20)*. A second RNase III enzyme located in the cytoplasm, Dicer *(21–24)*, together with transactivating response RNA-binding protein (TRBP) *(25,26)*, catalyzes the second processing step by cleaving the pre-miRNA at the base of the loop to generate an imperfect miRNA:miRNA* duplex of approx 21–23 nt, which will be incorporated into an effector ribonucleoprotein (RNP) complex *(27)*, such as the RNA-induced silencing complex (RISC) *(28)*. Dicer and TRBP have recently been shown to be part of a functional RISC, thereby coupling the initiation and effector steps of RNAi *(29)*.

A difference between siRNAs and miRNAs resides in base pairing. Although siRNAs show a perfect complementarity between the nucleotides of both strands, excluding the 2-nt 3' overhangs, miRNAs show a variable number of mismatches that may confer a certain degree of instability *(30,31)*. Based on the thermodynamic stability of the duplex, a strand selection process will determine the identity of the strand to be incorporated into a functional miRNA-containing RNP (miRNP) complex *(29,32–34)*. The miRNA strand with the less stable 5'-end pairing is loaded into the miRNP, whereas the miRNA*, also called the passenger strand, is usually destroyed *(33)*.

First identified in *Drosophila* S2 cells *(28)*, the RISC is the best-characterized RNP complex in RNA silencing. It has been reported to contain Argonaute 2 (Ago2) *(35)*, the staphylococcal nuclease Tudor *(36)*, the vasa intronic gene protein *(37)*, and the fragile X mental retardation protein *(37,38)*. Although the function of these proteins within the RISC remains unclear, Ago2 has been shown to play a central role in RISC activity *(39–41)*. The PAZ domain of Ago2, a domain also present in Dicer, recognizes and binds the 3'-end of single-stranded RNAs *(42–44)*, whereas the PIWI domain binds the 5'-end *(45)*. PIWI, which shows structural similarity to RNase H *(46)*, is responsible for the mRNA cleavage activity in the RISC *(47)*. Human Ago2 binding to a mature miRNA can lead to the cleavage or translational repression of the mRNA target *(48–50)*.

2. Potential Regulatory Roles for miRNAs

As of May, 2006, 462 different miRNAs have been identified in human, which corresponds to approx 2% of the genome (http://microrna.sanger.ac.uk/) *(51)*. Little is known about their biological functions, but they may regulate more than 30% of the genes *(52,53)*. miRNAs bind to a mRNA by an imperfect nucleotide base pairing. Generally, the critical miRNA:mRNA pairing region, referred to as the miRNA seed, is usually located in the 3' nontranslated region (NTR) of specific mRNAs and comprised of miRNA positions 2–8 in the 5' to 3' orientation. Perfect pairing of this miRNA region is a key parameter used by computational approaches that aim at predicting potential mRNA targets of miRNAs. Pairing of the miRNA 3' region appears to be less important, but may compensate a weaker binding of the 5' region *(54)*. In humans, mRNA regulation by miRNAs is believed to consist mainly in translational repression, although a recent study reported that miRNAs downregulate a greater number of transcripts than previously appreciated *(55)*. miRNA regulation of mRNAs is complex. For example, a given miRNA can regulate several different mRNAs. Conversely, a specific mRNA can be regulated by more than one coexpressed miRNA. This may allow for a finely tuned expression of a gene product whose levels are critical for normal cell function.

Experimental demonstration of a relevant miRNA:mRNA target interaction is arduous to achieve; only a few combinations have been experimentally validated thus far. A study of the let-7:lin-41 interaction in *Caenorhabditis elegans* by Vella et al. *(54)* has improved the understanding of the requirements for miRNA binding. The miRNA let-7 possesses six putative binding sites in the 3' NTR region of the mRNA lin-41. At least two sites are necessary for downregulation of lin-41 expression. The intervening 27-nt sequence also appears to be important for miRNA regulation *(54)*, suggesting that miRNA–mRNA interactions do not rely solely to the regions of complementarity. A better comprehension of the factors involved in mRNA recognition by miRNAs will help conceive better predictive methods that are useful to limit the number of potential mRNA targets to be investigated.

Prior to initiating studies aimed at characterizing a miRNA–mRNA interaction of interest, computational approaches remain the method of choice to identify mRNAs possibly subjected to miRNA regulation, or to identify miRNAs possibly regulating a mRNA. Several different algorithms have been created and each of them uses different parameters for the sequence requirement of a miRNA–target interaction. They are designed to search for the miRNA seed and to determine the free energy of the interaction. They can also look for phylogenetic conservation and for more than one miRNA binding site in a given 3' NTR. Some bioinformatic predictive tools are available on internet: Miranda (http://www.microrna.org) *(56)*, TargetScan (http://genes.mit.edu/targetscan/) *(57)*, and Diana MicroT (http://www.diana.pcbi.upenn.edu/) *(58)*. A new database web site, Argonaute (http://www.ma.uni-heidelberg.de/apps/zmf/argonaute/interface) *(59)*, provides to scientists relevant information on different predictive algorithms, miRNA identification, and RNAi pathway components.

3. miRNAs and Their Potential Involvement in Diseases

miRNAs have been shown to regulate an increasing number of cellular processes. They can regulate development, cell proliferation, apoptosis, and other important physiological processes, as reviewed by Ouellet et al. *(60)*. Given their recognized importance in gene regulation, a link between miRNAs and several major diseases is expected. Defects in miRNA-mediated regulation of mRNA translation may lead to overexpression of specific proteins, which accumulation may cause diseases (*see* **Fig. 1**). This may be the case for mutated miRNA or miRNA-binding site on the regulated mRNA that can lead to a loss of mRNA translational control.

Clinical situations of genomic instability have brought support for a role of miRNAs in oncogenesis, as human miRNA genes have been found in fragile sites involved in cancer *(61)*. In the highly malignant human brain tumor glioblastoma, a strong overexpression of miR-21 has been observed *(62)*. This miRNA has been found to suppress apoptosis in this tumor, thereby contributing to the tumorigenesis process *(62)*. In chronic lymphocytic leukemias, the genomic region containing miR-15a and miR16-1 is deleted or downregulated *(63)*. The absence of these regulatory miRNAs allows for the overexpression of the antiapoptotic Bcl2 protein, which helps evade apoptosis *(64)*. miR-143 and miR-145 are downregulated in various human cancer cell lines, particularly those established from colorectal tumors *(65)*. Potential targets of these miRNAs have been previously implicated in oncogenesis *(65)*.

miR-155, whose precursor (pre-miR-155) was initially found to be highly expressed in pediatric Burkitt lymphoma (BL) *(66)*, was recently shown to be absent in primary cases of BL *(67)*. Although the exact link between miR-155 and BL is unclear, changes in miR-155 levels may clearly influence expression of its target genes, which remain to be identified.

The miR-17-92 cluster is often overexpressed in tumor samples from B-cell lymphomas *(68)* and human lung cancer cell lines when compared to normal cell lines *(69)*. These studies revealed that the miR-17-92 cluster can act as a potential human oncogene. The targets for this miRNA cluster, as predicted by using TargetScan *(57)*, include tumor-suppressor genes, suggesting that miR-17-92 overexpression can downregulate expression of these suppressor genes, and favor tumorigenesis *(69)*.

Members of the let-7 miRNA gene family are deleted in different forms of cancers *(61)*, supporting their implication in oncogenesis. A reduction of let-7 expression has been observed in human lung tumor samples or cancer cell lines *(70)*. In this study, patients showing a reduced let-7 expression had the worst prognosis after a potentially curative resection. In *C. elegans*, let-7 regulates let-60, the orthologue of the human *RAS* oncogene. Bioinformatic analyses revealed that the three human *RAS* genes contain multiple let-7 binding sites, suggesting that let-7 may also regulate RAS expression in human. This is supported by an association between let-7 downregulation and an increased expression of RAS protein *(71)*, further implicating the loss of let-7-regulated RAS expression during the development of lung cancer.

Altered expression of a protein component of the miRNA-guided RNA silencing pathway may have a global impact on the expression of genes regulated by miRNAs. Indeed, a decreased expression of the RNase III Dicer was observed in nonsmall cell lung cancer (NSCLC) obtained from patients. This reduction is also associated with shorter postoperative survival *(72)*.

The emerging causal link between miRNAs and diseases suggest that health may lie on a delicate balance between the expression of miRNAs and that of the genes they are regulating. A shift in this balance may lead to a pathogenic downregulation or overexpression of the mRNA-encoded protein. Diseased organs or tissues may exhibit a unique set of miRNA expression profile, which could be used in improving diagnosis of diseases (*see* **Fig. 2**), such as cancer *(73,74)*.

In addition to cancer, cellular miRNAs can be implicated in host–virus interactions. miR-32 has been shown to restrict accumulation of the retrovirus primate foamy virus type 1 in human cells *(75)*. This virus encodes Tas, a protein inhibiting RNA silencing in mammalian cells, probably to attenuate the suppressive effects of miR-32.

As for miR-122, which is highly and specifically expressed in the liver, its sequestration caused a marked loss of autonomous replicating hepatitis C viral RNAs *(76)*. This miRNA was found to facilitate replication of hepatitis C viral by targeting the 5' NTR of its genome *(76)*.

Bioinformatical analyses aimed at identifying HIV-1 genes regulated by human miRNA targets yielded five potential targets: miR-29a and miR-29b may target the *nef* gene, miR-149, the *vpr* gene, miR-378, the *vpu* gene and miR-324-5p, the *vif* gene. Expression of these miRNAs was verified by microarray profiling of human T cells, hosts of HIV-1 infection *(77)*.

4. miRNAs as Potential Therapeutic Targets

The possible pathogenic consequences of a miRNA deregulation, associated with either miRNA downregulation or overexpression, makes them potential therapeutic targets. For example, in cases of BL cancer, miR-155 is highly overexpressed *(66,67)*. In this case, its neutralization by an antisense strategy using 2'OMe oligoribonucleotides perfectly complementary to the miR-155 sequence could be envisioned *(78)*.

It is known that viruses like Simian virus 40 *(79)*, Epstein–Barr virus *(80)*, and Kaposi's sarcoma-associated herpesvirus *(81)* encode viral miRNAs. These small RNAs may directly influence specific host and/or viral gene expression, possibly affecting antiviral host defenses or replication of the virus. Thus,

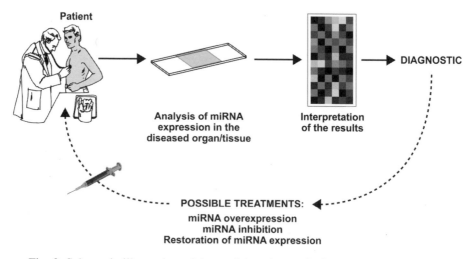

Fig. 2. Schematic illustration of the envisioned use of microRNA expression monitoring in personalizing diagnosis and medical treatment.

antisense 2'OMe oligoribonucleotides may also find applications as antiviral therapeutic agents.

In contrast, diseases, such as cancer, may also arise from a downregulated miRNA expression, as discussed for that of let-7 in the previous section. In that case, the objective would be the restoration of miRNA expression in the affected organ or tissue. Among the currently available approaches for such an intervention are the administration of miRNA duplexes, shRNA encoding cassettes, or even a viral vector encoding an shRNA.

Small-regulatory RNAs may also be used as therapeutic agents in treating non-miRNA mediated pathologies caused by overexpression of a specific gene. Here, approaches based on the administration of gene-specific siRNAs may be indicated.

Several obstacles that need to be surmounted before the launch of an RNAi-based therapy to fight genetic diseases are currently being addressed. For instance, the cost of an shRNA or siRNA therapy would be relatively high considering its relative instability, the amount required to achieve therapeutic levels in a 75-kg human being and the anticipated duration and frequency of the treatment. As for the use of viral vectors for stable expression of therapeutic RNAs in vivo, it may face uncertainties related to gene therapy, such as immunological issues and long-term undesirable effects.

In vivo delivery of therapeutic RNAs represents one of the key hurdles to the use of RNAi as a therapeutic approach. Several aspects of delivery, such as targeting of specific tissues, cellular uptake, and genomic integration, in addition to the issues of specificity, need to be either optimized or developed. Among the delivery methods being developed are cationic carriers, electroporation, and lentiviral-based approaches, as reviewed by Lu et al. *(82)*. From the intense research activities on the fundamental and therapeutic aspects of RNAi in the academia as well as in biotechnology firms, we can anticipate major and significant advances in the field of therapeutic RNAs in a near future.

5. Personalized Medicine Based on Monitoring miRNA Expression

Several studies have shown that some diseases, such as cancer, are associated with a change in miRNA expression levels *(63,70)*. But whether these changes are the cause or the effect of cancer remains to be determined. As for viral infections, miRNAs expressed from viruses like Epstein–Barr virus *(80)* and Kaposi's sarcoma-associated herpesvirus *(81)* may influence viral and host gene expression. These observations suggest that monitoring of miRNA expression levels in an affected organ or tissue may be used for diagnostic of a disease or an infection.

However, a clear link between an altered miRNA expression and a given disease first needs to be established. Comparative analyses require a "normal" range of miRNA expression in healthy organs or tissues to be defined. A number of methods that allow detection and quantification of the small miRNAs have emerged. A method to be useful for diagnostic purposes would need to be fast, reliable, reproducible, very sensitive (to detect miRNAs of lower abundance), and very specific, in order to discriminate between paralogous miRNAs that sometimes differ only from one nucleotide.

Northern blotting is a standard procedure to detect miRNAs. However, this method may not be sensitive enough, as some miRNAs are undetectable by Northern blot. In addition, it requires relatively large amounts of RNA, several separation and hybridization steps, and isotopic detection, which are far from ideal for clinical diagnostic. It is possible to improve the efficiency of Northern blot analyses by using locked nucleic acid (LNA)-modified oligonucleotide probes *(83)*, which improve sensitivity by 10-fold via enhanced hybridization properties, and by using digoxigenin-labeled RNA probes to allow rapid (minutes to hours) and nonisotopic detection of miRNAs *(84)*. LNA-modified oligonucleotides have also been used successfully to probe the presence of miRNAs in animal embryos *in situ* *(85)*, an approach that could be applicable to cancer diagnosis.

In 2004, Hartig et al. *(86)* published a method using signal-amplifying ribozymes to detect miRNAs. This method is sequence-specific and highly sensitive, with a detection limit of 50 fmol miRNA in the reaction mixture. The probes that were used had been designed for detection of nucleic acids in vivo. However, their stability must be improved to avoid ribonuclease-mediated degradation.

Another method to detect and quantify miRNAs is the primer-extension PCR assay *(87)*. In this assay, the first primer is used to convert an RNA template into cDNA in order to introduce a universal PCR binding site and to extend the cDNA to facilitate subsequent monitoring by quantitative PCR. The reverse primer is LNA-modified to increase hybridization affinity and improve amplification. This method is inexpensive, sensitive (in the femtomolar range) and allows discrimination between miRNA family members. Recently, a method to quantify miRNA gene expression with a single molecule, called the Direct miRNA assay, has been published *(88)*. It uses two LNA-DNA oligonucleotide probes hybridized to the miRNA of interest. Because these oligos are spectrally distinguishable, every single tagged molecule can be directly counted on a detection instrument. This assay is fast, sensitive, and specific.

All the methods previously described cannot be used to study the overall expression profile of miRNAs. For that purpose, a modified Invader assay can be used *(89)*. This method is based on the hybridization of a miRNA to two desoxyoligonucleotides (probe and invasive oligonucleodide) that generates a structure that is specifically cleaved by a 5' nuclease (Cleavase). The released invasive oligonucleotide serves in a second cleavage reaction, which involves a fluorescent-labeled oligonucleotide substrate linked to a dye quencher. Thus, the level of miRNA can be measured by a simple fluorometric assay. This assay can be performed in unfractionated detergent lysates, is fast (2–3 h incubation time) and allows sensitive and specific high-throughput screening analyses.

Finally, the sensitive and semiquantitative microarrays are also suitable for high-throughput detection of miRNAs. Several studies using this technique have been reported during the last few years, with some of them adapting the assay to make it more specific and sensitive *(90–92)*.

As illustrated in **Fig. 2**, we can imagine that, in a near future, monitoring of miRNA expression will be used as a routine test for diagnosis and treatment of diseases. The first step would be the sampling of the affected organ or tissue, either by biopsy or withdrawal of body fluids such as plasma, saliva, or semen. The next steps would be RNA extraction, if necessary, followed by monitoring and analysis of the results by comparison with a normalized miRNA expression profile, as deduced from data obtained from a bank of normal healthy tissues or fluids. Interpretation of the results would be useful to the physician for establishing a diagnosis and offering various therapeutic avenues to the patient. If the disease is caused by a virus, the treatment would possibly aim at neutralizing the function of viral miRNAs. Whereas if the disease is caused by an abnormal miRNA or gene expression, the treatment would consist either at restoring miRNA expression or targeting the mRNA of the disease-causing gene for degradation.

From all the evidences gathered thus far, we have all the reasons to be enthusiastic about the eventual use of regulatory RNAs in diagnosis and personalized therapy.

Acknowledgments

We are grateful to Gilles Chabot for graphic design. M.P.P. and L.-A.G. are supported by doctoral and master studentships from Natural Sciences and Engineering Research Council of Canada (NSERC), respectively. P.P. is a New Investigator of the Canadian Institutes of Health Research (CIHR) and The Arthritis Society. This work was supported by a Discovery grant from NSERC (262938-03) and a grant from Health Canada/CIHR (EOP-64706).

References

1. Elbashir, S. M., Harborth, J., Lendeckel, W., Yalcin, A., Weber, K., and Tuschl, T. (2001) Duplexes of 21-nucleotide RNAs mediate RNA interference in cultured mammalian cells. *Nature* **411,** 494–498.
2. Elbashir, S. M., Lendeckel, W., and Tuschl, T. (2001) RNA interference is mediated by 21- and 22-nucleotide RNAs. *Genes Dev.* **15,** 188–200.
3. Chiu, Y. L. and Rana, T. M. (2003) siRNA function in RNAi: a chemical modification analysis. *RNA* **9,** 1034–1048.
4. Lee, Y., Jeon, K., Lee, J. T., Kim, S., and Kim, V. N. (2002) MicroRNA maturation: stepwise processing and subcellular localization. *Embo. J.* **21,** 4663–4670.
5. Rodriguez, A., Griffiths-Jones, S., Ashurst, J. L., and Bradley, A. (2004) Identification of mammalian microRNA host genes and transcription units. *Genome Res.* **14,** 1902–1910.
6. Ying, S. Y. and Lin, S. L. (2005) Intronic microRNAs. *Biochem. Biophys. Res. Commun.* **326,** 515–520.
7. Lee, Y., Kim, M., Han, J., et al. (2004) MicroRNA genes are transcribed by RNA polymerase II. *Embo. J.* **23,** 4051–4060.
8. Cai, X., Hagedorn, C. H., and Cullen, B. R. (2004) Human microRNAs are processed from capped, polyadenylated transcripts that can also function as mRNAs. *RNA* **10,** 1957–1966.
9. Lee, Y., Ahn, C., Han, J., et al. (2003) The nuclear RNase III Drosha initiates microRNA processing. *Nature* **425,** 415–419.
10. Basyuk, E., Suavet, F., Doglio, A., Bordonne, R., and Bertrand, E. (2003) Human let-7 stem-loop precursors harbor features of RNase III cleavage products. *Nucleic Acids Res.* **31,** 6593–6597. ·
11. Zeng, Y., Yi, R., and Cullen, B. R. (2005) Recognition and cleavage of primary microRNA precursors by the nuclear processing enzyme Drosha. *Embo. J.* **24,** 138–148.
12. Filippov, V., Solovyev, V., Filippova, M., and Gill, S. S. (2000) A novel type of RNase III family proteins in eukaryotes. *Gene* **245,** 213–221.
13. Denli, A. M., Tops, B. B., Plasterk, R. H., Ketting, R. F., and Hannon, G. J. (2004) Processing of primary microRNAs by the Microprocessor complex. *Nature* **432,** 231–235.
14. Gregory, R. I., Yan, K. P., Amuthan, G., et al. (2004) The Microprocessor complex mediates the genesis of microRNAs. *Nature* **432,** 235–240.

15. Han, J., Lee, Y., Yeom, K. H., Kim, Y. K., Jin, H., and Kim, V. N. (2004) The Drosha-DGCR8 complex in primary microRNA processing. *Genes Dev.* **18,** 3016–3027.

16. Landthaler, M., Yalcin, A., and Tuschl, T. (2004) The human DiGeorge syndrome critical region gene 8 and Its D. melanogaster homolog are required for miRNA biogenesis. *Curr. Biol.* **14,** 2162–2167.

17. Bohnsack, M. T., Czaplinski, K., and Gorlich, D. (2004) Exportin 5 is a RanGTP-dependent dsRNA-binding protein that mediates nuclear export of pre-miRNAs. *RNA* **10,** 185–191.

18. Brownawell, A. M. and Macara, I. G. (2002) Exportin-5, a novel karyopherin, mediates nuclear export of double-stranded RNA binding proteins. *J. Cell. Biol.* **156,** 53–64.

19. Lund, E., Guttinger, S., Calado, A., Dahlberg, J. E., and Kutay, U. (2004) Nuclear export of microRNA precursors. *Science* **303,** 95–98.

20. Yi, R., Qin, Y., Macara, I. G., and Cullen, B. R. (2003) Exportin-5 mediates the nuclear export of pre-microRNAs and short hairpin RNAs. *Genes Dev.* **17,** 3011–3016.

21. Bernstein, E., Caudy, A. A., Hammond, S. M., and Hannon, G. J. (2001) Role for a bidentate ribonuclease in the initiation step of RNA interference. *Nature* **409,** 363–366.

22. Provost, P., Dishart, D., Doucet, J., Frendewey, D., Samuelsson, B., and Radmark, O. (2002) Ribonuclease activity and RNA binding of recombinant human Dicer. *Embo. J.* **21,** 5864–5874.

23. Zhang, H., Kolb, F. A., Brondani, V., Billy, E., and Filipowicz, W. (2002) Human Dicer preferentially cleaves dsRNAs at their termini without a requirement for ATP. *Embo. J.* **21,** 5875–5885.

24. Zhang, H., Kolb, F. A., Jaskiewicz, L., Westhof, E., and Filipowicz, W. (2004) Single processing center models for human Dicer and bacterial RNase III. *Cell* **118,** 57–68.

25. Haase, A. D., Jaskiewicz, L., Zhang, H., et al. (2005) TRBP, a regulator of cellular PKR and HIV-1 virus expression, interacts with Dicer and functions in RNA silencing. *EMBO Rep.* **6,** 961–967.

26. Chendrimada, T. P., Gregory, R. I., Kumaraswamy, E., et al. (2005) TRBP recruits the Dicer complex to Ago2 for microRNA processing and gene silencing. *Nature* **436,** 740–744.

27. Bartel, D. P. (2004) MicroRNAs: genomics, biogenesis, mechanism, and function. *Cell* **116,** 281–297.

28. Hammond, S. M., Bernstein, E., Beach, D., and Hannon, G. J. (2000) An RNA-directed nuclease mediates post-transcriptional gene silencing in Drosophila cells. *Nature* **404,** 293–296.

29. Gregory, R. I., Chendrimada, T. P., Cooch, N., and Shiekhattar, R. (2005) Human RISC couples microRNA biogenesis and posttranscriptional gene silencing. *Cell* **123,** 631–640.

30. Khvorova, A., Reynolds, A., and Jayasena, S. D. (2003) Functional siRNAs and miRNAs exhibit strand bias. *Cell* **115,** 209–216.

31. Schwarz, D. S., Hutvagner, G., Du, T., Xu, Z., Aronin, N., and Zamore, P. D. (2003) Asymmetry in the assembly of the RNAi enzyme complex. *Cell* **115,** 199–208.

32. Liu, Q., Rand, T. A., Kalidas, S., Du, F., Kim, H. E., Smith, D. P., and Wang, X. (2003) R2D2, a bridge between the initiation and effector steps of the Drosophila RNAi pathway. *Science* **301,** 1921–1925.

33. Matranga, C., Tomari, Y., Shin, C., Bartel, D. P., and Zamore, P. D. (2005) Passenger-Strand Cleavage Facilitates Assembly of siRNA into Ago2-Containing RNAi Enzyme Complexes. *Cell* **123,** 607–620.

34. Mourelatos, Z., Dostie, J., Paushkin, S., et al. (2002) miRNPs: a novel class of ribonucleoproteins containing numerous microRNAs. *Genes Dev.* **16,** 720–728.

35. Hammond, S. M., Boettcher, S., Caudy, A. A., Kobayashi, R., and Hannon, G. J. (2001) Argonaute2, a link between genetic and biochemical analyses of RNAi. *Science* **293,** 1146–1150.

36. Caudy, A. A., Ketting, R. F., Hammond, S. M., et al. (2003) A micrococcal nuclease homologue in RNAi effector complexes. *Nature* **425,** 411–414.

37. Caudy, A. A., Myers, M., Hannon, G. J., and Hammond, S. M. (2002) Fragile X-related protein and VIG associate with the RNA interference machinery. *Genes Dev.* **16,** 2491–2496.

38. Ishizuka, A., Siomi, M. C., and Siomi, H. (2002) A Drosophila fragile X protein interacts with components of RNAi and ribosomal proteins. *Genes Dev.* **16,** 2497–2508.

39. Liu, J., Carmell, M. A., Rivas, F. V., et al. (2004) Argonaute2 is the catalytic engine of mammalian RNAi. *Science* **305,** 1437–1441.

40. Rand, T. A., Petersen, S., Du, F., and Wang, X. (2005) Argonaute2 cleaves the anti-guide strand of siRNA during RISC activation. *Cell* **123,** 621–629.

41. Rivas, F. V., Tolia, N. H., Song, J. J., et al. (2005) Purified Argonaute2 and an siRNA form recombinant human RISC. *Nat. Struct. Mol. Biol.* **12,** 340–349.

42. Ma, J. B., Ye, K., and Patel, D. J. (2004) Structural basis for overhang-specific small interfering RNA recognition by the PAZ domain. *Nature* **429,** 318–322.

43. Song, J. J., Liu, J., Tolia, N. H., et al. (2003) The crystal structure of the Argonaute2 PAZ domain reveals an RNA binding motif in RNAi effector complexes. *Nat. Struct. Biol.* **10,** 1026–1032.

44. Yan, K. S., Yan, S., Farooq, A., Han, A., Zeng, L., and Zhou, M. M. (2003) Structure and conserved RNA binding of the PAZ domain. *Nature* **426,** 468–474.

45. Ma, J. B., Yuan, Y. R., Meister, G., Pei, Y., Tuschl, T., and Patel, D. J. (2005) Structural basis for 5'-end-specific recognition of guide RNA by the A. fulgidus Piwi protein. *Nature* **434,** 666–670.

46. Parker, J. S., Roe, S. M., and Barford, D. (2004) Crystal structure of a PIWI protein suggests mechanisms for siRNA recognition and slicer activity. *Embo. J.* **23,** 4727–4737.

47. Song, J. J., Smith, S. K., Hannon, G. J., and Joshua-Tor, L. (2004) Crystal structure of Argonaute and its implications for RISC slicer activity. *Science* **305,** 1434–1437.

48. Pillai, R. S., Artus, C. G., and Filipowicz, W. (2004) Tethering of human Ago proteins to mRNA mimics the miRNA-mediated repression of protein synthesis. *RNA* **10,** 1518–1525.

49. Pillai, R. S., Bhattacharyya, S. N., Artus, C. G., et al. (2005) Inhibition of translational initiation by Let-7 MicroRNA in human cells. *Science* **309,** 1573–1576.

50. Meister, G., Landthaler, M., Patkaniowska, A., Dorsett, Y., Teng, G., and Tuschl, T. (2004) Human Argonaute2 mediates RNA cleavage targeted by miRNAs and siRNAs. *Mol. Cell* **15,** 185–197.

51. Griffiths-Jones, S. (2004) The microRNA registry. *Nucleic Acids Res*, **32,** D109–D111.

52. Lewis, B. P., Burge, C. B., and Bartel, D. P. (2005) Conserved seed pairing, often flanked by adenosines, indicates that thousands of human genes are microRNA targets. *Cell* **120,** 15–20.

53. Xie, X., Lu, J., Kulbokas, E. J., et al. (2005) Systematic discovery of regulatory motifs in human promoters and 3' UTRs by comparison of several mammals. *Nature* **434,** 338–345.

54. Vella, M. C., Reinert, K., and Slack, F. J. (2004) Architecture of a validated microRNA:target interaction. *Chem. Biol.* **11,** 1619–1623.

55. Lim, L. P., Lau, N. C., Garrett-Engele, P., et al. (2005) Microarray analysis shows that some microRNAs downregulate large numbers of target mRNAs. *Nature* **433,** 769–773.

56. John, B., Enright, A. J., Aravin, A., Tuschl, T., Sander, C., and Marks, D. S. (2004) Human microRNA targets. *PLoS Biol.* **2,** e363.

57. Lewis, B. P., Shih, I. H., Jones-Rhoades, M. W., Bartel, D. P., and Burge, C. B. (2003) Prediction of mammalian microRNA targets. *Cell* **115,** 787–798.

58. Kiriakidou, M., Nelson, P. T., Kouranov, A., et al. (2004) A combined computational-experimental approach predicts human microRNA targets. *Genes Dev.* **18,** 1165–1178.

59. Shahi, P., Loukianiouk, S., Bohne-Lang, A., et al. (2006) Argonaute—a database for gene regulation by mammalian microRNAs. *Nucleic Acids Res.* **34,** D115–D118.

60. Ouellet, D. L., Perron, M. P., Gobeil, L. -A., Plante, P., and Provost, P. (2006) MicroRNAs in gene regulation: when the smallest governs it all. *J. Biomed. Biotech.* (in press).

61. Calin, G. A., Sevignani, C., Dumitru, C. D., et al. (2004) Human microRNA genes are frequently located at fragile sites and genomic regions involved in cancers. *Proc. Natl. Acad. Sci. USA* **101,** 2999–3004.

62. Chan, J. A., Krichevsky, A. M., and Kosik, K. S. (2005) MicroRNA-21 is an anti-apoptotic factor in human glioblastoma cells. *Cancer Res.* **65,** 6029–6033.

63. Calin, G. A., Dumitru, C. D., Shimizu, M., et al. (2002) Frequent deletions and down-regulation of micro- RNA genes miR15 and miR16 at 13q14 in chronic lymphocytic leukemia. *Proc. Natl. Acad. Sci. USA* **99,** 15,524–15,529.

64. Cimmino, A., Calin, G. A., Fabbri, M., et al. (2005) miR-15 and miR-16 induce apoptosis by targeting BCL2. *Proc. Natl. Acad. Sci. USA* **102,** 13,944–13,949.

65. Michael, M. Z., O' Conner, S. M., van Holst Pellekaan, N. G., Young, G. P., and James, R.J. (2003) Reduced accumulation of specific microRNAs in colorectal neoplasia. *Mol. Cancer Res.* **1,** 882–891.

66. Metzler, M., Wilda, M., Busch, K., Viehmann, S., and Borkhardt, A. (2004) High expression of precursor microRNA-155/BIC RNA in children with Burkitt lymphoma. *Genes Chromosomes Cancer* **39,** 167–169.

67. Kluiver, J., Haralambieva, E., de Jong, D., et al. (2006) Lack of BIC and microRNA miR-155 expression in primary cases of Burkitt lymphoma. *Genes Chromosomes Cancer* **45**, 147–153.
68. He, L., Thomson, J. M., Hemann, M. T., et al. (2005) A microRNA polycistron as a potential human oncogene. *Nature* **435**, 828–833.
69. Hayashita, Y., Osada, H., Tatematsu, Y., et al. (2005) A polycistronic microRNA cluster, miR-17-92, is overexpressed in human lung cancers and enhances cell proliferation. *Cancer Res.* **65**, 9628–9632.
70. Takamizawa, J., Konishi, H., Yanagisawa, K., et al. (2004) Reduced expression of the let-7 microRNAs in human lung cancers in association with shortened postoperative survival. *Cancer Res.* **64**, 3753–3756.
71. Johnson, S. M., Grosshans, H., Shingara, J., et al. (2005) RAS is regulated by the let-7 microRNA family. *Cell* **120**, 635–647.
72. Karube, Y., Tanaka, H., Osada, H., et al. (2005) Reduced expression of Dicer associated with poor prognosis in lung cancer patients. *Cancer Sci.* **96**, 111–115.
73. Lu, J., Getz, G., Miska, E. A., et al. (2005) MicroRNA expression profiles classify human cancers. *Nature* **435**, 834–838.
74. Jiang, J., Lee, E. J., Gusev, Y., and Schmittgen, T. D. (2005) Real-time expression profiling of microRNA precursors in human cancer cell lines. *Nucleic Acids Res.* **33**, 5394–5403.
75. Lecellier, C. H., Dunoyer, P., Arar, K., et al. (2005) A cellular microRNA mediates antiviral defense in human cells. *Science* **308**, 557–560.
76. Jopling, C. L., Yi, M., Lancaster, A. M., Lemon, S. M., and Sarnow, P. (2005) Modulation of hepatitis C virus RNA abundance by a liver-specific microRNA. *Science* **309**, 1577–1581.
77. Hariharan, M., Scaria, V., Pillai, B., and Brahmachari, S. K. (2005) Targets for human encoded microRNAs in HIV genes. *Biochem. Biophys. Res. Commun.* **337**, 1214–1218.
78. Cheng, A. M., Byrom, M. W., Shelton, J., and Ford, L. P. (2005) Antisense inhibition of human miRNAs and indications for an involvement of miRNA in cell growth and apoptosis. *Nucleic Acids Res.* **33**, 1290–1297.
79. Sullivan, C. S., Grundhoff, A. T., Tevethia, S., Pipas, J. M., and Ganem, D. (2005) SV40-encoded microRNAs regulate viral gene expression and reduce susceptibility to cytotoxic T cells. *Nature* **435**, 682–686.
80. Pfeffer, S., Zavolan, M., Grasser, F. A., et al. (2004) Identification of virus-encoded microRNAs. *Science* **304**, 734–736.
81. Samols, M. A., Hu, J., Skalsky, R. L., and Renne, R. (2005) Cloning and identification of a microRNA cluster within the latency-associated region of Kaposi's sarcoma-associated herpesvirus. *J. Virol.* **79**, 9301–9305.
82. Lu, P. Y., Xie, F., and Woodle, M. C. (2005) In vivo application of RNA interference: from functional genomics to therapeutics. *Adv. Genet.* **54**, 117–142.
83. Valoczi, A., Hornyik, C., Varga, N., Burgyan, J., Kauppinen, S., and Havelda, Z. (2004) Sensitive and specific detection of microRNAs by northern blot analysis using LNA-modified oligonucleotide probes. *Nucleic Acids Res.* **32**, e175.

84. Ramkissoon, S. H., Mainwaring, L. A., Sloand, E. M., Young, N. S., and Kajigaya, S. (2005) Nonisotopic detection of microRNA using digoxigenin labeled RNA probes. *Mol. Cell Probes* **20,** 1–4.

85. Kloosterman, W. P., Wienholds, E., de Bruijn, E., Kauppinen, S., and Plasterk, R. H. (2006) In situ detection of miRNAs in animal embryos using LNA-modified oligonucleotide probes. *Nat. Methods* **3,** 27–29.

86. Hartig, J. S., Grune, I., Najafi-Shoushtari, S. H., and Famulok, M. (2004) Sequence-specific detection of MicroRNAs by signal-amplifying ribozymes. *J. Am. Chem. Soc.* **126,** 722–723.

87. Raymond, C. K., Roberts, B. S., Garrett-Engele, P., Lim, L. P., and Johnson, J. M. (2005) Simple, quantitative primer-extension PCR assay for direct monitoring of microRNAs and short-interfering RNAs. *RNA* **11,** 1737–1744.

88. Neely, L. A., Patel, S., Garver, J., et al. (2006) A single-molecule method for the quantitation of microRNA gene expression. *Nat. Methods* **3,** 41–46.

89. Allawi, H. T., Dahlberg, J. E., Olson, S., et al. (2004) Quantitation of microRNAs using a modified Invader assay. *RNA* **10,** 1153–1161.

90. Nelson, P. T., Baldwin, D. A., Scearce, L. M., Oberholtzer, J. C., Tobias, J. W., and Mourelatos, Z. (2004) Microarray-based, high-throughput gene expression profiling of microRNAs. *Nat. Methods* **1,** 155–161.

91. Liang, R. Q., Li, W., Li, Y., et al. (2005) An oligonucleotide microarray for microRNA expression analysis based on labeling RNA with quantum dot and nanogold probe. *Nucleic Acids Res.* **33,** e17.

92. Babak, T., Zhang, W., Morris, Q., Blencowe, B. J., and Hughes, T. R. (2004) Probing microRNAs with microarrays: tissue specificity and functional inference. *RNA* **10,** 1813–1819.

17

Treatment Options and Individualized Medicine

Mouldy Sioud and Øyvind Melien

Summary

Although several drug targets are identified, current strategies in therapy do not take into account that patients vary in their response to drugs, both with respect to efficacy and toxic side effects. Whereas both clinical and histopathologic predictors of prognosis are established in some diseases, a better understanding of the molecular mechanisms that determine treatment response should play an important role in the development of individualized medicine. Treatment optimization will rely on the ability to adjust treatment algorithms for use in the individual patient based on the identification and validation of the factors that critically determine treatment outcomes, including diagnosis, disease phase and characteristics, organ functions, age, and gender. Although the analysis of a single genetic marker (e.g., CYP polymorphisms) may yield significant information that predicts drug response, the prediction obtained from the analysis of several genetic and epigenetic markers is potentially more powerful in selecting patients for effective therapy, whereas sparing those who would not respond or would suffer undesirable side effects. In this chapter, several relevant examples are presented.

Key Words: Individualized medicine; genomics; proteomics; gene profiling; genetic variations; polymorphisms; breast cancer; lymphoma; leukemia.

1. Introduction

Although several factors may influence individual drug responses, including age, gender, disease state, and organ function, there is increasing evidence that a large portion of variability in drug response is genetically determined *(1,2)*. In addition to DNA polymorphisms that represent common variation in a DNA sequence leading to either reduced or increased activities of the encoded protein *(3)*, gene expression profiling has enhanced our understanding of disease mechanism, classification of tumor stages, and prediction of treatment outcome *(4)*.

From: *Methods in Molecular Biology, vol. 361, Target Discovery and Validation Reviews and Protocols*
Volume 2, Emerging Molecular Targets and Treatment Options
Edited by: M. Sioud © Humana Press Inc., Totowa, NJ

Recent studies obtained with microarrays in several malignancies indicate that it is possible to predict with high precision diagnosis, prognosis, and response to therapy *(4)*.

It should be noted that despite the development of modern molecular tools for studying individual diseases in great detail, several pathologies remain poorly understood and the identification of the genetic markers or expression signatures that affect response to therapy will also provide clinical guidelines for prognosis and treatment. Also, these studies may also reveal novel molecular targets for therapeutic intervention. Relevant genetic differences between patients may include mutations altering the function of a protein involved directly (the real target of the drug) or indirectly in drug activity and metabolism, thus rendering the patients either more or less susceptible to treatment by the drug in question *(5)*. Genetic difference may also have an effect on the expression levels of nontarget genes and proteins in cells, which may be relevant to the mechanisms underlying unwanted toxic effects precipitated by drugs *(6)*.

2. Influence of Genetic and Other Factors on Drug Effects in Cancers

Cancer progression is characterized by the accumulation of multiple genetic mutations, chromosomal instabilities, and/or epigenetic changes that cooperate to drive malignancy *(7)*. Also, changes in gene expression are further affected by the microenvironment. Indeed, it is now well established that the microenvironment of the tumor–host interface plays a proactive role during malignant disease progression, including the transition from carcinoma *in situ* to invasive cancer, tumor cell dissemination, and metastasis *(8)*. In addition to the heterogeneity of stroma cells, tumor cells themselves are heterogeneous with respect to gene expression and genetic alterations. For example, breast cancer and lymphoma comprise several pathological subtypes, indicating the presence of numerous combinations of mutated and/or aberrant regulatory proteins that are sufficient to sustain cell proliferation *(8,9)*. Likewise, each individual patient's tumor may have a unique signature of molecular defects. It is also possible that each metastasis, originating from the same primary tumors, may have a unique expression profile. Thus, in addition to the genetic make up of the patient genome, the cellular composition of each tumor is a crucial determinant of both the biological and clinical feature of an individual's disease.

Regarding cancer therapy, there are several known genetic alterations or factors/markers that are expected to affect drug response. These include, drug transporter proteins, drug metabolizing enzymes that activate, inactivate, or detoxify drugs, and drug targets. The identification and understanding of these markers has the potential to allow clinicians to select appropriate therapy, and, therefore, avoid adverse drug reactions and therapeutic failures.

However, as with all biological systems, the complexity arises out of the existence of several genetic variations that may affect drug pharmacokinetics and pharmacodynamics.

Notably, the completion of the human genome sequence has led to a detailed exploration of the DNA sequence (the genome), genes that are transcribed into mRNAs (the transcriptome), and the translated proteins (the proteome). The role of the genome in drug effects is based on the premise that genetic variation plays a key role in cancer risk and disease outcome *(1,2)*. Polymorphisms represent common variation in a DNA sequence that may lead to reduced activity of encoded gene, but in some cases, also to increased activities *(3)*. Unlike somatic mutations, they are stable and heritable. Polymorphisms include single-nucleotide polymorphisms (SNPs), micro-, and minisatellites.

Because of their important roles in drug pharmacokinetics and pharmacodynamics, genetic polymorphisms in phase I (oxidative) and phase II (conjugative) enzymes are likely to represent some of the most common inheritable risk factors associated with common disease phenotypes, such as adverse drug reactions. Cytochrome P450 monoxigenases (CYPs) are phase I enzymes that catalyze the oxidation of endogenous and exogenous compounds, and are responsible for the metabolism of greater than 90% of clinically prescribed drugs *(10)*. CYPs can either detoxify anticancer drugs (e.g., epipodophyllotoxins, paclitaxel, *Vinca* alkaloids, and tamoxifen), or activate inactive prodrugs (e.g., cyclophosphamide). There are presently 57 genes in the human genome *(10)*, of which the CYP1A, CYP2B, CYP2C, and CYP3A subfamilies are involved in the metabolism of anticancer drugs. In addition to the roles of these enzymes in metabolizing drugs, there is also evidence suggesting that polymorphisms in the CYP genes may be associated with some human cancers *(11,12)*.

In addition to CYP genes, the situation is further complicated when one considers the impact of phase II enzyme on drug effects. These enzymes are involved in conjugating drug derivatives or the original parent drug for renal or biliary elimination. For example, glutathione-*S*-transferase (GST) conjugate glutathione to electrophilic molecules and oxidative metabolites *(13)*. GST genes are highly polymorphic and several SNPs in GST genes that affect response to cancer drugs have been identified. For example, breast carcinoma patient with the 105 VV in *GSTP1* gene exhibited an improved progression free survival. Similarly, 105 VV homozygotes colorectal cancer patients who received 5'-fluorouracil (5'-FU)/platinum chemotherapy showed a survival advantage when compared with heterozygotes and isoleucine homozygotes *(14)*.

A second important group of phase I enzymes is the UDP-glucuronosyl transferases (UGT), which catalyze the glucuronidation of several lipophilic drugs *(15)*. Irinotecan, a semisynthetic derivative of the cytotoxic alkaloid camptothecin, is approved worldwide for the treatment of metastatic colorectal cancer. Although it increases survival, it also causes severe diarrhea and neutropenia in 20–35% of patients treated. Notably, irinotecan is converted by liver esterases to an active metabolite, SN-38, a potent DNA topoisomerase I inhibitor that is primary inactivated UDT1A1 into SN-38 G, which is then excreted into bile and urine. However, reduced activity of UDT1A1 places patients at high risk for severe diarrhea and leucopenia induced by SN-38. Null mutations UDT1A1 lead to Criggler–Najjar syndrome, whereas less complete defects are associated with Gilbert's syndrome. The most common functional polymorphism is a A(TA)6TAA repeat in the promoter region of *1A1* variant. The most common form carries six TA repeats, whereas *UGT1A1*28* carries seven repeats that are associated with lower UGT activity.

In addition to genetic variations in drug metabolizing phase I and II enzymes, several other polymorphisms that are involved in drug response have been described *(16)*. 5'-FU adjuvant chemotherapy is now considered the standard treatment for stage III colorectal cancer. 5'-FU, an analog of uracil, is converted intracellularly into three main active metabolites, which inactivate the thymidylate synthase (TS). The effects of 5'-FU are counteracted by certain genetic variations in the tandem repeat sequences of the promoter enhancer region (*TSER*) of the thymidylate synthase gene, which is the case in the presence of the three repeat form *TSER*3* resulting in higher expression levels of TS *(17)*. Other enzymes such as dihydropyrimidine dehydrogenase (DPD) are also important in drug activity. Deficiency in DPD activity, however, leads to severe fatal toxicity following 5'-FU therapy *(18)*. Therefore, it is important to identify patients carrying defects or polymorphisms in the genes TS and DPD prior to starting therapy.

An important genetic variation, which has been related to drug effect is the CCND1 870A > G polymorphism in the gene for cyclin D1. The presence of this polymorphism has been reported to affect the outcome of childhood acute lymphopblastic leukaemia possibly by influencing the sensitivity to methotrexate treatment *(19)*. Furthermore, certain mutations in the epidermal growth factor receptor have been demonstrated to correlate with the response to tyrosine kinase inhibition exerted by gefitinib in a subgroup of patients with nonsmall-cell lung cancer *(20)*.

Of note, the most important downstream mechanism of cytostatic drug activity is the induction of apoptosis. Therefore, its deregulation may lead to drug resistance and survival of cancer cells despite that target proteins in cancer cells have been successfully targeted by anticancer drugs. Today, there are several active anticancer drugs and large number of combination therapies that are effective in both the adjuvant and metastatic treatments. However, no chemotherapy regimen is universally effective for all patients with the same tumor type. Although there are some available guidelines for selecting patients who are candidates for adjuvant chemotherapy, it is currently impossible to identify which of these regimens will work for a given patient before initiating therapy. Therefore, the question arises as to which particular drug and which combination of drugs is most suited for an individual tumor. In the case of breast cancer, steroid receptors and Her-2 are the tumor-based markers that are now accepted in clinical practice, having an established role in predicting hormone sensitivity or in Herceptin treatment, respectively *(21)*. The serine protease uPA and its endogenous inhibitor uPA are used in selecting node-negative patients who may not need to receive adjuvant chemotherapy *(22)*, thus avoiding toxic side effects of this treatment. uPA is implicated in cancer growth, invasion, and metastasis *(23)*.

Although clinical therapy failure of tumors is multifaceted, the acquisition of multidrug resistance in cancer cells is often associated with increased expression of ATP-binding cassette transporters, which protect cancer cells through the efflux of anti-cancer drugs *(24)*. About 50 genes encoding ATP-binding transporters, such as *ABCB1 (MDR1)*, *ABCC2 (MRP2)*, and *ABCC3 (MRP3)*, exist within the human genome, and several polymorphisms in *MDR1* gene have been identified *(25)*. Therefore, it is possible that specific haplotypes of the *MDR1* gene might determine the efficacy and toxicity of anticancer drugs.

Considering the multitude of molecular defects in tumor cells, it may be naive to expect that a single marker could provide a highly accurate response predictor. Therefore, instead of measuring individual markers, it is desirable to combine several markers, including gene expression profiles. With a microarray, the expression of tens of thousands of genes in a tumor biopsy can be determined simultaneously. Recent studies demonstrated that microarray could predict outcomes in cancer patients *(4*; *see* Chapters of 4 and 5, Volume 1).

2.1. Gene Profiling as Part of Drug Therapy

Today, the selection of treatment is not based on either DNA variations or the molecular characteristics of the tumor, but instead consideration of the patient's prior treatment history, disease state, general activity of the drugs and regimens in question, and their expected benefits for the patient as well as the familiarity of the physician with particular drugs. Because of these uncertainties, the individualization of chemotherapy selection based on molecular characteristics of the tumor is highly desirable. Recent technologies, such as microarrays and proteomics, now afford scientist and clinicians the ability to analyze gene expression for the complete coding sequences as well as to study genome-wide DNA sequence variation *(26)*. By providing complete genetic and genomic information, these molecular techniques, in particular microarrays will help clinicians to predict drugs that may increase effects and decrease side effects. A particular good example of this concept is in the diagnostic entity of diffuse large B-cell lymphoma (27), which has a very heterogeneous outcome pattern. Also, gene microarray studies have been able to subclassify several distinct gene expression patterns that correlate with distinct patient outcome patterns, including breast and hematologic malignancies (27–29). One of the aims of these studies is to develop signatures to distinguish tumors with a favorable prognosis from those with a poor prognosis. In this respect, several subtypes of acute myeloid leukemia that may require different treatment have been identified. In most, if not all, studies, the distinct groups identified via gene expression profiling are not apparent by traditional histopathological categorization or genetic analysis of the tumors. This molecular information should have relevance for diagnostic subclassification of tumors and more importantly provide valuable information for therapeutic targeting. Clearly, medical, legal, and economic issues all play a role in the implementation of prospective gene profiling at the bedside.

3. The Influence of Genetic Variations on Drug Effects in Other Diseases

The increasing focus on the role of genetic variation in drug targets and their downstream signaling pathways will extend the pharmacogenetic knowledge platform from the field of drug metabolizing enzymes into the clinically important target area. Thus, a number of genetic polymorphisms have been detected in drug targets and signaling elements, some of which have attained interest with regard to pharmacological treatment responses.

The group of G protein-coupled receptors (GPCR), of which there are approx 1000 different members, represent the molecular targets for at least 50% of current drugs and, thus, draw particular attention with regard to the significance of their genetic variation. Also, the heterotrimeric G proteins that are directly activated in response to GPCR stimulation contain SNPs, which appears to affect drug responses as well as some intracellular elements.

In the fields of cardiovascular diseases there are several examples of genetic variants affecting drug responses including polymorphisms in the genes for GPCRs such as β_1-adrenoceptors and angiotensin II receptors, G protein subunits and the angiotensin-converting enzyme (ACE). The use of β-adrenoceptor blockers is standard therapy in heart failure established on the basis of large clinical trials. There is, however, a variation in the response to this treatment, which appears, at least in part, to be related to polymorphisms in the β_1-adrenoceptor. The impact of genetic polymorphisms at codon 49 (Ser or Gly) and 389 (Gly or Arg) have been explored and recently it was reported that heart failure patients with the genotype Arg389Arg and Gly49 exhibited a more favorable response to β-adrenoceptor blockers than other patients when assessed as improvement in left ventricular ejection fraction *(30)*. Also, a polymorphism in the β_2-adrenoceptor has been reported to affect drug response in heart failure patients *(31)*. Thus, patients homozygous or heterozygous for the Glu[27] polymorphism responded better to karvedilol, a combined nonselective β-adrenoceptor blocker and α_1-adrenoceptor blocker.

Inhibitors of ACE also constitute a fundamental therapeutic strategy in cardiovascular disease; i.e., in heart failure, hypertension, as well as in diabetic and nondiabetic nephropathy. However, the response to these inhibitors varies and the role of the so-called insertion/deletion (I/D) polymorphism of the *ACE* gene *(32)*, denoting the presence (I) or absence (D) of a 287-bp element in intron 16 on chromosome 17, has been evaluated with relation to pharmacogenetics. Whereas the presence of the D allele has been linked to higher ACE activity *(33)* as well as increased mortality in heart failure *(34)*, it has been found that the ACE DD genotype appears to favor a beneficial effect not only of ACE inhibitors, but also in response to β-adrenoceptor blockers *(35)*.

Several polymorphisms in the genes for angiotensin II receptors have been described, and the SNP A1166C in the angiotensin II type 1 receptor has been associated with essential hypertension, myocardial infarction, and preeclampsia as well as other conditions. In addition, a role for the A1166C polymorphism with regard to pharmacological responses is suggested by studies of angiotensin II receptor 1 blockade *(36)*. Based on experiments infusing the active metabolite of the angiotensin II receptor 1 blocker losartan, EXP3174, in hypertensive patients, it was found that under conditions of a high-salt diet the systolic blood pressure was reduced by 6.6%; i.e., 12 mmHg, in the AA patients, whereas in the CC patients the reduction was only 1.3%, i.e., 2 mmHg.

Also a polymorphism at the level of heterotrimeric G proteins is reported to affect drug responses. The C825T polymorphism of the $G\beta_3$-subunit, which originally was found to be associated with hypertension, appears to enhance signaling mediated through the inhibitory G_i protein *(36)*. It was found that clonidine, a selective agonist acting on central α_2-adrenoceptors, and used as an antihypertensive drug resulted in a more pronounced reduction in systolic blood pressure in healthy individuals carrying the 825T allele *(37)*. This could be interpreted as based on a more efficient signaling elicited by clonidine through the α_2-adrenoceptors in the 825T allele individuals. Also the response to nitroglycerin assessed as venodilatation was reported to be more pronounced in young, healthy individuals carrying the 825T allele of the $G\beta_3$-subunit protein, thus suggesting that heterotrimeric G proteins are implicated in the pharmacodynamic mechanisms of this drug *(38)*.

Genetic polymorphisms on the receptors of blood platelets have been detected, and it is possible that some of these may influence drug responses.

Polymorphisms in the heterodimer glycoprotein (GP) IIb-IIIa ($\alpha_{IIb}\beta_3$), which is an integrin and fibrinogen receptor acting as the ultimate regulatory step preceding platelet aggregation and thrombus formation, has attracted particular interest as a target for antagonists like abciximab, tirofiban, and eptifibatide. The P1^A polymorphism affecting the glycoprotein IIb-IIIa receptor has been explored both as disease risk factor as well as a modifier of drug response not only for the antagonists of the GP IIb-IIIa receptor, but also for the effects of aspirin (39). The clinical and therapeutic significance of the P1^A polymorphism remains to be more precisely defined.

Therapy with 3-hydroxy-3-methylglutaryl-coenzyme A reductase (statins) decrease total and low-density lipoprotein cholesterol and has proven to be effective for cardiovascular risk reduction. However, considerable interindividual variation exits in response to therapy. Several SNPs across many genes known to affect cholesterol synthesis, absorption, and transport and statin metabolism were identified. Some gene variants seem to predict whether patient will benefit from treatment with statins (40).

As mentioned earlier, cytochrome p450 is a major drug-metabolizing enzyme that catalyzes the oxidative metabolism of several clinically used drugs, including some anticoagulant and antihypertensive drugs. An adenine to cytosine (A>C) transversion (CYP29*3) produce a protein variant with reduced activity for metabolizing warfarin, an anticoagulant. Individuals who are homozygous for CYP2C9*3 are more likely to experience bleeding events as compared to those with the wild-type genotype. Thus, screening for CYP2C9 variant may therefore allow clinicians to develop dosing protocols and surveillance techniques for reducing the risk of adverse drug effects in patients receiving warfarin or acenocoumarol for anticoagulant therapy (41). Recent discoveries have also identified variations in the gene for vitamin K epoxide reductase complex 1 (VKORC1) to affect warfarin responses (42), and a treatment algorithm including patient age and height in addition to CYP2C9 genotype and VKORC1 genotype has been shown to assess around 55% of the variability in warfarin dose level (43).

In the field of lung diseases the impact of pharmacogenetics has attracted considerable interest especially related to asthma therapy. The pharmacological strategies toward asthma are directed against bronchoconstriction as well as inflammation and genetic variations in key target molecules for drug action have been identified. Thus, SNPs in the genes for the β_2-adrenoceptor and adenylyl cyclase as well as changes in the promoter for the 5-lipoxygenase gene have been related to altered drug response. Patients homozygous for the Arg-16 genotype affecting the amino acid residue 16 in the β_2-adrenoceptor were reported to be more susceptible to asthma exacerbations and these patients improved when discontinuing the β_2-adrenoceptor agonist treatment and changed to ipratropium bromide *(44–46)*. The fact that several SNPs, at least 13, are present in the β_2-adrenoceptor gene attracted the attention to evaluate the role of haplotypes. The 13 SNPs was found to be organized into 12 haplotypes out of 8192 possible combinations *(47)* and comparisons of haplotype structures to SNPs showed a more prominent association between bronchodilation and haplotype than between bronchodilation and SNPs *(47)*. This may agree with the notion that evaluations of haplotype associations to drug responses can be more clinically relevant than assessments of the role of SNPs.

The β_2-adrenoceptor mediates its signaling through activation of adenylyl cyclase, and it was recently reported that the polymorphism Met772 in the adenylyl cyclase subtype 9 increased signaling exerted by the β_2-adrenoceptor under certain conditions *(48)*. In line with this it was found that the β-adrenergic induced bronchodilation was increased in human asthma in the presence of the Met772 polymorphism when corticosteroids was given concomitantly.

Leukotrienes are implicated in asthma and inhibitors of these mediators are established as therapeutic agents. 5-lipoxygenase (ALOX5) is one of the enzymes producing leukotrienes resulting in bronchoconstriction, and drugs that counteract ALOX5 pathways may improve asthma. However, this is not the case with all asthma patients, and it was hypothesized that a lack of response to inhibition of the ALOX5 pathway would reflect that leukotrienes could not be involved in the underlying pathogenetic mechanisms of asthma in these patients *(49)*. The promoter region for the ALOX5 gene has been shown to contain binding sites for transcription factors and genetic variations were detected in this area. In addition, it was reported that 6% of asthma patients did not have the wild-type ALOX5 core promoter locus and that patients belonging to this group did not respond to ALOX5 inhibition. These findings thereby illustrate how knowledge of individual genetic characteristics may have an impact on therapeutic strategies.

Genetic polymorphisms may also play a role for the effect of drug therapy in infectious diseases. In the case of infections with HIV-1 it has been found that the G protein-coupled chemokine receptors CCR5 and CXCR4 act as major coreceptors for virus cell entry. Furthermore, particular genetic polymorphisms detected in coreceptor genes are reported to cause resistance to HIV-1 infection and a delay of progression to AIDS *(50)*. Notably, a recent report also suggests that the presence of particular genetic polymorphisms in HIV patients, CCR2-64I or CXCL123'A, are beneficial for the response to highly active antiretroviral therapy *(51)*.

Heterotrimeric G proteins might somehow be involved in the susceptibility to the combination treatment of hepatitis C infection using interferon-α and ribavirin. The C825T polymorphism of the Gβ_3-subunit protein is reported to affect the response to this treatment in hepatitis C patients *(52)*. It was found

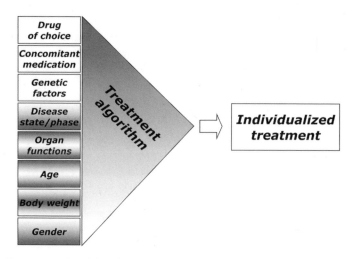

Fig. 1. Treatment algorithms in pharmacotherapy will depend on the development of models that can integrate relevant determinants with influence on drug response in combination with adjustments to the individual patient.

that patients with the GNB3 825 CC genotype did not respond the interferon-α/ribavirin treatment, albeit the explanation for this is unclear. However, it has previously been reported that the GNB3 825 CC genotype is associated with impaired immune function *(53)*. This observation may agree with recent findings that sudden infant death as a result of infection also appears to be associated with the GNB3 825 CC genotype *(54)*.

4. Toward Algorithms in Individualized Medicine

The efforts to establish a modern platform for individualized therapy is a demanding challenge to medicine. The evaluation of a rational approach to identify and handle a complex set of variable factors, which may influence drug treatment and responses, is critical. These factors include genetic variability of the drug metabolizing enzymes, drug transporters, drug targets and their signaling pathways, and as well drug–drug interactions and food–drug interactions in addition to disease state and phase, organ function/dysfunction, age, body weight, and gender. A future direction in pharmacotherapy might be to develop treatment algorithms (**Fig. 1**) for single drugs or drug regimens taking into account the relevant subset of critical determinants with adjustments to the single patient and further linked to practical implementable procedures. Algorithms aiming to integrate the premises of advanced pharmacological therapy can support a higher precision in individual treatment both with respect to optimize drug effects and to reduce the risks for unwanted toxic reactions.

The forces that can promote the previously described scenario are both the demands expressed by the patients themselves and the health authorities and in addition the results of ongoing scientific progresses, which continuously illustrate and update theses options. At the same time, it is essential to be aware of the gradual change in target molecule area for medical treatment and the impact these changes should have for establishing an individualized therapy. As a result of the last decades' intensive research and characterization of intracellular signaling pathways, there is an increasing number of novel drugs directed against molecular targets inside the cells. Several of these targets are key elements in cellular pathways in accordance with their potential of more pronounced therapeutic effects. However, because these key targets may be involved in other pathways that are also critical for different cell functions, there is a simultaneous risk for as pronounced deleterious effects. The success of using drugs acting on central intracellular molecules may thus depend on even more sophisticated and precise strategies to select the appropriate patients (based on diagnostic and disease phase criterias) and as well the ability to establish modes of specific cell delivery to ensure that the drugs predominantly reach the relevant targets. In other words, the progresses in signaling research, which contributes with novel and potentially powerful target options, may thereby further extend the challenge concerning a broad and long-term project for developing individualized therapy in medicine.

References

1. Bell, J. (2004) Predicting disease using genomics. *Nature* **429,** 453–456.
2. Meyer, U. A. (2004) Pharmacogenetics: five decades of therapeutic lessons from genetic diversity. *Nat. Rev. Genet.* **5,** 669–676.
3. Lai, E. (2001) Application of SNP technologies in medicine: lessons learned and future challenges. *Genome Res.* **11,** 927–929.
4. Huang, E., Cheng, S. H., Dressman, H., et al. (2003) Gene expression predictors of breast cancer outcomes. *Lancet* **361,** 1590–1596.
5. Wilkinson, G. R. (2005) Drug metabolism and variability among patients in drug response *N. Engl. J. Med.* **352,** 2211–2221.
6. Williams, R. S. and Goldschmidt-Clermont, P. J. (2004) The genetics of cardiovascular disease: from genotype to phenotype. *Dialogues in Cardiovasc. Med.* **9,** 3–19.
7. Dixon, K. and Kopras, E. (2004) Genetic alterations and DNA repair in human carcinogenesis. *Semin in Cancer Biol.* **14,** 441–448.
8. Liotta, L. A. and Kohn, E. C. (2001) The microenvironment of the tumour-host interface. *Nature* **411,** 375–379.
9. Staudt, L. M. (2002) Gene expression profiling of lymphoid malignancies. *Annu. Rev. Med.* **53,** 303–318.
10. Ingelman-Sundberg, M. (2005) The human genome project and novel aspects of cytochrome P450 research. *Toxicol Appl Pharmacol* **207,** 52–56.

11. Gajecka, M., Rydzanicz, M., Jaskula-Sztul, R., Kujawski, M., Szyfter, W., and Szyfter, K. (2005) CYP1A1, CYP2D6, CYP2E1, NAT2, GSTM1 and GSTT1 polymorphisms or their combinations are associated with the increased risk of the laryngeal squamous cell carcinoma. *Mut. Res.* **574,** 112–123.

12. Raimondi, S., Boffetta, P., Anttila, S., et al. (2005) Metabolic gene polymorphisms and lung cancer risk in non-smokers. An update of the GSEC study. *Mut. Res.* **592,** 45–47.

13. Efferth, T. and Volm, M. (2005) Gluthatione-related enzymes contribute to resistance of tumor cells and low toxicity in normal organs to artesunate. *In Vivo* **19,** 225–232.

14. Anderer, G., Schrappe, M., Brechlin, A. M., et al. (2000) Polymorphisms within glutathione S-transferase genes and initial response to glucocorticoids in childhood acute lymphoblastic leukaemia. *Pharmacogenetics* **10,** 715–726.

15. Efferth, T. and Volm, M. (2005) Pharmacogenetics for individualized cancer chemotherapy. *Pharmacology Therapeutics* **107,** 155–176.

16. Toffoli, G., Cecchin, E., Corona, G., and Boiocchi, M. (2003) Pharmacogenetics of irinotecan. *Curr. Med. Chem. Anti-Canc. Agents* **3,** 225–237.

17. Yamayoshi, Y., Iida, E., and Tanigawara, Y. (2005) Cancer pharmacogenomics: international trends. *Int. J. Clin. Oncol.* **10,** 5–13.

18. Van Kuilenburg, A. B., Muller, E. W., Haasjes, J., et al. (2001) Lethal outcome of a patient with a complete dihydropyrimidine dehydrogenase DPD deficiency after administration of 5'fluorouracil: frequency of the common IVS14+1G>A mutation causing dpd deficiency. *Clin. Cancer Res.* **7,** 1149–1153.

19. Costea, I., Moghrabi, A., and Krajinovic, M. (2003) The influence of cyclin D1 (CCND1) 870A>G polymorphism and CCND1-thymidylate synthase (TS) gene-gene interaction on the outcome of childhood acute lymphoblastic leukaemia. *Pharmacogenetics* **13,** 577–580.

20. Lynch, T. J., Bell, D. W., Sordella, R., et al. (2004) Activating mutations in the Epidermal Gorowth Factor Receptor underlying responsiveness of non-small-cell lung cancer to gefitinib. *N. Engl. J. Med.* **350,** 2129–2139.

21. Piccart, M. J., Di Leo, A., and Hamilton, A. (2000) HER2: a predictive factor ready to use in the daily management of breast cancer patient? *Eur. J. Cancer* **36,** 1755–1761.

22. Duffy, M. J. (2002) Urokinase plasminogen activator and its inhibitor, PAI-1, as prognostic marlers in breast cancer: from pilot to level 1 evidence studies. *Clin. Chem.* **48,** 1194–1197.

23. Andreasen, P. A., Kjoller, L., Christensen, L., and Duffy, M. J. (1997) The urokinase-type plasminogen activator in cancer metastasis: a review. *Int. J. Cancer* **72,** 1–22.

24. Efferth, T. (2001) The human ATP-binding cassette transporter genes: from the bench to the bedside. *Curr. Mol. Med.* **1,** 45–65.

25. Hoffmeyer, S., Burk, O., von Richter, O., et al. (2000) Functional polymorphisms of the human multidrug-resistance gene: multiple sequence variations and correlation of one allele with P-glycoprotein expression and activity in vivo. *Proc. Natl. Acad. Sci. USA* **97,** 3473–3478.

26. Lesko, L. J. and Woodcock, J. (2004) Translation of pharmacogenomics and pharmacogenetics: a regulatory perspective. *Nat. Rev. Drug Discov.* **3,** 763–769.

27. Margalit, O., Somech, R., Amariglio, N., and Rechavi, G. (2005) Microarray-based gene expression profiling of hematologic malignancies: basic concepts and clinical applications. *Blood Rev.* **19,** 223–234.

28. Sorlie, T., Perou, C. M., Tibshirani, R., et al. (2001) Gene expression patterns of breast carcinomas distinguish tumor subclasses with clinical implications. *Proc. Natl. Acad. Sci. USA* **98,** 10,869–10,874.

29. Stock, M. and Otto, F. (2005) Gene deregulation in gastric cancer. *Gene* **360,** 1–19.

30. Terra, S. G., Hamilton, K. K., Pauly, D. F., et al. (2005) β_1-adrenergic receptor polymorphisms and left ventricular remodeling changes in response to β-blocker therapy. *Pharmacogen. Genom.* **15,** 227–234.

31. Kaye, D. M., Smirk, B., Williams, C., Jennings, G., Esler, M., and Holst, D. (2003) β-Adrenoceptor genotype influences the response to carvedilol in patients with congestive heart failure. *Pharmacogen.* **13,** 379–382.

32. Rigat, B., Hubert, C., Alhenc-Gelas, F., Cambien, F., Corvol, P., and Soubrier, F. (1990) An insertion/deletion polymorphism in the angiotensin I-converting enzyme gene accounting for half the variance of serum enzyme levels. *J. Clin. Invest.* **86,** 1343–1346.

33. Ihnken, R., Verho, K., Gross, M., and Marz, W. (1996) Deletion polymorphism of the angiotensin I-converting enzyme gene is associated with increased plasma angiotensin-converting enzyme activity but not with increased risk for myocardial infarction and coronary artery disease. *Ann. Intern. Med.* **125,** 19–25.

34. Andersson, B. and Sylven, C. (1996) The DD genotype of the angiotensin-converting enzyme gene is associated with increased mortality in idiopathic heart failure. *J. Am. Coll. Cardiol.* **28,** 162–167.

35. McNamara, D. M., Holubkov, R., Postava, L., et al. (2004) Pharmacogenetic interactions between angiotensin-converting enzyme inhibitor therapy and angiotensin-converting enzyme deletion polymorphism in patients with congestive heart failure. *J. Am. Coll. Cardiol.* **44,** 2019–2026.

36. Spiering, W., Kroon, A. A., Fuss-Lejeune, M. J. M. J., and Leeuw, P. W. (2005) Genetic contribution to the acute effects of angiotensin II type 1 receptor blockade. *J. Hypertens.* **23,** 753–758.

37. Nürnberger, J., Dammer, S., Mitchell, A., et al. (2003) Effect of the C825T polymorphism of the G protein β3 subunit on the systolic blood pressure-lowering effect of clonidine in young, healthy male subjects. *Clin. Pharmacol. Ther.* **74,** 53–60.

38. Mitchell, A., Buhrmann, S., Seifert, A., et al. (2003) Venous response to nitroglycerin is enhanced in young, healthy carriers of the 825T allele of the G protein beta3 subunit gene (GNB3). *Clin. Pharmacol. Ther.* **74,** 499–504.

39. Rozalski, M., Boncler, M., Luzak, B., and Watala, C. (2005) Genetic factors underlying differential blood platelet sensitivity to inhibitors. *Pharmacol Reports* **57,** 1–13.

40. Schmitz, G. and Drobnik, W. (2003) Pharmacogenomics and pharmacogenetics of cholesterol-lowering therapy. *Clin. Chem. Lab Med.* **41,** 581–589.

41. Higashi, M. K., Veenstra, D. L., Kondo, L. M., et al. (2002) Association between CYP2C9 genetic variants and anticoagulation-related outcomes during warfarin therapy. *JAMA* **287**, 1690–1698.

42. Rieder, M. J., Reiner, A. P., Gage, B. F., et al. (2005) Effect of VKORC1 Haplotypes on transcriptional regulation and warfarin dose. *N. Engl. J. Med.* **352**, 2285–2293.

43. Sconce, E. A., Khan, T. I., Wynne, H. A., et al. (2005) The impact of CYP2C9 and VKORC1 genetic polymorphism and patient characteristics upon warfarin dose requirements: proposal for a new dosing regimen. *Blood* **106**, 2329–2333.

44. Israel, E., Drazen, J. M., Liggett, S. B., et al. (2000). The effect of polymorphisms of the beta(2)-adrenergic receptor on the response to regular use of albuterol in asthma. *Am. J. Respir. Crit. Care Med.* **162**, 75–80.

45. Taylor, D. R., Drazen, J. M., Herbison, G. P., et al. (2000) Asthma exacerbations during long term beta agonist use: influence of beta(2) adrenoceptor polymorphism. *Thorax* **55**, 762–767.

46. Israel, E., Chinchilli, V. M., Ford, J. G., et al. (2004) Use of regularly scheduled albuterol treatment in asthma: genotype-stratified, randomised, placebo-controlled cross-over trial. *Lancet* **364**, 1505–1512.

47. Drysdale, C. M., McGraw, D. W., Stack, C. B., et al. (2000) Complex promoter and coding region β_2-adrenergic receptor haplotypes alter receptor expression and predict *in vivo* responsiveness. *Proc. Acad. Natl. Sci. USA* **97**, 10,483–10,488.

48. Tantisira, K. G., Small, K. M., Litonjua, A. A., Weiss, S. T., and Liggett, S. B. (2005) Molecular properties and pharmacogenetics of a polymorphism of adenylyl cyclase type 9 in asthma: interaction between β-agonist and corticosteroid pathways. *Hum. Mol. Gen.* **14**, 1671–1677.

49. Drazen, J. M., Yandava, C. N., Dube, L., et al. (1999) Pharmacogenetic association between ALOX5 promoter genotype and the response to anti-asthma treatment. *Nat. Genet.* **22**, 168–170.

50. Ioannidis, J. P. A., Rosenberg, P. S., Goedert, J. J., et al. (2001) Effects of CCR5-Δ32, CCR2-64I, and SDF-1 3'A alleles on HIV-1 disease progression: an international meta-analysis of individual-patient data. *Ann. Intern. Med.* **135**, 782–795.

51. Passam, A., Zafiropoulos, A., Miyakis, S., et al. (2005) CCR2-64I and CXCL123'A alleles confer a favorable prognosis to AIDS patients undergoing HAART therapy. *J. Clin. Virol.* **34**, 302–309.

52. Sarrazin, C., Berg, T., Weich, V., et al. (2005) GNB3 C825T polymorphism and response to interferon-alfa/ribavirin treatment in patients with hepatitis C virus genotype 1 (HCV-1) infection. *J. Hepatol.* **43**, 388–393.

53. Lindemann, M., Barsegian, V., Siffert, W., et al. (2002) Role of G protein beta3 subunit 825T and HLA class II polymorphisms in the immune response after HBV vaccination. *Virology* **297**, 245–252.

54. Hauge Opdal, S., Melien, Ø., Rootwelt, H., Vege, Å., Arnestad, M., and Rognum, T. O. (2006) The G protein β3 subunit 825C allele is associated with sudden infant death due to infection, teta paediatre, in press.

Index

CANADA TODAY

1.

CANADA TODAY

A STUDY OF
HER NATIONAL INTERESTS
AND NATIONAL POLICY

By
F. R. SCOTT

Professor of Civil Law, McGill University

With a Foreword By
E. J. TARR

Prepared for the
BRITISH COMMONWEALTH RELATIONS CONFERENCE, 1938

OXFORD UNIVERSITY PRESS
LONDON   *TORONTO*   *NEW YORK*
1938

Issued under the auspices of the
Canadian Institute of International Affairs

PRINTED IN CANADA
BY THE HUNTER-ROSE CO. LIMITED, TORONTO

FOREWORD

THE first unofficial conference on British Commonwealth relations, held at Toronto in September 1933, met less than two years after the enactment of the Statute of Westminster. During that conference there were clear indications that a new approach to Commonwealth questions was emerging, an approach which involved a shifting of emphasis from discussion of the constitutional rights of the dominions to a search for useful fields of intra-Commonwealth co-operation.

The period from 1887, the date of the first Colonial Conference, down to 1931, the date of the Statute of Westminster, had been a period of significant constitutional development in intra-Imperial relations. The more important colonies had become self-governing dominions, and the greater part of Ireland had withdrawn from the United Kingdom to become a member country. The result was a group of autonomous states—in a word, Empire had become Commonwealth. The principal concern of Imperial conferences during that period, especially since the establishment of the Irish Free State, had been the settlement of constitutional questions. After 1931 most of the important constitutional questions that remained had become matters for individual action, if and when desired, rather than for group consideration. Such questions, which have already been dealt with by one or more of the members of the Commonwealth, are the creation of dominion great seals, the abolition of appeals to the Judicial Committee of the Privy Council, the establishment by the executive in a dominion of virtually complete control over the office of governor-general, and the removal from the domestic law of a dominion of the legal principle of the supremacy of the Imperial parliament. There doubtless remain subjects which can be more satisfactorily settled by mutual agreement. Of these the most pertinent seem to be

various aspects of foreign relations, of which some have
already been raised, such as the right to neutrality and the
right to secession.

Not only has the British Empire changed, but so has the
world in which it exists. When the Toronto conference was
held, Herr Hitler's appointment as chancellor was only of
seven months' standing. Since then we have witnessed the
rising power of Germany, Japan and Italy; the break-up of
the Paris peace settlement; the decline of the League; the
change in the balance of power in Europe and in the Far East.

In the light of these changes, both internal and external,
the emphasis must be not upon constitutional adjustments
as we formerly knew them, but upon another problem, that
of discovering to what extent there can be a unity of purpose
and action amongst all the members of the Commonwealth
or, in some cases, groups of members.

A number of questions then present themselves—questions
to which too little attention has been given in the past.
What are the members of the Commonwealth willing to
co-operate for? Is general co-operation of advantage to all
of them, or would their national interests and aspirations be
better fulfilled by a policy of national isolation, by membership in some regional grouping, or in a revised League of
Nations? Do these alternatives actually exist for all or any
member states of the Commonwealth? If the ultimate answers given to such questions by member states differ from
each other, can varying degrees of co-operation be developed
without threatening the underlying Commonwealth bond,
and if so, how?

In approaching such questions, the second British Commonwealth Relations Conference is to start with a realistic
discussion of the position of each member country. A paper
is being prepared in each country—in Great Britain, in
Eire, in India and in each Dominion—describing the most
important economic, political and social factors which determine its interests and sentiment, and analysing the movements of opinion amongst its citizens with respect to Commonwealth and international affairs. On the basis of these
statements it is hoped to discover, during the conference,

those fields of action in which future co-operation between
two or more or all members of the Commonwealth may be
most useful to the member countries, the Commonwealth,
and the world.

The Canadian Institute entrusted the task of writing the
principal Canadian paper to Professor F. R. Scott, of McGill
University. As he himself writes in his preface, his particular
aim has been "to show the relation between internal forces
and external policy". Thus it is that *Canada Today*, the
immediate purpose of which is to help in a re-examination of
Canada's relations with the other states in the Commonwealth, deals so largely with Canadian domestic policy.

The Canadian Institute of International Affairs, which is
affiliated with all the other Commonwealth institutes, is a
national organization with branches in sixteen of the principal Canadian cities. It is an unofficial and non-partisan
body, which aims to provide and maintain means of information upon Commonwealth and international questions and
to promote the study and investigation of these questions
by means of discussion meetings, study groups, conferences,
and the preparation and publication of books and reports.

None of the Commonwealth institutes is propagandist.
They endeavour to include in their memberships representatives of all important shades of opinion on Commonwealth and international affairs. They are precluded by
their constitutions from expressing an opinion on any aspect
of domestic, Commonwealth or international affairs. The
views expressed in this book, as in all Institute publications,
are purely those of the author or others quoted by him.

This volume is a condensed analysis of Canadian conditions and Canadian problems that have a bearing on
Canada's external relations. For a more detailed discussion
of similar questions the reader is referred to the publications
listed in the bibliography in this book and especially to
Canada Looks Abroad, by R. A. MacKay and E. B. Rogers,
which was published two months ago under the auspices of
the Canadian Institute by the Oxford University Press
(Toronto, London, New York). *Canada Looks Abroad* deals
with the geographic, economic and demographic background

of Canadian policy at greater length than does this volume. It then goes on to discuss the historical development of Canada's relations with other parts of the Empire, with the League of Nations, with the United States, the Far East and the U.S.S.R. One chapter deals with defence; a section is concerned with constitutional questions; one chapter describes the machinery through which external affairs are actually conducted; and others discuss the problems of parliamentary control of policy, the power of Canada to conclude treaties and give effect to them, and the question of neutrality. The final section is given to discussions of four alternative external policies: the present non-committal policy which has evolved slowly over a long period; non-intervention, or "isolation"; Commonwealth solidarity, or a "British front"; and collective security. The book also contains about sixty-five pages of documents expressing official policy on various aspects of external affairs and the views of political leaders on broad issues.

The National Council of the Canadian Institute of International Affairs wish to express their appreciation of the service rendered by Professor F. R. Scott in writing *Canada Today*. They also desire to record their gratitude for the invaluable assistance rendered by those many members of the Canadian and other Institutes who criticized the first draft of Mr. Scott's study.

E. J. TARR, *President,*
Canadian Institute of
International Affairs.

WINNIPEG, June 13, 1938.

AUTHOR'S PREFACE

THIS short survey of Canadian conditions and opinions was prepared at the request of the Canadian Institute of International Affairs as the principal Canadian paper for the second British Commonwealth Relations Conference, which is to be held at Sydney, Australia, in September 1938. My aim has been, following the conference agenda, to describe the most important economic, political and social factors which determine Canada's national interests and outlook, to distinguish the various schools of opinion within the country, and particularly to show the relation between internal forces and external policy. Limits of time and space have prevented a more extensive analysis of the many questions touched upon. Where popular opinions were being considered I have tried, though fully aware of the difficulties, to give a three-dimensional rather than a two-dimensional picture; to show, that is, not only what the alternatives are but also the degree of their support among the people and of their harmony or conflict with underlying forces. Throughout I have attempted to exclude common assumptions about Canada and the Commonwealth and to examine the facts objectively, but I am conscious that in the last resort even the so-called objective analysis rests unavoidably upon personal choice and estimate. The paper is a photograph of social facts rather than an attempt to answer the questions raised. Other points of view, and more detailed reports on special topics, will be presented to the conference in the Canadian supplementary papers.

The first draft of *Canada Today*, under the title "Canada and the Commonwealth", was written in the summer of 1937 and was circulated for comment to the branches of the Canadian Institute of International Affairs and to many individuals at home and abroad. I am greatly indebted to the study groups and to the individuals who read the draft—

their names are too numerous to mention—for their substantial assistance whether in the form of criticism or of new material. As far as possible I have embodied their suggestions in the text. In particular I wish to thank the members of the Research Committee and the secretariat of the Canadian Institute for their help in the work of revision and in the details of publication.

F. R. SCOTT.

McGILL UNIVERSITY,
Montreal, June 4, 1938.

CONTENTS

MAPS AND CHARTS

CHAPTER I

THE INFLUENCE OF GEOGRAPHY

CANADA'S geographical position and structure vitally affect her external relations as well as her internal organization. Externally the predominant factor is her isolation from every country save the United States; internally geography has divided the country into a number of distinct regions, widely separated and difficult to weld into a single political or economic framework.

BOUNDARIES

Canada occupies the northern half of the continent of North America, a total area of 3,694,863 square miles, or 27 per cent. of the area of the British Commonwealth. Her boundaries, except in the remote north, are now settled. Eastward lie the Atlantic and the "coast of Labrador", Newfoundland's mainland territory, the limits of which were defined by the Privy Council decision of 1927. To the south is the United States boundary, 3,987 miles long, of which 2,198 are on water and 1,789 on land.[1] To the west is the Pacific coast and the Alaskan boundary, the latter being some 1,500 miles of additional United States frontier. Northward Canada disappears in a sector of ice, the radii of which she has decided shall be the meridians of 60° and 141° west longitude. No formal international recognition has yet been given to the northern limits but neither has there been any challenge to the Canadian claims.[2]

For all practical purposes, Canada has frontier contacts with the United States alone. The Labrador boundary, the solitary land frontier not separating Canada from United States territory, runs through an uninhabited waste. The

[1]For a full description of the boundary see Wilgus, William J., *Railway Interrelations of the United States and Canada* (Toronto, 1937), p. 4.

[2]Norway, however, registered her general objection to the sector principle when admitting Canada's sovereignty over the Sverdrup Islands in 1930. See despatch in prefix to *Statutes of Canada*, 1931.

1

island of Newfoundland, which occupies a strategic position in the Gulf of St. Lawrence, is at the moment a British dependency, having given up its dominion status. Canadian intercourse with it is not extensive, though it furnishes essential supplies of iron ore to the steel mills of Nova Scotia, and is an important link in the chain of imperial communications as a landing-stage for trans-Atlantic cables and air-lines. Halifax, the easternmost large Canadian port, is 2,500 miles from Liverpool; Vancouver, the westernmost, is 4,200 miles from Yokohama.

The distance of Canada from Europe, however, has not meant an absence of world communications. The St. Lawrence to the east forms a national gateway through which travels a great part of Canada's total world trade. Vancouver has become an increasingly important outlet for trade not only with the Far East but with Great Britain and Europe via the Panama Canal. The Hudson Bay route, though still but slightly used as an outlet for grain to Europe, serves to remind Canadians that their fortunes are linked to the high seas. Only two out of the nine Canadian provinces are without coast.

INTERNAL GEOGRAPHIC DIVISIONS

Canada is a nation that in many respects has been built despite geography. The geographical obstacles she has had to overcome have been very serious. On the other hand it is often pointed out that the present Dominion is, in rough outline, a natural response to the geographical relationship between the interior continental plain, the Canadian Shield, and the vast waterways of the St. Lawrence River, the Great Lakes, the less known "great lakes" of the west and north and the connecting rivers. On this extraordinary system of water transport was based first the fur trade, next the eastern lumber trade, then the wheat trade. The oft-repeated statement that the "natural lines" of communication and trade for Canada run north and south and that the east-west structure is a costly piece of artificiality is true only in part. Most Canadian economists would say that the east-west communication has much in it that is "natural". Compass courses for trade are often irrelevant: there are many determinants, minor and major, and of these it is sufficient to point out the Great Lakes-St. Lawrence system as the chief. On it, despite geographical difficulties, has been forged the economic and political system of the country.

The inhabited part of the Dominion falls into five main divisions. To the east are the maritime provinces of Nova Scotia, New Brunswick and Prince Edward Island. They are a country of forests, hills and streams, with agricultural land suitable only for small-scale operations. Minor industries, lumbering, mixed farming and fishing constitute the principal economic interests of the population. The only large industrial undertakings are the coal mines and steel mills in Nova Scotia. The population is mostly British, and has a strong local patriotism. There are important French minorities, particularly in New Brunswick, where they constitute one-third of the population. These provinces are separated from the rest of Canada by ranges of mountains, and by the American boundary which cuts far north along New Brunswick to form a pronounced salient.

The St. Lawrence and Lower Lakes region covers the southern part of the provinces of Quebec and Ontario. Here is concentrated 60 per cent. of the population and 80 per cent. of the manufacturing activity of the Dominion.[1] Montreal and Toronto are the chief financial and industrial centres. In economic interests these two provinces are very similar, combining mixed agriculture with extensive operations in industry, water-power, forestry and mines, all within a comparatively short distance of the St. Lawrence waterways system and the Great Lakes. But in racial and religious background they are quite distinct, Quebec being 80 per cent. French and Catholic, while Ontario is 75 per cent.

[1]The following table shows the regional distribution of the population of Canada, according to the census of 1931:

	Inhabitants (1931)	Per cent. of Dominion Total
Maritime Provinces	1,009,103	9.73
Ontario and Quebec	6,305,938	60.77
Prairie Provinces	2,353,529	22.68
British Columbia	694,263	6.69
Yukon and Northwest Territories	13,953	.13

British and Protestant. In degree of development they also differ, industrial progress being much further advanced in Ontario, while Quebec has clung longer to her peasant agriculture.

The third section is the great prairie plain, the northern extension of the interior continental plain, out of which have been created the three prairie provinces of Manitoba, Saskatchewan and Alberta. This area is separated from eastern Canada by some 800 miles of sparsely inhabited country north of Lake Superior. It is still impossible to motor from Ontario to the west without going through the United States. The soil and climate here make the large-scale production of wheat the principal activity, though other field crops are of importance. A variable rainfall, particularly in southern Saskatchewan and Alberta, and uncertain factors such as frost, hail and insect pests make for large variations in the annual production. Wheat, which is the principal cash crop, has ranged from a record high of 566,726,000 bushels in 1928 to a low of 159,000,000 in 1937, with corresponding variability of income. The population in this area is the most mixed of any in the Dominion, having been augmented for the greater part by immigration during the earlier years of the present century; only about 49 per cent. are British by racial origin.[1]

The prairies are bounded on the west by the Rocky Mountains. On the Pacific slopes of the Rockies lies the fourth of the geographical divisions of Canada, British Columbia. This westernmost section consists mostly of mountains, with considerable forest, fishery and mineral resources, but with little agricultural land save in the valleys. Forestry, mining, fishing and farming are the main activities. The racial composition of the population is mostly British, but there are important Oriental minorities which are denied the franchise and constitute unassimilated groups.

To the north of the more inhabited portions of Quebec, Ontario, Manitoba and Saskatchewan lies the great Canadian Shield, sometimes called the Pre-Cambrian Shield. This is a vast outcropping of crystalline rock which stretches

[1] As shown in the 1936 census, *Canada Year Book*, 1937.

from Labrador to the Mackenzie River, covering an area of some 2½ million square miles, or 65 per cent. of the entire country. It is a great expanse of lakes, rivers, muskeg and forests, containing little arable land, but possessing, besides its forest resources of timber, pulp-wood and fur, large deposits of precious and base metals. Its uniform geological structure and natural resources provide a certain geographic and economic unity in northern Canada.

DISTRIBUTION OF POPULATION

The Canadian population has hitherto grouped itself in the first four of these main divisions for reasons which are largely physiographical. Nowhere does settlement extend northward to any great depth, so that the entire population has been strung out along the American border in a strip nearly 4,000 miles long. More than nine out of every ten Canadians live within 200 miles of the border, and more than half within 100 miles.[1] For many years it seemed as though this distribution of population would be permanent, and that Canadians would be unable to occupy more than the southern fringe of their vast domain. Two developments of recent years have to some degree caused a revision of this idea. The first is the opening up of the rich mineral deposits in the Canadian Shield. Great developments have occurred in these mining regions in the past ten years, and new towns have sprung into existence where formerly there was but empty wilderness. This has deepened the area of settlement, and caused a further shift in the economic balance away from agriculture. In a psychological sense it is tending to unify the country by giving a new outlet to the north for capital, ambition and talent; the old advice, "Go west, young man, go west", has become, "Go north, young man, go north". At the same time the Canadian Shield is unlikely to support a large permanent population. Hydro-electric works, the production of pulp and paper and the development of mineral resources will provide for a small fixed population; but any larger movements will be nomadic.

[1]MacKay, R. A. and Rogers, E. B., *Canada Looks Abroad* (Toronto and London, 1938), p. 12.

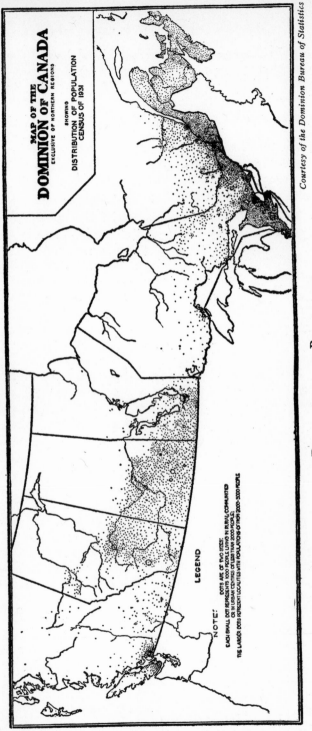

MAP OF THE
DOMINION OF CANADA
EXCLUSIVE OF NORTHERN REGIONS

SHOWING

DISTRIBUTION OF POPULATION
CENSUS OF 1931

LEGEND

NOTE:

DOTS ARE OF TWO SIZES:

EACH SMALL DOT REPRESENTS 1000 PEOPLE LIVING IN RURAL COMMUNITIES
OR IN URBAN CENTRES OF LESS THAN 2000 PEOPLE

THE LARGER DOTS REPRESENT LOCALITIES WITH POPULATIONS OF FROM 2000-3000 PEOPLE

DISTRIBUTION OF POPULATION

The other development which is having a similar effect on a smaller scale is the opening up of new areas of settlement in the Peace River district of Alberta and British Columbia, and in northern Saskatchewan. Here good soil extends far to the north, and temperature and rainfall are suitable for growth during the short summer season. The breeding of new types of wheat such as Marquis and Reward, which ripen early and so escape autumn frosts, has been one of the great achievements of the Department of Agriculture at Ottawa; it has made possible the continuous northward extension of agricultural settlement on the prairies.

Scientific agriculture and new mining fields are making Canadians look northward. The aeroplane and the radio make contacts with civilization possible for remote settlements. Canada as a thin ribbon of population across a continent is still a fact, but the opportunities for pioneering in the north are increasing and the awareness of their existence helps to develop and unify the national consciousness.

EFFECTS OF GEOGRAPHY

The geographical divisions of Canada are responsible for many of the economic, political and social characteristics of the Dominion. The building of national unity on such a long and narrow base would be a task of great difficulty even if additional divisive influences such as race, religion and historical tradition were absent. The Maritime Provinces had a longer history as separate British colonies than they have yet had as provinces of the Dominion. Their sense of identity, distinct from Canada, is still strong; their economic ties would naturally be more with their geographical neighbours, the New England states, than with central or western Canada. They do not feel they have received the full benefits of political union since Confederation, for the tariff wall has cut them off from their natural markets and forced them to become an outlying, almost remote, settlement of an economy concentrated to the west. Many of their sons and daughters have been forced to migrate south and west to find their livelihood: indeed, the Maritimes play the part of the Canadian Scotland, exporting talent which achieves a

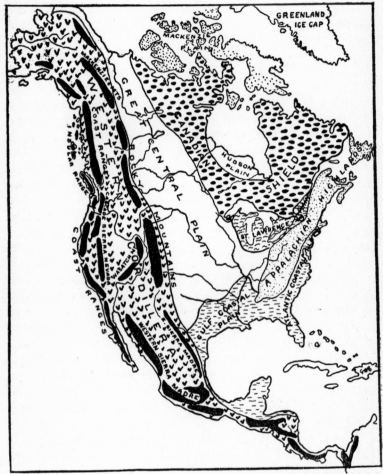

PHYSIOGRAPHIC DIVISIONS OF NORTH AMERICA

disproportionate share of important positions in Canadian (and American) political, educational and industrial life, but leaves behind a sense of stagnation and loss.

Geography gives Quebec and Ontario similar economic opportunities and interests which offset to some extent their racial and religious differences. Both provinces are the centres of protectionist thought, for in both live the manufacturers who benefit most from the tariff. The Prairie Provinces, predominantly suppliers of a single commodity which must be sold on a world market, are naturally inclined to free trade so as to be able to buy cheaply their agricultural machinery and domestic supplies; their dependence upon the eastern capital which controls railways and banks makes them lean to political radicalism and new experiments, particularly in times of depression. British Columbia, facing the Pacific, containing a considerable Oriental population, and separating the United States from her Alaskan territory, is most conscious of Canada's position in the Pacific and of the serious problems that would arise should war occur in that area, even if Canada were neutral.

Canada's climate, a consequence of her geographical position, affects the life, character and economic development of the country very greatly. The climate is bracing and healthy, but the variations of temperature and the long winters impose additional costs on transportation and construction; make for a short growing season and for problems of seasonal unemployment; and limit the agricultural produce to the range of north temperate fruits, grains and vegetables. Industrial processes requiring tropical or semitropical produce must thus rely on imports.

It was geography, as well as race, which made Canada a federal rather than a unitary state. No Dominion cabinet can be formed except on a federal basis, giving representation to each of the main divisions of the country. The Canadian Senate is composed of 24 senators from each of the four divisions of the Maritimes, Quebec, Ontario and the western provinces—a method which blends geography and race. Royal commissions must be appointed, the civil services staffed, and political patronage expended, in accordance with sectional and racial divisions. The twenty per cent. of the population which is neither British nor French, however, has little representation in the Dominion or provincial legislatures or administrative services.

Geography has laid upon the Canadian economy the inescapable burden of heavy transportation costs. The price the Dominion has had to pay to create an economic and political unity against great natural obstacles is to be seen in her 43,000 miles of railway, her canals, highways and telegraphs. Not all of this is chargeable against the effort to overcome geography: some of it, especially much of the railway mileage, is to be attributed to simple lack of intelligence in high places or in low, some of it to the recklessness of pioneer optimism and some to the corruption that always attends large-scale construction projects in a new country where the social controls are weak. However it has arisen, this overhead debt lies heavily upon the economy.

Geography, finally, makes Canada a North American nation. This simple and obvious fact has hitherto been an unconscious rather than a conscious influence upon Canadian life and thought, so strong have been the sentimental ties binding Canadians to Europe, particularly to Great Britain, and so live has been the fear that to turn attention from the old world would mean absorption by the United States. Today those ties are less strong and the fear less alive. The waves of immigration have ceased, and the children of immigrants have not the European memories of their parents. In 1911 a reciprocity treaty with the United States overthrew a government because the people believed it would mean annexation; in 1935 a new treaty, less extensive but of similar appearance, was negotiated with the approval of every political party in Canada. Canadians are beginning to talk of themselves as "North Americans", which formerly they seldom did.[1] Many factors have hastened the accep-

---

[1] See, e.g., *Canada, An American Nation* by J. W. Dafoe (New York, 1935), pp. 5-6. An editorial of March 13, 1938, in *Le Devoir*, a leading French-Canadian daily in Montreal, points out with approval the development of the North American viewpoint amongst English Canadians: "Un journal à sympathies conservatrices, à tendences impérialistes, le *Journal* d'Ottawa, n'écrivait-il pas ces jours-ci, au cours d'un article sur l'avenir du parti conservateur, une fois M. Bennett à sa retraite: 'L'héritage idéologique de ce continent nord-américain diffère du tout au tout de celui du continent européen?' En d'autres termes, nous sommes un peuple d'Amérique, nos problèmes sont d'Amérique, qu'on nous laisse la paix avec les problèmes particuliers de l'Europe: ces ont les siens, et nous avons les nôtres."

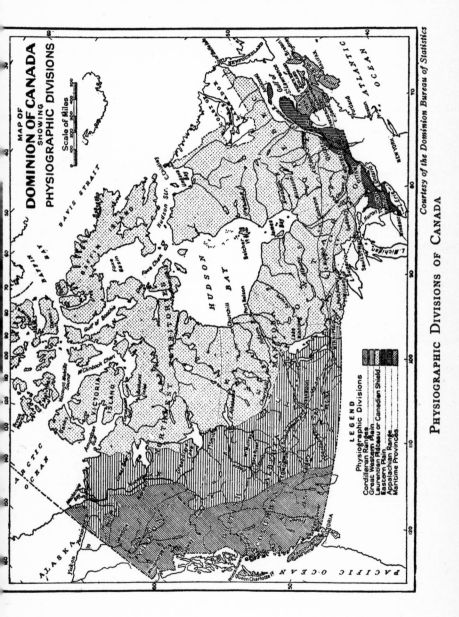

Courtesy of the Dominion Bureau of Statistics

PHYSIOGRAPHIC DIVISIONS OF CANADA

tance of this position, but the underlying influence has been geography. Moreover, in a world constantly on the verge of war, geographical isolation assumes an unwonted attraction.

CHAPTER II

THE POPULATION OF CANADA

CANADA on the average map appears as a large unbroken block of red, thus creating the impression that the country is both united and British. A closer inspection of physiographical features has shown how divided are the several sections of the country. An examination of the racial elements in the population will reveal a similar lack of unity.

GROWTH OF THE POPULATION

Of the aboriginal races, there are about 6,000 Eskimos and 123,000 Red Indians surviving. The two minorities are treated as wards of the Dominion, and do not possess citizens' rights.[1] The first European settlers were the French, many of whom came from Normandy and Brittany, ancestors of the French Canadians who now number approximately 3,300,000 or 30 per cent. of the population. British settlers (excluding the traders in Hudson Bay who came about the same time as the main wave of French Canadians) arrived first in Acadia, the original Nova Scotia, which was ceded to Great Britain by the Treaty of Utrecht in 1713 and which received a considerable influx of New Englanders prior to the American Revolution. That struggle sent to Canada large numbers of United Empire Loyalists, whose influx created the provinces of New Brunswick and Ontario, and the pro-British sentiment of whose descendants today often proves keener than that of many a later British immigrant. The first census after Confederation, taken in 1871, showed a population of 3,486,000, distributed racially as follows:[2]

British . . . . 60.55 per cent.
French . . . . 31.07 per cent.
Others . . . . 8.39 per cent.

[1] Unless, in the case of the Indians, they fought in the world war. Other disfranchised minorities under Dominion or Provincial laws, or both, are Doukhobors, Chinese, Japanese, and Hindus.

[2] This census covered only the four original provinces of Canada—Nova Scotia, New Brunswick, Quebec and Ontario. *Canada Year Book*, 1937, pp. 122-3.

Then came the building of the C.P.R., the opening of the Canadian west, and the adoption of a policy of attracting immigrants indiscriminately. Canada, like the United States, became a melting-pot into which were poured many kinds of human material. The process did not stop until the world depression began. The population grew to 5.37 millions in 1901 and 10.37 millions in 1931; today (1938) it is estimated at 11.2 millions. But now the racial proportions are altered; the British element has steadily declined since 1871, while the "Others" have increased. The process of change is shown by the following table:

	1871 per cent.	1881 per cent.	1901 per cent.	1911 per cent.	1921 per cent.	1931 per cent.
British.....	60.55	58.93	57.03	54.07	55.40	51.86
French....	31.07	30.03	30.71	28.51	27.91	28.22
Others.....	8.39	11.03	12.28	17.40	16.68	19.93

If the 1931 figures are broken down into the dominant racial groups, then we find that the French is the largest. The order is:

Origin[1]	Number (1931)
French......................	2,927,990
English......................	2,741,419
Scottish......................	1,346,350
Irish......................	1,230,808
German......................	473,544
Scandinavian..................	228,049
Ukrainian....................	225,113
Hebrew......................	156,726
Dutch......................	148,962
Polish......................	145,503
Indian and Eskimo............	128,890
Italian......................	98,173

[1] As the figures are based on paternity there is actually more intermixture than they suggest. See Hurd, W. B., *Racial Origins and Nativity of the Canadian People*, Census monograph No. 4 (Dominion Bureau of Statistics, Ottawa, 1938) (to be included in Vol. XII of the *Seventh Census of Canada, 1931*).

The population trend as indicated by the number of children under 1 year of age is as follows (1931):

	Total	Under 1 year	Per 1,000
British	5,381,071	86,202	16
French	2,927,990	73,000	25
German	473,544	10,066	21
Scandinavian	228,049	4,290	19
Ukrainian	225,113	5,229	22
Hebrew	156,726	2,192	14
Polish	145,503	3,375	23

It will be noticed how low is the British reproduction rate relative to that of other groups.

The distribution of the racial groups within the country varies greatly. The British elements are strongest in the Maritimes, Ontario and British Columbia: of those sections they constitute approximately 70 per cent., 75 per cent. and 70 per cent. respectively. Further, persons of British descent usually occupy the most influential positions in politics, religion and education, outside Quebec, and in finance and industry throughout the country. Their power to control the destinies of Canada is therefore very much greater than their numbers would indicate; also, their cultural influence on immigrants of other racial stocks is disproportionately strong. The French are concentrated largely in Quebec, of whose population they form 80 per cent.; but they are now spread far more generally throughout other provinces than was formerly the case, the principal settlements being in eastern and northern Ontario, New Brunswick, and the Prairie Provinces. Whereas in 1871 there were only 153,123 or 14 per cent. of the French Canadians outside Quebec, in 1931 there were 657,931 or 22 per cent.[1] This fact is a powerful deterrent to the separatist movement that has recently been revived by certain groups in French Canada. Of the

[1]See Anderson, Violet (ed.), *World Currents and Canada's Course* (Toronto, 1937), p. 121. It is also estimated that there are at least 1,500,000 French Canadians living in New England, thus showing that the north-south pull for French-Canadian emigrants from Quebec has been stronger than the east-west pull. In 1930 there were in the United States 264,361 French Canadians born in Canada.

2,067,725 persons of non-British, non-French extraction nearly 60 per cent. were confined to the three Prairie Provinces. The Oriental group, though small in number (Chinese 46,519; Japanese 23,342, 1931), are almost all on the Pacific coast and constitute a special minority since they are denied the franchise and are not treated on a plane of equality with other citizens. Finally, it is worth stressing the point that half the people of Canada today, if they look back to an ancestral "mother country", find it elsewhere than in the British Isles; the 51.86 per cent. British of 1931 have become less than 50 per cent. by 1938. Moreover, of the persons classified as British an unspecified number are American settlers of British extraction, other than United Empire Loyalists, whose mother country is really the United States. In 1931 only 14 per cent. of the total population had been born in the British Isles.[1]

RELIGIOUS AFFILIATIONS

To the internal divisions in Canada resulting from geography and race must be added those of religion. The following table shows the number of Canadians in each of the principal religious groups, and the proportion each group bears to the total population of the country:[2]

Religion	Total Population (1931)	Percentage of Total Population (1931)
Roman Catholic	4,285,388	41.3
United Church of Canada	2,017,375	19.4
Anglican	1,635,615	15.8
Presbyterian	870,728	8.4
Baptist	443,341	4.3
Lutheran	394,194	3.8
Jewish	155,614	1.5
Greek Orthodox	102,389	1.0
Others	472,142	4.5

[1]*Canada Year Book*, 1936, p. 118.
[2]*Ibid.*, pp 116-7. A more complete table is to be found in MacKay and Rogers, *op. cit.*, p. 64.

If the Protestant sects are classed together, they make up 54.9 per cent. of the total population, as against 41.3 per cent. Roman Catholic and 3.8 per cent. others. The Roman Catholics are 66.5 per cent. French Canadian, 8.9 per cent. Irish, 4.1 per cent. English, 3.6 per cent. Ukrainian and 3.5 per cent. Scottish.

Religion exerts a very large influence upon Canada's domestic and external affairs, particularly in these days when the "conflict of ideologies" brings everyone face to face in politics with fundamental moral and ethical alternatives. The Catholic and the Protestant interpretations of domestic and international events often differ widely. Thus the French Roman Catholic element in Canada was sympathetic to Italy in the Abyssinian War and Catholic opinion generally has supported Franco in Spain. Three delegates of the Spanish government were driven out of Montreal by organized bands of students when they attempted to speak in November, 1936, but the delegate of the rebels was officially received by the mayor in February, 1938. The Catholic Church is naturally very fearful of the power and influence of Moscow, and is no friend of a democracy which tolerates freedom of speech for those whom it calls "communists".[1] The authoritarian character of the Catholic Church makes it more lenient to the doctrine of fascism than the Protestant churches would be, and it is teaching a form of "corporatism" in Quebec, based on Papal encyclicals, as a remedy for social and economic ills. Because 66 per cent. of the Catholics in Canada are French Canadian, the Church tends to be isolationist in foreign policy and is inclined to be distrustful of the League of Nations.

These attitudes within Canadian Catholicism are frequently in sharp contrast to those adopted by the various Protestant Churches. The Protestant pulpits may vary in their emphasis on particular policies, and, in typical Protestant fashion, they speak with many voices, but their general influence in foreign affairs is against isolation and in

[1] In 1937, shortly after the Dominion parliament repealed the law making the Communist party illegal, the Quebec Legislature adopted the Padlock Act under which the Attorney-General can order the closing of houses of suspected Communists without judicial authorization, and can seize and destroy, also without judicial warrant, any communistic literature which is being printed or circulated.

favour of active Canadian support of the League and the Commonwealth. In domestic matters they emphasize, more than do the Catholics, the value of state control and social legislation to remedy economic evils, and oppose any changes in parliamentary government that savour of dictatorship from the "right" as well as from the "left". In some parts of Canada, as in the United States, an evangelical type of politico-religious revival can win much support; social credit was given to the people of Alberta in this manner through Mr. Aberhart's "Prophetic Bible Institute", and the British Israelite movement finds some support from certain elements in the population.

POPULATION AND IMMIGRATION

Recent studies of the effects of immigration upon the growth of Canada's population have led to some important, if tentative, conclusions.[1] While it would be dangerous to accept all the findings as final and complete they are sufficiently exact to render necessary a revision of the popular idea that every new immigrant means an increase of one in the size of the total population, or that Canada, because of her "vast resources" and "great open spaces", can readily absorb a large number of new immigrants.

Briefly, the facts appear to show that over the period 1851-1931 the total immigration was about equalled by the amount of emigration, mostly to the United States, so that in fact the net result was largely a substitution of foreign-born settlers (including British) for native-born Canadians. It has been demonstrated[2] that if there had been no emigration during those years the Canadian population would be at least as large as, and probably larger than, it is today, even if there had been no immigration from abroad at all. The following table gives some idea of the way the process worked during the decade 1921-1931:[3]

[1] A convenient summary of the evidence, with full references to sources, will be found in the Canadian Memorandum No. 1, presented to the International Studies Conference of 1937 by the Canadian Institute of International Affairs, on *Canada and the Doctrine of Peaceful Change*, edited by H. F. Angus. (Mimeographed.)

[2] See Angus (ed.), *op. cit.*, p. 63.

[3] *Canada Year Book*, 1936, p. 107.

Population, Census 1921   8,787,949
Natural Increase, 1921-1931 (est.)   1,325,256
Immigration, 1921-1931[1]   1,509,136

Total   11,622,341

Population, Census 1931   10,376,786
Emigration, 1921-1931 (est.)   1,245,555
Net Immigration, 1921-1931   263,581

In that decade, for every five persons coming into the country, four went out. At the same time unemployment in Canada increased by some 270,000.[2]

It would be improper to conclude that over the long period immigration was the sole cause of the emigration. There are many attractions in the United States, such as higher wages, which invite Canadians to move south, and Canadians have been exempted from the quota restrictions applicable since 1921 to other immigrants. Few immigrants settled in the Maritimes or Quebec, yet there was considerable emigration from these sections. It appears, however, that both migrations occurred together, and there is evidence to suggest that the relationship of cause and effect existed to some degree.[3] The waves of immigration are found to precede, not to succeed, emigration: the emigrants went largely from occupations reinforced by immigrants; the immigrants, being in large part single adult males between 20 and 35 years old, were better fitted for work at lower wage levels and hence were more attractive to Canadian employers seeking low costs.

This emigration of Canadians to the United States, it should be noted, is not all loss, from the Canadian point of view. The presence of so many people of Canadian antecedents in the States contributes to the understanding between the two countries. A good many Canadian emigrants hold positions of influence in American business and in the professions. The number of Canadian-born persons living in the United States in 1930 was 1,280,000: of these 264,361 were French Canadian.

[1]Including returning Canadians.
[2]Angus (ed.), *op. cit.*, p. 62.
[3]*Ibid.*, pp. 58-60.

PRESENT MOVEMENTS IN POPULATION

Emigration of Canadians to the United States was stopped partly by the depression, partly by the American legislation of 1930. The Canadian-born population must now stay in Canada and find employment at home. This it has to do in the face of a labour market depressed by the presence of large numbers of unemployed and drought victims.[1]

Immigration into Canada is now very restricted. Chinese immigration was ended by the Dominion Chinese Immigration Act of 1923; between 1925 and 1936 only 7 Chinese were admitted.[2] Japanese immigration is governed by the "gentleman's agreement" of 1907, as revised in 1928, under which the number of Japanese entering the country does not exceed 150 a year.[3] The total number admitted between 1929 and 1936 was 813.[4] Other immigration is governed by the new regulations laid down in the Order-in-Council of March 21, 1931, which limits immigration to the following four classes:[5]

1. A British subject entering Canada directly or indirectly from Great Britain or Northern Ireland, the Irish Free State, Newfoundland, the United States of America, New Zealand, Australia, or the Union of South Africa, who has sufficient means to maintain himself until employment is secured; provided that the only persons admissible under the authority of this clause are British subjects by reason of birth or naturalization in Great Britain or Northern Ireland, the Irish Free State, Newfoundland, New Zealand, Australia, or the Union of South Africa.

2. A United States citizen entering Canada from the United States who has sufficient means to maintain himself until employment is secured.

3. The wife or unmarried child under 16 years of age of any person legally admitted to and resident in Canada who is in a position to receive and care for his dependents.

4. An agriculturist having sufficient means to farm in Canada.

[1] The numbers on direct relief in recent years, including dependents, have been: November, 1932, 1,113,849; November, 1934, 1,063,592; November, 1936, 1,100,025; December, 1937, 951,000.
[2] *Canada Year Book*, 1937, p. 205.
[3] *Canadian Annual Review*, 1927-28, p. 145.
[4] *Canada Year Book*, 1937, p. 205.
[5] P.C. 695, March 21, 1931.

The annual immigration since this order took effect has been very small, averaging only about 12,000 annually for the past five years.[1] In spite of the preference for British immigrants revealed in the new regulations, nearly 80 per cent. of the new arrivals in Canada in the years 1931-1936 were from places outside the British Isles.

A noticeable movement of the population within the country in recent years has been the drift from country to town. Urbanization is not a purely Canadian phenomenon, but its development in the Dominion has been marked. Between 1891 and 1931 the proportion of the population living in rural centres decreased from 68.20 to 46.30 per cent.[2] In 1931, 41.74 per cent. of the people lived in cities or towns of 5,000 population and over.[3] The drift in the decade 1921-1931 was most noticeable in the provinces of Quebec and Ontario, and was several times greater in Quebec than in any other province—a fact which in part explains why the birthrate is declining rapidly in French Canada as well as in the Dominion as a whole. In that decade a net rural-urban movement occurred in Canada amounting to about 437,000, all ages.[4]

Moreover, even by 1931 it was apparent that the internal flow of population, which early in the century had been from east to west, had been reversed. The three Prairie Provinces by 1931 had not only ceased to absorb surplus population from the east, but were exporting part of their own surplus to the east. This movement has no doubt continued since 1931 owing to the various causes preventing a return of prosperous conditions to western agriculture. The prairies are thus proving unable to hold their own people under present conditions.[5]

The internal drift of the immigrant population shows the

[1]*Canada Year Book*, 1937, p. 194.

[2]Hurd, W. B., "The Decline in the Canadian Birth Rate", *Canadian Journal of Economics and Political Science*, February, 1937, p. 43.

[3]*Canada Year Book*, 1936, p. 125.

[4]See Hurd, W. B. and Cameron, Jean C., "Population Movements in Canada, 1921-1931: Some Further Considerations", *Canadian Journal of Economics and Political Science*, May, 1935, p. 226, note 3; Hurd, "The Decline in the Canadian Birth Rate", (*op. cit.*)

[5]See Hurd, "Population Movements in Canada, 1921-1931", in *Proceedings of Canadian Political Science Association*, 1934, Vol. VI, p. 224. In the five-year period, 1931-36, the population of the three Prairie Provinces increased by only 2.6 per cent.

same tendency to concentrate in cities, and cities in the east. "Despite continuous efforts on the part of the authorities to stimulate rural rather than urban settlement, the proportion of the current net immigration domiciled in towns and cities at the close of the decade (1921-1931) was three times greater than that found in the country. Whereas in 1921, only 56 per cent. of the foreign-born population in Canada was resident in urban centres, over 75 per cent. of the net foreign immigration during the last ten years found its way to towns and cities."[1] The cities and towns of Ontario and Quebec combined accounted for nearly 63 per cent. of the net increase in urban foreign-born over the ten-year period. Even rural immigrants did not prefer the prairies; Ontario alone absorbed 52 per cent. of the net rural immigration from abroad during the decade, while the four western provinces only accounted for 43 per cent.[2]

Other interesting features of Canadian population movements might be emphasized, but enough has been said to indicate how unreliable are many of the popular ideas about the "great open spaces" in Canada and their capacity to absorb large numbers of immigrants. Canada, in the present condition of her domestic and foreign markets, appears already overcrowded. If agriculture merely holds its own and other rural employment is not forthcoming, a rural surplus of 800,000 is quite possible by 1941.[3] To absorb the present natural increase in urban Canada, the estimated rural-urban migration, and the number of unemployed in 1931, would require a 45 to 50 per cent. increase in urban employment over the next decade.[4] There is little likelihood of this occurring. Canada would be more than able to supply her own population requirements for five or ten years to come if the rate of economic expansion obtaining during the period 1911-1931 were restored, and even if the boom conditions of 1901-1911 were repeated she would not need to draw more than a few thousand a year from abroad to reach the limit of her absorptive capacity.[5]

1Hurd and Cameron, op. cit., pp. 237-8.
2Ibid., pp. 233, 235.
3Hurd, "Population Movements in Canada, 1921-1931", (op. cit.), p. 231.
4Hurd and Cameron, op. cit., p. 232.
5Angus (ed.), op. cit., p. 70.

The foregoing estimates, based upon the most authoritative research that has been done in this field, are not generally known in Canada and are not accepted by all who do know of them. Some authorities contend that many more settlers can be supported in the Peace River district of Alberta, and that on the prairies themselves there may develop a type of self-contained peasant farm through a more scientific use of soils. Consequently the hope of revived immigration is one entertained by a number of individuals and institutions (such as transportation companies) which believe increased immigration will be a means of increasing the population, reducing the per capita debt burden and increasing the internal consuming power. The chief opposition comes from the French Canadians, who fear additions to the British majority, and labour organizations which take the view that the present immigration restrictions should be maintained "until the present unemployment and agricultural depression has disappeared".[1]

ASSIMILATION OF IMMIGRANTS

Assimilation is not a term easy to define nor a condition easy to measure. The French Canadian would use it differently from the English Canadian. If it means "to make Canadian", in the sense that the settler comes to accept Canada as the country of his primary allegiance and to feel at home there, then it occurs in nearly every instance. In this sense immigrants from the British Isles need to be "assimilated", for they do not have a Canadian viewpoint when they arrive. Acceptance of the English language and Canadian customs goes on steadily amongst most foreign-born immigrants. The new settlers seldom join the French-Canadian group. Perhaps the process of assimilation is best described by saying that everyone in Canada, except the French Canadian, sooner or later speaks some variant of the North American language and adopts North American habits, while keeping, in many instances, the language and culture of his forbears.

[1]See Trades and Labour Congress of Canada, "Representations to the Dominion Government, January 1938", *Canada Labour Gazette*, 1938, p. 144.

The assimilation of immigrants, in the form of intermarriage and a mixing of stocks, is slow. The "melting-pot" is not producing a racial alloy. Racial diversity is especially noticeable when a foreign group settles in a community, forms a "colony", and preserves its own language and customs, as do the Ukrainians, the Doukhobors, the Orientals, and some other peoples. Moreover, there is no national education system to unify the children's outlook rapidly. Each province has a separate educational programme, though there is some co-operation between provincial educational authorities, particularly in the western provinces. Separate schools for Catholics and Protestants exist by law in Ontario, Quebec, Saskatchewan and Alberta, and in practice education generally is divided on religious lines. The census of 1931 showed that the school system in Canada provided all but 7 per cent. of the children between the ages of 7 and 14 with schooling, but 34 per cent. of those between the ages 5-19 were not at school.[1] Of all children in Canada, only two-thirds go as far as the final year of elementary schools, one-fifth or more reach the final or matriculation year, one-tenth or more continue to a professional school or university, and about three per cent. obtain a university degree.[2] Besides this inadequacy of education, the fact that all newspapers are regional, and the almost total absence of popular periodicals which are read from coast to coast, tend to keep public opinion sectional, though the control of radio broadcasting is assisting in the development of a more national outlook.[3]

Assimilation in Canada thus has not meant cultural or linguistic uniformity, and permits of wide variations of behaviour and belief. The two major races, French and English, have approached each other remarkably little during

[1] *Canada Year Book*, 1936, p. 133; *Census of Canada*, 1931, Vol. IV, pp. 1354-5.

[2] Dominion Bureau of Statistics, *Cost of Education Bulletin No. 1*, 1934. The figures do not include Quebec and British Columbia.

[3] To connect the 53 stations making up a national network necessary to broadcast a single programme throughout Canada, takes over 8,000 miles of transmission lines (as opposed to less than 1,000 miles in Great Britain) and even then it only reaches 10 per cent. of the land area of the provinces of Canada and not more than 75 per cent. of the total population. The further facts that 30 per cent. of the people desire to hear broadcasts in their mother tongue, French; that Canada stretches through five time zones; and that all broadcasting is done in competition with American stations spending 50 times as much money, using 30 times as much power, covering the entire United States and at night more of Canada than the Canadian stations, illustrate the difficulties which have to be overcome in attempting to use the radio as an instrument for fostering national unity.

their long and close association. In the words of André Siegfried,[1] they have a *"modus vivendi"* without cordiality". This observation is not altogether true, for there are groups in the upper levels of professional and business life who know and respect each other; but it describes well enough the relations of the mass of each population, between whom is an almost impenetrable wall built of religion, race, language, education, history, geography and simple ignorance of one another's point of view. In times of political and economic calm the spirit of mutual non-interference permits each group to pursue its separate path with little disturbance, but every crisis reveals how wide is the gulf between them.

FUTURE GROWTH OF POPULATION

There are two kinds of estimates of Canada's future population—those made by speakers on public platforms, which receive wide publicity, and those made by academic students of the problem, which get buried in learned periodicals. The former predict a population by the year 2000 A.D. of anywhere from 50 to 200 million; the latter seem to agree that unless present trends are altered in a manner that is impossible to predict, the population will not be above 18 million by the end of this century, with a limiting population found ultimately somewhere between 20 and 35 million.[2]

Factors pointing to the lower estimates are the decline in the Canadian birth-rate, which, due to increasing urbanization and other factors, dropped 14.4 per cent. in the decade 1921-1931,[3] and has declined 23.3 per cent. since 1881; new statistics indicating that the extent of unoccupied land suitable for agricultural settlement in the Dominion is much less than was at first estimated;[4] a better understanding of the

---

[1]Siegfried, André, *Canada* (London, 1937), p. 255.

[2]See Angus (ed.), *op. cit.*, Chap. II, p. 41. All the authorities are there collected. The following are the most important; MacLean, M. C., and Hurd, W. B.,"Projection of Canada's Population on the Basis of Current Birth and Death Rates, 1931-1971", Canadian Paper for Yosemite Conference, Institute of Pacific Relations, 1936; Hurd, W. B., "The Decline of the Canadian Birth Rate", *Canadian Journal of Economics and Political Science*, February, 1937; MacKay and Rogers, *op. cit.*, pp. 55 ff.

[3]"Of this ten year decrease, slightly under 2.4 points or 16.7 per cent. seems to have been attributable to less favourable age distribution generally; slightly under 7.3 points or 50.7 per cent. to less favourable conjugal condition, and only something over 4.7 points or 32.6 per cent. to other causes including increased illegitimacy, birth control, abortion, infant mortality and so on." Hurd, W. B., "The Decline in the Canadian Birth Rate", (*op. cit.*), p. 57.

[4]See below, p. 45.

effects of immigration; and general considerations such as the world trend toward economic nationalism, which suggests that the expansion of Canadian foreign trade, and hence Canada's capacity to support new industries, is not likely to proceed as rapidly in the future as it has done in the past. It is always possible that new factors will enter in to upset these estimates, but in attempting to guess at future developments it would seem wiser to adopt the sober rather than the enthusiastic view. The rate of natural increase of population has declined from 17.8 per thousand population in 1921 to 10.6 in 1936.[1]

One interesting conclusion of these forecasts is that by 1971 the French-Canadian element in the population is likely to outnumber that of British descent. It is dangerous, however, to argue too much from this prediction. The French Canadians will still be concentrated very largely in a single province, and many of the non-British, non-French races in the country will by then be assimilated to those of British descent in attitudes and outlook, thus increasing the homogeneity of the non-French group. Moreover, the attitudes of the two races upon national questions may well grow more alike with the passage of time. Nevertheless, a progressive extension of the French influence in Canada is to be expected.

---

[1] *Canada Year Book*, 1937, p. 189.

CHAPTER III

THE NATURE OF THE CANADIAN ECONOMY

THE DEVELOPMENT OF THE ECONOMY

SINCE the earliest days of settlement in New France Canada has been a country depending largely upon foreign trade. Great wealth lay in her natural resources, but since population and markets were far away economic policy was concerned with extracting the wealth and exporting it to the markets. Despite the growth in manufacturing industries during the past fifty years, that description remains basically true of the present economy. Canada is built on the assumption that other people can and will buy her staple products.

Taken in historical order, the chief Canadian exports have been fish, in the early days of French settlement; furs, for the following two centuries; lumber, in the early and mid-nineteenth century; followed by wheat, with the opening of the west. Then industrial activity began to add its quota of products for export, such as flour, planks and boards, wood pulp and paper, and later automobiles. Mining has steadily increased its importance in the economy since the twentieth century began. The Pre-Cambrian Shield has supplied three of the principal sources of wealth, namely furs, forests, and minerals, and it also supplies the hydro-electric power which makes production possible in areas remote from other sources of energy. One measure of the success of this policy of staple production for export is the fact that Canada had, in 1935, the fifth largest export trade of any country in the world, and ranked sixth in total value of world trade.[1]

A picture of the principal divisions of production in Canada is given by the following table for the year 1935. The percentages are based on the net value of production in each division.[2]

[1]League of Nations figures, cited *Canada Year Book*, 1937, p. 501.
[2]Canada, Department of Trade and Commerce, *Survey of Production in Canada*, 1935

	Per cent. of Total Production for 1935
Division of Industry	
Manufactures........................	53.96
Agriculture..........................	26.01
Mining..............................	9.96
Forestry............................	9.50
Electric Power......................	5.22
Fisheries...........................	1.44
Construction, Custom and Repair.......	7.83

It will be noticed how far manufacturing is ahead of agriculture in terms of value of production. The figures for manufactures include some items also included under other heads (such as dairy factories, sawmills, etc.) but even when all duplication is removed manufactures count for about 40 per cent. of the total. The importance of manufacturing is reflected in the distribution of the population as between town and country; in 1931, 53.7 per cent. lived in urban, 46.3 per cent. in rural communities. In 1901 the proportions were the other way, 62.5 per cent. living in rural, and only 37.3 per cent. in urban communities. The change is another measure of Canada's growing industrialization. It is making the large metropolitan centres like Montreal, Toronto, Winnipeg and Vancouver of increasing importance as governmental and administrative units.

The net value of all goods produced in Canada in 1935 was estimated at $2,394,720,688, and total exports amounted to $756,625,925; thus 31.6 per cent. of the total production was exported.[1] This figure is emphatic proof of Canada's dependence on world markets. In many of the basic industries the home consumption is a small fraction of production. Moreover, when the export figures are analysed more closely they show that a comparatively few commodities constitute the great bulk of the exports; in 1937, for instance, the five staples—wheat and flour, pulp and paper, lumber, precious and base metals, and fish—accounted for two-thirds of the total. The extraction of a few staple products from the natural resources, and their shipment abroad, are, as has been

[1]Figures from *Survey of Production*, 1935, and *Canada Year Book*, 1937, p. 545.

NET PRODUCTION

1935

PROVINCIAL DISTRIBUTION

INDUSTRIAL DISTRIBUTION

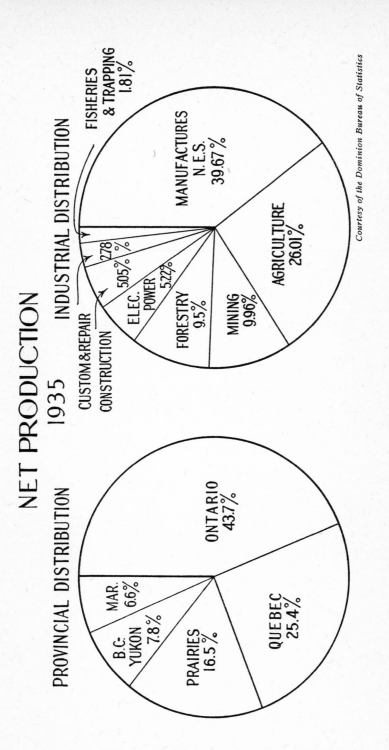

Provincial Distribution:
- ONTARIO 43.7%
- QUEBEC 25.4%
- PRAIRIES 16.5%
- B.C.-YUKON 7.8%
- MAR. 6.6%

Industrial Distribution:
- MANUFACTURES N.E.S. 39.67%
- AGRICULTURE 26.01%
- MINING 9.96%
- FORESTRY 9.5%
- ELEC. POWER 5.22%
- CONSTRUCTION 5.05%
- CUSTOM & REPAIR 2.78%
- FISHERIES & TRAPPING 1.81%

Courtesy of the Dominion Bureau of Statistics

said, dominant characteristics of the Canadian economy today.

If the figures for total net production are distributed amongst economic regions in Canada, the immense preponderance of the two central provinces is evident. Ontario accounted in 1935 for 43.7 per cent. and Quebec 25.4 per cent. of the total, or 69.1 per cent. between them. The three prairie provinces produced only 16.5 per cent., British Columbia 7.8 per cent., and the Maritimes together only 6.6 per cent. The importance and wealth of Ontario and Quebec, coupled with the nationalist sentiment in Quebec, tend to make these two provinces strong defenders of "provincial rights", while the other sections of the country, with fewer sources of revenue and more need of special attention, are apt to favour a reasonable assumption by the Dominion of essential social services.

Partly, no doubt, because of this dependence on foreign trade and because of the nature of her staple products, Canada is liable to a highly fluctuating national income. The demand for many of the staples is inelastic, and most of them are produced in other parts of the world. Wheat production is subject to the vagaries of nature at home and to rapid price changes in the world market. The depression of 1929, when the national income was cut 50 per cent. in four years,[1] revealed this weakness in the structure of the economy. Foreign trade dropped 65 per cent. in the same period. And because of the tariff and the regional grouping of many of the major economic activities (manufactures in Quebec and Ontario, wheat on the prairies, etc.) the changes in national income are very unevenly distributed throughout the economy, and set up within Canada political movements and claims for special treatment in depressed areas.

While historic economic tradition and the facts of geography have combined to make Canada so dependent on the direct exploitation of her natural resources and raw materials, it is nevertheless true that diversified manufacturing is steadily increasing in the country, and the percentage of manufactured exports to total exports is rising. No less than

[1]Innis, H. A. and Plumptre, A. F. W. (eds.), *The Canadian Economy and Its Problems*, (Toronto 1934), p. 181. The figures are for dollar values.

55 different kinds of commodities were exported in 1936 to a value of $2,000,000 or over.[1] Whereas in the early days of Canada's development the imports were made up chiefly of manufactured products and the exports of raw and semi-manufactured products, since the opening of the century this has been reversed. A considerable percentage of imports now consists of raw and semi-manufactured products for use in Canadian manufacturing industries, and the exports consist predominantly of products which have undergone some process of manufacture. In 1937, of the value of total imports 29 per cent. were raw materials, 9.8 per cent. partly and 61.2 per cent. fully manufactured; of total exports the raw materials were 35.9 per cent., partly manufactured goods 27.9 per cent., and fully manufactured goods 36.2 per cent.[2] The leading manufactures in Canada are, as might be expected, for the processing of raw materials. As the internal market expands so does the range of goods which may be profitably manufactured, and there are a number of industries in Canada serving the domestic and even foreign markets, using imported raw materials such as rubber, cotton and sugar. Canadian manufactures, however, are not being developed with a view to making Canada self-sufficient; their growth is entirely a matter of unplanned expansion determined by considerations of profitable investment.

Contemporaneously with the growth of manufacturing, an increased trend to monopolistic and semi-monopolistic control within the Canadian economy has taken place. In most of the large-scale industries, two, three, four or six corporations control from 75 to 95 per cent. of the output.[3] The

[1]*Canada Year Book*, 1937, p. 518.

[2]*Condensed Preliminary Report on the Trade of Canada*, 1936-37, p. 33. See also *Canada Year Book*, 1937, p. 519. The following table (*ibid*, p. 407) shows the rate of growth in industrial establishments:

Year	Capital	Employees	Salaries and Wages	Net Value of Products
1900	446,916,487	339,173	113,249,350	214,525,517
1910	1,247,583,609	515,203	241,008,416	564,466,621
1920	3,371,940,653	609,586	732,120,585	1,686,978,408
1930	5,203,316,760	644,439	736,092,766	1,665,631,771
1935	4,698,991,853	582,874	590,236,904	1,302,179,099

The technological improvement in manufacturing is evidenced by the small increase of employees as compared with the increase in the capital and net value of products. The number of establishments increased from 14,650 in 1900 to 25,491 in 1935.

[3]Innis and Plumptre (eds.), *op. cit.*, p. 182.

growth of the large corporation has proceeded more rapidly
than the growth of business in general. In 1932 the 100
largest non-financial corporations had 82 per cent. of the
assets of all Canadian companies publishing balance sheets,
including railways.[1] This concentration of economic power
in a few corporations has been accompanied by a concentration of control within the corporations themselves; the wide
distribution of share ownership, the use of such devices as
the holding company and non-voting stock, have tended to
vest the real direction of corporate affairs in the hands of
small managerial groups.

The trend toward monopoly is a factor of great importance
in contemporary Canada. It explains much that occurs in
the political and economic life of the Dominion. The powerful financial and industrial groups inevitably exert a continuous influence upon governmental policy. Indirectly, by the
opposition their power arouses amongst the people, they
have given rise to new political alignments. Monopoly has
brought class conflict into the political arena. All the minority parties that have either arisen or improved their position
since the depression—the socialist farmer-labour movement
known as the C.C.F.,[2] the Social Credit Party, Mr. Stevens's
Reconstruction Party of 1935, and the Communists[3]—have
derived their principal strength from the fact that they
organized the small man and the underdog against exploitation by the "trusts" and "big business". The same economic
conflict in part accounts for French-Canadian nationalism,
for the French Canadians feel that they are mere "hewers of
wood and drawers of water" in their own country, and resent
the fact that they are scarcely represented in the inner circles
of the large corporations.[4] Monopoly also brings the state
into economic life in an endeavour to protect the public
interest.

Most of the large Canadian firms are organized to do busi-

[1]*Report of the Royal Commission on Price Spreads*, 1935, p. 21. A detailed analysis of the
trend to monopoly is given in League for Social Reconstruction, *Social Planning for Canada*
(Toronto, 1935), Chap. III; see also Taylor, K. W., in Anderson, Violet (ed.), *World
Currents and Canada's Course*, p. 99.

[2]The abbreviation for "Co-operative Commonwealth Federation".

[3]The combined vote of these parties was approximately 25 per cent. of the total vote
at the 1935 general elections. See below, p. 66, n. 3.

[4]See Barbeau, Victor, *La Mesure de Notre Taille* (Montreal, 1936).

ness throughout the Dominion; they therefore provide unified structures reaching across provincial boundaries and tending to break down sectional and provincial barriers. The increasing accumulation of capital in these few hands is also responsible for the increasing investment of Canadian capital in foreign countries; the surplus funds made available by operations on a large scale seek the most profitable outlets, and if conditions look more promising elsewhere the money will be exported. Thus Canadians own large utilities in places as remote as Mexico and Brazil and have mining interests as far away as Rhodesia.

Besides its dependence on the export of staple products and its trend to monopoly, the Canadian economy today is noteworthy for its internal rigidities. The transportation costs in a country with Canada's geography and climate are inevitably high; large amounts of capital have been invested in permanent works in railways, roads, canals, harbours and terminals, and many of these are in full use for only a part of the year.[1] The very size of many corporations makes for high overhead costs and rigid organization. The tariff enables the prices of manufactured goods to be maintained at times when the prices for Canadian exports of wheat and raw materials are falling, thus causing slow adjustments and great inequities in the incidence, as between regions and classes, of the burdens of depression. Labour is rendered largely immobile by racial and geographical obstacles, as well as by trades union organization. Governmental, corporate and private debts are high,[2] and the costs of government (of ten governments, in fact) are heavy.

TRANSPORTATION SYSTEM

Canada is a land of great distances and widely separated economic areas. To make her development possible, she inevitably had to acquire a large and costly transportation equipment. Actually she provided herself with far more than

[1]Canadian transportation costs, it may be pointed out, are not all borne by producers and shippers. The average of Canadian rates is the lowest per ton mile in the world, the difference between high costs and low rates being made up by the tax-payer.

[2]See table of Dominion, provincial and municipal debts in Innis and Plumptre (eds.), *op. cit.*, pp. 62-4; D. C. MacGregor, "The Problem of Public Debt in Canada", *Canadian Journal of Economics and Political Science*, 1936, p. 167.

she needed. No less than three separate transcontinental railway systems were built—the Canadian Pacific Railway, completed in 1885, the Canadian Northern, built in the decade and a half just before the world war, and the Grand Trunk Pacific (with the government-built National Transcontinental), completed 1904-15. The Canadian Northern, the Grand Trunk and its subsidiary the Grand Trunk Pacific were taken over by the government between 1917 and 1921 and were merged with the Canadian Government Railways, being ultimately consolidated in 1923 under the descriptive title Canadian National Railways. The taking over was to prevent the bankruptcy which faced the private owners. One railway runs north to Churchill on Hudson Bay, providing a short, almost unused, route to Europe from the prairies during the brief season of navigation.[1] The main C.P.R. line to the Maritime Provinces runs through American territory in Maine, and both the C.P.R. and the C.N.R. are members of the Association of American Railroads. In freight and passenger rates, in equipment and in practice they are closely tied to United States lines. Canadian freight rates are set by the Board of Railway Commissioners on a basis determined by various factors such as cost, water competition, a desire to assist remote areas, and political considerations; five separate rate divisions exist, corresponding in some degree to the economic regions of the country.[2]

The manner of building of these lines, the extent of governmental grants and guarantees, the political consequences of the scramble for charters and privileges, constitute in the history of the Dominion a special chapter in which national vision blends with political corruption, the glamour of engineering achievement with the tragedy of waste and unnecessary duplication. Canada pays heavily today for the peculiar character of her rail system. Without a railway backbone, however, the Canadian body economic would never survive; these lines of steel enable prairie wheat to reach the Great Lakes or the Pacific, and the forest and mineral products of the Pre-Cambrian Shield to be brought

[1] Eight sea-going vessels cleared in 1936.
[2] Innis and Plumptre (eds.), *op. cit.*, pp. 71 ff.

within reach of markets. Railways are a primary factor in the unity of east and west as well as a major link in the chain of intra-Commonwealth communications.

In 1934 there were 42,916 miles of steam railways in Canada. It has been estimated that the debt incurred in respect of railways, including grants made to the C.P.R., accounts for more than half of the public debt of the Dominion.[1] In addition, some $300,000,000 have been spent on the canal systems, mainly in the St. Lawrence-Great Lakes area. The proposed St. Lawrence Waterways Treaty has not yet become effective owing to the rejection by the American Senate and the opposition of the provinces of Quebec and Ontario, and also to the uncertain distribution of legislative jurisdiction as between the Dominion and the provinces. Besides the Dominion canal systems there is the Panama Canal, which, by providing a direct connection between the east and west coast, open all year, has become an important factor in Canadian transportation development. Wheat from Alberta tends to move via Panama to Europe, and the competition of freight rates on this route exerts a powerful influence upon transcontinental railway rates in the Dominion.[2] The St. Lawrence route controls freight rates from Chicago to the Atlantic seaboard.

Highway construction in the Dominion is another part of the transportation problem. When the constitution of Canada was drafted railways were the predominant mode of commercial land transport, and power to control these was given to the Dominion. Highways were of local importance only, and fell under provincial or municipal management. Today the provinces, sometimes helped by the Dominion, have spent large sums on highway development, and the trucking services have become serious competitors of railways without having been brought under any co-ordinating authority. In 1937 a provincial Royal Commission was appointed by Ontario to investigate the problem.

Civil aviation is the latest mode of transportation to be developed, and is making steady progress. The first trans-

[1]MacKay and Rogers, *Canada Looks Abroad*, pp. 29-30.
[2]For a detailed discussion see Innis and Plumptre (eds.), *op. cit.*, Appendix V, by H. A. Innis.

Canada service opened in 1938. In 1937 began the test flights of Imperial Airways linking Canada with Great Britain by air. Aviation is proving most useful in opening and servicing the remote mining areas of the Canadian Shield; prospecting is aided, and machinery and supplies are carried into otherwise inaccessible regions.[1] The trial flights of the Soviet fliers over the pole in 1937 reminded Canadians that they are on the direct air route between Asia and North America.

Despite her dependence on foreign trade and her large system of inland waterways, Canada has not developed her own shipping fleet to any great extent. The net tonnage of all vessels registered in Canada at December 31, 1934, was 1,389,343.[2] Some 700,000 tons of this are in lake vessels,[3] and most of the remainder in coastal shipping. Few Canadian ships ply the high seas; the Canadian Pacific Steamships vessels, for instance, are registered in England and are mostly staffed by non-Canadians. The goods that leave Canadian shores in such abundance have in many cases already been sold to foreign purchasers, and are mostly loaded in non-Canadian ships. This fact does not make the trade any less important to Canada, but it is relevant to any discussion of Canada's providing naval protection for her foreign trade. The tonnage of freight entered outwards for the sea from Canadian ports for the fiscal year ending March, 1937, was about 16,000,000 tons, of which 8,000,000 tons were carried in British ships, 6,000,000 in foreign ships and 2,000,000 in Canadian vessels.

EXTERNAL DEBTOR AND CREDITOR POSITION

The development of Canadian resources and the increasing industrialization of the country have required large amounts of capital. It was natural for Canada to borrow that capital from the countries with which she had the closest connections —Great Britain and the United States. At first Great

[1] In 1936 more express and freight was carried by air in Canada than in any other country.—*Canada Year Book*, 1937, p. 709.

[2] *Ibid.*, p. 677.

[3] *Green's Register of Lake Tonnage*. Lloyds' list shows approximately 400,000 on the lakes and 840,000 coastal, but many vessels of the latter category are lakers which do a small coastal trade.

Britain supplied the bulk of the funds, but the outbreak of the world war in 1914 blocked that source and thenceforth Canada was compelled to look chiefly to the United States, and to herself. In 1913 the total British capital invested in Canada was some 2,570 millions of dollars, while American capital was only 780 millions; by 1937 British investments had risen to 2,727 but the American totalled 3,996. In the same period the investments of all other countries dropped from 180 to 131 millions.

The following table shows the foreign investments classified into main types, as at December 31, 1937[1] (in millions of dollars).

	Total	United Kingdom	United States	Other Countries
Government Securities....	1,696	516	1,177	3
Public Utilities:				
Railways............	1,626	1,060	546	20
Other...............	764	185	570	9
Manufacturing..........	1,389	383	990	16
Mining................	363	93	260	10
Merchandising and Service	228	75	149	4
Insurance..............	211	87	122	2
Finance and Mortgage Companies...........	296	162	97	37
Miscellaneous..........	275	160	85	30
	6,848	2,721	3,996	131

There were some 1,200 companies in Canada in 1934 controlled by, or definitely affiliated with, American firms, which manufacture for the Canadian market and for export markets made available either by the imperial preference or by arrangement with the parent company. In many cases foreign markets are assigned to branch plants by the parent companies in an attempt to reduce branch plant unit costs by increasing output.[2] Almost a fourth of the manufacturing in

[1]See Bulletin of Dominion Bureau of Statistics, January 27, 1938. *Estimated Balance of International Payments for Canada, 1937 (Preliminary Statement).*

[2]See Marshall, H., Southard, F. A., and Taylor, K. W., *Canadian-American Industry* (New Haven and Toronto, 1936), pp. 19, 242.

Canada is done by American-controlled or affiliated companies.

While the presence of this large amount of foreign capital influences Canadian policy in many ways, it must be viewed in relation to the total amount of capital in the country. It was estimated that in 1934 this sum was in the neighbourhood of 18,000 millions, and that of this amount 62½ per cent. was owned in Canada, 22 per cent. in the United States and 15 per cent. in Great Britain.[1] Moreover, Canada has for many years been an exporter as well as an importer of capital, and in 1937 was estimated to have no less than 1,694 millions invested abroad—a sum equal to about 25 per cent. of the foreign investments in Canada. It is interesting to note that 1,017 millions of this were in the United States, 624 in other countries and only 53 in Great Britain. Canada's net foreign indebtedness is thus 5,144 millions of dollars.[2] Owing to favourable conditions Canada was amortizing her foreign debt at the rate of about 3½ to 4 per cent. per annum during 1936-37.

The payment of interest on this debit balance is one of the major problems of Canadian economic policy. So long as world trade flourishes, Canadian exports will provide the necessary funds. In a world of shrunken trade and increasing tariff barriers the payment is rendered extremely difficult. The tariff policy of the Dominion must always keep in view this obligation of external payments, and must endeavour to secure for the Dominion as a whole an annual surplus sufficient to meet the obligation. In the past the principal surpluses have come from trade with Great Britain while the principal debts have been paid in the United States, the Canadian dollar having to be kept in a position of equilibrium relative to the pound sterling and the New York dollar.[3] The growth of the tourist trade[4] and the develop-

---

[1]*Canada Year Book*, 1936, p. 891.
[2]As at December 31, 1937. See the Bulletin, cited *supra*.

[3]In 1931-2 Canada was pinched between the depreciated pound and the appreciated dollar. From this painful situation she was relieved by Roosevelt's inflation policy. See Gibson, J. Douglas, and Plumptre, A. F. W., "The Economic Effects on Canada of the Recent Monetary Policy of the United States", in Canadian Papers for the Yosemite Conference, Institute of Pacific Relations, 1936; also chart showing relations of the pound and the dollar in Siegfried, *Canada*, p. 202.

[4]The net credit balance on tourist account was estimated at 170 million dollars in 1937. See below, p. 42.

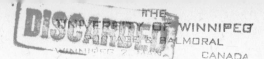

ment of new staples (pulp and paper, gold and other minerals) are helping considerably to facilitate payment on the external debt payable in the United States.

EXTERNAL TRADE

The importance of foreign trade to Canada has already been stressed. The direction and nature of that trade have also a great influence upon the Dominion's domestic and foreign policy. A simple picture of Canada's commercial dealings with foreign countries is given in the following tables.[1]

Canadian exports are distributed in the following percentages:

Fiscal Year	United Kingdom	Other British Empire	Total British Empire	United States	Other Foreign Countries	Total Foreign Countries
1896....	57.2	3.7	60.9	34.4	4.7	39.1
1916....	60.9	4.2	65.1	27.1	7.8	34.9
1926....	38.5	6.8	45.3	36.4	18.3	54.7
1932....	29.0	7.7	36.7	42.9	20.4	63.3
1937....	38.4	8.3	46.7	41.0	12.3	53.3

Canadian imports are derived from the following sources:

Fiscal Year	United Kingdom	Other British Empire	Total British Empire	United States	Other Foreign Countries	Total Foreign Countries
1896....	31.2	2.2	33.4	50.8	15.8	66.6
1916....	15.2	5.5	20.7	73.0	6.3	79.3
1926....	17.6	4.9	22.5	65.6	11.9	77.5
1932....	18.4	7.2	25.6	60.8	13.6	74.4
1937....	19.3	10.2	29.5	58.7	11.8	70.5

These figures show that Canada's most important economic relationships are with the United States. To that

[1]*Condensed Preliminary Report on the Trade of Canada*, 1936-37, p. 32. The figures represent dollar value.

country went 41 per cent. of Canada's exports in 1937, from it came 58.7 per cent. of the imports. The United Kingdom ranks a good second in economic importance, taking 38.4 per cent. of the exports and providing 19.3 per cent. of the imports; it also provides a very favourable balance for Canada. In terms of totals, Canada's trade with the United States was 729 million dollars in 1937, with the United Kingdom, 537 million dollars.

If Canada's trade is viewed with respect to its internal regional basis, the importance of foreign markets varies greatly. Certain parts of Canada, such as the prairies and the mining regions in northern Quebec and Ontario, could not live at all without foreign trade; other parts, such as the rural districts of Quebec and the Maritimes, are more self-sustaining. For British Columbia and the Prairie Provinces the export trade with Great Britain is of paramount importance, whereas Ontario imports more from the British Isles than she exports to them. The principal consuming markets of Canada are in Ontario and western Quebec, where population and wealth are concentrated.

The United States and Great Britain accounted for nearly 80 per cent. of Canada's total foreign trade in 1937. During the world depression Canada's commercial relationships with the United States declined while those with the United Kingdom increased; between 1929 and 1934 the proportion of Canadian exports to and imports from the United States fell from 37 to 33 and 69 to 54 per cent. respectively, while exports to Britain rose from 31 to 43 per cent. and imports from Britain from 15 to 24 per cent.[1] This was due to various causes amongst which may be mentioned the tariff increases in the United States and Canada, the greater intensity of the depression in the United States as compared with Great Britain, the Ottawa Agreements, and the fact that a large part of Canadian trade with the United States is in capital goods and in manufacturers' raw materials, the demand for which is particularly affected by a depression.[2] The improvement in conditions since 1933, however, and particularly the

[1]*Condensed Preliminary Report on the Trade of Canada*, 1936-37, p. 32.
[2]See Gibson and Plumptre, *op. cit.*

Reciprocity Treaty with the United States which came into force on January 1, 1936, have tended again to increase the United States' share of Canada's total trade.

Since 1935 a significant change has come over Canada's trade relations with the United States. Formerly the visible trade balance was unfavourable to Canada; in 1929 the debit balance was as high as $363,800,000.[1] This difference was made up by the surplus of exports to Great Britain and other countries, and by other items of exchange such as tourist expenditures. In 1936 and 1937, however, the trade with the United States (including gold exports) showed a favourable balance of considerable proportions. This change is making Canada less dependent on trade in Europe as a means of meeting her debt charges in the United States, though the permanence of the change may be open to doubt.[2]

In 1937 Canada's trade with countries outside Great Britain and the United States was about evenly divided between other parts of the British Empire and other foreign countries. Exports to the latter were as high as 24 per cent. of total exports in 1929. Trade with other British Empire countries has grown while trade with other foreign countries has relatively declined in recent years. Belgium and Japan are Canada's best customers amongst non-British countries, apart from the United States. The trade with Japan in certain raw materials increased rapidly as the Sino-Japanese dispute of 1937 became acute; exports to Japan of nickel, scrap iron, lead, copper, aluminium, zinc and sulphite rose from 8½ million dollars in 1936 to 17½ million dollars in 1937.[3] It is clear that Japan, like Great Britain, looks to Canada as a source of supply of raw materials in time of war.

The gross value of Canada's external trade varies greatly with world conditions. The high point of 1929 showed exports at $1,368,000,000 and imports of $1,266,000,000. By 1933 these had fallen to $528,000,000 and $406,000,000, or declines of 61.5 per cent. and 67.9 per cent. respectively.[4] By 1937 the exports had reached a value of $1,061,181,000

[1]Condensed Preliminary Report on the Trade of Canada, 1936-37, p. 31.
[2]The most recent figures seem to suggest a revival of the adverse balance.
[3]Calendar years. In the same period Japan's purchase of Canadian foodstuffs declined.
[4]Canada Year Book, 1937, pp. 528-9.

and imports a value of $671,875,000.[1] These variations are
reflected rapidly in the Canadian economy, though, as has
been said, the internal rigidities may distribute the effect of
the changes very unevenly.

The distribution of Canadian trade by continents is of importance, because of its bearing on the possibility of regional
economic and political arrangements. In the fiscal year
1936-37, the continental percentages of Canadian imports
and exports were:[2]

	Imports	Exports
North America, Total............	61.3	43.4
{ United States................	58.7}	41.0}
{ Other......................	2.6}	2.4}
Europe, Total...................	25.5	46.0
{ United Kingdom.............	19.3}	38.4}
{ Other......................	6.2}	7.6}
Asia..........................	5.3	3.4
South America.................	4.2	1.3
Oceania.......................	2.6	3.8
Africa........................	1.1	2.1

These figures show again Canada's predominant dependence upon North America; they also indicate the very small
degree of trade with South America.

The above analysis shows the visible trade items. Amongst
the invisible items the tourist trade is of great importance;
it might be described as a major industry of the Dominion.
In 1929 the net income from this source reached 187 million
dollars, deduction being made of Canadian tourist expenditure abroad; in the years 1935-37 it was 123, 156 and 170
millions respectively. Nearly all of this comes from the
United States, and helps to adjust the balance of trade with
that country in Canada's favour. To stimulate the influx of
tourists large amounts of money are being spent improving
highways, developing summer and winter sport resorts, and
opening up scenic regions.

[1]*Condensed Preliminary Report on the Trade of Canada*, 1936-37, p. 31.
[2]*Ibid.*, p. 16.

CANADIAN TRADE AGREEMENTS

The principle on which the Canadian tariff has been built since 1907 is that there are three categories of duties—the general, the intermediate and the British preferential. The general tariff provides a maximum rate for countries with which Canada has no commercial treaty relationships; the intermediate is for countries which the Dominion wishes to treat more favourably; the British preference, initiated in 1897, gives a lower rate for any part of the British Empire to which the Canadian government may wish to extend it. According to the practice in the Commonwealth, concessions under the British preference are not available to foreign countries with which Canada has most-favoured-nation treaties.

This broad tariff structure is modified by numerous individual agreements with particular countries. Canada, with a few exceptions, adopts in practice the unconditional most-favoured-nation principle, and hence tariff concessions to one country (excluding British preferential rates) are automatically extended to all other countries with which Canada has treaty arrangements. Easily the most important trade agreements are those regulating Canada's dealings with her two biggest customers—the United States and Great Britain.

The trade agreement between Canada and the United States came into effect on January 1, 1936. Canada secured reduced duties on some 60 commodities representative of the main fields of Canadian production. Concessions by Canada included the extension to the United States of the intermediate tariff in its entirety,[1] and reductions in 88 items below existing favoured-nation rates. Unconditional most-favoured-nation treatment in respect of customs matters was mutually agreed upon.[2]

The trade relations between Canada and Great Britain are governed by the Ottawa agreements of 1932, modified by the changes which took effect on September 1, 1937. The

[1]This concession means that the general tariff has ceased to be of great importance in the Canadian tariff structure; practically all Canadian trade is governed now by the intermediate or by the British preferential rates.

[2]See Feis, H., "A Year of the Canadian Trade Agreement", *Foreign Affairs*, July, 1937; Bidwell, Percy W., "The Prospects for a Trade Agreement with the United Kingdom", *Foreign Affairs*, October, 1937.

principal Canadian exports benefitted were wheat, timber, hams and bacon, fisheries products, milk products, copper, lead and zinc; British manufactures given lower rates in the Canadian market were mostly in the groups of iron and steel, drugs and chemicals, textiles and leather goods. Under the agreement revisions of duties may be sought by the British government before the Dominion Tariff Board. So far these have resulted in only modest changes of former schedules, and little additional preference for the British manufacturer.

Canadian trade with both the United States and Great Britain has increased very greatly since these agreements went into effect, but it is not easy to decide how far the increase was due to these or to other factors. Total trade between Canada and Great Britain, both exports and imports, increased by approximately $143,000,000 from March, 1933, to March, 1937, but in the same interval total trade with the United States increased $371,000,000, though the reciprocity treaty had only been in effect 15 months while the Ottawa agreements had been operating for nearly four and a half years.[1]

Besides these two principal agreements, Canada has trade treaties with other British dominions such as Australia, South Africa, New Zealand, Southern Rhodesia and the Irish Free State. There is an agreement with France, and special arrangements have been made with Germany, Poland and Japan. Altogether most-favoured-nation treatment is accorded some 32 foreign countries.[2]

NATURAL RESOURCES

That Canada has been endowed by nature with very considerable natural resources is an undoubted fact. She possesses unoccupied land, large forests, rich coal and mineral deposits, undeveloped water powers. The natural basis for a prosperous community seems to be present. The easy assumption is too often made, however, that nothing is lacking save population to make this wealth useful and available.

[1]*Condensed Preliminary Report on the Trade of Canada*, 1936-37, p. 31.   See also Taylor, K. W., "The Effect of the Ottawa Agreements on Canadian Trade", in Canadian Papers for the Yosemite Conference, Institute of Pacific Relations, 1936 (C.I.I.A., Toronto).
[2]See summary in *Canada Year Book*, 1937, pp. 487 ff.

What has already been said about population problems will suggest there is a fallacy in this conclusion.

Moreover, a closer inspection of Canada's resources makes them appear less alluring. The most obvious possession of the Dominion is land, yet by far the greater part of the land is unsuited for agricultural settlement. The Dominion Bureau of Statistics estimates that only 27.5 per cent. of the land area of Canada is "potential" agricultural land (352,000,000 acres), of which total 46.3 per cent. (163,000,000 acres) is occupied, leaving some 189,000,000 still unoccupied.[1] Of the "occupied" land possibly as much as 40,000,000 acres is either rough bush land, unfit for production of anything but timber, or semi-arid. The maximum area under field crops was reached in 1930, with 62,214,000 acres. Since then this figure has slowly declined. The official figure for "potential" agricultural land as given above is unreliable; a competent authority has called it a gross exaggeration.[2] It does not rest upon a scientific analysis of soil, and makes no allowance for remoteness of markets. Thus for the province of Nova Scotia, whose settlement began over 200 years ago, the official figures give a total area of some 17,000,000 acres, an area "occupied" as farm land of some 4,000,000 acres and an area of "estimated possible farm land" of some 8,000,000 acres. There is little doubt that every piece of land in Nova Scotia that would sustain life on any reasonable scale was long ago taken up. Indeed, some land from which people are trying to make a living today is so poor that it probably ought to be abandoned.

The official figures for the other provinces are almost as misleading. In the three Prairie Provinces the most recent surveys suggest that in 1931 there were only another 20,-000,000 acres or so available and suitable for occupation: if these were filled with settlers in accordance with existing agricultural practices it would only increase the population of the area by 600,000 or 700,000 persons.[3] This assumes too

[1] *Canada Year Book*, 1936, p. 38.

[2] See Mackintosh, W. A. in Bowman, Isaiah (ed.), *Limits of Land Settlement* (New York, 1937), p. 71. I am indebted to Prof. A. R. M. Lower for this general criticism of the official figures.

[3] Angus, H. F. (ed.), *Canada and the Doctrine of Peaceful Change*, pp. 53-4; Mackintosh, W. A., *Prairie Settlement: The Geographical Setting* (Toronto, 1934) (*Canadian Frontiers of Settlement*, Vol. I), pp. 232-4.

that there would be a market for the additional wheat grown. In a great part of the west it is "wheat or nothing". Only one-third of what is needed to support life on the prairies can be produced there, owing to the specialized nature of western agriculture. The size of farms has been increasing and the density of rural population decreasing, thus reducing the degree to which agriculture can stimulate immigration.[1] The Attorney-General of Saskatchewan declared before the Royal Commission on Dominion-Provincial Relations that at present (1937) of economically free land (i.e. land that it would pay under present conditions to settle) there is in Saskatchewan none.

Natural resources in Canada are frequently the sole source of livelihood in their area. Much of the mining country in the Pre-Cambrian Shield will produce nothing but minerals; the soil is second or third rate in quality and uneven in occurrence, and will seldom support independent agricultural communities. Increased supplies of minerals are not needed for present domestic consumption. Unless, therefore, these resources can be extracted and sold abroad, or a larger market can be provided at home, they are not resources at all. "The millions of tons of bituminous coal underlying the province of Alberta are no more natural resources *under existing conditions* than is the nitrogen in the atmosphere overlying that province."[2] If conditions change, particularly if world trade develops, Canada will be able to employ more persons in the development of her wealth, but in the present Canadian economy the "value" of the resources is largely determined by foreign demand over which Canada has little control.

Certain raw materials are found in small quantity only or are lacking altogether. The petroleum supply is meagre, though the Turner Valley fields of Alberta are showing considerable promise. Because of the lack of a market for the natural gas overlying this oil field, it has been disposed of for many years by the simple process of burning it off at the rate of 225,000,000 cubic feet per day.[3] Canada has little

[1]Bowman (ed.), *Limits of Land Settlement*, p. 72.
[2]Angus (ed.), *op. cit.*, p. 55.
[3]Alberta's first attempt to control this huge wastage was prevented by the courts. See Spooner Oils case, Canada, *Supreme Court Reports*, 1933, p. 629.

anthracite and imports virtually all her supplies; about half the bituminous coal used is imported, owing to the distance of the Nova Scotia and Alberta fields. Iron ore is found in a number of places but not rich in quantity or quality; consequently supplies are imported from the Wabana deposits of Newfoundland and the Mesabi range of Minnesota. Aluminium and tin are absent. Tropical and semi-tropical products—rubber, cotton, silk, sugar, cocoa, coffee, tea and oils—must be imported.

Canada's large foreign trade, her accumulation of capital equipment and her ability now to service her foreign debt, all are proof that her natural resources have been effectively developed and that the money invested in her has been, on the whole, put to profitable use. At the same time the numbers of her unemployed and the difficulties she has experienced in her public finance during and since the world depression, serve as reminders that a proper utilization of her resources calls for an improvement in her internal economic organization as well as in the state of world markets. Many Canadians feel, indeed, that even without waiting for world improvement Canada could, by appropriate internal reforms (about which there is much difference of opinion) increase her consuming power and provide a larger home market for her own produce, while many see a similar possibility in intra-Commonwealth economic co-operation.

THE STATE AND ECONOMIC LIFE

The state has played a very large part in the development of Canadian industry and commerce. Canadians possess many of the individualistic traits common to a people with a strong pioneering tradition, but at the same time they have not hesitated to employ the power of the state to achieve results which could not be obtained by individual action. The construction of canals and railways was the first economic undertaking to engage the attention of Canadian governments on a large scale. The three transcontinental lines all received ample, at times too ample, state aid in the form of direct subsidies, grants of land or guarantees of bonds. Today the Canadian National Railway System functions as a state-owned public corporation, with approximately 24,000 miles of track, or 57 per cent. of the total Canadian mileage. The Canadian Pacific Railway, though privately owned, is governed as to rates, the construction of branch lines and certain other aspects of administration, by the Dominion Board of Railway Commissioners. Many other transportation facilities come under public control. All harbours and canals belong to the Dominion; harbours are managed by a centralized National Harbours Board and the canals by the Department of Transport. A system of telegraphs, a number of hotels and an express delivery service belong to the Dominion as part of the Canadian National Railways. The Post Office is a Dominion government department, and radio broadcasting is licensed and controlled by the Canadian Broadcasting Corporation, modelled after the British Broadcasting Corporation, and reaching many Canadians with its own stations. From the period of the war until 1936 the Dominion government operated a merchant marine, but in the latter year the ships were sold and the service discontinued; the only shipping service now carried on by the state is that connecting with the West Indian ports in conformity with the Canadian-West Indian Trade Agreement Act of 1926, and consisting of a fleet of 11 vessels. Dominion control over air transport has been secured by the enforcement within Canada of the Convention Relating to Aerial Navigation of 1919; the subject of aerial navigation was held by the Privy Council in 1932 to be within Dominion jurisdiction. In 1937 a corporation known as Trans-Canada Air Lines, the shares of which are owned by the Canadian National Railway Company, was created to develop the transcontinental air service.

Besides these national services, the Dominion government controls economic policy through a number of agencies. The maintenance of a tariff is the best example of a type of state interference with business, which has always received the hearty support of Canadian manufacturers. The use of the tariff to achieve a political rather than an economic objective is seen in the system of imperial preferences, in force since 1898. Adjustments in the tariff can be effected through the instrumentality of the Tariff Board to which may be referred proposals for alterations of schedules.

Since 1935 Canada has had a central bank partly state-controlled from the first, and now state-owned, which allows of increased control over the internal credit situation and foreign exchange movements.[1] A Dominion Trade and Industry Commission was created by Mr. Bennett in 1935 with authority to control unfair trade practices and enforce commodity standards; this legislation was upheld by the Privy Council but the Commission has been little employed since the King government took office. A National Employment Commission existed from 1936 to 1938 for the purpose of collecting information regarding unemployment and advising as to the best measures to improve and co-ordinate relief administration throughout the country; unemployment relief generally, however, is managed by the provinces and municipalities with Dominion financial assistance.

Government control of marketing has been experimented with to some degree. Mr. Bennett established a Wheat Board with power to fix prices to producers and to market the entire wheat crop, and he enacted the first Natural Products Marketing Act to control, in co-operation with the provinces, the marketing of many primary products. Mr. King repealed the former legislation and the Privy Council invalidated the latter, but the Wheat Board was replaced by one with less extensive powers, and the provincial marketing acts are still in operation to a limited extent.

Turning to the provincial services, the best known is the Ontario Hydro-Electric Power Commission, which produces and distributes electric power in Ontario. The distribution, and in some cases the production also, of electric power is provided in part by provincial commissions in Nova Scotia, New Brunswick, Manitoba and Saskatchewan. Road building is a major provincial service; in 1935 the funded provincial debt for highways stood at close to 500 million dollars. The telephone system is publicly owned in the three provinces of Manitoba, Saskatchewan and Alberta; by this means remote areas and sparsely populated districts are

[1] See special article on the Bank of Canada in the *Canada Year Book*, 1937, pp. 879-86.

provided with telephone communication which private enterprise would never have brought them. The retail sale of alcoholic beverages is a state enterprise in all provinces but Prince Edward Island, which enjoys prohibition.[1] In addition to these provincial services, many municipalities have their own systems for electric light and power, gas, water and street railways.

The state in Canada has also intervened in the economic sphere on behalf of industrial workers and certain other unprotected classes, by adopting various forms of social legislation. It would be impossible in brief compass to analyse in detail this large body of law. It is mostly provincial in character because of the constitutional allotment of powers; in consequence it varies greatly in different parts of the country. Dominion legislation is small in quantity. There is no national labour code. The Dominion assists in the payment of old age pensions, which are now in force in every province on a non-contributory basis; it also pays a share of the money distributed by the provinces in unemployment relief. There is a Dominion Department of Health, but it has exercised little direct administrative authority save over certain health services of minor importance. A Dominion Industrial Disputes Investigation Act makes possible the creation of voluntary arbitration and conciliation boards in certain types of industrial dispute. A pensions service for the blind was begun in 1937. A Farmers' Creditors Arrangement Act provides machinery for debt adjustment between creditors and debtors.[2] The Dominion co-operates with the provinces in the establishment and operation of Employment Service Offices.

Provincial legislation provides workmen's compensation in all but one of the provinces, payable in most instances out of an insurance fund created by compulsory contributions from employers only. Mothers' allowances exist in seven provinces. Minimum wages for women are set by boards

---

[1]*Canada Year Book*, 1937, p. 626.

[2]See Easterbrook, W. T., "Agricultural Debt Adjustment", *Canadian Journal of Economics and Political Science*, 1936, p. 390. Several provinces have also adopted measures designed to protect farmers and householders against dispossession by creditors.

for certain industries in seven provinces. New Brunswick has a Fair Wage Act, enabling a board to fix in any trade, industry or business wages and hours where these are found, on inquiry, to be unfair. Legislation providing for enforcement and extension of collective labour agreements exists in Nova Scotia, Quebec, Ontario and Alberta, and minimum wages of male employees are thus fixed by piecemeal arrangement in a considerable number of industries. The state does not set minimum male wages generally save in British Columbia and Alberta. Health insurance has been enacted in British Columbia, but has not yet been put into operation; it exists nowhere else in Canada, though some provinces provide payment for medical services to the unemployed. Municipal doctors are fairly common in the prairies especially in Saskatchewan, and experiments in voluntary co-operative health service organization on a city or county basis, are being encouraged in Ontario. Every province regulates hours of labour to some degree, but the 48-hour week is by no means general. The Eight-Hour-Day Convention of 1919 was ratified by Canada in 1935; but the legislation enacted by the Dominion Parliament in 1935 to give effect to it was declared *ultra vires* by the Privy Council in 1937. Compulsory education exists in every province except Quebec.

No unemployment insurance exists in Canada, Mr. Bennett's legislation of 1935 having been set aside by the Privy Council. The King government in 1937 proposed an amendment to the B. N. A. Act to give jurisdiction over this head to the Dominion; only five out of the nine provinces have agreed to the proposal, and so far there has been no further action taken to secure the change. There is no national system regulating hours or wages, and no health insurance or holidays with pay. State aid to assist housing development is extremely meagre. There is little uniformity in the provincial regulations on the various matters covered by social legislation.[1] Since the impetus to reform given by the

[1] In 1933 the total expenditure of all provinces on general factory and minimum wage inspection was only 8.5 cents per non-agricultural worker, which was less than that spent in the state of New Hampshire, which ranked thirty-fourth amongst the American states. *Report of Royal Commission on Price Spreads*, 1935, p. 129.

depression there has been some improvement in the administration of the provincial social services, but no forward movement can be expected until the financial relations and distribution of constitutional powers between the Dominion and the provinces are placed on a sounder basis.

STANDARDS OF LIVING

The standard of living of the Canadian people is generally rated high. The enquiry conducted by the League of Nations in 1929 into comparative living standards ranked Canada second after the United States.[1] This investigation was based on rather limited data, however. Moreover in a country divided like Canada into economically distinct areas no single description will do for the whole territory. The Prairie Provinces of Canada, exposed as they have been to the double scourge of low prices for wheat and prolonged drought, have had their standard of living lowered further during the depression and raised less during the recovery than have the industrialized sections of the country. The standard in Quebec is lower than that in Ontario, a fact vividly revealed by contrasting the vital and health statistics for the two provinces.[2] There are, too, factors of taste and value which are impossible to include in any quantitative analysis. The French Canadian, because of the character of his religious education, tends to believe that a high standard of living is a proof of "materialism" and a dangerous influence on society. All that will be attempted here is to give some statistics out of which a general picture of Canadian conditions may emerge.

The average earnings disclosed by all wage-earners during the twelve months prior to the last three censuses were as follows:[3]

[1]See *International Labour Review*, 1929, pp. 580, 876. The order of the first seven countries was (Great Britain—100), U.S. 191, Canada 171, Australia 143, Denmark 104, Sweden 101, Irish Free State 98. Indices of real wages and cost of living have not varied sufficiently since 1929 to alter this ranking to any great extent.

[2]See also table in *Submission by the Government of Saskatchewan to the Royal Commission on Dominion-Provincial Relations* (1937), p. 297, showing that Ontario in 1931 with a population of 3.4 millions had about three times as many automobiles, radios and telephones as Quebec, whose population was 2.9 millions.

[3]*Canada Year Book*, 1937, p. 789.

AVERAGE EARNINGS OF ALL WAGE-EARNERS TEN YEARS
OF AGE OR OVER

	Male	Female
1911	$ 593	$313
1921	1057	573
1931	927	559

The same statistics show that in 1930 there were 60 per cent. of the male workers and 82 per cent. of the female workers receiving less than $1,000 a year. This was, however, a year of declining revenues, and these figures include individuals of all ages, as well as employments which provide some remuneration in kind. Some attempt has been made by the Dominion Bureau of Statistics to calculate earnings per family for average families in selected cities; in 17 cities studied the modal group (1930) was in the $1,200-$1,399 or the $1,400-$1,599 income class.

These figures may be compared, with some caution, with calculations of minimum budgets. A budget of minimum requirements for a family of five produced by the Montreal Council of Social Agencies in 1926 placed the amount of necessary income at $1,102. Corrected for variations in the cost of living index, this works out at $1,059 for 1930. This would seem to indicate that average wages of individuals would not enable them to support a family of five on a minimum budget, but that in families where there are several wage-earners the average is likely to be above the minimum.[1]

The 1931 census showed that for Canada as a whole 54.5 per cent. of urban householders lived in rented dwellings. Land owning amongst farmers is high, four-fifths of the number of farms being owned by those who work them. Figures for acreage, however, show that more than one-third of the acreage is worked by tenants and another third is mortgaged to an average of 40 per cent. of its value. Between 1921 and 1931 tenant acreage increased 34 per cent., part tenant acreage 111 per cent., while the fully owned

[1]Further statistics, particularly with regard to unemployed, will be found in Marsh, L. C., *Health and Unemployment* (Toronto, 1938), Chap. 20.

acreage actually decreased. This tendency to concentration of ownership in land has continued since 1931, at least on the prairies, as appears from the figures presented by the Saskatchewan government to the Rowell Commission.[1]

The income tax in Canada begins for single persons at $1,000, and for married persons with two children at $2,800. In 1936 there were 199,102 Canadians who paid income tax. Less than 12 per cent. of these were getting more than $5,000 per year. An estimate made of the distribution of total national income amongst all wage and salary earners, based on census and income tax returns for 1931, shows the following picture:[2]

Size of Income	Number of Persons Male and Female	Per cent. of Total	Income (Millions of dollars)	Per cent. of Total Income
Under $1,000.......	1,526,000	56.2	790.0	25.4
$1,000—$1,500.....	643,000	23.7	805.0	25.9
$1,500—$3,000.....	448,000	16.5	896.0	28.8
$3,000—$10,000....	85,000	3.2	401.0	12.9
$10,000—and over..	11,000	0.4	219.0	.7.0
Totals.........	2,713,000	100.0	3,111.0	100.0

This table shows that the 11,000 income receivers at the top had as large a total income as 400,000 at the bottom of the social scale. Almost half the total earnings went to 20 per

[1]See *Submission* (*op. cit.*), p. 145. The figures are:

LAND TENURE IN SASKATCHEWAN, 1901-1936

Year	Land		Farms		
	Owned	Rented	Owners	Tenants	Owner-Tenants
	Per cent.	Per cent.	Per cent.	Per cent.	Per cent.
1901..........	96.1	3.9	96.1	1.6	2.3
1921..........	80.5	19.5	77.6	10.8	11.6
1931..........	70.5	29.5	66.5	15.4	18.1
1936..........	65.2	34.8	60.7	20.4	18.9

See also *Brief Submitted by the Government of Ontario to the Royal Commission on Dominion-Provincial Relations*, Vol. I, p. 20, where it is shown that 14,948 or 5 per cent. of the farm owners own 26,098,771 acres or 23.07 per cent. of the "occupied" farm acreage of the Prairie Provinces.

[2]Woodsworth, J. S., *Distribution of Personal Income In Canada*, cited League for Social Reconstruction, *Social Planning for Canada* (Toronto, 1935), p. 16.

cent. of the earners. Statistics for bank deposits for 1935 indicate a similar maldistribution of wealth: 92.5 per cent. of the four million depositors have accounts averaging only a little over $100; the top 1 per cent. of depositors own 35 per cent. of total deposits.[1] An insurance company has calculated (1937) that of every 100 Canadian men starting life at 25, by age 65 "36 have died, 1 is wealthy, 4 are well-to-do, 5 live on earnings, 54 are no longer self-supporting".[2]

In 1934 the Royal Commission on Price Spreads made an extensive examination of economic conditions in the country, and many Canadians, accustomed to believe that all workers in the Dominion enjoyed a high standard of living, were shocked at the disclosures of extremely low wages and poor working conditions in a number of Canadian industries. In some instances the offenders were industries enjoying monopoly power and high protection. "The evidence before the Commission proves that, in certain industries, the sweat shop still survives in Canada and that, more generally, unemployment and low wages have reduced many workers to a state of abject poverty."[3] A great many men and women were found to be working for rates of ten cents per hour or less. At the same time there were (November, 1934) 1,149,063 Canadians dependent on direct relief.[4] A family of five on relief in Montreal was receiving $39.48 per month; this had reached $42.23 by 1936. Other "black patches" undoubtedly exist in the country: even in 1937 the Chevrier Commission on Transportation found truck drivers receiving $15 to $18 per week of 65 hours in Ontario. A proposed minimum wage ordinance for unskilled labour in Quebec in February, 1938, suggested hourly rates ranging from 15 to 25 cents, which were an advance on current rates of from 5 to 20 per cent.

From the depression figures there has, of course, been some recovery. Relief expenditures have dropped considerably, though in part this is due to drastic cutting of relief rolls and

[1]*Canada Year Book*, 1937, p. 902. The 1 per cent. includes corporation as well as individual accounts.

[2]Cited, League for Social Reconstruction, *Democracy Needs Socialism* (Toronto, 1938), p. 13.

[3]*Report of Royal Commission on Price Spreads*, 1935, p. 107.

[4]*Report of Dominion Commissioner of Unemployment Relief*, March 30, 1935, p. 22.

a maintenance of grants at bare subsistence levels. Provincial regulation of wages and hours has improved, and doubtless has eliminated some of the worst conditions disclosed by the Price Spreads Inquiry. Mr. Bennett's attempt to deal nationally with Canadian economic and social problems failed, however, and there is no possibility that the unco-ordinated provincial action can deal adequately with the situation. Minimum wages for experienced women workers under existing regulation in Ontario and Quebec are $12.50 per week of 48 to 54 hours. There are still 951,000 persons dependent on direct relief.[1] Another depression could easily reproduce, in intensified form, the suffering of the last crisis. A growing militancy amongst Canadian trades unions in 1936-37, moving even the usually tranquil Catholic Syndicates in Quebec to carry on strikes, is an indication of a feeling amongst the industrial workers in Canada that legislatures have failed to assist them and that self-help is necessary to improve their living standards.

An interesting contrast between the living conditions in two different areas in the country, the prairies and Ontario, is provided by the following analysis made of the 1931 census material:

When the census was taken in the summer of 1931 a period of relative prosperity enjoyed by western agriculture had just drawn to a close. The census gives a total of 288,000 farms for the three Prairie provinces and 192,000 for Ontario, and contains a brief record of farm facilities in all the provinces. Of the 288,000 farms of the Prairie provinces, 5,036 have water piped in the kitchen; or one out of every 57.20 farms in western Canada in contrast with one out of every 9.54 in Ontario. In the West one out of every 72.8 has water piped in the bathroom (it would be interesting to know how many have a bathroom of any kind) as compared with one out of 15.76 in Ontario. One out of every 34.44 Western farmhouses is lighted by gas or electricity as compared with one out of 5.95 in Ontario. In proportion to farms Ontario has more than twice as many rural telephones and over 40 per cent. more rural automobiles than western Canada. Of these automobiles four out of five in Ontario, four out of seventy-six in Western Canada, may travel on paved or gravelled highways, or, 20 per cent. of Ontario

---

[1]December, 1937. This includes 551,000 non-agricultural and 400,000 agricultural persons receiving aid. *Labour Gazette*, February, 1938, p. 124.

farms and 94.7 per cent. of all western farms are located on dirt roads."[1]

Canada shows many of the characteristics of an older industrial community as regards standards of living and the distribution of income. It reveals a great concentration of wealth, the social counterpart of the trend to monopoly, while not only amongst the unemployed but also amongst a considerable section of industrial and agricultural labourers the standard of living is low. In the intermediate brackets there is an average standard lower than that of equivalent groups in the United States but considerably higher than that in Europe. Even the better paid Canadian employees, however, are without the social security provisions which most European workers enjoy.

LABOUR AND FARMER ORGANIZATIONS IN CANADA

(A) Labour Organization.

By comparison with most democratic countries the Canadian labour movement is in the earlier stages of development. The total membership in Canadian unions in 1931 was only 310,544 out of a total wage-earning group of 2,570,000. Even excluding from this latter figure the professional and higher-paid salaried workers, there would remain at least 2,000,000 whom a trades-union movement might hope to organize. This means that more than 85 per cent. of the workers were unorganized.[2] In 1936 union membership had only risen to 322,473,[3] which is less than it was in 1919-20 despite the increase in population.

Not only are most Canadian workers unprotected by trades unions, but such unions as exist are divided against each other. The Roman Catholic Church in Quebec, fearful of losing its hold over the industrialized French-Canadian workers, organized the Federation of Catholic Workers of Canada in 1921. These Catholic Syndicates, as they are

[1]Innis and Plumptre (eds.), *op. cit.*, p. 110.

[2]*Social Planning for Canada*, p. 114. Canada was ranked twenty-third amongst the nations by the International Federation of Trades Unions in 1925; Brady, A., *Canada* (Modern World Series) (London, 1932), p. 257.

[3]*Annual Report on Labour Organization*, 1936.

called, have a priest as chaplain to every local, and seldom move without clerical advice.[1] They have hitherto been more concerned with carrying on struggles against communism and the international unions than against employers for better wages, though in 1937 they conducted several inconclusive strikes. Their membership in 1936 was 45,000.

The principal non-sectarian unions are divided between the "international" unions and the "national" unions. The international unions are affiliates of the American Federation of Labor or the Committee on Industrial Organization, to which they pay dues. Part of these dues, however, is remitted to Canada to finance the Trades and Labour Congress of Canada, the co-ordinating authority for the Dominion. In 1936 the Congress, representing 66 organizations, had a membership of 149,398, the total membership of international unions being 174,769. The split between the A. F. of L. and the C. I. O. has not been permitted to invade Canada, and most C. I. O. unions are still members of the Trades and Labour Congress. Indeed it seems that the principal support of the Trades and Labour Congress comes from unions which have split from, or have never been in, the A. F. of L. in the United States.[2]

The national unions in Canada are organized in the All-Canadian Congress of Labour which has a membership (1936) of 31,883. It favours the industrial rather than the craft union. Its members constantly exploit the patriotic appeal in their fight against the international unions. In addition to this organization there exist some smaller organizations, like the Canadian Federation of Labour, which split from the All-Canadian Congress (membership, 1936, 25,081), and the once powerful One Big Union (membership, 24,000, in 1935) which operates in the western provinces. Total membership in Canadian unions, excluding the Catholic unions, was about 100,000.

Many reasons may be given for the backward condition

[1] The constitution of the Federation contains this clause: "The F.C.W.C. is a frankly and openly Catholic organization. It affiliates with itself Catholic organizations alone, it adheres to the whole doctrine of the Church and it promises always and in everything to follow the directions of the Pope and of the Canadian bishops." Quoted Latham, A. B., *The Catholic and National Labour Unions of Canada* (Toronto, 1930), p. 99.

[2] Ware, Norman J. and Logan, H. A., *Labor in Canadian-American Relations* (Toronto, 1937), p. 68.

of Canadian labour organization. Race, religion and geography make union difficult. Workers in mines and forests may be hundreds of miles from the nearest urban centres. Often they are in "company towns". The individualist philosophy pervades North America, and a belief in steady financial progress as the inevitable reward for honest toil continues to dominate the outlook of the people, making even those inside the unions poor proselytizers and those outside blind to the need for co-operation. The constant addition of new immigrants to the Canadian labour market up to 1930 provided employers with cheap labour willing to work hard to establish itself in its new home, and liable to deportation at the hands of administrative tribunals if it ran foul of the law. Between 1930 and 1934, when there was considerable labour unrest due to the depression, more immigrants were deported than in the previous 27 years, many for acts arising out of their connection with radical movements. Moreover, the lack of a common background in the workers has been an additional factor in enabling large-scale industrial enterprises to oppose trade unionism very effectively. When the premier of the largest industrial province in Canada can enter an election with a policy of preventing Canadian workers from choosing their own unions freely, it would seem to indicate, even though his threats were not implemented by legislation, that the public have not moved very far in the political direction travelled by New Zealand, Australia and Great Britain.[1]

Labour's lack of organization is reflected also in the absence of a consumer's co-operative movement in Canada. Some beginnings have been made, but the total membership in retail co-operative societies affiliated with the Co-operative Union of Canada was only 11,000 in 1935, and the total number of societies was 34.[2] These figures, however, do not include the credit unions in Quebec known as the "Caisses Populaires", which have a considerable membership. An interesting experiment in co-operation is being carried on in

---

[1]Mr. Hepburn bitterly fought the C.I.O. when it first became active in Ontario. See Ware and Logan, *op. cit.*, pp. 63 ff. He interpreted his victory in the election of 1937 as an endorsation of his anti-C.I.O. policy. (See Montreal *Gazette*, October 7, 1937.)

[2]*Canada Year Book*, 1937, p. 767.

Nova Scotia and Prince Edward Island under the direction of St. Francis Xavier University.

(B) Farmer Organization.

By contrast with Canadian labour, the Canadian farmers, particularly in the western provinces, have shown great initiative. Both on the side of economic and of political organization they have been active. Whereas total sales in the retail co-operatives amounted to less than $4,000,000, total business in the agricultural co-operatives amounted to over $158,000,000 in 1935, while their membership was 367,000. The biggest and best-known of these societies are the wheat pools of western Canada. Despite their losses during the depression the pools have survived as co-operative elevator companies and in 1936 handled approximately 50 per cent. of the total wheat crop of the Dominion.

From the farmers also have come the most successful independent political movements in Canada. The Ontario farmers captured the provincial legislature in 1919, and the United Farmers of Alberta were successful in the provincial elections of 1921. In 1922 Manitoba returned a farmer government. Sixty-six "Progressives", as these farmer groups were generally called, were elected to the Dominion Parliament in 1921, twenty-four from Ontario and forty-one from the western provinces.[1] All these groups lost ground as the boom period of the 1920's gathered momentum. They had no political philosophy to differentiate them from traditional liberalism, and to that fold they mostly returned. The United Farmers of Alberta survived the longest until, due to the depression and internal difficulties, they were overwhelmingly defeated by William Aberhart and his Social Credit followers in 1935.

[1]Brady, *Canada*, p. 110.

CHAPTER IV

POLITICAL PARTIES

THE party system in Canada is a convention of the constitution, as it is in England. The law does not require it, but the present working of the governmental machinery depends upon it. There are two major parties in the Dominion field, Liberals and Conservatives, which have alternated in office since Confederation with the single exception of the Union government of 1917-21. Parties of the same names, though not always with the same policies, contest provincial elections and have generally controlled provincial politics. There are also a number of minor parties, which rise and fall with the varying stimuli to political action and which have hitherto been more successful in the provincial than in the federal arena.

LIBERAL

The Liberal Party, led by Mr. Mackenzie King, now forms the Dominion government, with the largest majority in the House of Commons since Confederation, though a minority in the Senate.[1] The party is also in power in every province except Quebec and Alberta. It last wrote a programme at a convention held in 1919, but programmes count for little in Canada except amongst the minor parties before they attain power. In general it has stood for nationalism in its political relations with the Commonwealth and other countries, and internationalism in trade. It has been responsible for most of the initiative in the development of Canadian autonomy within the Commonwealth since 1921, for it held office from that year until 1930, except for a brief interval in 1926. Its

---

[1]The Canadian Senate being nominative and not elective, a victory at the polls does not change the composition of the upper house until vacancies caused by death can be filled by new nominations.

tariff policy has always been more moderate than that of the Conservatives, though it does not favour free trade. It has advocated social legislation in principle, but since it has also supported "provincial rights" it has been either unable or unwilling to implement these principles in the Dominion field save in a comparatively small degree. It is opposed to all attempts to control production or marketing, and inclines to view the state as the traditional policeman standing on the edge of the open market to see that competition is fair. The progressive disappearance of the open market has not altered its attitude. It draws its support from all parts of the country and all classes of people; the name 'Liberal' unites ultra-conservative protectionist French Catholics from Quebec (most of whom have voted Liberal for years) and progressive free-trade British Protestants from the western provinces. Imperial preference was the invention of the Liberal party; the Ottawa agreements, though loyally observed by it, run counter to its aim of freeing the channels of world trade generally.

CONSERVATIVE

The Conservative party has traditionally been a party of imperial co-operation abroad and economic nationalism at home—an inconsistency the exact reverse of that found in Canadian Liberalism. Its pro-imperialist leaning, however, has not excluded a growing acceptance of the idea of Dominion autonomy. Sir Robert Borden, in fact, took the lead among Dominion prime ministers in pressing for a definition of Dominion status. The party has never professed a belief in state interference with business, but under Mr. Bennett, who was appointed leader in 1927 and who held office from 1930 to 1935, the party programme took such a sudden shift to the "left" that it made the Liberals appear far more conservative than the Conservatives. A glance at the Dominion statutes of 1933-35 will reveal how active was the Conservative leader in the promotion of social reform and state control of the economy. Mr. Bennett nationalized the radio, created a central bank, established a national system of marketing boards for primary products, pegged the price of wheat and placed the whole wheat export trade under a Wheat Board, negotiated a St. Lawrence Waterways Treaty with the United States, entered into the Ottawa agreements, initiated the new reciprocity agreement with Washington, extended the criminal law to prohibit unfair trade practices, created a Trade and Industry Commission to enforce the new prohibitions, and adopted Dominion legislation to deal with unemployment insurance, minimum wages, maximum hours, and the weekly day of rest. In the face of this political *tour de force* it is difficult to know how to describe the political philosophy of the Conservative party in Canada today. It is certainly not Tory, not *laissez-faire* liberal, and not the same as appears from its previous programme of 1927. The party is in partial eclipse; it holds but 37 seats at Ottawa and controls no provincial legislature; Mr. Bennett has announced his retirement; a new leader is to be chosen and a new programme written. Whoever the leader may be, it is likely that the party will continue at least moderately progressive in its programme and will seek to attract the younger men who are dissatisfied with the lack of action and leadership in the present Liberal party. It is likely also that there will be a further move toward nationalism in foreign affairs; already the party name has been changed from Liberal-Conservative (the double title derives from a distant past) to National-Conservative. The change is a reflection of the shift in Canadian opinion generally, and also a bid for French-Canadian support.

It must always be remembered, however, that the two major parties in Canada, like any parties, need campaign funds, and neither of them depends upon membership fees for its principal support. They consequently rely for the most part upon the contributions of well-to-do individuals and corporations. Such help sets immediate limits to the kind of political action which may be expected from them.[1] So long as this relationship between private and corporate

[1]Sometimes this help is given in return for specific concessions. Any student who wishes a realistic view of Canadian politics should read "After Beauharnois—What?", by R. A. MacKay, in *Maclean's Magazine*, Oct. 15, 1931, reprinted in Dawson, R. MacG., *Constitutional Issues in Canada, 1900-1931* (London, 1933), p. 208. Other articles on Canadian political parties will be found in the latter volume. For a good historical analysis, see "The Development of National Political Parties in Canada", by F. H. Underhill, *Canadian Historical Review*, 1935, p. 367.

wealth and the two major parties exists, so long will it be
true that neither of them will sponsor anything approaching
a labour or social-democratic programme; nor will either
interfere greatly with the tariff structure behind which
Canadian industry has grown up.

An acute observer of Canadian affairs, M. André Siegfried, has left a description of the Liberal and Conservative
parties as he saw them in 1906.[1] It still is relevant despite
the passage of a generation. The parties are constituted,
he points out, on the British model with British names, but
their methods of controlling constituencies and the tone of
their polemics are derived from the United States. They are
quite detached from the principles which gave them birth,
and tend to become mere associations for the securing of
power. Whichever side succeeds, it is well known that the
country will be governed in much the same way. Canadian
statesmen stand in fear of great movements of opinion, and
seek to lull them rather than to encourage them and bring
them to fruition. They fear that the unity of the Dominion
will be endangered if vital questions are raised, and exert
themselves to prevent the formation of homogeneous parties
divided according to creed or race or class. The result is
that Liberals and Conservatives differ very little in their
opinions upon crucial questions, since they are both made up
of the same varied elements; employers and labourers,
townsmen and farmers, French and English, Catholics and
Protestants.[2] Despite this similarity of programme and behaviour, the parties are sacred institutions to be forsaken
only at the risk of one's reputation and career. It is rarely
indeed that a Canadian politician shifts his party allegiance.

While this situation is open to attack by the political
scientist, it is understandable in view of the varied elements
and interests within Canada. The major parties provide a
political façade which covers up the ill-joined sections under-
neath, and by so doing create a certain spirit of unity, sometimes more apparent than real, even where there is little

[1]Siegfried, A., *The Race Question in Canada* (London, 1907), pp. 141 ff.

[2]The Liberal programme of 1919 and the Conservative programme of 1927 are to be
found in Dawson, *op. cit.* Their similarity is striking.

basis for it. At times the cracks are evident even through the façade.

SOCIAL CREDIT

In 1935 Social Credit suddenly became a force in Canadian politics. With no previous record of steady growth and little warning of its coming power, it placed Mr. Aberhart in office in Alberta in the provincial elections of 1935, and sent seventeen members to the Dominion House of Commons to become the third largest group at Ottawa. It has attempted to spread its doctrine into other western provinces, with some slight success; two Saskatchewan constituencies were won in the federal elections of 1935 and 5 Manitoban seats in the provincial elections of 1936. The party, however, failed to elect a member in the British Columbia elections of 1937, and, despite an organized "invasion" from Alberta, won only two seats in the recent Saskatchewan elections.[1]

The economic proposals of Social Credit have been found impossible of application in Alberta. Its opponents ascribe this to their inherent falsity; Mr. Aberhart ascribes it to the opposition of the eastern bankers and their "tools" at Ottawa. The disallowance of three Albertan statutes by the Dominion government in 1937, and the setting aside of three others in 1938 by the Canadian Supreme Court,[2] indicate that both Liberal party policy and the B. N. A. Act stand in the way of any thorough attempt at this particular economic experiment in a single Canadian province.

It would be unwise, however, to assume that either Mr. Aberhart or Social Credit is politically finished by this rebuff. The movement is at bottom an agrarian revolt in the west against the financial and commercial policies of the east (Montreal and Toronto). "It is the fundamental feeling of dissatisfaction with national fiscal policies which have placed burdens upon agriculture for the benefit of secondary

[1]Results of the Saskatchewan election of June 8, 1938, in 50 of the 52 seats, were:

	Liberal	C.C.F.	Social Credit	Conservative	Other
Number of members......	36	10	2	0	2
Percentage of vote........	46	19	15	12	8
Percentage of vote, 1934...	48	24	0	27	1

[2]On the ground that the laws infringed the exclusive Dominion power to regulate banks and banking, currency, and interprovincial trade and commerce. An appeal has been taken to the Privy Council. See (1938) 2 D.L.R., p. 81.

industry; and it is also the deep agrarian hatred of high interest rates, mortgages and debt."[1] These underlying causes are not removed by disproving the A plus B theorem. Mr. Aberhart is capable of reviving a lagging support by adopting a new line of attack, as he did in 1936 with his debt reduction legislation; he is not likely to be displaced until some other party appears equally concerned to protect the farmers' interests.

CO-OPERATIVE COMMONWEALTH FEDERATION

In 1932 an attempt was made to unite farmer and labour movements in Canada under one political banner. Their common interests vis-à-vis an economic system becoming increasingly monopolistic were growing clear to many of their supporters, and a conference in Calgary in that year succeeded in forming an alliance between delegates representing nearly all the local farmer and labour parties of the four western provinces.[2] The name Co-operative Commonwealth Federation was chosen, to symbolize a federation of parties working together for a Canadian co-operative commonwealth. The leadership was placed in the hands of J. S. Woodsworth, veteran social reformer and labour representative from Winnipeg. In 1933 a number of "white-collar" and professional people joined the movement and a party manifesto was issued with a programme calling for a regulated economy based on wide public ownership of financial institutions and industries. The C.C.F. takes as its models the labour parties of other parts of the Commonwealth and of the Scandinavian countries.

The party has had some electoral success. It polled 400,000 votes in the general election of 1935,[3] despite the sudden emergence into the political arena of two new protest parties—Social Credit and the Reconstruction party. It is

[1]Ferguson, G. V., "Economic and Political Outlook of the Canadian West", in Anderson, Violet (ed.), *World Currents and Canada's Course*, p. 115.

[2]The original groups represented at the Conference which launched the C.C.F. were the United Farmers of Alberta, the United Farmers of Canada (Saskatchewan section), the Canadian Labour Party of Alberta, the Independent Labour Party and Co-operative Labour Party of Saskatchewan, the Independent Labour Party of Manitoba, the Socialist Party of Canada (British Columbia) and the Canadian Brotherhood of Railway Employees.

[3]In that election the Liberals polled 47 per cent. of the popular vote, the Conservatives 30 per cent., the C.C.F. 9 per cent., the Reconstruction party 9 per cent., and the Social Credit party 4 per cent.

the official opposition in Saskatchewan and was for three years in British Columbia, though in each case the groups were small. Twenty-seven C.C.F. members were sitting in Canadian legislatures in 1937, of whom seven were at Ottawa. The party suffered, however, at first from internal dissensions and later, when these were overcome, from its lack of ability to create an organization and to raise funds. The inability of most international trades unions to take part in politics bars this form of support,[1] and the Catholic clergy in Quebec have warned their flock against the C.C.F. on the ground that no one can be both a Catholic and a socialist, thus making progress in Quebec almost impossible. At the present moment the movement is largely western, being strongest in British Columbia, Saskatchewan and Manitoba, with small organized groups in Ontario, Quebec and New Brunswick.

OTHER GROUPS

The Communist party has been organized in Canada since 1924. It became nationally important after its eight leaders were imprisoned in 1931, but since their release has made little headway. Its existence provides Quebec authorities with an excuse for adopting reactionary laws, although its programme of activity at the moment is of the popular front variety. Its influence, particularly amongst the foreign-born worker group in Canada, however, has been considerable. Only one Communist has every succeeded in getting elected to a Canadian legislature,[2] although Tim Buck, the national secretary, always polls a substantial vote in the civic elections in Toronto.

The Reconstruction party was organized by the Honourable H. H. Stevens just before the 1935 elections, with a programme of progressive Conservatism much like that of Mr. Bennett. Mr. Stevens had been Mr. Bennett's Minister of Trade and Commerce but resigned in 1935 after a dispute with his chief. Though polling a substantial vote, the party returned its founder as its sole representative to Ottawa. Since then it has not functioned as a political machine, and the split with the Conservative party is likely to be healed.

[1]There are signs that this attitude is changing in Canada as in the United States.
[2]In Manitoba.

Another important political movement in Canada is the *Union Nationale* in Quebec. But this is part of the wider subject of French-Canadian nationalism, and will be dealt with in the following chapter.

*   *   *   *   *

The political situation in Canada is not stable. Its two outstanding characteristics at the moment are the uncooperative attitude of the provincial governments of Quebec, Ontario and Alberta, and the inactivity of the Dominion authorities in face of grave national problems. The three provincial premiers "steal all the headlines", while Ottawa is waiting for reports from its numerous Royal Commissions. So far has sectionalism developed that the Royal Commission on Dominion-Provincial Relations, faced with the most important national task of any public body in Canada since confederation, has not been able to secure even a promise of co-operation from all the provinces. The absence of a firm leadership from Ottawa leaves the sense of national unity voiceless and unorganized against the attacks of provincial autonomists. Between the *laissez-faire* Dominion government on the right wing and the scattered forces of the political left, is a wide area of dissatisfied citizens not knowing where to turn. A sense of direction is wanting, and none can predict whence it will come.

CHAPTER V

THE NATIONALIST MOVEMENT IN FRENCH CANADA

THE French Canadians in Canada now number about 3,300,000. They form the most homogeneous and united group in the country, for they are not divided by religion or racial origin, and their upper governing class is not in control of great wealth and hence far removed from the mass of the people. Moreover, their sense of being ringed round by an alien civilization makes them subordinate their inner differences to the single racial purpose of self-preservation. Their home is the province of Quebec, where 78 per cent. of those in Canada live (the number in the United States is variously estimated at 1½ to 3 millions); but the spread into other provinces is proceeding steadily. In 1871 only 14 per cent. of the French Canadians lived outside Quebec; in 1931, 22 per cent. did. Their percentage of the provincial populations in 1931 was: Quebec, 79; New Brunswick, 33.5; Prince Edward Island, 14.7; Nova Scotia, 11; Ontario, 8.7; Manitoba, 6.7; Saskatchewan, 5.5; Alberta, 5.2; British Columbia and territories, 2.2. These figures show the strong eastern concentration of the race.

BASIS OF FRENCH-CANADIAN NATIONALISM

The French Canadian in a real sense is the truest Canadian. He has lived on the soil for three hundred years, and the family ties with another world have long been broken. To Canada alone does he feel attached, for England conquered him and France first deserted him and then travelled a political and spiritual road his clergy have taught him to abhor. He sees no help coming from without; he knows he must build upon his own resources. And when he thinks of "Canada", he seldom, like the English Canadian, pictures a "dominion stretching from sea to sea"; rather he looks to the province of Quebec and the valley of the St. Lawrence, the part of North America to which the word "Canada" was first applied. To the English Canadian this is mere provincialism; to him, it is nationalism and true patriotism.[1] He builds outward from his securely held position and does not attempt to embrace the rest of a continent where now there are only a few outposts of his race.

Because of this basis to his politics, the French Canadian looks upon both the Commonwealth connection and confederation in much the same way; they are both political ties with the English which are part of his historic destiny. He cannot avoid them; he does not, at the moment, wish to break them, but they do not command his warm allegiance. Both represent a *mariage de convenance*. The British connection is valuable to him in helping to fend off Americanization, and the monarchic tradition is naturally dear to a priesthood fearful of democracy. Confederation was the best bargain that he could make at the time with a Protestant majority; to him the B. N. A. Act is as much a "treaty between races" as a political constitution.[2] In the historic evolution of his relationship with English Canada, which he views as a continuous development, the confederation arrangement is neither evocative of particular loyalty nor suggestive of great permanence.[3] His political status has already been changed five times—by the cession of 1763, the Quebec Act of 1774, the Constitutional Act of 1791, the Act of Union of 1840 and the B. N. A. Act of 1867. Whenever the next change comes, he is determined that it will result in no loss of privileges or autonomy for himself.

Such is the general character of French-Canadian nationalism, and it will be recognized as the natural aspiration of a people who believe in themselves and who are determined to survive with their language, their traditions and their religion. From time to time, however, and more particularly of recent years, there has arisen an extremer form of nationa-

[1] A leader of the more moderate nationalists, Mr. L. M. Gouin, K.C., has said "We Quebecers . . . do not put Ottawa above Quebec. . . . If we have to choose between the Confederation and our own nationality, we refuse to sacrifice the soul of our race either to the Dominion or to the Empire". Anderson, Violet (ed.), *World Currents and Canada's Course* (Toronto, 1937), p. 124.

[2] See Brossard, R., "The Working of Confederation", *Canadian Journal of Economics and Political Science*, 1937, p. 335.

[3] See Siegfried, *Canada*, pp. 258, 263; Hudon, Théophile, *Est-ce la Fin de la Confédération?* (Montreal, 1936), pp. 18 ff.

list fervour, which resembles closely the movements which have swept over Ireland and other European countries where there is a racial group struggling for freedom. This spirit manifests itself in economic as well as political forms; it seeks immediate steps toward independence for the race, and it is intolerant of alien groups and alien rights. In Quebec such a movement is now running strong.[1] It has been stimulated by the world depression, which caused great unemployment amongst French Canadians; by the growing awareness of the extent to which Quebec is dominated by English-Canadian and American "trusts" and financiers; by the fear of another imperialist war, and by the decadence of the old Liberal party machine which had governed the province without a break from 1896 to 1936. To some degree also it was fostered by certain of the clerical authorities, who saw in a revival of nationalism a means of fending off social unrest which might easily turn radical and begin to question the utility of the wealth and privileges possessed by the Roman Catholic Church in Quebec.

UNION NATIONALE

Politically the nationalist movement has taken the form of the creation of a new provincial party, the *Union Nationale*, which has been in power since 1936, and which is pledged to give to the French Canadian the place in Confederation which he feels has been denied him. Its leader is Maurice Duplessis, formerly leader of the provincial Conservative party, who was politically astute enough to ride to power on the new wave of feeling which has swept the province in the past few years. His activities since taking office have been varied but always colourful. He and his fellow premiers, Mr. Hepburn of Ontario and Mr. Aberhart of Alberta, provide the only vigorous—if erratic—leadership to be found in Canadian politics today.

Out of the *Union Nationale* has come some needed reform in the social legislation of the province. Collective labour

[1]See "Nationalism in French Canada", *Round Table*, December, 1936; Lower, A. R. M., "External Policy and Internal Problems", *University of Toronto Quarterly*, April, 1937, p. 3; Bovey, Wilfrid, "French Canada and the Problem of Quebec", *Nineteenth Century*, January, 1938, p. 731; Angus, H. F. (ed.), *Canada and Her Great Neighbor* (Toronto and New Haven, 1938), *passim*.

agreements are favoured, co-operative institutions are being promoted, and collaboration with Ontario on minimum wage rates has been sought. The nationalist feeling has found expression in the attempts that have been made to give pre-eminence to the French language in the interpretation of laws,[1] to frighten workers away from the international unions, and to obstruct all efforts to amend the British North America Act. Behind the attack on international unionism, however, many people see something quite different from nationalism; a deeper motive seems to be the desire to prevent "communistic" ideas from entering the province and disturbing the religious and political views of the population. The "Padlock Act" and the growing censorship of films and literature are other weapons in the same offensive.

In achieving its economic objectives French-Canadian nationalism is meeting great difficulties. It is only in recent years that the economic aspect of their position has engaged the attention of the nationalist leaders; the older generation, men like Bourassa and Lavergne, were concerned chiefly with political and religious affairs. The world depression shifted the emphasis to the economic. In Quebec the natural resources in mines, forests and water power, the banks and financial houses, are largely owned and exploited by English-Canadian or American capital; the French Canadian provides the cheap labour, usually lacking trades union protection. The nationalists of today are determined that this situation shall change, and that in their own province they shall not be restricted to exercising a political power rendered helpless by the existence of concentrated economic power in other hands. With this determination many English Canadians, only too aware of the situation in Quebec in regard to living standards and social legislation, would warmly sympathize. The difficulty is to decide upon a practical policy for effecting a change, and here the nationalists are at the moment baffled. A straightforward socialist programme would give them the control they want, for the state could

---

[1] By a statute adopted in 1937 the French version of statutes and codes was made to prevail whenever it differed from the English. The law was repealed in 1938 because of its unsettling effect on the established interpretation of the law and because of its doubtful constitutionality in view of section 133 of the B.N.A. Act.

then expropriate the "foreign" (i.e. non-French) capital and place French Canadians in charge of their own state-controlled utilities. But socialism at the moment stands condemned by the clergy of Quebec. Consequently the nationalist movement is in an impasse; it must risk clerical censure or else continue to submit to economic inferiority. So far it has avoided the first alternative, and has had to content itself with such measures as compelling foreign corporations developing natural resources to take out provincial charters, beginning a tentative programme of hydro-electric development under state control, supporting "*la petite industrie*" in the small towns in the province, and stimulating the "*achat chez nous*" which is the French-Canadian equivalent of a "buy British" campaign. It is impossible to predict how long these slender achievements will satisfy the demand for action. The drive against "communism" in Quebec, sponsored by the clergy, is a powerful deterrent to any proposals that the government should expropriate existing investments, for the accusation of "communist" would at once be hurled at any daring advocate of such an idea.[1]

The political and economic situation in Quebec is transitional. Much will change before a new equilibrium is found. The increasing urbanization and hence industrialization of the French-Canadian people, and the exploitation of their workers by corporations which they do not control, are producing fertile soil for a more radical movement among the masses than has yet appeared. For that reason the other parts of Canada are viewing with some alarm the growth of a fascist movement in the province, and the denial by the authorities of long-established constitutional rights of freedom of the press, of speech, and of public meeting. The "Padlock Act", aimed only at an undefined "communism", is being enforced though communism in Quebec is in fact almost non-existent, while organized fascist parties are drilling members and distributing extreme anti-semitic propaganda without interference of any sort. The mass of the

[1]Mr. Duplessis, for example, was charged with following Russian and Mexican tactics by the Liberal opposition leader in Quebec simply because he ventured to remove some of the tolls from an important private bridge leading to the island of Montreal.

people, there seems little doubt, do not favour the fascist movement, yet there are enough idle young men in the cities to give it considerable support, and enough approval by authorities in church and state of strong action against suspected "reds" to provide an atmosphere in which fascism can flourish.[1] Whatever may be the outcome, it will profoundly affect the whole Dominion, for the French exert an extremely powerful political influence at Ottawa. No national policy can long be followed which does not receive considerable support from Quebec.

[1]See "Embryo Fascism in Quebec", by "S.", *Foreign Affairs*, April, 1938.

CHAPTER VI

CONSTITUTIONAL PROBLEMS

WHEN the Dominion of Canada was created in 1867 the federal form of government was preferred to the unitary state. The choice was due to the insistence of the French Canadians upon the preservation of their own laws, customs and traditions, and also to the strong local patriotism of the Maritime Provinces, which were sceptical of the wisdom of confederation. Racial divisions and sectional feelings thus became embedded in the governmental structure. The constitution as adopted, however, was more centralized than its American model, for civil war was raging to the south when the British North America Act was being framed, and the cause of the conflict seemed to the Canadian statesmen to lie in the doctrine of "states' rights". The United States had reserved to the states or to the people the residue of legislative power, leaving the central government with specified powers only. For Canada the reverse principle was consequently adopted; the federal parliament was given the residuary power over all matters of common interest to the whole country, leaving merely local matters to the provinces. It was expected that the Dominion would develop a greater unity on matters of national concern as time passed, and a greater uniformity even in the provincial laws relating to property and civil rights, in all the provinces except Quebec.[1]

JUDICIAL REVOLUTION

This original concept, which is found clearly expressed in the writings and speeches of the framers of the constitution, was entrusted, after 1867, to the keeping of the courts. They had no easy task to perform. The vision of the statesmen

[1]This was the purpose of Sec. 94 of the B.N.A. Act, which has never been made use of since it was drafted. The opinions of various Canadian leaders of 1867 about the nature of Canadian federalism will be found collected in the brief presented by the League for Social Reconstruction to the Royal Commission on Dominion-Provincial Relations, January, 1938.

had to be perceived in the dry language of the lawyers, and a just balance maintained between the growing needs of the central authorities and the legitimate autonomy of the provinces. The problem was comparatively simple with subjects which fell within the more clearly defined sections of the B. N. A. Act, under such headings as "solemnization of matrimony", "banking", "telegraphs" or the "constitution of the courts". It became very difficult with the new subjects of legislation which emerged as the state embarked more and more upon schemes of social security and economic control. How are statutes dealing with minimum wages, unemployment insurance, marketing, old age pensions, to be classified? They were not enumerated in the original document, drafted in the heyday of *laissez-faire*. They had to be placed within some of the more general phrases in the Act. Of these, three were the most likely receptacles—the Dominion residuary power over matters affecting the "peace, order and good government of Canada", the Dominion power to regulate "trade and commerce", and the provincial jurisdiction over "property and civil rights in the province". None of these powers is precise; the legal interpretation might just as well have favoured any one as any other. Yet ever since the end of the last century the courts, led by the Privy Council, have favoured the solitary provincial power, with few exceptions. Thus laws relating to insurance, controlling the distribution of liquor, regulating provincial marketing and price fixing, providing arbitration in industrial disputes, fixing minimum wages, maximum hours and conditions of employment, establishing unemployment insurance, controlling the production of natural gas, and even giving effect to international conventions relating to provincial matters, have all been held to fall within the "property and civil rights" clause. The Dominion trade and commerce clause has never yet, by itself, supported a single piece of Dominion legislation. The Dominion residuary clause has been narrowed down almost to the vanishing point by the development of the judicial doctrine that it could be invoked only amidst war, pestilence or famine. It can now be said that the residuary power in Canada is vested in the provinces, except in a national emergency more grave than anything experienced during all the calamities of the world crisis which began in 1929.

So great an alteration of the original statute would scarcely have taken place had the final authority for interpreting the constitution been a Canadian court. Canadian judges were living in the environment out of which the B. N. A. Act grew; they knew its purpose, and understood the meaning of its terms. When the Supreme Court of Canada was created in 1875 it was hoped that few if any appeals would be taken thereafter to the Judicial Committee of the Privy Council, but events were to prove the contrary. The appeal of right from the new Supreme Court was barred, but appeals by special leave, or prerogative appeals, were continued. The Minister of Justice and most members of the Dominion parliament who took part in the debate on the Supreme Court Bill were in favour of abolishing all appeals, but it was recognized that this would require imperial legislation.[1] A British court thus became the arbiter of Canadian constitutional growth. The early decisions of the Canadian judges and of the Supreme Court on the Canadian constitution were imbued with a spirit of national unity quite at variance with the concept of the Dominion as a loose federation of sovereign states which later prevailed in the Privy Council, and which has perforce come to be the accepted, because it was the final, statement of the law. By an historical accident, the reverse of that which gave a John Marshall to the American Supreme Court, the Judicial Committee was dominated for two periods totalling thirty years by two men who consistently favoured provincial sovereignty— Lords Watson and Haldane. Of Lord Watson, Lord Haldane himself has written: "He completely altered the tendency of the decisions of the Supreme Court. . . . In a series of masterly judgments he expounded and established the real constitution of Canada".[2] Of Lord Haldane it can be said

---

[1] The clause barring the appeal as of right was strongly objected to by the imperial law officers, but the Canadian government refused to withdraw it and the Bill was not disallowed. See article by Lucien Cannon, K.C., in 1925 *Canadian Bar Review*, 455.

[2] See *Juridical Review*, 1899, p. 279. Lord Haldane repeated his praises of Lord Watson's creative work for Canada in his *Education and Empire* (1902), pp. 138-9, and in an article in the *Cambridge Law Journal*, 1922, cited 1930 *Canadian Bar Review*, p. 438. See also speeches of Hon. C. H. Cahan and Rt. Hon. Ernest Lapointe, Canada, *House of Commons Debates* (unrevised), April 8, 1938, pp. 2336-53.

that he followed faithfully in the Watsonian tradition. The actual number of overrulings of the Canadian Supreme Court are not many, but they occur in matters of crucial importance; many important cases also have gone direct to London from provincial courts of appeal. It was the Judicial Committee which (1) made the Dominion residuary clause an emergency power only, (2) reduced the trade and commerce clause to a secondary position, (3) gave provincial corporations capacity to do business throughout the country, (4) set aside the Dominion Industrial Disputes Investigation Act, (5) gave treaty legislation in part to the provinces. Moreover, the Supreme Court, once the Privy Council has decided, must follow the decision as best it can in future cases. The constitutional difficulties in which Canada finds herself today are due less to defects in the original constitution than to a persistent pro-provincial bias which has permeated, with few exceptions, the English interpretations of the Canadian constitution.[1]

DIVERGENCE BETWEEN CONSTITUTIONAL LAW AND NATIONAL DEVELOPMENT

The disturbance in the legal equilibrium established in 1867 has produced a parallel disturbance in the Dominion-provincial financial relations which were built upon that equilibrium. Under the original constitution it seemed that the provinces would need only moderate incomes since all matters of national import were allotted to the Dominion; the taxing powers of the provincial authorities were consequently limited to "direct" taxation, and they were given annual subsidies to be paid from Dominion revenues and intended to be fixed for all time. The increase in provincial powers, however, coming at a time when the people were demanding more and more services from governments, meant that the provinces had to assume the new duties and hence involved large increases in provincial expenditures. Today the Canadian provinces, having won the constitutional battles, find themselves overburdened with charges which many of them can no longer meet out of revenues. In

[1] The principal exceptions are aeronautics and radio.

their keeping now are the sick, the unemployed, the aged poor, the needy mothers, the orphans and the industrially exploited, as well as control of trade and commerce in the province.

Each province decides for itself how far it will meet these burdens. The Dominion cannot control provincial spending. On the other hand it can scarcely allow any of the provinces to go bankrupt. The situation is thus most unsatisfactory. Several Dominion-provincial conferences met to deal with the problem but disbanded without reaching a settlement. The Liberal government in 1936 introduced a bill to amend the B. N. A. Act by creating a "loan council" after the Australian model, but withdrew it later in face of provincial opposition. Meanwhile, temporary escape from the necessity of a solution was found in the extension of Dominion "loans" to needy provinces; these had reached a total of $132,000,000 by March 31, 1937.[1] Finally, a Royal Commission under the chairmanship of the Hon. N. W. Rowell was appointed in the summer of 1937 to study and report generally on the relations between the Dominion and the provinces. When its report is ready Canada will have to decide in which constitutional direction she wishes to travel—toward greater centralism or toward a looser federalism. She has not yet faced her constitutional difficulties as boldly as have her two sister federations, the United States and Australia.

From the point of view of Canada's international position the most serious consequence of the legal interpretations of the B. N. A. Act has been the splitting asunder of the Dominion's treaty-making power. The decision of the Privy Council in 1937 on this point virtually destroyed the achievements of the previous twenty years of nation building. Canada has now the *right* to act as an independent nation in the world society, but the *power* to fulfil that role has been denied her. She can make treaties, but may not be able to enforce them, unless they can be classed as "empire" treaties under Section 132 of the B. N. A. Act, and this appears to be a highly restricted category. Other treaties must now be allotted to the Dominion or provincial parliaments, like

[1]*Canada Year Book*, 1937, p. 36.

ordinary statutes, in accordance with the judicial ideas as to the nature of the subjects covered by them. No other autonomous country is so handicapped. Canadian plenipotentiaries appointed by Ottawa, or by London on Ottawa's advice, may still meet foreign diplomats to plan international action but cannot give binding assurances that the treaty arrived at will be enforced, since the enforcement in some cases rests with the provinces. No doubt some classes of treaty will seem clearly to fall within the Dominion field, but there will always be an element of doubt which only the courts can clarify. It would be necessary for plenipotentiaries from each of the nine provincial governments to be present at negotiations in order to be certain that the Dominion would not be left in default, as she is at the moment in regard to the three labour conventions ratified by Mr. Bennett but the implementing of which has been declared by the Privy Council to rest with the provinces.[1]

The hopes of the statesmen of 1867 for a strong united Canada have been only partially fulfilled. In the realm of material things their faith was justified. Large commercial, industrial and financial undertakings now operate on a national scale within the free trade area of the Dominion. Railways, banks, insurance companies and the principal agencies of manufacture and distribution, have their head offices in Montreal or Toronto and an administrative organization that reaches from coast to coast. They cover the geographical and racial diversities with an economic uniformity. The inhabitants of Halifax, Montreal and Vancouver draw cheques on the same banks, buy the same insurance policies, mortgage their houses to the same trust companies, ride in the same cars, drink the same whisky, eat the same canned goods and smoke the same cigarettes. But while Canadian economic concentration has been developing, her constitutional unity has been steadily deteriorating as a result of legal interpretation. The business

[1]On the effects of Privy Council decision (*A. G. for Canada* v. *A. G. for Ontario*, [1937] A. C. 326) see articles in *Canadian Bar Review*, June, 1937; the *Canadian Journal of Economics and Political Science*, May, 1937; the *Round Table*, September, 1937; also Daggett, A. P., "Treaty Legislation in Canada", *Canadian Bar Review*, March, 1938; Jennings, W. Ivor, "Constitutional Interpretation—The Experience of Canada", *Harvard Law Review*, November, 1937; brief submitted to the Rowell Commission by League of Nations Society, January, 1938.

leaders and modern science have been subduing geography
while the judges have been expanding provincial sovereignty.

Hence there is a conflict between the economic and the
legal realities in Canada. The large corporations cannot be
effectively controlled in the public interest by nine provincial
legislatures, while their efficiency is hampered by the multitude of varying and vexatious laws and taxes to which they
are subject. The Dominion, on the other hand, is incom-
petent to meet concentrated economic power with an equal
political authority, or to provide remedies for economic
problems which are essentially national in scope. This failure of the Dominion to act produces, by a curiously inverse
process, a greater degree of provincialism and sectional
feeling, for the economic policies formulated by the financiers
and industrialists in the east have borne heavily upon the
extremities of the Dominion and upon the agricultural exporters, who complain they are sacrificed to the money power
and who blame Ottawa for tolerating the exploitation. Thus
is the vicious circle complete: less power at Ottawa means
more power to big business in the east; this results in less
attention to the needs of the Maritimes and the west, which
creates sectional demands for compensation and encourages
attempts at local solutions. In the long run the "depressed
areas" may come to realize that their only hope lies not in
local but in national action, which will subordinate the interests of eastern industry to the needs of the national
economy; but a suspicion that Ottawa will always be
dominated by the east undermines confidence in so-called
"national" policies and hence in national powers.

Thus to the separatist and divisive influences of geography,
race and religion must now be added the disintegrating force
of provincial sovereignty. Canada has made slow progress
in the task of nation-building, and in recent years has lost
constitutional ground. To the Quebec nationalists, the
Privy Council has been a fairy godmother; they can now
ask for an increase in French minority rights in return for a
surrender of their new provincial autonomy. Only recently,
because of the greater need for governmental action, has the
seriousness of the constitutional situation been appreciated,

but already the sectional feeling is so strong that the political problem of securing amendments to the B. N. A. Act appears almost insurmountable. Bold leadership and a statesmanlike appeal for co-operation will be needed if sectionalism is to be overcome, and of these there is at the moment little indication.

CHAPTER VII

THE GROWTH OF CANADIAN NATIONAL FEELING

PREVIOUS chapters in this volume have disclosed the divisions within Canada. These have been emphasized because they provide a key to the understanding of most Canadian problems. Nevertheless Canada, the single country, is still a fact. Over the longer period a sense of national unity has been steadily growing within the Dominion, despite the many obstacles which it has had to overcome. It is shown in innumerable ways, some visible to the outsider, others felt and understood only by those who have lived and travelled in the country. The historical background to Canadian life is both rich and deep, and its record of endeavour and achievement makes for a community of feeling between different sections and groups. A native art movement, springing from the "Group of Seven" who started painting just before the world war, has made the beauty of the Canadian landscape part of the national consciousness. The radio, the aeroplane, the railways, the motor-car and the telephone have reduced the vast size of the country to manageable proportions. There are numbers of organized movements and associations, from political parties to learned societies, from chambers of commerce to athletic clubs, which operate on a national basis within the Dominion. All these are symptoms of nationhood. Canada's participation in the world war, and subsequently in the work of the League of Nations and in the achievement of Dominion status, stimulated very greatly the sense of nationality. The economic depression gave it a setback by creating internal strains and accentuating sectional and class differences; a Social Credit Alberta and a nationalist Quebec appear less integrally part of Canada than were those sections before these political changes occurred. Few people believe, however, that such sectionalism as now exists, strong though it undoubtedly is, creates any real threat to the continued existence of confederation.

The attitude of Canadians toward the United States is a gauge of their own sense of national solidarity. It is when Canadians feel most insecure that they are most fearful of the American influence. A very considerable suspicion, even dislike, of the United States and its constant "Americanization" of Canada exists in certain sections of Canadian opinion. The more Catholic and the more British parts of Canada in particular look upon the United States as a "materialistic" nation whose luxury and extravagant behaviour are in danger of tempting the honest Canadian away from his simple and sober manner of living. Sometimes special interests exploit this antipathy to achieve a particular object, as when high protectionists fought the reciprocity treaty in 1911 on the ground that they were saving Canada from annexation, or employers wishing to preserve the open shop attacked Mr. Lewis and the C. I. O. in 1937 under the guise of helping Canadian labour to save itself from American domination. The anti-American feeling has declined in recent years, however, and the decline is an indication that Canadians have matured to the point where they no longer fear the loss of their identity on the American continent.

The feeling of a Canadian nationality is shared in some degree by most of the French Canadians. For many of them (as has been pointed out) the concept does not extend beyond their own race, even their own province. Even these, however, unless they are separatists, accept the idea of a common Canadian nationality, with a dual language and a dual culture, as a proper basis of association with their English-speaking fellow-citizens. The French Canadians, indeed, were the first to make this idea a normal part of their political thinking. English Canadians have been inclined to look upon Canada as an entirely British country with "one language and one flag" (in fact it has neither) and to think of French Canada, whenever they considered it at all, as an unavoidable and geographically restricted exception to the otherwise happy uniformity. In recent years this attitude has begun to change. A number of English-speaking Canadians have moved closer to the French-Canadian position. Imperialist sentiment of the old sort has declined while the concept of Canada as an autonomous North American nation has grown. This concept is equally valid for both French and English. As the French Canadian expands his vision to include the whole of Canada and not merely the province of Quebec, and as the English Canadian ceases to think of Canada simply as the British part of North America and accepts it, with all its racial variation, as his prime allegiance, they both find they tread on common ground. In a real sense it is true that only in so far as Canada obtains full control over her own foreign policy can she become a united country internally. "The only common denominator [between French and English] seems to be a common allegiance to a common country."[1]

These factors explain why the possibility of another world war, in which Canada might be expected to take part on the side of Great Britain, contains so great a danger for Canadian national unity. The French Canadian feels no obligation or desire to take part in any European wars. His fear that because he is part of the Dominion he will inevitably be dragged into all such wars makes him view his political connection with English Canadians with the greatest suspicion, and makes him feel that the English Canadian is not a true Canadian at all.[2] The Conscription Act of 1917 was not applied in Quebec without bloodshed, and any future attempt to force French Canadians overseas to fight will be resisted much more strongly, particularly if by some chance Great Britain were to be fighting against Italy or with Soviet Russia as an ally. Nor will such resistance be confined by any means to French Canadians. A very large proportion of the 2,000,000 Canadians who are neither French nor British do not understand an allegiance divided between Canada and the Commonwealth. Not even all the British blood in Canada will wish to fight abroad, unless the issue at stake is something deeper than a balance of power in

[1]Lower, A. R. M., in *Canada, The Empire and the League* (Proceedings of Canadian Institute on Economics and Politics, Lake Couchiching, Ontario, 1936) (Toronto, 1936), p. 111.

[2]It is significant that the French word for English-Canadian is *"Anglais"*; for himself, it is *"Canadien"*.

Europe. An increasing number of Canadians of all racial origins are coming to the belief that Canada must have the constitutional right to complete neutrality in future British wars, so that whatever course will best preserve the unity of the country may be freely taken. The growth of this idea is another indication of the growth of the Canadian national consciousness.

CHAPTER VIII

CANADA'S DEFENCE PROBLEM

THE defence of a country is both a political and a military problem. On the political side it means the maintenance of good relations with other countries so as to avoid conflicts if possible and to settle those that arise before they reach the stage of war. This should be the first aim of defence policy in any state not determined upon a programme of aggressive expansion. Military force enters principally when diplomacy has failed, though between states which distrust one another military force will exert a potent influence upon diplomacy and may have a deterrent effect on hostile aggression. Once the military have taken charge of operations, defence becomes a matter of defeating any opposing forces likely to be met on the field of battle.

DIPLOMATIC DEFENCES

Canada has not yet developed her machinery for the conduct of international affairs to the same point as other self-governing nations. She has diplomatic representatives in three foreign countries only—the United States, Japan and France.[1] She has a High Commissioner in London, and an Advisory Officer at Geneva. Canadian relations with other states, such as Germany, Italy, Poland, the Soviet Union and China, are conducted through the British Foreign Office and its diplomatic and consular channels, or through foreign consuls in Canada. Canada is better able to supervise her commercial relations, since Canadian trade commissioners exist in twenty-five countries.[2] In the countries where Canada has a minister of her own she has the machinery for settling disputes by negotiation. Where she has no minister her relations with a country depend largely on the attitude of the British government and its representative,

[1] At the time of writing, the government is proposing to establish legations at Brussels and The Hague with a single minister in charge of both.
[2] See list in *Canada Year Book*, 1937, pp. 495-7.

87

who has other than Canadian interests to protect. Even where Canada has her own representatives she cannot by diplomatic action avoid wars if, as seems to be the case, she has no right to neutrality in the event of Great Britain deciding to resort to war. The Canadian minister at Tokyo, for example, might succeed in preventing any dangerous issue arising between Japan and Canada, and yet if the British ambassador to Tokyo were withdrawn and an Anglo-Japanese war begun the Canadian minister would have to be recalled and Canada exposed immediately to attack on the Pacific coast. In countries like Germany, where there is no Canadian representative, the recall of the British Ambassador would leave Canadian citizens totally unprotected regardless of whether Canada was directly concerned in the dispute or not. Canada can, it is true, bring some influence to bear upon the British government as to the conduct of its policy (an influence perhaps commensurate with the degree of responsibility Canada is prepared to assume), but the principle of equality of status has not yet been fully applied to the conduct of foreign affairs. Canadian diplomatic defences are thus incomplete.

MILITARY DEFENCE OF CANADIAN TERRITORY

The problem of military defence for Canada is being actively discussed at the present time. It will be considered here, first from the point of view of home defence, and secondly from the point of view of co-operation in wider defence arrangements with other powers.

The traditional view of the problem of defence, still widely held in Canada, is that the British navy is Canada's protection against external aggression. More recently it has become usual to point to the United States navy and the Monroe Doctrine as safe-guarding Canadian soil, particularly from attack across the Pacific. Both these views are obviously true in part, for while these fleets command the north Atlantic and the north-east Pacific they are bars to any large-scale invasion of Canada from Europe or from Asia; nevertheless, they suffer from over-simplification. It is more nearly correct to say that, by providing herself with coastal defences well within her own capacity to maintain, Canada can defend herself against any scale of attack which can reasonably be anticipated at the present time without having to rely upon other people's aid. What the distant future may bring is, of course, another matter.

Canada's security from the danger of armed invasion depends on two factors—the present international situation and the natural advantages derived from geography. In most discussions of defence insufficient attention is paid to the first factor. Yet defence cannot be discussed in the abstract; defence means defence against particular powers or combinations of powers. It so happens that there are no powers which threaten to invade Canada. No South American power is planning her conquest. It is no longer a part of Canadian defence policy to contemplate war with the United States: hence the famous undefended frontier. No Asiatic power except Japan is in an expansive and aggressive mood. Japan has both an "historic mission" and an actual commitment on the Asiatic mainland (besides the very real threat from the Soviet Union) sufficient to keep her occupied for an indefinite period. China is now defending Canada on the Pacific by keeping Canada's only potential invader fully engaged.

Europe is the only remaining continent from which an attack might be expected. Italy's ambitions are clearly Mediterranean; if she ever looks to America, it will more likely be to South America. Germany is left. What are Germany's ambitions? The *Drang nach Osten* is Canada's immediate defence from that quarter. Not even *Mein Kampf* suggests Canada as a part of greater Germany. In any case Germany must establish an hegemony in Europe before she can safely begin any trans-Atlantic adventures; this means she must first dispose of the balance of power against her. Hence Russia and France are part of Canada's defence at the present moment, quite as much as is Great Britain (whose recent policy, indeed, appears to many Canadians to be one of encouragement for Germany's expansion). Only if Germany and her fascist allies win the next European war and are not themselves destroyed by the victory would it be necessary for Canadian defence policy to contemplate the still remote possibility of an attack in force from Europe.

Mr. Mackenzie King, in his statement to the House of Commons on foreign policy on May 24, 1938, expressed himself as follows on this point:

If we are unlikely of our own motion to take part in wars of conquest or wars of crusade, it is equally unlikely that at the moment, with the world as it is today, any other country will single out Canada for attack. The talk which one sometimes hears of aggressor countries planning to invade Canada and seize these tempting resources of ours is, to say the least, premature. It ignores our neighbours and our lack of neighbours; it ignores the strategic and transportation difficulties of transoceanic invasion; it ignores the vital fact that every aggressor has not only potential objects of its ambition many thousands of miles nearer which would be the object of any attack, but potential and actual rivals near at hand whom it could not disregard by launching fantastic expeditions across half the world. At present danger of attack upon Canada is minor in degree and second-hand in origin. It is against chance shots that we need immediately to defend ourselves. The truth of this is recognized in every country. What may develop no one can say.[1]

In addition to these political reasons why Canada is comparatively secure at the moment, there are unusual geographical obstacles in the path of any invader. Three thousand miles of Atlantic and four thousand of Pacific Ocean are the beginnings of his difficulties. Both the Atlantic and the Pacific coasts lend themselves to home defences. The St. Lawrence is not navigable in winter, and with buoys removed and mines laid would be exceedingly difficult to utilize for transport purposes in summer. Canada would be bound to have lengthy warning of any attempted attack in force.[2] The eastern points most in need of protection are the harbours of the Maritimes, such as Halifax, Sydney and St. John; an army in control of these, however, is still separated from Montreal by 800 miles of barren country. The physical features of the Pacific coast are even more discouraging to the landing of any large force, though

[1]Canada, *House of Commons Debates* (unrevised), May 24, 1938, p. 3439.
[2]See *Canadian Defence Quarterly*, cited in MacKay and Rogers, *op. cit.*, p. 181.

they would lend themselves, if undefended, to the planting of bases for raiding.[1]

Military experts in Canada are consequently of the opinion that Canadian defence policy does not need to prepare for armed invasion. The utmost that need be expected at the moment are "minor attacks by combined sea, land and air forces, to destroy something of strategic or commercial value, or to secure an advanced base of operations, and this applies to coasts, to focal sea areas and to the preservation of Canadian neutrality", and also "sporadic hit and run raids by light cruisers or submarines to destroy our main ports and focal sea areas".[2]

To deal with these minor attacks and sporadic raids, Canada is already preparing her coastal defences, both east and west. The technical details need not be considered here: in general the need is for fixed coastal batteries and anti-aircraft defences at such points as Halifax and Sydney on the Atlantic, Vancouver and Esquimalt on the Pacific; sea and air forces capable of searching out and destroying hostile craft and their temporary bases; and supporting infantry units ready to move quickly to threatened zones. Under the new and enlarged defence plans now being carried out these will be provided within the next three or four years. It is therefore true to say that Canada is preparing to meet and is fully capable of meeting her local defence requirements at the present time out of her own financial resources. It is also true, however, that her armaments industry is not yet able to manufacture the heavier equipment needed, and she must therefore purchase supplies from outside sources. At present most of the orders have been placed with English firms—with the consequence that the rapidity of defence development has been impeded by British rearmament plans.

Thus far, it will be observed, no reliance has been placed on those two particular guarantees of Canadian defence— the British navy and the Monroe Doctrine. Obviously their

[1]For a more extended discussion of these points see MacKay and Rogers, op. cit., Chap. XI.

[2]Hon. Ian Mackenzie, Minister of National Defence, House of Commons Debates (unrevised), March 24, 1938, p. 1793; see also, "Canuck", "The Problems of Canadian Defence", Canadian Defence Quarterly, April, 1938, p. 269.

existence is a still further safeguard for Canada. The analysis just given makes these two additional factors, however, of more potential than immediate utility. When Japan has completed her campaign in China it is conceivable that she might be insane enough to look across the Pacific; at that moment the Monroe Doctrine and the American navy would become vitally important. That moment, however, is not in sight. The same is true of a threat from Germany. As for the British navy, it no doubt operates as a powerful check upon Hitler's ambitions in Europe. So also does the French army, the Russian airfleet and whatever other European forces may be expected to line up against Germany in the next European war. The Royal navy is one element in a far wider picture.

There are, it is true, individuals in Canada, many of them sincere, who are frightened by the current wave of militarism and who feel that an invasion of Canada is a real danger. The Toronto *Star* in February, 1938, published a doctored photograph of planes bombing the city of Toronto. It was not felt to be necessary to suggest whose planes they were or how they might be expected to return, Toronto being 4,000 miles from Europe. Such propaganda makes the increase in defence estimates politically easier. Mr. King, despite his recent statement that Canada is under no threat of invasion, said in a radio address, on his return from the Imperial Conference of 1937, "Never imagine that to the overpopulated countries and under-nourished peoples of other continents, the countless attractions and limitless possibilities of Canada are unknown; or that, in some world holocaust, our country would escape the 'terror by night' or 'the arrow that flieth by day'."[1] In this atmosphere of vague impending doom, the general public seldom stops to ask which people are eyeing Canada, or how they plan to transport themselves to her shores.

It is sometimes said that Canada is vitally concerned with keeping open the trade routes of the Atlantic, on account of her large overseas trade. The statement is obviously true

---

[1]*Crown and Commonwealth: An Address on the Coronation, the Imperial Conference, and visit to the Continent of Europe*, delivered over the national network of the Canadian Broadcasting Corporation, Ottawa July 9, 1937 (Ottawa, King's Printer, 1937), p. 15.

up to a point. Canada's foreign trade is essential to the economic welfare of the country, given the continuation of Canada's present economic policy. But this trade is not essential in the sense that without it Canadians would starve to death. There is food and shelter for all within the country, and it might be cheaper to reorganize the economy during the period of cessation of the trade than to engage in a war to preserve it. A recent study group of the Canadian Institute of International Affairs on the subject of defence unanimously agreed that "few of the great trading countries have in practice defended their shipping on the high seas, and it seemed to be clear that Canada's defence policy could not be designed with the object of defending her goods, even those which might be carried far from home in her own ships". Moreover, it has been shown[1] that in actual fact there is very little "Canadian" trade on the Atlantic. A sort of de facto "cash and carry" principle prevails; Canada sells her produce to European importers in Canada, and they collect it in their own ships at Canadian ports. It is their trade, rather than Canada's, on the high seas. They are more vitally concerned to import it than is Canada to export it, and they are only too anxious to see it continue, not for Canada's sake, but for their own. No one in Canada has ever taken seriously the suggestion that she should "blast her way into the markets of the world"; present defence plans contemplate the protection of "focal sea areas" (a vague term in current use amongst the military experts) apparently as a part of coastal defence and as a protection of overseas shipping only as it converges on Canadian ports.

If Canada were to remain neutral in a war in which the United States were involved it might be necessary to defend that neutrality against violation. For example, if Japan and the United States were at war, Japan might wish to use the British Columbia coast as a base of operations, or the United States might want to transport troops and equipment across Canadian territory into Alaska. In either case Canada would have to protect her neutrality, for fear of becoming

[1]See above, p. 36.

involved as an ally of one of the belligerents. Coastal defences of the kind already described, when completed, will take care of submarine bases or temporary landing parties. If the United States were determined to use Canadian territory, there is nothing Canada could do to prevent it.

PREPARATION FOR DEFENCE OF THE COMMONWEALTH
OR OF THE LEAGUE

The immediate defence of Canada, then, is not beyond the capacity of Canadians acting alone, provided they are content simply to safeguard their own territory. From the purely national point of view Canada needs no military alliances in the present world. If Canadian foreign policy includes the idea of intervention in Europe or elsewhere on behalf of the Commonwealth or the League, however, other considerations at once arise. The character of Canadian defence forces must be altered, and preparation for joint action begun. To protect Canada, as has been shown, fixed coastal batteries, mine sweepers, aircraft and possibly a few submarines are necessary, with a small supporting infantry force at each coast. To prepare for an expeditionary force to Europe, the emphasis must be placed on mobile and mechanized units, trained and equipped for immediate integration with the British army. These units must be supplied with machine guns, tanks, bombing-planes, and all the paraphernalia of modern warfare, much of which is superfluous, either in kind or quantity, for the defence of Canada alone. This type of army, on a modest scale, is contemplated and is in fact being organized in Canada.[1] The possibility of co-operation in war abroad has always been a dominant factor in Canadian defence policy, since until comparatively recently most Canadians have accepted without question the military alliance implicit in the former empire relationship,

[1]Canada has a permanent active militia of 4,000 men, a non-permanent militia with a peace establishment of 100,000 but an actual strength of about 45,000, and a paper reserve militia. The naval forces consist of four destroyers, with two on order (four to be placed on the Pacific and two on the Atlantic coasts) and a number of mine sweepers; total personnel (March, 1938) 119 officers and 1,462 ratings, with a volunteer reserve of 77 officers and 1,344 ratings. The Air Force consists of an authorized permanent personnel of 1,730 and a non-permanent force of 1,064; 102 aircraft are being secured, and landing fields have been constructed across the country to permit of rapid concentration. See MacKay and Rogers, op. cit., pp. 192 ff., and speech of the Minister of Defence (Hon. Ian Mackenzie) on March 24, 1938, cited above, p. 91, n. 2.

and empire wars have not been fought in North America for over a century. Even today the ratio of defence expenditures as between land, sea and air is 2: 1: 1, whereas a purely national defence policy would place both naval and air expenditures ahead of those devoted to the infantry.[1] In addition, Canada is under contractual agreement with Great Britain to permit the use of Halifax and Esquimalt harbours by the British fleet, and has always co-ordinated her training and equipment with British practices. There is thus a difference between local defence requirements and present defence policy, a difference representing Canada's recognition of the possibility of having to take part in an overseas war.[2]

Because of the growing isolationist sentiment in the country the government spokesmen have tended recently to emphasize the home defence needs and to deny any "commitments" to or preparations for war abroad. To do this without unduly offending imperialist and other sentiment requires no little verbal ingenuity. An example of the kind of statement that is made is seen in the following extract from Mr. King's speech on February 19, 1937, justifying the increase in the Canadian defence estimates:

. . . In the course of this debate it has been necessary at different times from this side of the house to repeat that what we are doing we are doing for Canada and for Canada alone. That has been necessary for the reason that an impression had been created that what we were doing had relation to some expeditionary force which would be sent overseas. When we say that what we are doing we are doing for Canada alone, we mean we are doing it for the defence of our country within the territorial waters of the coasts of our country, and within Canada itself for the defence of Canada. But I hope it will not be thought that because we have laid emphasis on the fact that what we are doing we are doing for Canada, we are not thereby making some contribution towards the defence of the British Commonwealth of Nations as a whole, or that we are not making some contribution towards the defence of all English-speaking communities, that we are not making some contribution towards the defence of all democracies,

[1]See Glazebrook, G. de T., *Canada's Defence Policy*, Report of Round Tables of Conference of Canadian Institute of International Affairs, 1937, p. 16.

[2]In the past Canada's contributions to imperial defence have been military rather than naval, and the habit of spending more on the military has continued. Many regiments which came back from the last war continued in existence. They became social and recreational centres; the winter quarters were club rooms and the summer camps cheap holiday outings. It was politically wise to maintain them.

that we are not making some contribution towards the defence of all those countries that may some day necessarily associate themselves together for the purpose of preserving their liberties and freedom against an aggressor, come from wherever he may.[1]

The latter part of this double-barrelled statement is addressed to the body of opinion which feels strongly that Canada must prepare to meet the challenge of any aggressive powers, in order to preserve the same institutions and principles for which the empire took part in the last world war. As already indicated, Canadian defence arrangements already take this into account, though not to the extent this opinion would wish. The following note contributed by a Canadian expresses this point of view: it is given here in full and without comment to show how its adherents see the defence problem.

There is only a very slight chance of Canada becoming involved in war arising out of any local issue. There is every chance of our becoming involved because of issues in which we are concerned along with every other free country. It is therefore the world issue that must dominate our consideration of defence policy. Canada's first line of defence, like Britain's, is on the Rhine.

The nations of the world of our time are divided into three groups,— the Fascist states, governed by dictators, believing in war, ambitious and dissatisfied with their shares of empire; the Communist state, which may at any turn be added to by proletarian revolutions; and the Liberal and Democratic states, which are satisfied with the status quo which they secured partly by their greater progress in the nineteenth century and partly by their victory in the late war. The only possibility of a war affecting Canada or any other part of the Commonwealth arises from the determination of the Fascist states to redress the balance, and the certainty that they will attempt to do so by war, unless the armed forces of the free nations are so strong and united as to foredoom the attempt to failure. If war does come Canada will again have to be defended on the fields of Flanders and in co-operation with the British Navy. If those fail Canada will have no option but to submit to whatever terms the Nazis dictate.

The defence of the mainland of Canada from invasion can be so easily provided for that no nation on either side of us would attempt it. Nor would they have the slightest need to do so. If the British Navy were out of the way it would be a very simple matter for Germany to

[1]Canada, *House of Commons Debates*, February 19, 1937, p. 1058.

seize the island of Cape Breton and use it as a base from which to destroy all our Atlantic trade or for Japan to seize Vancouver Island and destroy our Pacific trade. Without export trade Canada cannot do more than exist. Exports take up so large a proportion of our production, both agricultural and industrial that their cessation would disrupt our whole economic structure and cause unemployment so great as to be beyond our power to cope with. It is nonsense to talk of the trade not being Canadian trade because it is carried from our shores in ships of foreign registry or owned by foreign purchasers. An enemy nation which secured control of the oceans could get all the supplies it needed from other countries and our trade would come to an end.

It is natural and right that our defence policy should be directed first of all to our own defence and, since such defence will cost all that we can at present afford to spend, our Government is taking the right course in making such defence its sole present aim. But as our people come to realize the world situation more clearly they will insist on our being prepared to do our part, if it becomes necessary. That can only be done by co-operation first with Great Britain, then with the other parts of the Empire and the United States, and ultimately in a League of the Free Nations for the defence of our common liberties and interests.[1]

---

[1]This is a point of view held by a considerable body of opinion in the United States. Its best expression is perhaps to be found in Walter Lippmann's article in *Foreign Affairs*, July, 1937, "Rough-hew Them How We Will". He sees the hand of a divine Providence in the American neutrality legislation giving effect to the "cash and carry" principle, since it will assist the democratic powers.

CHAPTER IX

CANADA'S EXTERNAL ASSOCIATIONS

CANADA'S external associations are primarily with the British Commonwealth and the United States, for obvious historic and geographical reasons; but her development as a supplier of international markets and a member of the League has brought her into wide contact with the world at large.

ASSOCIATIONS WITH THE COMMONWEALTH

Canada's associations with the Commonwealth are in all essential respects the same as those of her sister dominions. The formal link of the Crown is apparent in all the functions of government, both Dominion and provincial. High Commissioners are exchanged between Ottawa and London, and the Union of South Africa now has an accredited representative at Ottawa—the first to come from any dominion. All Canadians enjoy the common status of British subjects, though British subjects from other parts of the Commonwealth require five years residence before they can be classed as "Canadian citizens" or "Canadian nationals" under certain Canadian laws.[1] The Privy Council remains the final court of appeal for Canada, much criticized but not yet abandoned.[2] Canadians participate in various organs of Commonwealth co-operation set up under the Imperial Conferences, such as the Imperial Economic Committee and other joint bodies. Canadian officers are sent for training to

[1] E.g. under the Immigration Act, the Foreign Enlistment Act, etc.

[2] In the 1938 session of the Canadian Parliament, the Hon. C. H. Cahan, Secretary of State in the Conservative administration, 1930-35, introduced a bill to abolish appeals to the Privy Council "in relation to any matter within the competence of the Parliament of Canada". Mr. Lapointe, the Minister of Justice, in his speech supporting the bill, expressed the opinion that the Canadian Parliament had the power to do away with all appeals. Mr. Cahan then stated that he would be very glad to see an amendment in committee to that effect (Canada, *House of Commons Debates*, unrevised, April 8, 1938, p. 2353). The bill was later withdrawn to permit of further study by law associations and other interested bodies throughout the Dominion. Mr. Cahan has stated that he hopes Mr. Lapointe will re-introduce a similar bill on behalf of the government at the next session. If not, he will himself re-introduce the bill. The wide measure of support given the bill is indicative of the movement of opinion against the use of appeals to the Privy Council.

the Imperial Staff College. But Canada has consistently opposed the creation of any central Commonwealth organization which would possess executive power or which might give the impression that a new system of control was being established in London. There is no likelihood that this attitude will change.

Canada's trade relations with Great Britain and other members of the Commonwealth have already been described. 46.7 per cent. of Canadian exports went to empire countries in 1937 and 29.5 per cent. of her imports came from them. This considerable trade, second only to that between Canada and the United States, is the result both of historic commercial relationships and of the imperial preferences. There is no doubt that Canada's trade with the Commonwealth is based to some extent upon political considerations, and that should her political objectives change in this regard the importance of the empire in her economy would gradually diminish. The political factor, however, does not appear to be of great importance in the total picture. Great Britain's need for foodstuffs and raw materials makes trade with Canada very natural.

It is not easy to assess the cultural and sentimental ties that join Canada to the Commonwealth. They have their roots in language, literature and religion; in respect for the Crown and in parliamentary democracy; in a common history and in family relationships. These ties are strong in some sections of Canada, weak in others. They are strongest in the Maritimes, Ontario and British Columbia; less evident in the Prairie Provinces where the non-British immigrants are mostly settled; and weakest in Quebec. Canadians with a pro-British attitude occupy most of the important positions in the Protestant churches, in public affairs, in education, in business and in the press. In an emergency, they would act with considerable unanimity. Nevertheless, imperialist sentiment amongst the general population has declined in recent years. For half the Canadians the "British tradition" is something which they found existing in the country of their adoption, or else, as in the case of the French Canadians, something which was imposed

upon them. These people are Canadians first, members of
the Commonwealth after. This does not mean that many,
perhaps most of these Canadians have not a great respect
for the British Commonwealth and its traditions. Their
loyalty to Canada includes unquestionably a certain loyalty
to the British connection. The degree of the latter loyalty,
however, is obviously much less than would be found
amongst Canadians of British origin. And even large numbers of the British Canadians have transplanted the greater
part of their loyalty.

In the matter of imperial defence Canada has always followed an apparently independent course. At the moment of
crisis in the past she has not stinted her expenditure (witness
South Africa and the world war) but in times of peace she
has been suspicious of joint efforts for imperial defence. She
has never contributed to the British navy,[1] and recently has
given a distinctly cold reception to the "peregrinating imperialists" who from time to time suggest that she should.
Most Canadians are convinced that the British navy, even
admitting its deterrent effect on aggressors, is no larger than
it would be if the Dominion were totally independent.[2]
Great Britain quite properly builds for her own defence
rather than for Canada's. She must protect the North
Atlantic trade routes, for she needs foodstuffs and raw
materials both from Canada and the United States. At the
same time it has already been pointed out that Canada has
never ceased to prepare for possible joint action with Great
Britain. The principle of "no commitments" is now advanced as the corner-stone of Canada's defence policy, at the
same time as officers are being exchanged with British units,
equipment is being made uniform with the latest British
models, and a military force is contemplated of a kind different from that required for purely domestic needs. To most
imperialists, Canada's co-operation in defence matters seems
pitifully inadequate; to those who support a policy of neutrality Canada seems to be preparing already for another
intervention in Europe whenever Britain calls.

[1]Though in 1912 she would have done so but for the opposition of the Senate.
[2]". . . If Canada dropped out of the Empire tomorrow Great Britain could not reduce
her armed strength by one war-ship, aircraft or man."—"Canuck", "The Problems of
Canadian Defence", *Canadian Defence Quarterly*, April, 1938, p. 268.

In considering Canada's attitude to the Commonwealth a distinction must be made between the desire for neutrality and the desire for secession. Even those Canadians who wish Canada to have the right to neutrality when Great Britain or any other part of the Commonwealth is at war, do not wish to secede from the Commonwealth. According to some imperialists neutrality means secession; others challenge this assumption. It is important to remember, however, that people who believe neutrality is possible in an empire joined merely by a personal union under the Crown are not, in their hearts, aiming to destroy the Commonwealth. Despite the increasing tendency to independent action in international affairs, the vast majority of Canadians hope the Commonwealth will continue and that Canada will remain a member of it. Even many of the French-Canadian nationalists have said that they do not desire to quit the Commonwealth altogether; their independent republic would remain a dominion under the Crown. None of the movements of opinion within Canada which conflict with the concept of a strongly united Commonwealth must be taken to indicate the growth of a secessionist movement.

A further distinction that needs to be made is that between a right to neutrality and a policy of neutrality. A right to remain neutral is an adjunct of autonomy, a necessary constitutional power if Canada is to have full control over her own foreign policy. A policy of neutrality is the exercise of that right in a particular event. Some people who ask for the right wish to adopt the policy, but many others wish Canada to have the right so that she may really be free to adopt a policy of neutrality or not, according to her own decision when the next war comes. It is the automatic belligerency at some one else's choice which is objected to even though that belligerency be purely technical at the outset.

There is also in Canada a considerable body of opinion which would place the importance of the maintenance of Commonwealth unity ahead of the right to neutrality in time of war. Such people would put first the preservation of the Commonwealth association, hoping at the same time that neutrality might still turn out to be possible. Although they would maintain Canada's freedom of action as to participation in the conduct of overseas wars, and would always impress the Canadian point of view upon the British government as to any matter affecting Canada's interests, they would take for granted Canada's technically belligerent status in any British or Commonwealth war. They think that a neutral Canada would be virtually certain, in a conflict involving great powers, to have her neutrality challenged in such a way as to present the alternatives of accepting belligerency or breaking the Commonwealth connection. By many of this group the relationship with Great Britain is accepted as including a tacit military alliance.[1]

The British connection has left, as need scarcely be said, a permanent mark on Canadian social and political institutions. It is seen most noticeably in the parliamentary nature of the Canadian government, in the structure of the courts, in the organization of the military forces, and in religious and educational traditions. But in spite of this tutelage the greater number of Canadian institutions and activities are now North American or just plain Canadian. The parliamentary tradition has been blended with a federalism which is American in origin. Political behaviour is often American despite the forms of government. History relates Canada to Great Britain, but the daily contacts of Canadians are with the United States. It has been estimated that some 30,000,-000 crossings of the Canadian-American boundary were made in the year 1931-32.[2] Canadian sports and amusements are American. Only small groups in the principal Canadian cities read English periodicals, though English books are more widely distributed. Most English-speaking Canadians read some American magazines, which have a greater total circulation in Canada than have the Canadian publications. Every Canadian with a radio may tune in at any time to a variety of United States programmes, and their constant influence affects his outlook even though he may occasionally

[1]An estimate of the relative strength of the various groups of opinion in Canada is made below, pp. 135 ff.

[2]See address by R. H. Coats on "The Two Good Neighbours" in *Proceedings of Conference on Canadian-American Affairs*, 1937, edited by Trotter, R. G., Corey, A. B., and Mc-Laren, W. W. (Boston, 1937), pp. 106 ff.

rise at a special hour to hear a coronation service from London or some other empire broadcast. Cultural diffusion east and west is difficult within the Dominion; it is relatively easy north and south across the international boundary. The natural affiliations of the Maritime Provinces are with the New England states; many more Quebec French Canadians have emigrated to the United States than to other parts of Canada; Ontario's business and labour connections are predominantly American; the Prairie Provinces are highly Americanized; while British Columbia is an integral part of the Pacific slope.[1] Thus does the United States press upon Canada in a way that Great Britain cannot, and though the British traditions continue, and provide a kind of psychological counterweight which is very powerful, the other influence is the more insistent. The Commonwealth provides the Sunday religion, North America the week-day habits, of Canadians.

British institutions are now thoroughly incorporated into Canadian life and blended with American elements adapted to Canadian needs. Their continuation in Canada may be expected, regardless of the continuance of the Commonwealth relationship. England's contribution to Canada is kept alive now not so much by the existence of the Commonwealth as by the voluntary adherence of Canadians themselves to the traditions with which their national life began. On the other hand the existence of these traditions largely guarantees Canada's continued membership in the Commonwealth.

ASSOCIATIONS WITH THE UNITED STATES

In the formal political sense, the United States is a foreign country to Canadians, one of the three foreign countries to which a Canadian minister has been accredited. In actual fact the United States is not regarded as a foreign country at all. When the Canadians talk about the "foreigners" in the population, they are not thinking of American settlers.[2] A

[1]See Ware, N. J. and Logan, H. A., *Labor in Canadian-American Relations* (Toronto, 1937), p. 3.

[2]Mr. Hepburn called the C.I.O. organizers "foreign agitators", but Canadian politicians welcome American financiers with open arms if they have money to invest in Canada.

very special relationship exists between the two countries, as unlike ordinary international intercourse as are the dealings of the British countries one with another. The existence of this relationship makes Canada unique in the British Commonwealth, for no other member has similar associations with any country outside the Commonwealth.

Throughout the preceding analysis of the basic factors in Canadian life, the influence of the United States has inevitably appeared, and there is no need to repeat what has already been said. Trade and commerce, radio, the films, newspapers and periodicals, sports, tourist visits and family connections, maintain the constant intercourse. When disputes arise and adjustments must be made between the governments, little difficulty is ever experienced: witness the settlement of the *I'm Alone* case, and the steady achievements of the International Joint Commission regulating boundary waters. Perhaps it would be wrong to attribute all the American characteristics of Canadian life to the influence of the United States. Men and women, whether north or south of the American boundary, derive from the same racial stocks, live on the same continent, and have to abstract a living from a very similar physical environment; it is not surprising that in the process of time their social and economic institutions have come to have great similarities. When a Canadian talks of Canada as an American nation, he does not mean that he wants to become a citizen of the United States, or hopes Canada will enter the American Union; he means that he recognizes now, and is not afraid to face the fact, that his destiny and chief interests lie in North America.[1]

Events that occur in the United States have immediate repercussions in, and seem closely related to, Canada. Dramatic English events, particularly those touching the Crown, awake great interest in Canada, but the internal social and political developments in England seem remote. The election of President Roosevelt, and the stimulus which his personality and programme have given to social and political

---

[1] It has been suggested that the proper reply for a Canadian to the question frequently addressed to him in England, "Are you an American?", is, "Yes, I am a Canadian". Due to the fact that "United States" is a noun from which no adjective can be made, the word "American" must do a double duty.

changes within the United States, have had a great influence upon Canadian policy in the past five years. Mr. Bennett's legislative reforms of 1935 were not improperly called in Canada, "Mr. Bennett's 'New Deal' ". Recovery in the United States preceded and promoted Canadian economic improvement. The sudden rise of Lewis and the C. I. O. stirred Canadian trades unions into more militancy and activity than they had shown since the world war. Mr. Roosevelt's visit to Buenos Aires in 1936 made the Pan-American Union a topic of discussion in the Canadian Institute of International Affairs, if not in the country at large. It is generally true that every important development in the United States is followed with a varying time lag by a similar development in Canada. Only occasionally are English changes followed in Canada; possibly the introduction of new divorce legislation into the Canadian parliament following A. P. Herbert's divorce bill is a recent example, as is also the structure of the Canadian Broadcasting Corporation, which was modelled on the B. B. C.

CANADA AND THE LEAGUE OF NATIONS

Since 1920 Canada's membership in the League of Nations has been an important factor amongst her external associations. It has affected to a considerable degree both her relationship with the United States and with the British Commonwealth.

The idea of the League of Nations was attractive to Canadians for two reasons. In the first place the creation of the League gave an opportunity for Canada to appear before the world as an independent nation. Canada, it has been said, was born in an ante-room at Geneva. In the second place, Canadians along with other British peoples can be easily aroused to international co-operation by an idealistic or humanitarian appeal. The ideals and work of the League of Nations evoked considerable enthusiasm amongst certain sections of the Canadian people, and made them desire to shape a Canadian foreign policy in accordance with the requirements of a world collective system. This was particularly true in later years, for at first the League was not understood. While this loyalty to the League did not destroy a sense of loyalty to the Commonwealth, it made the latter appear less important to many people.

The history of Canada's participation in League activities shows a decided opposition to the idea of the League as a body with power to enforce its decisions. Canadian delegates at Geneva have generally been willing to co-operate on minor international matters but unwilling to promote or support schemes for mutual assistance in the event of war. In this respect Canadian official action has often been less co-operative than some sections of public opinion would have wished. Canada opposed the Italian suggestion of an inquiry into raw materials in 1920, and supported the British government in its rejection of the Treaty of Mutual Guarantee of 1923 and the Protocol of 1924. Canada moved for the deletion of Article X of the Covenant, and when this failed was instrumental in obtaining the interpretative resolution of 1923 which recognized that the Council, in recommending military measures in consequence of aggression, should take into account the geographical situation and the special conditions of each state. The Canadian representative at the time of the Manchurian incident went fully as far as Sir John Simon in suggesting caution and minimizing the aggression of Japan. Mr. Mackenzie King in his speech in the Canadian House of Commons on June 18, 1936, and in his speech at the League Assembly on September 29, 1936, declared that Canada had no absolute commitments to apply military or even economic sanctions against an aggressor named by the League; that it was for the parliament of Canada (not the League Council or Assembly) to decide in the light of the circumstances of each case how far Canada would participate in any form of compulsion.[1] Yet he had applied the sanctions against Italy without waiting for parliamentary approval, so strong was the opinion in the country.

While thus making clear to the League that she would not give definite commitments in advance, Canada nevertheless took part in the general work of the League in the same

[1] A full analysis of Mr. King's various statements in this connection is given by Escott Reid in "Mr. Mackenzie King's Foreign Policy", *Canadian Journal of Economics and Political Science*, February, 1937.

manner as her sister dominions. She adopted the Optional
Clause and the General Act for the Pacific Settlement of
International Disputes. She has attended the sessions of the
I. L. O.; but the lack of an effective labour party, the influence of the employer and agricultural classes in Canada,
and constitutional difficulties, have prevented the Dominion
from implementing more than four of the fifty-seven draft
conventions of the International Labour Conference.[1] An
attempt was made by Mr. Bennett in 1935 to implement
three other conventions, but the Privy Council invalidated
the legislation. None of the provinces has shown any in-
clination to use the exclusive legislative power in this regard
which the courts have recognized as vested in them; their
legislatures are generally dominated by agricultural representatives and include very few labour spokesmen.[2]

Canada's willingness to participate in the application of
sanctions at the outset of the Italo-Abyssinian war, and the
almost complete unanimity with which this policy was approved, at least in English-speaking Canada, indicated that
when loyalty to the Commonwealth and to the League were
combined the majority of the Canadian people were willing
to undertake very considerable commitments in world
affairs. At the same time the more cautious attitude, the
North American suspicion of all European politics, is always
present in the country. The French Canadians in particular
are suspicious of the League, which many of them look upon
as the creation of freemasons and atheists.[3] The Dominion
government's repudiation of special responsibility for the
Canadian representative's motion, in the Committee of
Eighteen, to apply the oil sanction, gave expression to the
isolationist feeling. In spite of the League's virtual disappearance as an instrument of collective security a belief in
this idea has not died in the Dominion. The disillusionment
and disappointment of recent years, however, have made

[1]As of January 1, 1937. See *Canada Year Book*, 1937, p. 740.

[2]British Columbia is the sole exception: the Eight Hour Day Convention was put
into force by provincial law. In a number of cases, although the provincial legislatures
have not specifically implemented the conventions, nevertheless they have enacted legislation covering many of the points dealt with by them.

[3]See Bruchési, Jean, in *Canada: The Empire and the League* (Proceedings of the Canadian Institute on Economics and Politics, Lake Couchiching, Ontario, 1936) (Toronto,
1936), p. 143.

most of the League supporters profoundly sceptical of the possibility of building again an effective world organization at Geneva until the European nations settle some of their own differences by their own action. In consequence, most Canadians today look upon Europe as being in a condition indistinguishable from that which existed at the beginning of this century.

Outside Quebec, sentiment in Canada toward the League has thus moved from early indifference through a short period of enthusiasm and active support (Abyssinia) to almost complete disillusionment. This disillusionment has spread its influence into the field of Commonwealth affairs. Manchuria, Abyssinia, Spain, China, Austria—these milestones on the road of international disintegration have alienated the sympathies of considerable sections of English-Canadian opinion towards the Commonwealth connection. These events have had the contrary effect on numerous other English Canadians.

The former group contend that an inkling of what would occur were the League to disappear was perceived at the first British Commonwealth Relations Conference,[1] and that its fears have been amply justified. The influence of recent international events has reacted in three ways to the detriment of the Commonwealth association. In the first place, the policy of the British government since 1931 has steadily estranged those Canadians who believe it prefers power politics of the pre-League type to the principles established by the Covenant. The spectacle of a British Foreign Secretary going to Geneva, by private agreement with a covenant-breaker, to beg the powers to recognize a conquest acquired by barefaced aggression against a fellow member of the League, is one which these Canadians cannot

[1]"If a breakdown of the attempt to establish a humane and reasonable world-order ever did bring these diverse regional factors into active play, who could tell how far the countries now associated in the British Commonwealth might drift apart on their way to encounter their diverse fates, whatever these fates might respectively prove to be? To a well attuned ear, the proceedings at the British Commonwealth Relations Conference which met at Toronto in September 1933 had a tragic as well as an assuring note." A. J. Toynbee, in *British Commonwealth Relations* (Proceedings of the first British Commonwealth Relations Conference) (London, 1934), p. 14. Further opinion of a similar sort was expressed at the first annual Studies Conference of the Canadian Institute of International Affairs, held in May, 1934; see the report published by the Institute and distributed privately to members.

view without a sense of bitterness and shame, however much Canada herself may be open to criticism for her attitude toward sanctions. Distrust of British policy very naturally breeds a dislike of the idea of the Commonwealth being asked to back the new policy should it result in the expected war. In the second place, even many imperialists feel disturbed at the long refusal of Great Britain to take a firm stand against the threats of the dictators; while approving her rearmament programme, they feel that the toleration of fascist expansion is jeopardizing the trade routes of the Empire and inviting future aggression at a time when the strategic position of Great Britain will be far weaker. Lastly, and perhaps most seriously, the revival of an armaments race on a huge scale, the return of the struggle for the balance of power in Europe, and the growing belief that a useless repetition of the world war is almost certain to occur sooner or later, make numbers of English Canadians turn to a policy of North American isolation and self-defence, and confirm the French Canadians in their determination not to allow themselves to be involved again. If Europe has reverted to her former state of armed anarchy, there seems to these Canadians little use in intervention if there is any possibility of staying out.

The trend of events has had a very different effect on another group of English Canadians. Such people may or may not have approved recent British policy, but their opinion of what Canada's policy should be now is determined by the plain fact that Great Britain is in danger. To them the preservation of the Commonwealth is a fundamental article of faith. When the security of the Commonwealth was reasonably assured they took the association as a matter of course; but now that that security is threatened, they urge Canada to rally to the support of the "mother country". Today they are more determined in their support of Great Britain than at any time since 1919. The divergence of opinion on the question of Canada's place in the Commonwealth is thus becoming more marked, and is increasing the strain on national unity.

ASSOCIATIONS WITH OTHER COUNTRIES

Canada's international relations, apart from those with the Commonwealth, the United States and the League of Nations, are principally of a commercial nature. It might be thought that relations with France would be particularly close, owing to the fact that so many Canadians are of French origin. The French Canadian, however, has little attachment to his mother country. The sentimental tie has been effectively broken, partly by the absence of political association for 175 years, but more particularly by the fact that France has turned anti-clerical while the French Canadian has remained a staunch believer and an ultramontane. Only to a slight extent, amongst a few intellectuals, does modern French thought or policy influence the thinking or attract the attention of the French Canadian. Nevertheless a certain formality of interest is maintained; Canada has appointed a minister to France, and on important historic occasions French representatives visit Quebec and make appropriate speeches.

While the influence of France in Canada is slight, the influence of the Papacy is considerable. The final decision in regard to the appointment of Roman Catholic bishops in Canada is made in Rome. At one period of Canadian history (during the religious conflict over the Manitoba School Act of 1890) it was pressure from the Apostolic delegate, Mgr. Merry del Val, which eased the agitation in French Canada. The Catholic Church, as M. Siegfried has pointed out, has interests in North America far wider than the aspirations of French-Canadian nationalism.[1] The publication of the *Ne Temere* decree in 1908 precipitated a Canadian conflict over the marriage question.[2] The teaching of "corporatism" in Quebec today is a consequence of the social doctrine contained in recent Papal encyclicals. Because of the Vatican influence in Canada, the influence of Italy is also, at the moment, considerable. French Canada approves the Italian policy in Spain though this is inimical to the interests of France.

[1] Siegfried, André, *Canada*, pp. 69-70.

[2] A Marriage Bill was introduced into the Dominion Parliament to overcome the effects of the decree, but it was declared *ultra vires* by the courts. See *In Re Marriage Legislation* [1912] A.C. 880.

The presence of a Canadian minister in Tokyo is evidence of Canada's commercial and political concern with the Far East. Canadian trade with far eastern countries is only a small part of her total foreign trade, but is by no means a negligible quantity. In particular, as has been pointed out, Canada's trade with Japan has increased considerably in recent years. Canada has also been interested in the political arrangements for maintaining peace in the Pacific. She was largely instrumental in persuading Great Britain to abandon the Anglo-Japanese alliance in 1921 out of concern for American feeling. She became a party to the Nine Power Treaty and the Four Power Treaty adopted at the Washington Conference as a basis for future relations between the countries bordering on the Pacific. Canadians were amongst the founders of the unofficial Institute of Pacific Relations. Canada has never attempted, however, to bring any pressure to bear upon other signatories to the Washington treaties to compel them to stand by their engagements. She has left the initiative here, as in Europe and in the League, to powers which are more closely involved in the disputes which have arisen. It is noteworthy that the Canadian government refused to apply against the belligerents in the Sino-Japanese conflict the provisions of the neutrality legislation adopted in 1937.[1] Canadian exporters are being permitted to make their increased profits out of the demand stimulated by war in the east, though they were prohibited from similar commercial transactions with the rebels and the government forces in Spain. Canada's general policy of moving when Britain and the great powers move and not moving when they do not fitted in here very well with the Catholic opinion which did not wish any help to reach the Spanish government and the commercial opinion which wanted to seize the opportunity of greater trade with Japan.

Canadian connections with Latin-American countries are very slight. There is no diplomatic representative accredited to any Central or South American state. Trade commissioners, however, have been appointed for the Argentine Republic, Brazil, Cuba, Mexico, Panama and Peru. The

[1]See below, pp. 125-6, for its description.

total Canadian exports to South and Central America amounted to only $17,000,000 in 1936, less than Canada's exports to Australia. In part this diminutive trade may be due to the absence of a determined attempt on the part of Canada to develop markets, but the prevailing opinion in Canada holds that no very great commercial development is likely until the standard of living in those countries is materially raised.[1] If, however, one thinks of the two Americas together, then their importance from the Canadian point of view, even with the undeveloped South American trade, is at once appreciated. In 1937 they absorbed 45 per cent. of Canadian exports and supplied 65 per cent. of her imports.[2]

[1]See the discussion of this and other aspects of Canada's relations with Latin America in *Canada and the Americas*, a report of the Round Table Conference of the Canadian Institute of International Affairs held at Hamilton, May, 1937, by F. H. Soward; also, MacKay and Rogers, *op. cit.*, Chap. VIII.
[2]See table on p. 42, above.

CHAPTER X

SOME ADVANTAGES AND DISADVANTAGES OF MEMBERSHIP IN THE COMMONWEALTH

IT WOULD be impossible to find agreement in Canada about the advantages and disadvantages of membership in the Commonwealth, since different groups would disagree as to what constituted an "advantage". The Orangeman in Ontario and the Catholic in Quebec look at the British connection from fundamentally different points of view. Instead of attempting, therefore, to form two lists of the consequences of membership, one labelled "advantages" and the other "disadvantages", the more objective method will be followed of considering what seem to be the principal results, leaving the reader to form his own estimate as to their utility for Canada.

Membership in the Commonwealth means that Canada has always been a partner in a world-wide political organization. This has made the inhabitants of the Dominion more conscious of their place in international affairs, more concerned with world movements, than they would have been as citizens merely of a North American state. It has lessened to some extent the provincialism and sectionalism to which the country is only too addicted. This effect of the Commonwealth association, however, has of late years lost some of its force. Canadian foreign trade is so extensive, her relationships with other countries so wide, that complete isolation from the rest of the world is no longer possible. The lumberman in British Columbia, the farmer on the prairies, the miner in central Canada, know what a world market is. Modern methods of communication keep all parts of Canada in constant touch with important world events.

If the imperial ties were broken, Canada would at once have to increase her diplomatic services to enable her to conduct her affairs with foreign states. The right of Canadians to use the British diplomatic and consular services has thus saved Canada the necessity of creating and paying for these services herself.[1] Every Canadian, by his possession of the status of British subject, can make use of a ready-made system of protection throughout the world. He travels and trades with status. On the other hand the absence of official Canadian representatives in most countries has meant that Ottawa has had to rely upon non-Canadian sources of information for much of its knowledge of world affairs.[2] Copies of despatches sent to London from British diplomats may be forwarded to Ottawa, but these will not contain the same kinds of information, or even the same interpretation of events, as would be selected by a Canadian who was viewing foreign developments from the Canadian point of view.

In the international world, Canada as a British dominion can speak with an authority she would hardly possess were she an independent country of eleven million people. Canada has shared to some extent in the prestige and the power of the whole Commonwealth. It is not easy, however, to measure "prestige". It would be of more use to Canada today were she a country trying to force her will upon weaker nations; in so far as she deals with foreign countries on terms of mutual benefit and goodwill the potential power behind her is of no special value. Other relatively unarmed countries, many with valuable raw materials as in South America, do not appear to suffer any particular handicap in their foreign relations. Canada's most important affairs are with the United States and the British Commonwealth, and here "prestige" is of no value today, however useful it may have been in dealings with the United States during the nineteenth century, and however useful it may again become in a changing world.[3]

The fact that Canada began its life as a colony quite naturally has produced in many Canadians an attitude of mind which can best be described as "colonialism". This outlook continues to dominate a certain number of people, despite

[1]The British consular services, however, on the whole are self-supporting.

[2]Canadian representatives in London, Washington, Paris, Tokyo and Geneva are able to supply the government with a great deal of very useful information; but these sources are incomplete.

[3]See Trotter, R. G., "Which Way Canada? An Inquiry Concerning Canadian-American Relations and Canada's Commonwealth Policy", *Queen's Quarterly*, XLV, 3, Autumn, 1938.

the growth of Dominion autonomy. It produces a distrust of things Canadian, a sense of inferiority, and a tendency to follow borrowed traditions blindly rather than to think out and act upon a native policy. Sometimes, to compensate for the inner weakness, an ostentatious patriotism appears based more on narrow loyalty than reasoned faith. Canada will not be a nation in the full sense until Dominion status has become a psychological fact as well as a political reality.

One of the commonest ideas held about Canada's membership in the Commonwealth is that through it she has been provided with defence. Prior to the establishment of the Dominion and its extension to the Pacific the burden of Canada's border defence was borne in large measure by the British government. In 1870, however, British forces were withdrawn from Canada, except for the garrisons at Halifax and Esquimalt, which were maintained until 1905. Up till confederation expansionist agitation in the United States would have repeatedly threatened Canadian independence had not the United States realized that northward aggression would face the military power of Britain. On the other hand it must be remembered that some of the agitation for annexation of Canadian territory was an appeal to anti-British rather than to anti-Canadian prejudices.[1]

So far as an invasion from Europe or Asia is concerned, at no time in the past 100 years is it reasonable to suppose that any power would have contemplated such an attack, whether the British navy or the Monroe Doctrine existed or not. Japan did not become a modern state until the end of the nineteenth century, and her expansion has since then been quite naturally toward the Asiatic mainland. Russia, after the sale of Alaska in 1867, paid no more attention to America. Germany and Italy did not become united until 1870 and have been engrossed since in European and African affairs. The Germany of 1914, had it been victorious in the world war, would no doubt have contemplated further colonial expansion, conceivably at the expense of Canada; if this is so, the Dominion was defended by France, Russia

[1]See Trotter, R. G., "The Canadian Back Fence in Anglo-American Relations", *Queen's Quarterly*, XL, 3, August, 1933.

and the other allied powers fighting Germany just as much as by England and the United States. Canada would be better defended today by a strong League of Nations, or even by a strong alliance between England, France and Russia, than she ever can be by the British Commonwealth alone.

As regards the problem of defence in the future, it would appear that neither Commonwealth aid nor the Monroe Doctrine is immediately essential, though both are important. It has been shown how Canada will be able to defend her own coasts from any expected scale of attack, when her present defence plans are completed. Geography and international political alignments give her, at the moment, all the defence she needs in addition to her own strength. In the contemporary world the only place where Canadians are likely to die violent deaths on the field of battle is in Europe. Were it not for the Commonwealth connection Canada would certainly be as isolationist as all the other American states. It is true that a number of Canadians consider Great Britain the principal supporter of peace in Europe; they believe that if she should be defeated in a war it would be only a matter of time before Canada was subject to a serious threat of invasion which could only be avoided by alliance with, followed by political subjection to, the United States; that the preservation of Canadian independence therefore requires participation in the major struggles of Britain wherever they may be. In short, they think that defending England is defending Canada in a very real sense, quite apart from questions of sentiment or of moral obligation.[1] The same long-range argument, of course, would lead Mexico and the South American republics to defend themselves by fighting in Europe, since they are equally liable to invasion; it would mean also that Canada should help France and China, both of which can be relied on to oppose Germany and Japan, Canada's principal potential enemies.

It has been pointed out that the Canadian defence forces are equipped and trained according to English standards.

[1]An argument tending to support this view is presented in Trotter, R. G., "Which Way Canada? An Inquiry Concerning Canadian-American Relations and Canada's Commonwealth Policy", *loc. cit.*

This is clearly an effect of the Commonwealth association. It results in Canada having to rely to a great extent on Great Britain for supplies. If the Atlantic sea route were blocked during a war, Canadians might find it impossible to maintain the coastal batteries at Halifax and Esquimalt, equipped with English guns. A defence policy based on purely Canadian needs would more naturally follow United States practices, since supplies are more likely to be available from that country. The danger of Canada being cut off through the application of the United States neutrality laws is less than the danger that air and submarine attacks may make impossible any transport across the Atlantic. It is in the interest of the United States that Canada should be able to defend her neutrality against, and to repel invasion by, a non-American aggressor.

Another consequence of Commonwealth membership, already pointed out, is that Canadian defence policy has emphasized military at the expense of naval and air power. A concern solely with local defence needs would have resulted in expenditure devoted much more to coastal defences and much less to the militia.

Canada's relations with the United States have grown steadily closer with the industrial development of the Dominion, despite Canada's membership in the Commonwealth. Yet most Canadians would feel that the process of Americanization in Canada would have proceeded further and more rapidly had Canada been an independent state. Certainly the links with Great Britain and the other dominions, the position of the Crown, and innumerable other British influences have tended to make Canadians feel they were different from Americans even when the other influences of geography and commercial intercourse were making the two countries more and more alike. Had it not been for membership in the Commonwealth, Canada would probably have joined the Pan-American Union. It would be a comparatively simple matter, from the military point of view, to create a league of American nations whose pooled defence forces would be impregnable against outside attack. Yet even today the sense of being a "British" country is still

strong enough to make most Canadians unwilling to take
this step, and the idea of such a league shows no sign of
entering the realm of practical politics.

Turning to matters of trade, it would seem that the existence of the Commonwealth has not affected the development of the Canadian economy to any preponderant extent
since the repeal of the Corn Laws in 1846. After that date
Canada went her own economic way. The British preference,
it is true, and the Ottawa agreements, have diverted more
Canadian trade into imperial channels than would have gone
in that direction for purely economic reasons. Canada might
have had fewer American branch factories had they not
sought the benefit of imperial preferences. But Canada
possesses raw materials which many countries, particularly
Great Britain, need and must purchase on the world market.
Canadian nickel must be bought because scarcely any other
nickel exists; the best Canadian wheat will find a market
because no better wheat is produced. Canadian foreign trade
would no doubt be more widely spread were it not for the
spirit of economic nationalism which operates within the
Commonwealth, but it is doubtful how far the Commonwealth increases the total volume of that trade. Moreover,
in so far as special economic arrangements between Commonwealth countries have the appearance, to outside nations, of
creating a British economic bloc and a market closed to
foreigners, they increase the world struggle for raw materials
and thus add to the general political unsettlement and to
Canada's insecurity.[1]

It would be impossible to trace all the effects of membership in the Commonwealth on the internal development of
the Canadian people. Their attitudes toward government,
politics, law, religion, and indeed most other fields of human
activity, have been profoundly coloured by the British connection. The sectional variations in the strength of this influence, its counter-action by other influences of racial mixture and geography, its decline in the face of the growing
national consciousness of Canadians, have already been noted.

---

[1]Dr. Raymond Leslie Buell has remarked that the result of the Ottawa agreements
"has been not only to demoralize still further world trade as a whole, but to make the
Empire the object of envy of the overcrowded dictatorships". See *Canada, The Empire
and the League* (*op. cit.*), p. 54.

Two other effects of membership in the Commonwealth already touched upon deserve emphasis. In the first place, Canadians of British origin, no matter how much they might be separated by the sectional divisions of the country, have been in the past united in their sense of loyalty to the Commonwealth. Up to a point this common bond overcame sectional divisions. At the same time the force that tended to unite the English Canadians tended also to keep them apart from the French. French Canadians have felt that English Canadians were merely Englishmen in Canada and not properly Canadians, believing (without full warrant) that the latter placed loyalty to the Commonwealth ahead of loyalty to the interests of Canada.[1] Were Canada not a part of the Commonwealth Canadians would be more inclined to place the interests of their own country first, and a similar loyalty would tend to unite the two races in a way that has not occurred in the past.

The second of these consequences is found in the progressive deterioration of the Canadian constitution as a result of the Privy Council decisions. Mention has been made of the way in which judicial interpretation has altered the nature of the original federal structure, giving Canada in effect a constitution under which the central government has a limited number of powers and the residue remains with provincial authorities.[2] It was sentiment and colonial status which prevented the Canadian Supreme Court from being made the final court of appeal; from this point of view membership in the Commonwealth has greatly retarded the development of Canadian unity. It is fair to add, however, that most Canadians have accepted these decisions without much criticism until recently, when the seriousness of the Dominion's position has come to be recognized. If anything is to be done now, the responsibility rests upon Canada.

---

[1] The history of English-speaking Canada for more than a century has displayed a persistent Canadianism which has been willing to use the imperial connection for class or sectional aims and which has frequently sacrificed imperial interests. The annexation manifesto of 1849 was supported for reasons of commercial interest by a class which had just been claiming a monopoly of genuine loyalty. The imperialist sentiment of Canadian manufacturers at the Ottawa Economic Conference of 1932 was not very noticeable.

[2] See above, pp. 75 ff.

CHAPTER XI

THE PROBLEM OF NEUTRALITY

IN the preceding discussion of Canada's position in the Commonwealth, the question of neutrality has frequently arisen. As the international situation deteriorates and another world war seems to draw closer, the rights and duties of Canada in time of war are increasingly being discussed by Canadians.

EMERGENCE OF THE PROBLEM

Historically, Canada has always felt free to keep out of minor wars in which Great Britain might be engaged, but not free to keep out of major wars. Sir John Macdonald refused to lend Great Britain aid during the Khartoum incident in 1884, and in an interesting letter to Sir Charles Tupper he put forward the sensible proposal that "the reciprocal aid to be given by the colonies to England should be a matter of treaty deliberately entered into and settled on a permanent basis".[1] Sir Wilfrid Laurier distinguished between the "life and death struggle" and the "secondary wars" of England, holding that Canada was obliged to engage in the former only.[2] Mr. King took an isolationist stand, implying a right to non-participation, in the Chanaq affair in 1922. Events since then have shown that England may have obligations of a major kind in Europe which Canada does not share. Impliedly Canadian non-participation in a major war in which Great Britain might be involved was admitted in the Locarno Treaty. The Imperial Conference declaration in 1926, that the members of the British Commonwealth were *"autonomous Communities within the British Empire, equal in status, in no way subordinate one to another in any aspect of their domestic or external affairs, though united by a common allegiance to the Crown, and freely associated as members of the British Commonwealth of Nations"*, logically contained within

[1]Cited MacKay and Rogers, *Canada Looks Abroad*, p. 73.
[2]See below, p. 136, n. 1.

it the concept of neutrality in any war. The Statute of Westminster in 1931 legalized Dominion legislative independence and set the seal on the new constitution of the Commonwealth. But as it dealt with legislative and not executive power, and as it gave Canada no capacity to amend the B. N. A. Act, it did not clarify the specific issue.

In 1933, at the first British Commonwealth Relations Conference, the question of neutrality was side-stepped by the ingenious device of suggesting that it was "academic" and "unprofitable" to consider "legal conceptions as to war and neutrality appropriate to the pre-League world".[1] Already in that year, however, a formal political declaration of a policy of neutrality for Canada was enunciated by the newly-organized farmer-labour party, the Co-operative Commonwealth Federation, in its party manifesto. Many people in Canada were making up their minds to neutrality while the more bashful Commonwealth representatives were refusing to consider the problem. It was obvious by that date that the "pre-League" world had become the post-League world. Since then the repeated assertions by the Canadian government that Parliament is "free to decide" the question of participation in empire wars when the moment arises, is at once a recognition of the strength of this opinion in Canada and also an implied assumption that the freedom is unfettered by commitments. No serious discussion of the future of the British Commonwealth can now avoid facing squarely the problem of neutrality for its members.

The question that now presents itself is not peculiar to Canada. It requires, indeed, an answer from every member of the Commonwealth, though it is not essential that these answers should be all the same, since Australia and New Zealand might well feel that their geographical position and interests compel them to a different solution from that which

[1]Toynbee, A. J. (ed.), *British Commonwealth Relations*, p. 181. Three classes of people in Canada describe talk of neutrality as "academic": those who do not want the subject discussed at all; those who, like Prof. F. H. Underhill, (see Anderson, Violet (ed.), *World Currents and Canada's Course*, p. 130) feel that the Canadian people will be denied any choice when war starts by reason of existing commitments to intervene; and others who believe that, however legally Canada might assert her neutrality, the chance of maintaining it against potential foes would be negligible. It seems clear, however, that if a country ever wishes to remain neutral, the existence or otherwise of the right is a matter of some practical importance.

might be suitable for South Africa or Canada. The answer involves a choice between differing concepts of Commonwealth. Is the Commonwealth necessarily and for every member an offensive-defensive alliance?[1] Must every dominion support ultimately by armed force the foreign policy of the British government regardless of whether there is any possibility of controlling that policy? To put it more simply for 1938, has the Conservative party of Great Britain the power to declare war for every dominion? Or is the Commonwealth to be thought of as fulfilling the terms of the definition of 1926, namely, a free association of states completely independent in every matter of domestic and foreign policy? If the Balfour formula means what it says, it means that the right to neutrality is necessarily a part of the concept of the modern Commonwealth. Certainly the dominions cannot be equal to Great Britain if the government of that country can put them into a war, while their own governments have no such power.

It is not proposed to argue here whether or not the right to neutrality exists for Canada as a matter of law. The point is contentious, but the overwhelming weight of authority takes the view that legally the state of technical belligerency is created in the Dominion by a British declaration of war.[2] The argument for Canada's immediate commitment is stronger than that made out for dominions like Eire and the Union of South Africa, which have adopted legislation enabling them to control fully their own foreign affairs; the former country has even got rid of the special privileges for British naval vessels in its harbours. In any case, domestic changes within the Commonwealth as to how the royal prerogative may be exercised can have no effect on the international community, and unless the right is recognized

[1]Even the term "alliance" is improper to describe the existing situation. An alliance presupposes sovereign states, voluntarily entering into a compact. The present obligation of the dominions to take part in British wars is not a matter of agreement between equals but a relic of colonial status. A colony is necessarily at war when its governing authority declares it to be so.

[2]See MacKay and Rogers, *Canada Looks Abroad*, chap. XV. See also Kennedy, W.P. M., *The Constitution of Canada*, 2nd ed. (Toronto, 1938), pp. 540 ff.; Corbett, P. E.,"Isolation for Canada", *University of Toronto Quarterly*, 1936, p. 120; Keith, A. B., *The Governments of the British Empire* (London, 1935), p. 99, *Constitutional Law of the British Dominions* (London, 1933), p. 70; Hancock, W. K., *Survey of British Commonwealth Affairs*, vol. I, (London, 1937), p. 305; Scott, F.R.,"Canada and the Outbreak of War", *Canadian Forum*, June, 1937. Contra, Ewart, J. S., 1932 *Canadian Bar Review*, 495; Burchell, C. J.,in MacKay and Rogers, *op. cit.*, pp. 241 ff.

abroad it is of little value. Nothing has been done officially by the Commonwealth to bring the existence of dominion autonomy in peace and war to the attention of foreign governments.

CONFUSION OF OPINION IN CANADA

Most people in Canada at the present moment are divided on, and confused about, the question of neutrality. They have not been taught to distinguish between the right to neutrality and a policy of neutrality, while the subtle differences between passive and active belligerency escape them altogether. A great many either do not see that the achievement of the right is an essential prerequisite for the exercise of a free choice—a choice that may just as easily be in favour of supporting Great Britain as of neutrality—or else they believe they already have the right and think that further discussion is an attempt to tie Canada to a permanent policy of neutrality. The political leaders have generally refrained from clarifying the issue, and have used language that is capable of contradictory interpretations. Mr. King has been most explicit, yet every statement he has made implies the existence of the right to neutrality, without discussing how it has been achieved or how it may be exercised. His attitude is succinctly expressed in this sentence: "It will be for this parliament to say in any given situation whether or not Canada shall *remain neutral*."[1] A state which "remains" neutral until parliament decides obviously is not made a belligerent by action of the British government. Again, on his return from the Imperial Conference of 1937, Mr. King said that the "full and untrammelled responsibility of the Canadian parliament for decision on the vital issues of foreign policies and defence was completely maintained throughout. It was made clear in the conference discussions that Canada was not committed to joining in any Imperial or any league military undertakings, and equally, that there was no commitment against such participation."[2] Despite the ambiguity of the term "participation" the whole tenor

[1] Canada, *House of Commons Debates*, January 25, 1937, pp. 249-50. Italics added.
[2] July 19; cited, Canada, *House of Commons Debates*, April 1, 1938 (unrevised), p. 2092.

of the statement implies that Canada has control over the declaration of war.

Against these statements of the Prime Minister are, as has been said, the opinions of nearly all the constitutional authorities. Moreover, Mr. Lapointe, the Minister of Justice, has acknowledged that Canada is automatically committed to a state of passive belligerency.[1] He has not, however, explained how "active" passive belligerency must be. For, assuming that no right to neutrality exists, Canada's legal relations with the enemy state are drastically changed without Canada's consent by a British declaration of war. The decision to send troops may be discretionary, but other vital matters are not. Automatic and complete economic sanctions against England's enemy legally go into force, for example, even before the Canadian parliament meets to decide its course of action. It would be illegal for any Canadian to trade with the enemy after the outbreak of war, since trading with the enemy is a crime. This is surely "active participation", yet it has never been so much as mentioned in any governmental statement of policy. Canada has also undertaken to allow the British government the use of the harbours of Halifax and Esquimalt for naval purposes, and this agreement is inconsistent with a neutral position.[2] Passive belligerency would thus, in the opinion of most people, be certain to become active participation. For this reason the present Canadian policy of *laissez-faire* as regards the right to neutrality would work out as a continuation of the traditional policy of participation.

Some Canadians who admit that this analysis is probably correct would reply that it is mostly irrelevant, since even if the right to neutrality were conceded and Canada tried to remain neutral, she would inevitably be dragged in, like the United States in 1917, if the war continued for long. There is no doubt much force in this contention. It is not safe to assume, however, that attempts at neutrality armed with

[1] He has said: "There is all the difference in the world between neutrality, and participation or non-participation, which we shall be always free to declare, in the event of any war. . . . But neutrality is quite different. . . . This question as to the right of the dominions to be neutral is one of the questions yet to be solved. . . ." Canada, *House of Commons Debates*, February 4, 1937, p. 547.

[2] The text of the Canadian government's undertaking is given in House of Commons, *Sessional Papers*, 1937, No. 285; also in MacKay and Rogers, *op. cit.*, p. 299.

more detailed legislative support than has existed hitherto will be useless in the future. And the real importance of the right to neutrality, from the Commonwealth point of view, is psychological. If Canada is involved in a war at its outset just because of the legal ties and their consequences, a great number of Canadians will vent their indignation upon the Commonwealth connection, whereas if they are dragged into the war otherwise they will have only themselves and the world situation to blame. A concession of the right would thus appear to be a safeguard for Commonwealth as well as for Canadian unity.[1]

Various factors, amongst which the creation of the Spanish Non-Intervention Committee in 1936 was perhaps the chief, led the Canadian government in 1937 to arm itself with wide powers for keeping Canadians from participating in foreign (i.e. non-British) wars or civil wars which might involve the peace of the country. Two statutes were passed by the Dominion parliament in that year, containing permanent provisions capable of application in any future situation. The first was the Foreign Enlistment Act.[2] This substantially re-enacted for Canada the provisions of the imperial Foreign Enlistment Act of 1870, and gave the Dominion government power to prohibit the enlistment of Canadians in foreign armies either during a war or a civil war. The second amended the Customs Act[3] so as to give the government discretionary power in peace or war to "Prohibit, restrict or control the exportation, generally or to any destination, directly or indirectly, or the carrying coastwise or by inland navigation, of arms, ammunition, implements or munitions of war, military, naval or air stores, or any article deemed capable of being converted thereinto or made useful in the production thereof, or provisions or any sort

[1]Some Canadians believe that foreign countries would refuse to recognize Canadian neutrality. Obviously the decision of enemies of Great Britain would be based on their conception of their own interest. Normally it would be to their interest to be at peace with Canada, though they would probably wish to interfere with trade coming from Canada and such interference might well lead to war unless Canada were content to submit quietly, like the Scandinavian countries from 1914 to 1918. Here again it is well to remember that 50 per cent. of Canadian trade is carried in British vessels, 37½ per cent. in foreign and 12½ per cent. in Canadian vessels.

[2]Statutes of Canada, 1937, cap. 32. It is interesting that the Canadian government introduced a Foreign Enlistment Act in 1875, but later withdrew it.

[3]Statutes of Canada, 1937, cap. 24, sec. 10.

of victual which may be used as food by man or beast . . . ". The Dominion government exercised its new powers under this legislation in the summer of 1937 when the acts were made applicable to Spain.

The present policy of Canada is a threefold one of emphasizing Parliament's freedom of choice without explaining what it means, providing legislation to assist neutrality in non-British wars, and proceeding with military preparations which lend themselves to some form of participation in the next war in which the Commonwealth is engaged. This policy appears acceptable to most Canadians, since the imperialists believe it gives them what they want and most of the others fail to perceive the degree to which it leaves them committed. If one looks for indications of opinion in the country, however, it is evident that a great body of opinion would favour the possession by Canada of the right to neutrality, so that the Canadian parliament could decide on each occasion what foreign policy it should pursue in the event of any war. Certainly French Canadians take this view, and they constitute 30 per cent. of the population. Of the remaining 70 per cent. another 20 per cent. is of non-British origin, and can scarcely feel a sentimental obligation to take part in every British war. In numerous bodies and associations representing different groups of English-Canadian opinion (farmer and labour groups, trades union meetings, university student conferences, etc.[1]) during the past few years, resolutions have been adopted either calling explicitly for the right or else advocating a foreign policy which implied that the right existed.

It appears reasonable to assume that a considerable majority of the people of Canada believe either that the Dominion has or that it should have the right to remain neutral whenever it so desires. There would not be so strong a support as this for a definite *policy* of neutrality, which would tie the hands of the government in advance, although,

[1]See, for instance, C. C. F. statement, cited MacKay and Rogers, *op. cit.*, p. 387; resolution of United Farmers of Ontario, 1936, and petition of 13,000 university students in 1937 asking for clarification of the legal situation. The Trades and Labour Congress of Canada voted in 1937 in favour of holding a referendum before Canada takes part in any future wars.

as pointed out below, isolationist sentiment has grown greatly in strength during the past seven years.[1]

ADVANTAGES OF CLARIFICATION

The right to neutrality is inherent in the principle of equal status. It may well be argued that the time seems to have arrived when this principle should be given its full effect in the international sphere, for it is now abundantly clear that no collective system of international security exists to render neutrality obsolete. Already constitutional writers are beginning to picture the state of affairs which would prevail were the dominions to acquire this further attribute of sovereignty. A single Crown common to all the members, but acting for each on the advice of the particular government concerned whether in peace or in war, would be the basis of the Commonwealth constitution. The citizens of each member country, while possessing the common status of British subjects for certain purposes of intra-Commonwealth cooperation, would also possess a separate nationality for purposes of international intercourse. Such ideas are not new to the Commonwealth; to extend them to situations of peace and war is merely to develop existing practices to a further point.

From the point of view of Canada, the change would require an abandonment of the present agreement regarding the use of the harbours of Halifax and Esquimalt by British naval vessels, an extension (though not necessarily to every country) of the Canadian diplomatic service, and the transfer of the remaining imperial prerogatives over foreign affairs from London to Ottawa. For the Commonwealth as a whole the change would best be effected after an agreement arrived at in an Imperial Conference, followed by formal notification to every foreign government of the new situation. The right having been established, individual dominions could then make separate agreements with Great Britain or with one

[1]See page 135, below. Mr. J. S. Woodsworth's motion in the House of Commons in 1937 calling for a policy of neutrality would have left the government no option but one of isolation in the event of war; its defeat therefore did not involve a parliamentary decision as to the advisability of acquiring the right of neutrality. See Canada, *House of Commons Debates*, January 25 and 28, and February 4, 1937.

another on matters of defence if they so desired. The regional grouping and interests of dominions would find effect within the Commonwealth according to the natural geographic and economic inclinations of the different members. Even those dominions which gained the right of neutrality but entered into no new commitments for defence, would still be as free as they are now to participate in Commonwealth wars. The Commonwealth would not be disrupted; it would, on the contrary, have achieved a peaceful change according to the best democratic tradition, and clarified a constitutional situation which is now clouded with doubt and uncertainty. It would have made a decision calmly and without ill-feeling which may otherwise have to be made in the stress of a sudden emergency. Thenceforth the Commonwealth as a whole could not be imperilled, as it can be at present, through the pursuit by a particular British government of a foreign policy which might involve England in war and yet meet with the strong disapproval of some or all of the dominion governments.

Those who argue that to discuss and plan for neutrality is to invite disruption of the Commonwealth, are repeating today an argument that has been steadily used to oppose or postpone every application of the democratic principle to the government of the former British colonies.[1] It is, on the contrary, highly dangerous to leave so delicate a question to be decided under threat of hostilities. A claim to the right of neutrality advanced at the beginning of a war, without general consent and when emotions were strongly aroused, might well be interpreted as secession. Even under the serious though less critical international situation which exists today, were Canada to make a *unilateral* declaration it would be interpreted in some quarters, no doubt, as implying a more complete withdrawal from the Commonwealth orbit than is intended by many of those who advocate acquisition of the right of neutrality. Such interpretations have been made of other steps toward dominion autonomy.

[1]The argument that greater freedom for the dominions strengthens rather than weakens the Commonwealth is well expressed in *The British Empire* (Royal Institute of International Affairs Study Group Report) (London, 1937), pp. 230-1. As was said by B. K. Long in Willert, (Sir) A., Hodson, H. V., and Long, B. K., *The Empire in the World* (London, 1937), p. 125, "Discussion and recognition of the most far-reaching dominion rights can only do good".

An agreement about neutrality reached by *Commonwealth* discussion in time of peace, however, need not involve any such threat of secession. Nor need constitutional changes in Canada, by which Ottawa secured the same degree of control as have South Africa and Eire over all kinds of treaties and documents affecting them to which the King's name must be appended, produce any more disturbance in the Commonwealth than occurred when those dominions added these functions to their powers of self-government, which many claim to have made neutrality legally possible.

CHAPTER XII

PRESENT OBJECTIVES OF CANADA'S EXTERNAL POLICIES

POLITICAL

THE student of Canadian affairs who understands the mixed nature of the Canadian population, the world-wide distribution of Canadian foreign trade, and the conflicting pulls of British sentiment and North American geography, will not be surprised to find that Canadian foreign policy lacks a clear and positive direction. Any government at Ottawa which must make decisions on international affairs is speaking for a political party which represents every section of the country and of the people, and therefore every principal difference of opinion. In no field of political life is André Siegfried's comment on Canadian statesmen more true, that they "fear great movements of opinion, and seek to lull them rather than to encourage them and bring them to fruition". Politicians must find a policy which will be supported, in its main lines, not only by a majority of the people of Canada, but by a majority of the members of each of the two major racial groups in Canada. Too definite a stand, it seems evident, will simply transfer every international quarrel to Canadian shores and produce two antagonistic camps within the country, as happened with the attempt to enforce conscription in 1917. In short, the internal political situation is such that instead of hammering out a policy at party caucuses or conventions and then putting it before the public for their acceptance or rejection, Canadian politicians have preferred to let the event, at the last moment, determine the policy.

A consequence of this fear in the political leaders is that the Canadian public is largely ignorant of, and confused about, questions of foreign policy. This is less true of the French Canadians; they are not better informed, but they have at least a clear, simple policy of isolation from all foreign wars and entanglements. The majority of English-speaking Canadians have not, except in some quarters and quite recently, given conscious thought to the question of what foreign policy Canada should follow. Even the members of parliament devote little time to the problem. The Prime Minister, with all his other duties, is still carrying the responsibilities of the Secretary of State for External Affairs, and there is no effective parliamentary committee for detailed discussion of policy. Most of the debates that have occurred in the past three years have been due to pressure from the small C. C. F. group or other independents in the House of Commons.[1] Undoubtedly such bodies as the Canadian Institute of International Affairs, the League of Nations Society, and the Canadian Broadcasting Corporation through its discussions and nation-wide broadcasting of lectures, coupled with the seriousness of the threat of war, are helping in the building of an informed opinion, but the subject can still be kept well in the background of political issues.

At the same time a certain kind of foreign policy, though not consciously planned and selected, is given to Canada ready-made by facts of history, race, geography and economics. Proximity to the United States, constitutional and sentimental ties with Great Britain, geographic isolation from centres of world conflict, the necessity for extensive foreign markets, and more recently membership in the League of Nations, are basic influences determining the direction in which she is likely to move.[2] The absence of a nationally chosen foreign policy, therefore, does not mean the absence of a foreign policy, but rather it means a policy of drift in whatever direction these forces may impel the country at a given moment. Prior to 1914 the colonial status of Canada made the empire tie the predominant factor in every critical situation; the unity of the empire meant that in practice Canadian policy was inevitably what the British Foreign Office determined it should be on every major issue.

[1] On this whole question see Chapters XII and XIII in MacKay and Rogers, *op. cit.*

[2] See Scott, F. R., "The Permanent Bases of Canadian Foreign Policy", *Foreign Affairs*, July, 1932.

The insistence upon separate membership in the League of Nations, and the insistence on the progressive evolution of dominion status, were the first occasions on which Canada asserted a policy which might be called original. Yet once in the League Canada tended to follow rather than to lead, her only distinctive contribution being the early attempts to water down the obligations of the covenant as to sanctions. Now that Geneva has ceased to be a centre of major world affairs Canada is thrust back more upon her own initiative; the covenant gives little guidance upon policy, and theoretically the British Foreign Office makes no binding commitments for Canada. Thus, for the first time in her history, Canada is now faced with the full responsibilities of an autonomous state in a world of international anarchy.

In face of this new situation, the full implications of which are only beginning to be realized, certain fairly well defined groups of opinion can be discerned in Canada, centering around the three possible policies of non-intervention in foreign wars, imperialism or a British front policy, and collective security. These groups, it should be noticed, by no means differ on all points of foreign policy. They are all agreed that Canada must continue to trade in world markets—this means that there are no economic isolationists or "autarchists" in Canada. Again, nearly all their supporters are agreed that friendly relations with the United States, membership in the Commonwealth, and membership in the League should continue, though the non-interventionists insist that neither membership should involve commitments. The differences between these groups narrow down to questions of emphasis in policy and particularly to the problem of economic and military action in wars abroad.[1]

The non-interventionists (who generally call themselves isolationists though they do not envisage breaking all ties with foreign countries) are opposed to Canada's participating in overseas wars, whether for the League or for the Commonwealth. Canada's contribution to world peace, they feel,

[1]Canadian writers vary in their estimate of the number of these groups. Mr. J. W. Dafoe listed three in 1936 (*Foreign Affairs*, January, 1936) but five in 1937 (*World Currents and Canada's Course*, p. 144). Hon. Ian Mackenzie, Minister of National Defence, names five (*House of Commons Debates*, March 24, 1938). Prof. Underhill boils them down to two—those who want to take part in the next European war and those who don't.

is best made by her staying quietly at home and minding her own business. Her work for humanity is to develop her resources and to make them available to all in the markets of the world. She has no enemies, save those which the British connection or League obligations may make for her. People who want her raw materials can buy them freely enough. She can provide for her own defence, and can go peacefully on her own way, they feel, with every bit as much safety as any other American nation. Some non-interventionists would be isolationist as against Europe and the Far East only; they would welcome a development of Pan-American-ism for the better co-operation of all people in the two Amer-icas, believing that here a regional security system is both feasible and desirable.

The imperialist or "British front" school believe that the Commonwealth is still a unit as far as primary issues of policy are concerned. Whether the relationship between the mem-bers be called an alliance, an entente or a partnership, it requires, they feel, that the dominions and Great Britain should stand or fall together in any emergency, and pur-sue parallel policies on major world issues. This opinion tends to view the United States with suspicion (though some would hope to see an "Anglo-Saxon front" emerge) and to dismiss the League of Nations as an impossible dream in a world of hard realities. There are shades of opinion within this imperialist camp, however, and many who formerly supported a League policy for Canada have reverted to the imperialist position, either because they believe a strong Commonwealth is the best alternative to a League, or be-cause they think that the Commonwealth may be the foundation on which the collective system can be rebuilt in the future. Sometimes, making the best of both worlds, the spokesmen for a British front policy speak of "collective security within the Empire".[1]

The third policy for Canada, which still has many ad-herents despite its vanishing chances of realization, is a policy based on the idea of a revived League of Nations, leading eventually to the re-establishment of the collective

[1]E.g. Senator Griesbach, in *Queen's Quarterly*, Spring, 1937.

system of security. The supporters of this policy would hold that peace is indivisible and cannot be maintained by armed alliances, British or other. They believe that nothing has failed at Geneva except the statesmanship of the great powers, amongst which they would include Great Britain as a chief offender. British foreign policy ever since the National government took office in 1931 seems to them to have displayed the worst features of the old, secret diplomacy and imperialist "power politics" which they thought the English people had renounced when they subscribed to the covenant. The toleration of Japanese aggression in Manchuria in 1931, the indifference to Hitler's rearmament programme in 1933 and to his remilitarization of the Rhineland in 1936, the making of a private naval treaty with Germany in 1935, the cold-blooded nature of the Hoare-Laval Treaty regarding Abyssinia and the backing-down over sanctions, the farce of non-intervention in Spain and Mr. Chamberlain's new policy of collaboration with the League's arch-enemies, have produced in them a profound distrust of British influence in the present international situation. Canadian policy in the past they recognize also as having been short-sighted and selfish at Geneva but her greater remoteness from the issues and the small weight that her voice can carry, while not excusing her from blame, free her in their eyes from any major responsibility for the League *débâcle*. Many people, formerly of this collectivist opinion, their faith in a revived League being dead, have turned to a temporary isolationism rather than to imperialism as the present best policy for Canada. Having once raised their loyalty to the height of a world system they cannot accept as a substitute an empire alliance based merely on race and history and constantly intriguing to keep itself on the stronger side of a European balance of power. Other League supporters are hoping against hope that a positive alliance between existing League members, committed first to a stopping of further aggression and then to the progressive strengthening of the various organs of League co-operation, may yet arise out of the present chaos. To this they would wish Canada to lend her full support.

These three groups and their subdivisions include all those parts of the population which have thought about foreign affairs. There is in addition a large number of individuals who have not accepted any of these positions, and who drift along without positive direction, capable of being driven into one or another of the camps by the trend of the news and the pressure of popular feeling. This unattached opinion is content that Canada should continue playing the minor part she now plays, and believes she is reserving her own freedom to act as seems best when the moment for action comes. It is the way this opinion swings which will largely determine Canada's course of action should a war occur; those who can control the swing will probably control the bulk of opinion.

Estimates of public opinion are risky undertakings, but the association of particular policies with particular racial groups in Canada enables one to arrive at some sort of approximation of the numbers supporting an isolationist position at the present time. The French Canadians are almost wholly isolationist. Probably half of the 2,000,000 other persons of non-British origin are still too alien to British ideas or too opposed to British policy to favour European commitments. This makes approximately 4,000,000, or nearly 40 per cent. of the total population. To these must now be added an unnumbered but substantial group of people of British origin who, partly through the disillusionment following the last war and the breakdown of the League, partly through longer associations with North America, and for other reasons,[1] have moved into the isolationist position. In terms of mere numbers, it is not unreasonable to place in this group today fully half the population of Canada.[2] Many in the other half will turn isolationist if British policy continues during the next few years to be what it has been since 1931. Whereas up to 1914 the official attitude of Canada, should Great Britain be involved

[1]Left-wing political groups, apart from Communists, are inclined to isolationism. Then there are nearly 400,000 Irish Catholics in Canada, a fair portion of whom have no fondness for the British connection.

[2]Senator Molloy estimated 90 per cent. of the Canadian people to be isolationist in 1937; see quotation in Soward, F. H.,"Canada and Foreign Affairs", *Canadian Historical Review*, June, 1937, p. 189.

in a major war in Europe, was "Ready, aye, ready",[1] today
it is one of "No commitments", either for or against intervention. This is the political recognition given to isolationist
sentiment.

Yet once again it must be remembered that the strength of
the imperialist position is not in its surface showings but in
its underlying controls. Its real power is found partly in its
instinctive appeal to the ancient loyalties of the British half
of Canada, partly in its occupation of those offices in government, industry, finance, the army, the church and the press
which will enable it to crystallize opinion and formulate
policy when a decision must be made, and partly also in that
complex of relationships—constitutional ties, absence of the
right to neutrality, co-operation in defence arrangements,
adaptation of Canadian industry to British armament requirements, etc.—which contains within it by implication
the whole of the imperialist policy, and which Canada can
scarcely be expected suddenly to scrap when the moment of
crisis has arisen. Against these pulls the arguments of the
isolationists are likely to be of little avail. There will be no
referendum at that moment to discover the opinion of the
human beings who inhabit Canada; critical decisions will be
made in a number of places outside of parliament where
imperialist sentiment prevails; and inside parliament, where
the major decision must be taken, the total French-Canadian
and foreign group which is most isolationist holds only about
25 per cent. of the seats.

This analysis of Canadian sentiment toward foreign affairs
has been given as a background against which can be set the
present official policy of the Canadian government. Since
1937 it has been comparatively easy to outline the basic
points of Mr. King's foreign policy, for in that year Mr.
Escott Reid, national secretary of the Canadian Institute of

---

[1]"If there were an emergency, if England were in danger—no, I will not use that expression; I will not say if England were in danger, but simply if England were on trial with
one or two or more of the great powers of Europe, my right hon. friend might come and ask,
not $35,000,000, but twice, three times, four times $35,000,000. We would put at the dis-
posal of England all the resources of Canada; there would not be a single dissentient voice."
Sir Wilfrid Laurier, Canada, *House of Commons Debates*, Dec. 12, 1912, cited Dawson, R.
MacG., *The Development of Dominion Status, 1900-1936* (London, 1937), p. 167. Compare
Sir W. Laurier's statement in the House of Commons, Feb. 5, 1900, cited Dawson, *op. cit.*,
p. 135: ". . . If England at any time were engaged in struggle for life and death, the
moment the bugle was sounded or the fire was lit on the hills, the colonies would rush to the
aid of the mother country."

International Affairs, made a summary of the policy as he
found it in Mr. King's speeches and decisions on international
affairs,[1] and Mr. King remarked in parliament that the summary was "a very good statement of some of the features of
Canada's foreign policy". The principles enumerated were:

1. The guiding principle in the formulation of Canada's foreign
policy should be the maintenance of the unity of Canada as a nation.

2. Canada's foreign policy is, in the main, not a matter of Canada's
relations to the League, but of Canada's relations to the United
Kingdom and the United States.

3. Canada should, as a general rule, occupy a back seat at Geneva
or elsewhere when European or Asiatic problems are being discussed.

4. Canada is under no *obligation* to participate in the military
sanctions of the League or in the defence of any other part of the
Commonwealth.

5. Canada is under no *obligation* to participate in the economic
sanctions of the League.

6. Before the Canadian government agrees in future to participate
in military or economic sanctions or in war, the approval of the parliament or people of Canada will be secured.

7. Canada is willing to participate in international inquiries into
international economic grievances.

Mr. King's only criticism of this statement was that "possibly it stresses too much what has to do with possible wars
and participation in war, and does not emphasize enough . . .
what has been done in the way of trade policies and removal
of causes of friction between this and other countries". It
would therefore seem proper to add to the last principle Mr.
Reid's own amendment[2] to the effect that "Canada should
pursue, within the measure of its power, 'the attempt to
bring international trade gradually back to a sane basis, to
lessen the throttling controls and barriers'". This endeavour
is one that Mr. King has pursued with some success. Finally,
to complete the summary of present policy, there should perhaps be added an eighth principle deducible from Mr. King's
attitude during 1937, that whenever Great Britain and other
powers chiefly interested agree to plans for localizing a war

[1] "Canada and the Threat of War", *University of Toronto Quarterly*, January, 1937, p.
243, quoted in Soward, "Canada and Foreign Affairs" (*op. cit.*), p. 195. Mr. Reid discussed
the policy further in "Mr. Mackenzie King's Foreign Policy, 1935-36", *Canadian Journal
of Economics and Political Science*, February, 1937, p. 86.

[2] In the last quoted article, at p. 97.

between states or a civil war, the Canadian government is willing to accede to such proposals provided they fall short of military commitments.[1]

It will be observed how this policy takes account of the permanent factors in Canada's background and environment, and how it gives expression to the important groups of opinion in Canada without offending those of opposite views. The "maintenance of the unity of the nation" means that Ottawa cannot embark upon a foreign policy which will so divide French and English, or Catholic and Protestant, as to threaten the existence of the federal union; foreign policy must always be tested by its effect on domestic unity, just as much as by its effect on Commonwealth unity or League unity. The second principle states a fact resulting from history and geography; Canada's relations with the United Kingdom and the United States (both considered, be it noted, as "foreign" policy) are of prime importance, and her policy at Geneva must not strain these relationships too far. The proposition that Canada should occupy a "back seat" at Geneva with regard to Europe and Asia is in line with the growing feeling that Canada is essentially a North American nation which should follow rather than lead in the solution of problems in remote continents. The fourth, fifth and sixth principles are a declaration of complete freedom from commitments to sanctions of any sort in any war; they conform to the rising tide of sentiment in Canada which is convinced that whatever decision is made on such vital matters should be one freely entered into to secure the best interests of Canada when all the factors, domestic as well as foreign, are considered. The seventh principle, the willingness to seek economic co-operation, is a prime necessity for any country as heavily committed as Canada to external trade. Finally, the participation in schemes to localize war means that in general such plans, when initiated by other powers, are likely to receive Canadian support.

While thus showing clearly the motives from which it springs, this present Canadian foreign policy, like that of most democratic nations today, shows a lack of positive

[1] A description of the new neutrality legislation is given above, p. 125.

direction and of long-range vision. It is principally one of preserving traditional relationships while subtracting their commitments,[1] and of a "wait and see" attitude for the future. It is a policy which enables politicians to postpone the evil day of decision, which may seem a good thing for the politicians but is a poor one for the people, since it is the negation of the democratic method and means that when the decision must be made a foreign policy dictated by blind forces instead of conscious purposes will prevail. It has already been pointed out how slight Canada's freedom of choice may turn out to be in so far as British wars are concerned, unless she takes steps in advance to make alternative courses possible.

ECONOMIC

The present objectives of Canadian economic policy spring from the nature of the Canadian economy. That economy, as has been pointed out, requires a large export market for a comparatively few staple products, and at the same time has developed a number of secondary industries which demand continued tariff protection. The interests of the primary producers, particularly the wheat grower, call for a policy of freer trade, but the manufacturing interests are politically stronger and have never been seriously challenged in their tariff stronghold. Present Canadian commercial policy, seeking as it must for ever-widening export markets, is thus unable to make concessions to foreign countries which would dislocate existing industries to any considerable extent. Two foreign markets are especially important to Canada—the United Kingdom and the United States; in both Canada holds a preferred position under the Ottawa agreements of 1932 and the trade treaty of 1935, and the maintenance of this position is the bed-rock on which her policy rests.

Because of the individualistic nature of the Canadian economy, economic policy is only in part, perhaps only in

[1]It is to be noted that the "policy of no commitments" differs from the old imperial relationship and also (probably) has altered Canada's obligations toward the League. As Mr. J. W. Dafoe has said, "The Canadian government's only admitted 'vital interest' is the defence of Canada—beyond that it will consider what it is prudent and necessary to do when decisions can no longer be deferred. This is rejection, not only of League engagements, but of any obligation, legal, moral, implied or advisable towards the Commonwealth of British Nations or any nation member of the Commonwealth". See Anderson, Violet (ed.), *World Currents and Canada's Course*, pp. 147-8.

small part, the creation of the government which the people elect. Canada exercises no control over her foreign trade in the sense that New Zealand does, where the government itself markets a considerable proportion of the exports through state boards. Every Canadian corporation is free to sell abroad where it will and at any prices it is able to get. Canadian financiers may invest Canadian funds in areas of their own choosing. For example, Canadian trade policy in the Far East has recently been to increase very rapidly the sale of such essentials to Japan as scrap iron, copper, nickel, lead and zinc, but this decision was not a government decision though it makes Canada an important factor in the Sino-Japanese dispute. So, too, there has been no parliamentary decision that Canada is to turn her resources to the manufacture of British armaments, though this is very definitely increasing Canada's commitments in Europe, as did the manufacture of supplies for the Allies by United States manufacturers from 1914 to 1917 increase American commitments. In considering the objectives of Canadian economic policy, this distinction between what the Canadian government decides and what independent Canadian exporters decide must be borne in mind, for frequently Canadian policy in fact will be determined by the exporters rather than by the government. Foreign policy proper has been socialized, is decided upon by the cabinet and is carried out by government agents. Economic policy in the international field is a resultant of the combined effects of governmental action on the one hand and the trade agreements, cartelizations, marketing agreements and sales policies of Canadian corporations on the other. Once economic policy (public and private) has turned in a certain direction, foreign policy cannot easily take a different course.

There is nothing isolationist in Canadian economic policy, however her foreign policy may show a trend in this direction. The only instance of the "no commitment" doctrine in the economic sphere is in regard to Spain, to which country, as has been pointed out, the government applied its neutrality legislation in the summer of 1937. Mr. Bennett went partially isolationist against the Soviet Union in 1931 when he placed an embargo on certain Russian imports, but Mr. King removed that embargo in 1936. Canadian industry is developing steadily, but not in the direction of economic self-sufficiency since its dependence on foreign trade increases rather than declines. The question whether it is possible to be politically isolationist while the economy is so largely geared to the war preparation requirements of great powers in Europe and the Far East is one which has received little attention in Canada, even from the isolationists themselves.

So far as internal economic policy is concerned, it is difficult to define any "national" objective. Giving a free hand to business but checking its worst abuses, while protecting workers and farmers against certain economic and social hazards, contains about all that can safely be put into such a phrase. Individual initiative and the profit motive are the dominant impulses to economic action. That these incentives, operating amidst Canada's natural resources, will continuously raise the standard of living of an increasing population is the belief of a great majority of the people and proposals for national planning on a socialist scale are confined to left-wing minority political parties.[1] The idea that the first duty of the state is to see that the economy provides a basic standard of decent living for every citizen is not a political idea which either of Canada's major parties has yet espoused. Mr. Bennett adopted part of this philosophy in his election campaign of 1935, but the economic policy of the succeeding government has been of a more *laissez-faire* variety. Canada has experienced nothing like so great a movement for social reform during the past decade as has, for instance, swept over the United States. Such reform parties as have been at all successful politically have been provincial rather than national, like Social Credit in Alberta and the *Union Nationale* in Quebec, which undoubtedly came to power by capturing the demand for change.

---

[1]The League for Social Reconstruction has outlined its planning proposals in two books: *Social Planning for Canada* (Toronto, 1935), and *Democracy Needs Socialism* (Toronto, 1938).

CHAPTER XIII

CO-OPERATION IN THE COMMONWEALTH

WHEN people form a political association they do so with some object in view. They may wish to unite against enemies, to escape from tyranny, to improve their economic condition, to glorify a race or a religion. Political unity may also be the obligatory unity of conqueror and conquered. Association may be less than complete unity, as in treaties of alliance or trade. Whatever form it may take, a political relationship expresses some definite purpose or aim. What the British Commonwealth is feeling for today is a new definition of its own purpose, which will be valid for its nationally autonomous members under modern world conditions.

In the early days of the British Empire its growth and development were the result of racial expansion. The British peoples took to the sea and to foreign trade. They explored, conquered and settled in various parts of the world, some uninhabited, some inhabited. They sent their sons and daughters to build new homes in the new lands. The motives of the individual settlers were various, but the venture as a whole was a national venture. In a world of independent national states, where force was the ultimate arbiter of international disputes, this process of expansion and aggrandizement was purpose enough in itself. It brought prestige and power and by its mere existence made Britain great.

This centralized empire could not last. It could not last because centralized government, under early conditions of transport and communication, was necessarily unrepresentative of the distant territories, and the British people have never long tolerated autocratic government. Dominion autonomy was the inevitable product of the parliamentary British tradition. No person trained in that tradition could submit to having his life and destiny shaped by a government which he could not control, not even when it was a British government. The same spirit which made Englishmen behead one king and expel another in the seventeenth century, turned the colonies into autonomous dominions in the twentieth century. Independence of action proved that the dominions were British in spirit, not that they were anti-British. It was failure to recognize their own characteristics when displayed by Englishmen outside England which lost the English their American colonies.

Today the old ideas of empire are dead in so far as the majority of Canadians are concerned. True, a strong body of imperialist tradition exists in Canada, which hankers after, perhaps believes in, the simple, old certainties of size and strength. But the continued enlargement of the empire, it need hardly be said, cannot be a part of dominion foreign policy. The sense of racial superiority which may come from seeing a map coloured largely in red or in thinking of the hundreds of millions of British subjects and of the unsetting British sun, is a feeling that any adult mind will want to eliminate rather than foster. Nor can the primitive slogan, "What we have we'll hold", act as a unifying principle for nations anxious to establish peace on a permanent foundation. The possibility that the Commonwealth, as it now exists, contributes to international insecurity through its failure to deal with the problems of colonies and raw materials must be frankly faced by every member. Appeals for joint action in matters of defence are equally inadequate as the basis of future co-operation; defence is only an instrument of policy, and not a policy in itself. Moreover, for Canada, the special assistance of the Commonwealth in defence matters is not at the moment essential. The principles on which the Commonwealth can continue to co-operate in the future will have to be principles different in kind and quality from those which sufficed in the past. What, then, are such principles?

In approaching this critical question care must be taken to avoid vague generalities. Since empire became Commonwealth, the preservation of peace has always been advanced as an aim of the Commonwealth association. So, too, has the maintenance of democracy. It is not questioning the sincerity of these pronouncements to point out that they do not necessarily produce co-operation. Whose peace is to be preserved? Peace in Canada may best be secured in the opinion of many by avoiding all European wars. Democracy is further advanced in the Scandinavian countries which remained neutral in 1914 than in any of the countries which fought to make the world safe for democracy. The objectives of peace and freedom are undoubtedly objectives for the Commonwealth; the difficulty is that dominions may legitimately differ as to the best way of achieving these objectives.

It will be simplest in exploring the possibilities of Commonwealth co-operation from the Canadian point of view to start with the easier problems. It is beyond question a useful thing, both for the members of the Commonwealth and for the world, that between these members war is extremely improbable.[1] The practice of settling intra-Commonwealth disputes by negotiation and compromise is of great value to the partners in the association, and no doubt a good example to their fellow nations. The Commonwealth, by its mere existence as a large area of peace and peaceful change, performs a valuable function in a world society possessing too little of either.

Within the Commonwealth there is at the moment a great deal of co-operation on a multitude of technical matters, each of considerable importance in its own field. This "quiet co-operation"[2] covers such things as copyright, statistics, customs, patents, education, cable and wireless communications, workmen's compensation, oil pollution of navigable waters, forestry, and merchant shipping. Laws have been harmonized, standards developed, research planned and information exchanged. These forms of co-operation are extremely useful, and the fact that they can occur more easily amongst a number of nations because of the Commonwealth tradition makes the Commonwealth itself of value.

Underlying these various kinds of joint effort is the general idea of the progressive improvement of social and scientific

[1]The term "unthinkable", though frequently used, should perhaps be limited to relations between the Anglo-Saxon communities in the Commonwealth.

[2]See a useful survey of it in *The British Empire*, a report by a study group of members of the Royal Institute of International Affairs (London, 1937), chap. XII; also Palmer, G. E. H., *Consultation and Co-operation in the British Commonwealth* (London, 1934).

conditions in Commonwealth countries. Each dominion government is endeavouring to solve its local problems, many of which are affected by conditions in some other part of the Commonwealth. Wherever this is so, co-operation becomes valuable. Co-operation with other foreign states may be equally valuable; the Commonwealth promotes co-operation because the will to mutual aid is stronger.

In so far as the raising of the internal standard of living is a common objective for dominion governments, the existence of the Commonwealth is potentially of the greatest importance. A freer exchange of goods and services, a more co-operative and scientific development of Commonwealth resources and markets, can be made to benefit every member. British preference is a recognition of the common purpose of economic co-operation. There is, however, a danger lurking in any such scheme, the danger that a short-term benefit for the members may be secured at the expense of co-operation with foreign states. Nothing would be of less use to Canada, and it would seem to the Commonwealth as a whole, than an attempt to create an economic bloc out of the dominions, Great Britain and her dependencies. It has been pointed out that the Ottawa agreements have already evoked criticism from American and other sources. Economic co-operation remains a valuable principle of Commonwealth action if it is for the purpose of raising the general standard of living in Commonwealth countries (and not merely for the purpose of raising prices through production control) and if, in addition, it creates no obstacles to wider forms of world economic co-operation. If empire agreements are intended for the purpose of producing a bargaining power which can break down other nations' trade barriers, they might lead eventually to an increase of world trade, but the difficulty of changing the direction of the trade they stimulate makes such results highly doubtful.

In the matter of immigration, it has been shown how difficult is Canada's position. An unexpectedly long period of prosperity might produce a demand for employment which Canada could not fill from her own population. If this occurs, immigration will revive of its own accord. But this condition has not yet occurred, save possibly in certain skilled trades, and the lack of labour here is due to the Dominion's own short-sightedness in not carrying on technical training amongst the unemployed. No new attempt to foster immigration by official action is likely to be expected from Canada at the present time. There is clearly no gain, from the Canadian point of view, in permitting individuals to transfer from the dole in England to the dole in Canada. State-aided schemes for shifting population from the British Isles to Canada belong to long-range planning rather than to immediate policy; indeed, Canada is having to face the problem of internal shifts away from her drought areas in the west to more suitable localities.

A majority of the human beings who constitute the population of the empire are not yet full citizens enjoying self-government. Viewing the empire as a whole, the right to select the governing authority and hold it responsible to the will of the people is a right possessed by a minority of British subjects. So long as this remains true, and accepting democracy as a Commonwealth ideal, the British nations have a large task to perform, a task that might perhaps be described as that of progressively eliminating the remnants of empire from the Commonwealth. The more politically advanced parts of the Commonwealth are thus under an obligation to co-operate for the purpose of raising the political, educational and economic level of the subject peoples. Perhaps the Commonwealth is nearing the time when it will accept the principle that the improvement of the condition of the native population is the first charge to be met out of the economic development of any area. Canada is not as directly concerned in this problem as some other parts of the Commonwealth, yet she has her minorities to whom she has not accorded full citizenship, and in this respect she faces an unfulfilled obligation. The British Commonwealth has not yet evolved what might be termed a "nationalities policy", which aims to achieve a progressive improvement in the cultural and economic advancement of native races.[1]

[1] A clear realization of the need for such a policy will be found in *The Alternative to War*, by C. R. Buxton (1936). See also Hancock, W. K., *Survey of British Commonwealth Affairs*, vol. I (London, 1937), p. 506.

In most of these various fields useful forms of co-operation can be developed or expanded, without the danger of offending organized groups of opinion. Greater difficulties begin to arise when the most important field of all is entered—that of foreign policy and its allied subject, defence. Even here the area of uncertainty can be narrowed through the existence of well-understood ideas. Imperial federation is dead forever, at any rate with Canada as a federating unit. Canadian foreign policy will remain autonomous, and no delegation of executive authority to a central imperial cabinet is conceivable. The existing centralization of the right to declare peace and war is being questioned because it conflicts with this principle of self-determination. It follows that there is a right to differ as to foreign policy. Members of the Commonwealth have agreed they will not take any international action likely to affect the interests of other members without previously giving an opportunity to each member affected to make its interests known, and "that neither Great Britain nor the Dominions [can] be committed to the acceptance of active obligations except with the definite assent of their own Governments".[1] Thus in place of formal machinery for reaching a united decision there exists merely an understanding, called by some writers a constitutional convention, that every government has the right to express its views in relation to the foreign policy being pursued by any other Commonwealth government, if in its opinion its interests are affected by the pursuit of that policy.[2] There is also a vague

[1] *Summary of Proceedings, Imperial Conference, 1926*, Cmd. 2768, cited Dawson, *op. cit.*, p. 342.

[2] The Imperial Conference of 1930 approved a three-point summary of the main recommendations made at previous Imperial Conferences "with regard to the communication of information and the system of consultation in relation to treaty negotiations and the conduct of foreign affairs generally".

The first point was, "Any of His Majesty's Governments conducting negotiations should inform the other Governments of His Majesty in case they should be interested and give them the opportunity of expressing their views, if they think that their interests may be affected." The report later makes it clear that this point does not apply merely to treaty negotiations: "The application of this is not, however, confined to treaty negotiations. It cannot be doubted that the fullest possible interchange of information between His Majesty's Governments in relation to all aspects of foreign affairs is of the greatest value to all the Governments concerned."

The second point was, "Any of His Majesty's Governments on receiving such information should, if it desires to express any views, do so with reasonable promptitude. . . . It is clear that a negotiating Government cannot fail to be embarrassed in the conduct of negotiations if the observations of other Governments who consider that their interests may be affected are not received at the earliest possible stage in the negotiations. In the absence of comment the negotiating Government should, as indicated in the Report of the 1926 Conference, be entitled to assume that no objection will be raised to its proposed policy."

The third point was "None of His Majesty's Governments can take any steps which might involve the other Governments of His Majesty in any active obligations without their definite assent." (*Summary of Proceedings, Imperial Conference, 1930*, Cmd. 3717, cited Dawson, *op. cit.*, pp. 403-4).

recognition that the purpose of these arrangements is to help
to co-ordinate the foreign policies of the various governments.[1] Canada is not likely to promote any change in this
situation, and the Canadian government in practice inter-
prets the relevant resolutions of the Imperial Conferences
to mean that its failure to express dissent from a United
Kingdom policy of which it has knowledge must not be
interpreted as meaning assent to that policy or a willingness
to support it.[2]

What applies to foreign policy applies also to defence. Co-
operation and consultation exist, but, in so far as Canada is

[1]"During the discussions [at the Imperial Conference of 1937] emphasis was laid on the
importance of developing the practice of communication and consultation [on questions of
foreign affairs] between the respective Governments as a help to the co-ordination of
policies. . . . Being convinced that the influence of each of them in the cause of peace was
likely to be greatly enhanced by their common agreement to use that influence in the same
direction, they declared their intention of continuing to consult and co-operate with one
another in this vital interest and all other matters of common concern." (*Summary of
Proceedings, Imperial Conference, 1937*, Cmd. 5482, pp. 13-4).

[2]The views of the Canadian government on this point were set forth on a number of
occasions during the parliamentary session of 1938.

(a) On March 17, Mr. T. L. Church asked the following question:
"Has any action been taken by the government to assure His Majesty's government of
Great Britain of Canada's moral support, interest, co-operation and aid in the present foreign
situation, and will any papers relating thereto be tabled?"

Mr. King replied as follows:
"Mr. Speaker, the answer to the question as drafted is in the negative. As already
indicated in answer to a question by the member for Rosetown-Biggar (Mr. Coldwell) on
March 1, the government has been receiving from the United Kingdom government certain
communications relating to the international situation. Such communications are continuing. As indicated in that answer and in answer to a question by the member for Winnipeg
North Centre (Mr. Woodsworth), on February 25, these communications are in the nature
of information rather than consultation upon policies. As such, they are helpful to the
Canadian government in assisting it to understand the actual facts of the current situation."

(b) In reply to a question asked by Mr. M. J. Coldwell on March 1, subsequent to the
resignation of Mr. Anthony Eden and the ensuing debates in the British parliament, Mr.
King said:
"The Canadian government has been furnished with full summaries of recent statements
made in the British House of Commons by the Prime Minister of the United Kingdom and
the former Secretary of State for Foreign Affairs. In addition, it has received a brief
report of a conversation with a representative of a foreign government. These communications, as is usually the case, are in the nature of information rather than consultation. The
Canadian government has not offered any opinion on the statements in question."

(c) The following excerpt from the debate on the defence estimates on April 1 is also
instructive:
"Mr. COLDWELL: . . . The Prime Minister of Great Britain has stated in the house
that the dominions have been consulted and that to some extent recent pronouncements in
regard to Czechoslovakia are in part due, it is said, to the attitude of the self-governing
dominions.
"Mr. MACKENZIE KING: Consulted, did my hon. friend say?
"Mr. COLDWELL: Yes, consulted.
"Mr. MACKENZIE KING: I do not believe the Prime Minister of Great Britain has
used that word. I may be wrong, but my recollection is that the Prime Minister said that
we had been kept informed of what had taken place. But that we had been consulted, or
that any advice had been given by the government, was not, I think, suggested.
"Mr. COLDWELL: I think in certain press dispatches the word 'consulted' was used.
I know that when I was thinking of what I was going to say I took that word 'consulted'
from one of the dispatches. But if the right hon. gentleman says that that is not the word
that should have been used, I take it that the government has been kept informed, and if
there has been any actual or implied advice with respect to that information I think we
should be given to understand what that advice may have been, if any has been given.
"Mr. MACKENZIE KING: I can assure my hon. friend right away that no advice
has been asked and none has been given by the present government."
(Canada, *House of Commons Debates*, unrevised, March 1, 1938, p. 994; March 17,
1938, pp. 1530-1; and April 1, 1938, p. 2104).

concerned, stop short of an express understanding equivalent to a military alliance. The nature of the present defence policy of Canada has already been analysed, and it has been pointed out that, far from excluding the possibility of war in conjunction with Great Britain, Canadian defence plans take such an emergency into account while the government clings to the principle of parliamentary decision on each situation as it arises. In this matter also the policy of Canada is unlikely to change in the near future, given the divisions of opinion within the country. At the same time, on the economic side Canada is co-operating to a considerable extent through the acceptance by various industries of large orders for the manufacture of war equipment. This co-operation, as has been shown, is operating as one of the powerful underlying forces linking Canadian foreign policy ever closer to that of Great Britain, despite the surface retention of the "no commitment" policy.

If the problem of intra-Commonwealth co-operation on foreign policy could be based on an active League of Nations, then at once the situation would be clarified. Postulating a functioning collective system, Commonwealth foreign policy is replaced by League policy on the vital issues of war, and neutrality disappears. The first British Commonwealth Relations Conference was correct in its statement that in such a world the purely Commonwealth problem becomes academic. Theoretically, the ideal solution—if not the only solution—is a world system for the maintenance of law and justice in which the Commonwealth members have agreed to the nature of their commitments. The creation of such a system, in the opinion of many Canadians, thus remains as the ultimate and the most unifying principle of co-operation for Commonwealth members. Every form of co-operation inconsistent with that ultimate aim is dangerous and injurious to the welfare of the world and hence the Commonwealth. For though the great powers may have destroyed the effectiveness of the League they have not succeeded in destroying the effectiveness of the education in international behaviour carried on by the League. Unless every lesson learned since 1914 has proved false, power politics, balance of power diplomacy, armed alliances unrelated to generous and sincere offers of settlement to opposing forces, are not steps towards peace, but are simply preparations for another war which in turn will create more problems than it solves.

The present world, however, has no such League. No great power is advocating an attempt to re-establish it. Its achievement has ceased to be (if it ever was) a leading principle of British foreign policy; if Britain and France were to win another war, can it be said that a new League with any greater chances of success than the last would be created? Today the dominating motive actuating Commonwealth members in international affairs is that of postponing immediate war and preparing to be on the winning side when hostilities begin. In such a world, co-operation between the dominions and the United Kingdom must necessarily be chiefly concerned with defence matters. Here the attitude of the dominions will vary in accordance with their national sense of need and commitment. Canada's share in defence co-operation will not be likely to change in the next few years. In the ultimate event of a European war involving Great Britain some Canadian contribution, even if only economic, is certain; its extent, particularly in a military sense, will depend on unpredictable factors both foreign and domestic. One thing can be said with safety: the degree of Canada's willing participation will be greatly increased if British policy leans to the principles of collective security.

The fields in which Commonwealth members may pursue joint policies are important. They are being developed to some extent now: their further expansion along proper lines is desirable. But no group of nations scattered about the world like the British nations, comprising within their borders a multitude of races, religions and economic areas, has any difficulties unlike those which are shared by mankind in general. The Commonwealth must seek the solutions to its problems, not apart from other peoples, but in conjunction with them.

For Canada at the present moment grave internal problems, economic, racial and constitutional, dominate all other issues. Commonwealth co-operation can be of some, but probably not of great, assistance to her in solving these domestic difficulties. Canadians must first make up their own minds as to what kind of society they want and how they propose to get it; then only will they see clearly how to harmonize their foreign and domestic policies. Canada is searching for a new basis on which to re-establish her national unity, and until she finds it she has no accepted internal criterion with which to measure her external obligations. When she knows her own mind on her national objectives she will know better what contribution she can make toward international and intra-Commonwealth co-operation.

BIBLIOGRAPHY

For more extended bibliographies on Canadian affairs the reader is referred to: *Canada looks abroad*, by R. A. MacKay and E. B. Rogers (published under the auspices of the Canadian Institute of International Affairs by the Oxford University Press, Toronto, London and New York, 1938); the *Selected bibliography* prepared by Miss Margaret Cleeve, of the Royal Institute of International Affairs, for the British Commonwealth Relations Conference, 1938; the bibliography in *Select documents in Canadian economic history, 1497-1783*, edited by H. A. Innis (Toronto, 1929); and the bibliographies published in the *Canadian journal of economics and political science* and the *Canadian historical review*.

I. Sources

A mass of information is to be found in the briefs submitted by provincial governments and by various organizations to the Royal Commission on Dominion-Provincial Relations (the Rowell Commission) in 1937 and 1938. The report of the Commission is expected in 1939. Eight volumes of a series of books on Canadian-American relations, sponsored by the Carnegie Endowment for International Peace, have already been published, and more are forthcoming; several of them have been referred to in foot-notes. The nine volumes in the series entitled *Canadian frontiers of settlement* are invaluable (particularly vol. I, Mackintosh, W. A., *Prairie settlement, the geographical setting*; vol. VII, Dawson, C. A., *Group settlement: ethnic communities in western Canada*; vol. IX, Lower, A. R. M. and Innis, H. A., *Settlement and the forest frontier in eastern Canada*, by A. R. M. Lower, *Settlement and the mining frontier*, by H. A. Innis. Among recent government reports the following will be found useful: *Report of the Royal Commission to inquire into railways and transportation in Canada* (Ottawa, 1932); *Report of the Royal Commission on banking and currency* (Ottawa, 1933); *Report of the Royal Commission on price spreads and mass buying* (Ottawa, 1935); *Final report of the National Employment Commission* (Ottawa, 1938).

Useful documents are to be found in R. MacGregor Dawson's two volumes, *Constitutional issues in Canada, 1900-1931* (London, 1933) and *The development of dominion status, 1900-1936* (London, 1937). *Canada looks abroad*, by MacKay and Rogers, contains about 65 pages of speeches and other documentary material and, on page 389, a list of other sources. The *Canada year book*, published annually by the Dominion Bureau of Statistics, is invaluable, as is also *The encyclopedia of Canada* (6 vols.), edited by W. S. Wallace (Toronto, 1935-37).

II. Books on Canadian Affairs

Anderson, Violet, (ed.), *World currents and Canada's course*, Lectures given at the Canadian Institute on Economics and Politics, 1937 (Toronto, 1937).

ANGUS, H. F. (ed.), *Canada and the doctrine of peaceful change* (published by the Canadian Institute of International Affairs (Toronto, 1937) (mimeographed).

ARMSTRONG, ELIZABETH H., *The crisis of Quebec, 1914-1918* (New York, 1937).

BARBEAU, VICTOR, *La mesure de notre taille* (Montreal, 1936).

BRADY, A., *Canada* (Modern World Series) (London, 1932).

Canada, the empire and the league, Lectures given at the Canadian Institute on Economics and Politics, 1936 (Toronto, 1936).

Canadian constitution, The, Series of broadcasts by C.B.C. (Toronto, 1938).

Canadian papers, 1933 (published by the Canadian Institute of International Affairs, Toronto, 1933).
(Mackintosh, W. A., "Canadian tariff policy"; MacDonald, James M., "Statistical outlines of Canada's transpacific trade"; and other papers.)

Canadian papers, 1936 (published by the Canadian Institute of International Affairs, Toronto, 1936) (mimeographed).
(Gibson, J. D., and Plumptre, A. F. W., "The economic effects on Canada of the recent monetary policy of the U.S.A."; Hurd, W. B., and MacLean, M.C., "Projection of Canada's population on the basis of current birth and death rates"; Taylor, K. W., "The effect of the Ottawa agreements on Canadian trade"; and other papers.)

Conference on Canadian-American affairs, Canton, New York, 1935, *Proceedings* (Boston, 1936).

Conference on Canadian-American affairs, Kingston, Ontario, 1937, *Proceedings* (Boston, 1938).

DAFOE, J. W., *Canada: an American nation* (New York, 1935).

Democracy needs socialism (published under the auspices of the Research Committee of the League for Social Reconstruction, Toronto, 1938).

GLAZEBROOK, G. DET., and BENSON, W., *Canada's defence policy*, Report of round tables of annual conference, 1937, Canadian Institute of International Affairs (Toronto, 1937) (pamphlet).

INNIS, H. A., and PLUMPTRE, A. F. W. (eds.), *The Canadian economy and its problems* (published by the Canadian Institute of International Affairs, Toronto, 1934).

INNIS, MARY QUAYLE, *An economic history of Canada* (Toronto, 1935).

JACKMAN, W. T., *Economic principles of transportation* (Toronto, 1935).

KELSEY CLUB OF WINNIPEG, *Canadian defence: what we have to defend*, A series of broadcast discussions (Ottawa, 1937).

KENNEDY, W. P. M., *The constitution of Canada, 1534-1937*, 2nd. ed. (Toronto, 1938).

MACGIBBON, D. A., *The Canadian grain trade* (Toronto, 1932).

MACKAY, R. A., and ROGERS, E. B., *Canada looks abroad* (published under the auspices of the Canadian Institute of International Affairs, Toronto, 1938).

MACKINTOSH, W. A., *Economic problems of the prairie provinces* (Toronto, 1935).

MARSHALL, H., SOUTHARD, F. A., and TAYLOR, K. W., *Canadian-American industry* (Toronto, 1936).

SÉBILLEAU, PIERRE, *Le Canada et la doctrine de Monroe* (Paris, 1937).

SIEGFRIED, ANDRÉ, *Canada* (London, 1937).

Social planning for Canada (published under the auspices of the Research Committee of the League for Social Reconstruction, Toronto, 1935).

SOWARD, F. H., *Canada and the Americas*, Report of round table of annual conference, 1937, Canadian Institute of International Affairs (Toronto, 1937) (pamphlet).

STRANGE, WILLIAM, *Canada, the Pacific and war* (published under the auspices of the Canadian Institute of International Affairs, Toronto, 1937).

WITTKE, CARL, *A history of Canada*, rev. ed. (New York, 1933).

WRONG, GEORGE M., *The Canadians: the story of a people* (Toronto, 1938).

III. PERIODICALS

Canadian banker (Toronto, quarterly).

Canadian bar review (Ottawa, monthly).

Canadian defence quarterly (Ottawa).

Canadian forum (Toronto, monthly).

Canadian historical review (Toronto, quarterly).

Canadian Institute of International Affairs: reports of annual conferences (Toronto).

Canadian journal of economics and political science (Toronto, quarterly).

Dalhousie review (Halifax, quarterly).

Financial post (Toronto, weekly).

Foreign affairs (New York, quarterly).

International affairs (London, every two months).

League of Nations Society in Canada: reports of annual conferences (Ottawa).

Maclean's magazine (Toronto, bi-monthly).

Pacific affairs (New York, quarterly).

Queen's quarterly (Kingston).

Revue trimestrielle canadienne (Montreal, quarterly).

Round table (London, quarterly).

Saturday night (Toronto, weekly).

University of Toronto quarterly (Toronto).

The following are some of the more important articles that have appeared recently in the foregoing and other periodicals:

BOVEY, WILFRID, "French Canada and the problem of Quebec", *Nineteenth century*, CXXIII, 731 (January, 1938).

BREBNER, J. B., "Canada, the Anglo-Japanese alliance and the Washington conference", *Political science quarterly*, L, 1 (March, 1935).

BROSSARD, ROGER, "The working of confederation: a French-Canadian view", *Canadian journal of economics and political science*, III, 3 (August, 1937).

BRUCHÉSI, J., "Defence—and French Canada", *Maclean's magazine*, June 15, 1937.

———————— "Canadian unity and the French Canadians", *Revue trimestrielle canadienne* XXIV, 94 (June, 1938).

CAHAN, C. H., "Canada and/or commonwealth loyalty", *United empire*, XXIX, 21 (January, 1938).

———————— Speech on appeals to the judicial committee of the privy council, Canada, *House of commons debates* (unrevised), April 8, 1938, pp. 2336 ff.

"Canada and imperial defence", *Canadian defence quarterly*, XII, 2 (January, 1935).

Canadian bar review, June, 1937. Special number on constitutional questions.

"Canuck", "The problems of Canadian defence", *Canadian defence quarterly*. April, 1938.

DAFOE, J. W., "Canada's interest in the world crisis", *Dalhousie review*, XV, 4 (January, 1936).

Economist, The, special supplement, "The dominion of Canada", January 18, 1936.

FEIS, H., "A year of the Canadian trade agreement", *Foreign affairs*, XV, 4 (July, 1937).

FERGUSON, G. HOWARD, "Canada must arm", *Maclean's magazine*, April 15, 1937.

GREEN, J. F., "Canada in world affairs", *Foreign policy reports*, June 15, 1938.

GRIESBACH, W. A., "A united empire front", *Queen's quarterly*, XLIV, 1 (Spring, 1937).

KEENLEYSIDE, H. L., "Department of external affairs", *Queen's quarterly*, XLIV, 4 (Winter, 1937-38).

LOWER, A. R. M., "America and the Pacific", *Dalhousie review*, XVIII, 1 (April, 1938).

———————— "Canada can defend herself", *Canadian forum*, January, 1938.

MARTIN, DAVID, "Canada: our military ward", *Current history* (June, 1938).

MARVIN, D. M., "The bank of Canada", *Canadian banker* (October, 1937).

"Nationalism in French Canada", *Round table*, No. 105 (December, 1936).

NOBLE, S. R., "The monetary experience of Canada during the depression", *Canadian banker* (April, 1938).

REID, ESCOTT, "Canada and the threat of war: a discussion of Mr. Mackenzie King's foreign policy", *University of Toronto quarterly*, VI, 2 (January, 1937).

———————— "Mr. Mackenzie King's foreign policy, 1935-6", *Canadian journal of economics and political science*, III, 1 (February, 1937).

"S", "Embryo fascism in Quebec", *Foreign affairs*, XVI, 3 (April, 1938).

SCOTT, F. R., "The permanent bases of Canadian foreign policy", *Foreign affairs*, X, 4 (July, 1932).

———————— "Canada's future in the British commonwealth", *Foreign affairs*, XV, 3 (April, 1937).

SOWARD, F. H., "Canada and the league of nations", *International conciliation*, No. 283 (October, 1932).

"T", "Canada and the Far East", *Foreign affairs*, XIII, 3 (April, 1935).

TARR, E. J., "Canada in world affairs", *International affairs*, XVI, 5 (September-October, 1937).

———————— "Defence and national unity", *Maclean's magazine*, July 1, 1937.

TROTTER, R. G., "The Canadian back fence in Anglo-American relations", *Queen's quarterly*, XL, 2 (August, 1933).

———————— "Which way Canada?", *Queen's quarterly*, XLV, 3 (Autumn, 1938).

UNDERHILL, F. H., "Keep Canada out of war", *Maclean's magazine*, May 15, 1937.

INDEX